Allergy and Allergic Diseases

Allergy and Allergic Diseases

Editor: Kevin Parker

FOSTER ACADEMICS

www.fosteracademics.com

www.fosteracademics.com

FOSTER ACADEMICS

Cataloging-in-Publication Data

Allergy and allergic diseases / edited by Kevin Parker.
p. cm.
Includes bibliographical references and index.
ISBN 978-1-63242-525-6
1. Allergy. I. Parker, Kevin.
RC584 .A45 2018
616.97--dc23

Foster Academics,
118-35 Queens Blvd., Suite 400,
Forest Hills, NY 11375, USA

ISBN 978-1-63242-525-6 (Hardback)

Printed and bound in China.

Contents

Preface

This book was inspired by the evolution of our times; to answer the curiosity of inquisitive minds. Many developments have occurred across the globe in the recent past which has transformed the progress in the field.

The diseases that are caused by the hypersensitivity of the immune system towards organisms or elements present in the environment are known as allergies or allergic diseases. These diseases can cause severe to mild damage in different people based on their immune system. Most common allergies found in humans are food allergies, allergic asthma, hay fever, anaphylaxis, atopic dermatitis, etc. The objective of this book is to give a general view of the different aspects of allergic diseases. It is a valuable compilation of topics, ranging from the basic to the most complex researches in the field of allergic diseases. It will prove to be immensely beneficial to students and researchers in this field.

This book was developed from a mere concept to drafts to chapters and finally compiled together as a complete text to benefit the readers across all nations. To ensure the quality of the content we instilled two significant steps in our procedure. The first was to appoint an editorial team that would verify the data and statistics provided in the book and also select the most appropriate and valuable contributions from the plentiful contributions we received from authors worldwide. The next step was to appoint an expert of the topic as the Editor-in-Chief, who would head the project and finally make the necessary amendments and modifications to make the text reader-friendly. I was then commissioned to examine all the material to present the topics in the most comprehensible and productive format.

I would like to take this opportunity to thank all the contributing authors who were supportive enough to contribute their time and knowledge to this project. I also wish to convey my regards to my family who have been extremely supportive during the entire project.

Editor

Oral Peanut Challenge Identifies an Allergy but the Peanut Allergen Threshold Sensitivity Is Not Reproducible

Susanne Glaumann[1,2]*, Anna Nopp[3], S. G. O. Johansson[3], Magnus P. Borres[4,5], Caroline Nilsson[1,2]

1 Department of Clinical Science and Education, Södersjukhuset, Centre for Allergy Research, Karolinska Institutet, Stockholm, Sweden, 2 Sach's Children's Hospital, Södersjukhuset, Stockholm, Sweden, 3 Department of Medicine, Clinical Immunology and Allergy Unit, Karolinska Institutet, Stockholm, Sweden, 4 Thermo Fisher Scientific, Uppsala, Sweden, 5 Department of Pediatrics, Institute for Clinical Sciences, The Sahlgrenska Academy at the University of Gothenburg, Sweden

Abstract

Background: Double-blind placebo-controlled food challenge, DBPCFC, the gold standard for diagnosing food allergy, is time-consuming and potentially dangerous. A basophil allergen threshold sensitivity test, CD-sens, has shown promising results as a diagnostic tool in food allergy.

Objectives: To evaluate the reproducibility of oral peanut challenge and compare the outcome to CD-sens in peanut-sensitized children.

Methods: Twenty-seven children (4–19 years) underwent a DBPCFC followed by a single-blind oral food-challenge. The peanut challenges (1 mg to 5 g) were evaluated by severity scoring. Blood samples were drawn for CD-sens before the two first challenges.

Results: Thirteen children (48%) did not react at any of the challenges. Fourteen reacted at both peanut challenges but not to placebo. Only two of these children reacted at the same threshold dose and with the same severity score. All other children scored differently or reacted at different doses. For children with a positive challenge the geometric mean of the ratio of the doses was 1.834 ($p = 0.307$) and the arithmetic mean of the difference between the severity scores was 0.143 ($p = 0.952$). No association was obtained between the two peanut challenges regarding severity score ($r_s = 0.11$, $p = 0.71$) or threshold dose ($r_s = 0.35$, $p = 0.22$). Among the children positive in peanut challenge, 12 were positive in CD-sens. Two were low-responders and could not be evaluated. Geometric mean of the ratio of CD-sens values in children with a positive challenge was 1.035 ($p = 0.505$) but unlike for the severity score and the threshold dose the association between the two CD-sens values was strong ($r_s = 0.94$, $P < 0.001$).

Conclusions: For a positive/negative test the reproducibility is 100% for both peanut challenge and CD-sens. However, a comparison of the degree of allergen threshold sensitivity between the two tests is not possible since the threshold dose and severity scoring is not reproducible.

Editor: Anthony Peter Sampson, University of Southampton School of Medicine, United Kingdom

Funding: This work was supported in part by the Foundation "Mjölkdroppen", Sweden; Swedish Asthma and Allergy Associations Research Foundation, Sweden; Centre for Allergy Research, Karolinska Institutet, Sweden; Hesselman Foundation, Sweden; Foundation "Samariten", Sweden and Princess Lovisa's Association for Childrens Medical Care, Sweden. The funders had no role in study design, data collection and analysis, decision to publish, or preparation of the manuscript.

Competing Interests: MPB is employed at Thermo Fisher Scientific. All other authors have declared they have no conflict of interest.

* E-mail: susanne.glaumann@sodersjukhuset.se

Introduction

Peanuts are one of the most common foods causing allergic reactions in children [1,2]. The severity of the reactions vary but can be life threatening [3] and lead to a decreased quality of life [4,5]. Peanut allergy is usually diagnosed by case history, skin prick test (SPT) and/or immunoglobulin E antibody (IgE-ab) determination. However, the diagnosis often needs to be confirmed by a food challenge. Double-blind placebo-controlled food challenge (DBPCFC) is considered the gold standard [6,7] and is an attempt to mimic real life exposure under standardized conditions. In addition, DBPCFC is the accepted reference test for food allergy when new diagnostic methods or therapies are evaluated [8]. However, DBPCFC is time consuming and associated with risks of severe allergic reactions. It is also difficult to objectively evaluate if a DBPCFC is positive or negative or to determine the severity of the allergy [9]. Besides, placebo reactions may occur in up to 13% of the DBPCFC [10].

The reproducibility of the severity of the reactions and the threshold doses at DBPCFC has to our knowledge so far not been properly documented. A score system for low dose DBPCFC for peanut integrating both symptoms and dose (<100 mg peanut protein) has earlier been published but the peanut challenges were

Table 1. Symptom score according to Astier [20] to evaluate clinical reactions in DBPCFC.

Symptom score	Symptoms
0	**no symptoms**
1	abdominal pain that resolved without medical treatment, rhino conjunctivitis or urticaria <10 paplers, rash
2	**one organ involved,** *abdominal pain requiring treatment, *generalized urticaria, *non laryngeal angioedema, *mild asthma (cough, fall of peak expiratory flow <20%)
3	**two organs involved** (of symptoms mentioned under 2)
4	**three organs involved** (of symptoms mentioned under 2) **or asthma** requiring treatment or laryngeal edema, or hypotension
5	**cardiac and respiratory symptoms requiring hospitalization in the intensive care unit**

not repeated to evaluate the reproducibility [11]. In addition there is no worldwide accepted score system available to evaluate both the severity of the reactions and threshold doses making it hard to compare the results from different studies.

New promising diagnostic tools like basophil allergen threshold sensitivity tests have been evaluated in allergy [12,13,14,15]. A basophil activation test represents the IgE-mediated inflammatory pathway of the allergic response [16,17]. In IgE-mediated allergy tissue mast cells and basophils in the blood are sensitized with IgE-ab against the allergen to which the individual reacts. By stimulating the basophils in vitro with decreasing doses of the allergen, the smallest amount of allergen stimulating the cells can be detected by determination of CD63 up-regulation by flow cytometry. This is designated as the basophil allergen threshold sensitivity, CD-sens [18] and the method has been shown to be an alternative to complex allergen in-vivo challenges. A good correlation has been found between CD-sens and SPT-titration [12] and allergen challenge tests in allergic rhino conjunctivitis [12] and allergic asthma [15] suggesting that CD-sens is a relevant marker of in vivo allergen sensitivity.

The aim of this study was to evaluate the reproducibility of oral peanut challenges for the determination of the allergen threshold sensitivity and to compare it to CD-sens to peanut.

Methods

Study Population

This study includes 27 children who were part of a previous study (n = 38) where peanut allergy was confirmed by double-blind placebo-controlled food challenge (DBPCFC) [13]. The children, aged 4–19 years old, were referred to Sach's Children's Hospital, Stockholm for an oral peanut challenge. All children had a suspected peanut allergy, IgE-ab to peanut (≥0.35 kU_A/L) in serum (ImmunoCAP®Thermo Fischer Scientific, Uppsala, Sweden) and/or a positive skin prick test (SPT) (≥3 mm) to peanut (Soluprick 1/20, ALK, Copenhagen, Denmark) at inclusion. Exclusion criteria were antihistamines or oral steroids taken 4 days prior to the challenge or a history of previous anaphylactic reactions to peanut. A DBPCFC followed by a single-blind oral food-challenge (SBOFC) was performed. The SBOFC was blinded for the child and the parents. In children reacting with severe allergic symptoms at the first peanut challenge the SBOFC was not performed due to ethical reasons. Thus, among 38 children 27 underwent two peanut and one placebo challenge and were included in the present study. All three challenges were planned to take place within one month. The median number of days between the two peanut challenges was 14 (range 7–126). For five children this interval was rather long due to common illness or for social reasons. Of these, three children were negative in both food challenges and CD-sens. For the other two the time between the challenges was 56 (patient J2) and 126 (patient J17) days, respectively.

Ethics Methods

The study was approved by the local ethics committee (Dnr 2008-1001-31/2) and the parents provided written consent.

Challenge Testing

The challenges were performed using a challenge medium with 11% peanut and 7% fat [19]. Increasing doses of peanut were given every 30 minutes in up to 5 steps from 1 mg to 5 g; dose 1 = 0.001 g, dose 2 = 0.01 g, dose 3 = 0.1 g, dose 4 = 1 g and dose 5 = 5 g. The smaller increase between dose 4 and 5 is based on the experiences from our routine DBPCFC because most children are unable to eat 91 g of the challenge medium, chocolate ball. A negative test was defined as no allergic symptoms during two hours after challenge completion. All children stayed at least 2 hours after the challenge and longer if needed. Symptoms were scored according to Astier et al. [20] (Table 1).

Blood Sampling

After preparation of the skin with local anaesthesia, a peripheral venous catheter was provided. Before the two first challenges a blood sample was drawn and stored at +4°C for a maximum of 24 hours for CD-sens analyses.

Basophil Analyses

Basophil allergen threshold sensitivity, CD-sens [12,18] was calculated by stimulating the cells with decreasing concentrations of peanut extract. The same batch of peanut raw material was used in all oral challenges and CD-sens analyses. The stock solution, 1/20 weight/volume, was further diluted 1/50 and designated 1 000 arbitrary units per mL (AU/mL). Each sample was tested with 0.1–1000 AU/mL. In summary, anti- FcεRI (Bühlmann Laboratories AG, Schönenbuch, Switzerland) and N-formyl-methionyl-leucyl-phenylalanin (fMLP) (Sigma Chemilcal Co, St. Louis, Missouri, US) were used as positive controls and RPMI as negative control. Leucocytes were stained with CD63 (Immunotech, Marseille, France) and CD203c (Immunotech) and counted in a Navios flow cytometer (Beckman Coulter, Inc., Fullerton, CA, USA). The cut-off determining a positive allergen test was set to 5% of CD63-positive basophils [12,18].

Individuals with basophils, which after anti-FcεRI stimulation, i.e. the positive control, responded with 0–5% CD63-upregulation were regarded as non-responders. For individuals with a response between 5–16% (low-responders) the results should be interpreted with caution. The cut off 16% was calculated from the positive

			[1st] peanut challenge			[2nd] peanut challenge		
Patient	sex	Age (years)	Symptoms	Severity score	peanut (g)	Symptoms	Severity score	Peanut (g)
J2	female	12.7	urticaria, stomach-ache mouth-itch	3	1.1	asthma, skin-itch, rhinitis, urticaria, stomach-ache	4	6.1
J8	male	15.4	stomach-ache mouth-itch	2	0.1	conjunctivitis, rhinitis, stomach ache	2	1.1
J15	female	17.4	stomach-ache, mouth-itch	2	0.1	mouth-itch, stomach-ache, urticaria, rhinitis	3	1.1
J17	female	14.0	tiredness, mild asthma, mouth-itch	4	6.1	tiredness, stomach-ache, vomiting, conjunctivitis	2	6.1
J19	male	9.8	mouth-itch	1	0.01	mouth-itch, stomach-ache	1	3.6
J22	male	5.4	stomach-ache	1	4.1	conjunctivitis, stomach-ache, tiredness	2	6.1
J24	female	17.6	tiredness, vomiting, mouth- itch, stomach-ache	3	6.1	mouth-itch	1	1.1
J28	male	7.6	stomach-ache	1	6.1	erythema, stomach-ache, tiredness	1	6.1
J31	male	19.0	mouth-itch, urticaria, cough, stomach-ache, tiredness, erythema	4	1.1	mouth-itch	1	0.01
J33	female	12.2	mouth-itch	1	0.01	stomach-ache, tiredness	2	0.1
J36	male	18.4	mouth-itch, stomach-ache, tiredness	2	0.01	mouth-itch, stomach-ache	2	0.001
J38	female	7.9	cough, tiredness	2	0.01	hoarseness, cough, mouth-itch, conjunctivitis, rhinitis, vomiting, stomach-ache, tiredness, urticaria	4	6.1
J39	male	5.9	mouth-itch , stomach-ache tiredness	2	1.1	mouth-itch, asthma	4	1.1
J41	female	11.8	mouth-itch, stomach-ache, tiredness	2	0.1	mouth-itch, stomach-ache, tiredness	2	0.1

Figure 1. Age, sex, symptoms and Astier severity score [20] in children with two positive peanut challenges.

controls (mean 76%, −3SD) of an in-house reference material of 264 allergic children and adults [13].

Basophil allergen threshold sensitivity was measured as the lowest allergen concentration giving 50% (LC50) of maximum CD63 up regulation. CD-sens is defined as the inverted value for LC50 multiplied by 100 and describes the degree of the patient's allergen threshold sensitivity, that is a positive relation between the CD-sens value and the degree of the patient's allergen sensitivity. [18].

Statistics

In patients reacting at both challenges, Wilcoxon Signed Rank Test was used to test differences between the first and the second challenge for Astier score, threshold dose and CD-sens. The values for threshold dose and CD-sens were tested on log-transformed values, thus testing the relative change. The differences between the first and the second challenge are presented in Bland-Altman plots and the associations between first and second value were assessed with Spearman rank order correlation (r_s). No adjustment

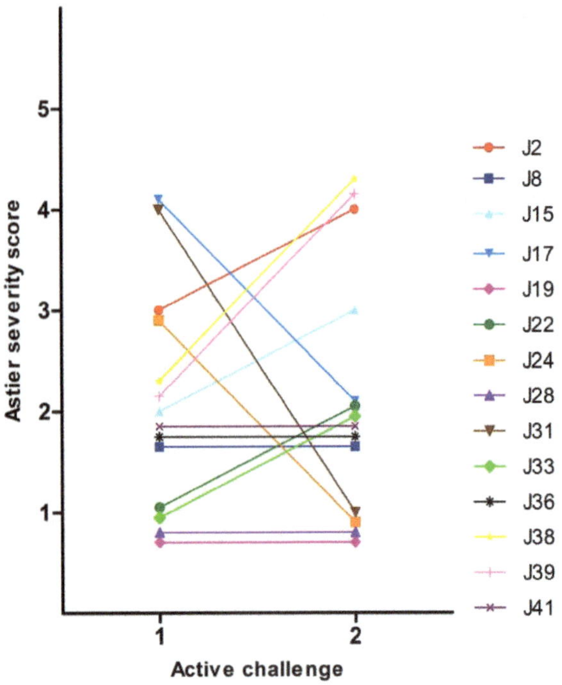

Figure 2. Severity scores according to Astier [20] in the same child at the two peanut challenges.

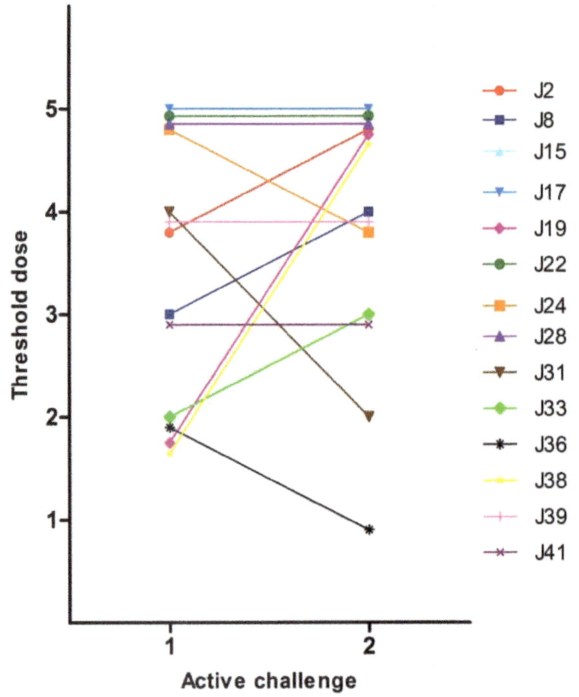

Figure 3. Threshold doses of peanut in the same child at the two peanut challenges. The amount peanut eaten were divided into 5 dose steps: Dose 1 = 0.001 g; Dose 2 = 0.01 g; Dose 3 = 0.1 g; Dose 4 = 1 g; Dose 5 = 3.6–5 g.

for multiple testing has been performed. Thus, significant results should be regarded as descriptive and explorative. Statistical analysis was carried out using IBM SPSS Statistic 20.0, Chicago, Ill, USA. A p-value <0.05 was considered significant.

Results

Patient Characteristics

The median age of the 27 children in the study was 12.2 years (range 5.4–19) and 48% were girls. All 27 children had a diagnosis of peanut allergy and where IgE-sensitized to peanut. Thirteen children had a clinical convincing history of peanut allergy and the other fourteen children were diagnosed with peanut allergy due to results of tests performed in routine clinical work-up.

Oral Food Challenge

The severity of the reactions was scored according to Astier et al. [20] (Table 1). Fourteen children (52%) reacted with allergic symptoms at both peanut challenges, but not on placebo, and were considered as positive (Figure 1). Two children (J28, J41) reacted at the same severity score and had the same threshold dose at the two peanut challenges while all other children (n = 12) scored differently or reacted at different threshold doses (Figure 2 and 3). Thirteen children (48%) did not react at any of the three challenges. All children negative in the challenges consumed full doses (6.1 g peanut). In children with a positive challenge the arithmetic mean of difference in the severity scores (challenge 2 - challenge 1) was 0.143 ($p = 0.952$) (Figure 4) and the geometric mean of the ratio of the doses (challenge 2/challenge 1) was 1.834 ($p = 0.307$) (Figure 5). No association was obtained between the first and the second peanut challenge regarding severity score ($r_s = 0.11$, $p = 0.71$) or threshold dose ($r_s = 0.35$, $p = 0.22$).

CD-sens

CD-sens was performed on blood drawn before the first and second challenges in all children (n = 26) except one. In this child, blood was collected at the second and third challenges due to a misunderstanding. All children with a positive CD-sens at the first challenge where also CD-sens positive at the second challenge. The peanut CD-sens values are presented in figure 6 and 7. Twelve of 14 children with positive challenges were positive in CD-sens to peanut. The remaining two could not be evaluated since they were low responders i.e. had a too low response to the

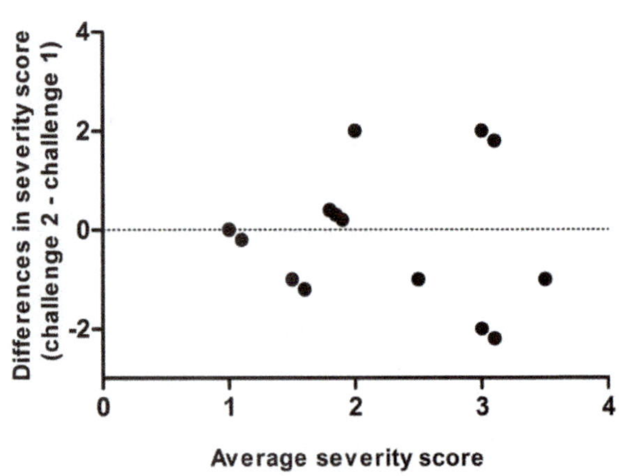

Figure 4. The differences in severity score (challenge 2–challenge 1) in each child with positive peanut challenges, presented as a Bland-Altman plot. The arithmetic mean of the difference between the severity scores was 0.143.

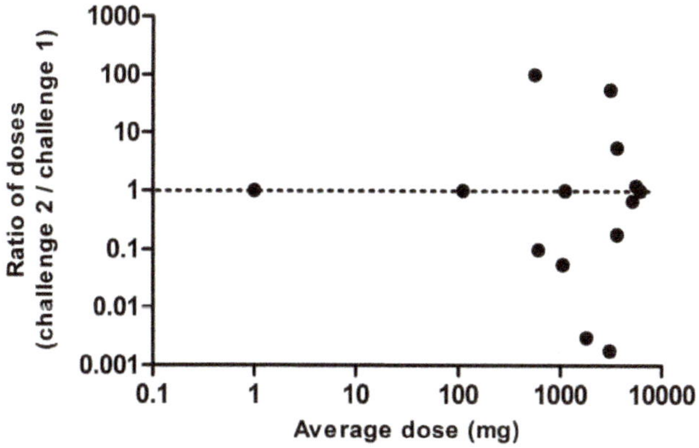

Figure 5. The differences in the ratio of the dose, mg (challenge 2/challenge 1) in each child with positive peanut challenges, presented as a Bland-Altman plot with logarithmically transformed data. The geometric mean of the ratio of the doses was 1.834.

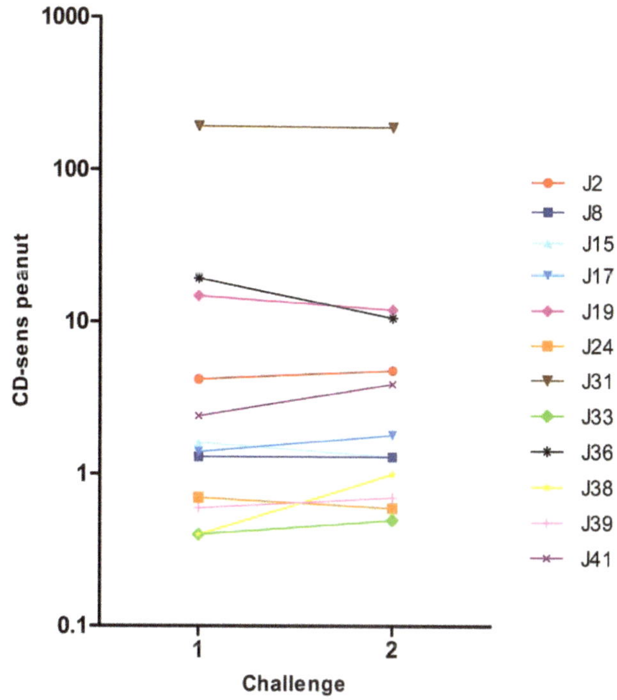

Figure 6. Peanut CD-sens values in the same child at the two peanut challenges.

positive control anti-FcεRI (<16%). Three children had slightly positive values in CD-sens (0.3–0.5) but were negative in challenge. However, all 10 children negative in CD-sens were also negative at both peanut challenges. The geometric mean of the ratio of CD-sens values (challenge 2/challenge 1) in children with a positive challenge was 1.035 ($p = 0.505$) (Figure 8) and the association between the two CD-sens values was strong ($r_s = 0.94$, $P<0.001$).

Discussion

The aim of this study was to evaluate the reproducibility of oral peanut challenges (DBPCFC and SBOFC) for the determination of the allergen threshold sensitivity and to compare it to CD-sens to peanut. However, in contrast to CD-sens it was not possible to quantitatively estimate the allergen threshold sensitivity with oral peanut challenge in a reproducible way. Thus, a comparison of the degree of allergen threshold sensitivity obtained by oral peanut challenge with CD-sens, was not possible to achieve.

The DBPCFC is an attempt to mimic real life exposure under standardized conditions and is today the gold standard for the diagnosis of food allergy [21,22]. However, it is difficult to evaluate the reactions at DBPCFC [9] and each research group is using its own severity scores [11,23,24]. Besides, there are several factors affecting the outcome of a food challenge in addition to the amount of allergen given during challenge, for example aversion to the tested food and the evaluation of subjective symptoms [9]. Thus, reactions to placebo at the DBPCFC have been reported in a significant number [10]. This is in contrast to our study where no positive reactions to placebo occurred.

In the present study all children but two reacted with a different severity score or at another dose when the peanut challenge was repeated. Several studies have tried to determine the threshold dose in peanut allergic patients to predict the clinical sensitivity [24,25,26]. Van der Zee and colleagues [24] aimed to evaluate if the presence of risk factors for a severe allergic reaction to peanut is associated with the patient's clinical sensitivity by determine the eliciting dose of peanut in a DBPCFC and thereby predicting the severity of the allergic reaction. However, they were not able to find a relation between the threshold dose in DBPCFC and the severity of a previous reaction at home. Besides, Skirpak and colleagues [27] evaluated a 23 weeks oral immunotherapy to milk with DBPCFC before and after treatment. The outcome of the food challenge was based on the lowest dose causing a reaction and not from changes in the severity of the reactions. In that study 29% of the patients in the placebo group ($n = 7$) did not react at the same dose at the second DBPCFC. Although the numbers of patients in that study was low, the results indicate that food challenges can be difficult to reproduce [27]. These findings are in line with our observations showing that the severity of the clinical reaction of an oral peanut challenge is not reproducible.

A food challenge can tell you if a patient is allergic or not [13] but when we in this paper investigated the allergen threshold sensitivity and its reproducibility we could not demonstrate a reproducibility of the peanut challenges for determination of allergen sensitivity.

In CD-sens the correlation between the two CD-sens values was strong. A good correlation does not always mean that there is a high reproducibility, but with a high reproducibility there should be a good correlation. For the peanut challenge we could not demonstrate any statistical differences or correlations for doses or symptoms between the two challenges. Thus the low correlation support that the reproducibility was poor for dose and severity score. Difficulties to determine allergen thresholds doses at food challenges have also been noted by others [28]. This is in contrast to CD-sens where we did not find any significant differences but a significant and strong correlation between the two CD-sens occasions. This is supporting that CD-sens measured at different time-points strongly are associated.

Since the CD-sens value is directly related to the allergen concentration of the preparation used and since allergen extracts are not satisfactorily standardized the CD-sens values cannot be compared between different allergens [15]. In this study we used, for the CD-sens analyses, an extract of the same raw material used at the oral challenges. However, since we were not able to determine the patient's allergen threshold sensitivity by oral

	1st challenge		2nd challenge	
Patient	CD-sens Peanut	LC50 (AU/mL)	CD-sens Peanut	LC50 (AU/mL)
J2	4.2	23.6	4.8	21.1
J8	1.3	77.2	1.3	74.5
J15	1.6	62.4	1.3	78.4
J17	1.4	69.4	1.8	56.0
J19	14.8	6.8	12	8.3
J22	Low responder	Low responder	Low responder	Low responder
J24	0.7	149.7	0.6	166.4
J28	Low responder	Low responder	Low responder	Low responder
J31	192	0.5	188	0.52
J33	0.4	263.0	0.5	220.0
J36	19.2	5.2	10.6	9.4
J38	0.4	272.0	1.0	96.0
J39	0.6	162.0	0.7	136.0
J41	2.4	41.7	3.9	25.5

Figure 7. Peanut CD-sens values in children with two positive peanut challenges.

challenge we could not compare the severity of the peanut challenge reaction with CD-sens to peanut.

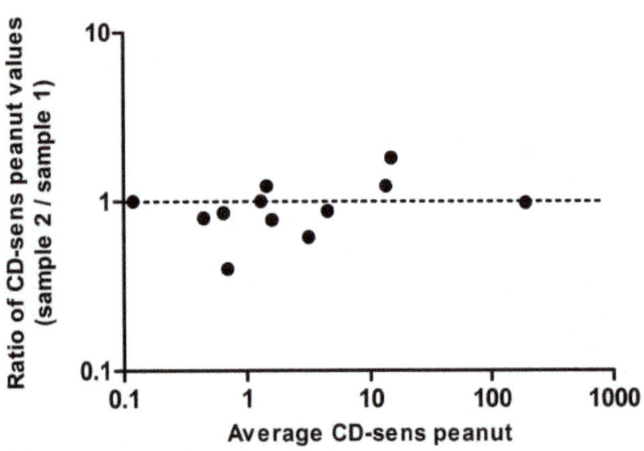

Figure 8. The differences in the ratio for peanut CD-sens values (challenge 2/challenge 1) in each child with positive peanut challenges, presented as a Bland-Altman plot with logarithmically transformed data. Geometric mean of the ratio of CD-sens values was 1.035.

CD-sens has previously been shown to have a good correlation with clinical tests of allergen sensitivity e.g. SPT-titration [12] and allergen challenge in rhino-conjunctivitis [12] and allergic asthma [15]. Interestingly, in allergic asthma there was an excellent correlation between CD-sens and the allergic inflammation behind the bronchial sensitivity but not between CD-sens and the non-specific bronchial hyper-reactivity [12]. Thus, we propose that CD-sens can be used in food allergy to predict the patient's basic allergen sensitivity. CD-sens allows evaluation and monitoring over time of the degree of allergen sensitivity with no risk for the patient. In addition, CD-sens is also, cost effective and time saving.

The strength of the present study is that all oral peanut challenges were performed in the same clinic with the same experienced senior physician grading the patient's clinical reaction and symptom score. An error introduced by performing the second peanut challenge as SBOFC, e.g. that the nurse performing the test was aware of the results of the first challenge, would have resulted in a falsely too good correlation. However, no correlation was found.

Since this is a rather small study the results should be interpreted with caution. Another limitation is that all children with severe anaphylactic reaction at the first peanut challenge were excluded for clinical and ethical reasons when the study was planned, we expected a severe reaction to re-occur. It should also be noted that the blood samples for CD-sens analyses were drawn at the first two challenges and not at the two peanut challenges.

To our knowledge there is no published study investigating the reproducibility of oral food challenge regarding both severity score and dose. Thus, clinical trials using DBPCFC for testing the outcomes of treatments [24,27] can only be correctly evaluated if the study includes information about the reproducibility of the challenges.

We conclude that we were not able to determine the severity of an allergic reaction to peanut since the children reacted at a different dose or with another severity score when the challenge was repeated. However, for a positive/negative test result, the concordance between the two CD-sens values and the two peanut challenges were 100% respectively, but comparison of the degree of allergen threshold sensitivity between the two tests was not possible to achieve since the threshold dose and severity scoring were not reproducible.

If DBPCFC should continue to be used as gold standard for the diagnosis of a food allergy and to predict the severity of a potential clinical reaction, its precision and reproducibility must be documented and improved. Besides, it is of great importance to develop a scoring system integrating both the symptom severity grade and the allergen dose and which can be used world-wide. CD-sens shows promising result with only small variations between the two test occasions but further studies of the role of CD-sens in food allergy diagnosis and treatment trials are most urgent.

Acknowledgments

We would like to thank all children and their parents for participating in the study. We are also very grateful to Ann-Charlotte Sundqvist and the nurses at the Allergy Department, Sachs' Children's Hospital for skilful participation in oral peanut challenges. We wish to acknowledge Åse Olerud and Justus Adédoyin for help with basophil analyses and serological tests and Magnus Rudengren for statistical help. Finally a special thanks to Gunnar Lilja and Malin Berthold for valuable advice in the writing process of the manuscript.

Author Contributions

Conceived and designed the experiments: AN SGOJ CN MPB. Performed the experiments: CN SG AN. Analyzed the data: SG AN. Contributed reagents/materials/analysis tools: SGOJ MPB CN. Wrote the paper: SCG CN AN SGOJ MPB.

References

1. Osborne NJ, Koplin JJ, Martin PE, Gurrin LC, Lowe AJ, et al. (2011) Prevalence of challenge-proven IgE-mediated food allergy using population-based sampling and predetermined challenge criteria in infants. J Allergy Clin Immunol 127: 668–676 e661–662.
2. Chafen JJ, Newberry SJ, Riedl MA, Bravata DM, Maglione M, et al. (2010) Diagnosing and managing common food allergies: a systematic review. JAMA 303: 1848–1856.
3. Sampson HA, Mendelson L, Rosen JP (1992) Fatal and near-fatal anaphylactic reactions to food in children and adolescents. N Engl J Med 327: 380–384.
4. Cummings AJ, Knibb RC, Erlewyn-Lajeunesse M, King RM, Roberts G, et al. (2010) Management of nut allergy influences quality of life and anxiety in children and their mothers. Pediatr Allergy Immunol 21: 586–594.
5. Ostblom E, Egmar AC, Gardulf A, Lilja G, Wickman M (2008) The impact of food hypersensitivity reported in 9-year-old children by their parents on health-related quality of life. Allergy 63: 211–218.
6. Bock SA, Sampson HA, Atkins FM, Zeiger RS, Lehrer S, et al. (1988) Double-blind, placebo-controlled food challenge (DBPCFC) as an office procedure: a manual. J Allergy Clin Immunol 82: 986–997.
7. Bock SA (2000) Evaluation of IgE-mediated food hypersensitivities. J Pediatr Gastroenterol Nutr 30 Suppl: S20–27.
8. Gellerstedt M, Bengtsson U, Niggemann B (2007) Methodological issues in the diagnostic work-up of food allergy: a real challenge. J Investig Allergol Clin Immunol 17: 350–356.
9. Niggemann B (2010) When is an oral food challenge positive? Allergy 65: 2–6.
10. Vlieg-Boerstra BJ, van der Heide S, Bijleveld CM, Kukler J, Duiverman EJ, et al. (2007) Placebo reactions in double-blind, placebo-controlled food challenges in children. Allergy 62: 905–912.
11. Hourihane JO, Grimshaw KE, Lewis SA, Briggs RA, Trewin JB, et al. (2005) Does severity of low-dose, double-blind, placebo-controlled food challenges reflect severity of allergic reactions to peanut in the community? Clin Exp Allergy 35: 1227–1233.
12. Nopp A, Johansson SG, Ankerst J, Bylin G, Cardell LO, et al. (2006) Basophil allergen threshold sensitivity: a useful approach to anti-IgE treatment efficacy evaluation. Allergy 61: 298–302.
13. Glaumann S, Nopp A, Johansson SG, Rudengren M, Borres MP, et al. (2012) Basophil allergen threshold sensitivity, CD-sens, IgE-sensitization and DBPCFC in peanut-sensitized children. Allergy 67: 242–247.
14. Rubio A, Vivinus-Nebot M, Bourrier T, Saggio B, Albertini M, et al. (2011) Benefit of the basophil activation test in deciding when to reintroduce cow's milk in allergic children. Allergy 66: 92–100.
15. Dahlen B, Nopp A, Johansson SG, Eduards M, Skedinger M, et al. (2011) Basophil allergen threshold sensitivity, CD-sens, is a measure of allergen sensitivity in asthma. Clin Exp Allergy 41: 1091–1097.
16. Sabato V, van Hengel AJ, De Knop KJ, Verweij MM, Hagendorens MM, et al. (2011) Human basophils: a unique biological instrument to detect the allergenicity of food. J Investig Allergol Clin Immunol 21: 179–184.
17. Shreffler WG (2006) Evaluation of basophil activation in food allergy: present and future applications. Curr Opin Allergy Clin Immunol 6: 226–233.
18. Johansson SG, Nopp A, van Hage M, Olofsson N, Lundahl J, et al. (2005) Passive IgE-sensitization by blood transfusion. Allergy 60: 1192–1199.
19. van Odijk J, Ahlstedt S, Bengtsson U, Borres MP, Hulthen L (2005) Double-blind placebo-controlled challenges for peanut allergy the efficiency of blinding procedures and the allergenic activity of peanut availability in the recipes. Allergy 60: 602–605.
20. Astier C, Morisset M, Roitel O, Codreanu F, Jacquenet S, et al. (2006) Predictive value of skin prick tests using recombinant allergens for diagnosis of peanut allergy. J Allergy Clin Immunol 118: 250–256.
21. Lieberman JA, Sicherer SH (2011) Diagnosis of food allergy: epicutaneous skin tests, in vitro tests, and oral food challenge. Curr Allergy Asthma Rep 11: 58–64.
22. Nowak-Węgrzyn A, Assa'ad AH, Bahna SL, Bock SA, Sicherer SH, et al. (2009) Work Group report: Oral food challenge testing. Journal of Allergy and Clinical Immunology 123: S365–S383.
23. Codreanu F, Collignon O, Roitel O, Thouvenot B, Sauvage C, et al. (2011) A novel immunoassay using recombinant allergens simplifies peanut allergy diagnosis. Int Arch Allergy Immunol 154: 216–226.
24. van der Zee T, Dubois A, Kerkhof M, van der Heide S, Vlieg-Boerstra B (2011) The eliciting dose of peanut in double-blind, placebo-controlled food challenges decreases with increasing age and specific IgE level in children and young adults. J Allergy Clin Immunol 128: 1031–1036.
25. Eller E, Hansen TK, Bindslev-Jensen C (2012) Clinical thresholds to egg, hazelnut, milk and peanut: results from a single-center study using standardized challenges. Ann Allergy Asthma Immunol 108: 332–336.
26. Flinterman AE, Pasmans SG, Hoekstra MO, Meijer Y, van Hoffen E, et al. (2006) Determination of no-observed-adverse-effect levels and eliciting doses in a representative group of peanut-sensitized children. J Allergy Clin Immunol 117: 448–454.
27. Skripak JM, Nash SD, Rowley H, Brereton NH, Oh S, et al. (2008) A randomized, double-blind, placebo-controlled study of milk oral immunotherapy for cow's milk allergy. J Allergy Clin Immunol 122: 1154–1160.
28. Assa'ad AH, Bahna SL (2012) Food allergy: diagnosis and beyond. Ann Allergy Asthma Immunol 108: 289–290.

2

Poor Reproducibility of Allergic Rhinitis SNP Associations

Daniel Nilsson[1,2], Anand Kumar Andiappan[3,4], Christer Halldén[2], Chew Fook Tim[3], Torbjörn Säll[5], De Yun Wang[6], Lars-Olaf Cardell[1*]

1 Division of ENT Diseases, Department of Clinical Science, Intervention and Technology, Karolinska Institutet, Stockholm, Sweden, 2 Biomedicine, Kristianstad University, Kristianstad, Sweden, 3 Department of Biological Sciences, National University of Singapore, Singapore, Singapore, 4 Singapore Immunology Network (SIgN), Singapore, Singapore, 5 Department of Cell and Organism Biology, Lund University, Lund, Sweden, 6 Department of Otolaryngology, National University of Singapore, Singapore, Singapore

Abstract

Replication of reported associations is crucial to the investigation of complex disease. More than 100 SNPs have previously been reported as associated with allergic rhinitis (AR), but few of these have been replicated successfully. To investigate the general reproducibility of reported AR-associations in candidate gene studies, one Swedish (352 AR-cases, 709 controls) and one Singapore Chinese population (948 AR-cases, 580 controls) were analyzed using 49 AR-associated SNPs. The overall pattern of *P*-values indicated that very few of the investigated SNPs were associated with AR. Given published odds ratios (ORs) most SNPs showed high power to detect an association, but no correlations were found between the ORs of the two study populations or with published ORs. None of the association signals were in common to the two genome-wide association studies published in AR, indicating that the associations represent false positives or have much lower effect-sizes than reported.

Editor: Michael Edward Zwick, Emory University School of Medicine, United States of America

Funding: The Swedish Research Council funded the study. The funder had no role in study design, data collection and analysis, decision to publish, or preparation of the manuscript.

Competing Interests: The authors have declared that no competing interests exist.

* E-mail: lars-olaf.cardell@ki.se

These authors contributed equally to this work.

Introduction

Allergic rhinitis (AR) is the most common allergic disease affecting more than 500 million people worldwide and is characterized by nasal symptoms including sneezing, rhinorrhea and nasal blockage. AR is also associated with an IgE-mediated immune response against allergens [1]. The development of AR is due to a complex interaction between both environmental and genetic factors. The heritability for AR has been estimated to be as high as 70–90% [2,3].

In AR a number of case-control and family-based association studies as well as linkage studies have identified a number of SNPs and chromosomal regions potentially associated with the disease. Until 2010 an absolute majority of the genetic studies of AR were candidate gene studies. The few exceptions were cases of classical linkage analysis. In 2011 a genome-wide association study (GWAS) [4] and a GWAS meta-study [5] were published in addition to a number of candidate gene studies. Thus, the current list of implicated SNPs is clearly dominated by results from early candidate gene studies. In total, this has resulted in more than 100 single nucleotide polymorphisms (SNPs) reported as associated with AR. However, the investigations that have resulted in this list of SNPs are very heterogeneous with respect to sample sizes, type of study populations and phenotype definitions.

Case-control association tests have become a very popular method to search for genetic variants in linkage disequilibrium with risk factors (http://www.wtccc.org.uk). Today, a large number of traits/diseases have been investigated using this technique e.g. diabetes, schizophrenia, coronary diseases and various forms of cancer. Over the past 15 years standards have shifted towards larger sample sizes of both cases and controls. It has also become apparent that an association can only be considered reliable if it has been properly replicated. In a study based on self-reported data on 50 medical phenotypes from a cohort of more than 20 000 genotyped individuals, approximately 75% of expected associations were successfully replicated [6]. One observation was that different traits and diseases varied drastically with respect to their reproducibility of reported associations, probably reflecting inflation of the effects in some reports and differences among diseases in the likelihood of proper disease classification. In a systematic investigation aiming for replication of reported risk-associated polymorphisms in prostate cancer, 18 out of 50 SNPs were successively replicated [7], whereas only 10 out of 93 and 5 out of 44 SNPs were replicated in two different replication studies in asthma [8,9]. Thus, in the ongoing investigation of a disease it is of importance to monitor the general reproducibility of reported associations. In AR no such evaluation has previously been performed.

In this study we have investigated the general reproducibility of reported SNP associations from previous candidate gene studies using two different study populations, one Swedish and one Singapore Chinese. The result shows poor reproducibility of AR SNP associations.

Results and Discussion

To investigate the reproducibility of reported associations from previous candidate gene studies in AR, two study populations, one from Sweden (352 AR-cases, 709 controls) and one from Singapore (948 AR-cases, 580 controls), were analyzed using a set of 49 SNPs reported as associated with AR. These SNPs constitute a subset of a total of 116 AR-associated SNP markers compiled from 52 different studies (Table S1 and S2). The present study investigates the same phenotype (AR) and the same SNP markers that were reported in the initial studies.

Association test results are summarized in Table 1, Table S3, S4, S5 and S6. In the Singapore Chinese population (CP), 45 SNPs were analyzed. The distribution of *P*-values showed a very good fit to the expected distribution in the absence of an effect. The lowest *P*-value was 0.003 for rs3761547 in the *FOXP3* gene and no SNP showed a false discovery rate (*Q*-value) below 0.1. The 49 SNPs analyzed in the Swedish population (SP) also showed a good fit to the expected distribution of *P*-values in the absence of an effect. There was, however, a slight overrepresentation of *P*-values below 0.01. The lowest *P*-value ($P=0.00084$, $Q=0.033$) was found for rs4732416 in *CCL24* when testing for genotypic effects. However, in the corresponding test of allelic effects the *P*-value was 0.75 and two additional SNPs in this gene showed no significant associations. In the *FOXJ1*-gene the rs880213 SNP showed *P*-values below 0.01 both at the allele and genotype levels. The corresponding *Q*-values were 0.28 and 0.085. Significant *P*-values were observed in both populations for rs20541 in *IL13* and for rs13340504 in *CCL24*. In both cases, however, significant *P*-values were observed for the association test in CP and the skin prick test (SPT) in SP. Thus, the overall pattern of *P*- and *Q*-values in the present study indicates that very few if any of the SNPs are associated with AR.

The lack of replication can have several explanations: the previously reported effects may simply not be present in the populations investigated here, the original reports may be false positive associations (type I error), or the reported odds ratios (ORs) may be inflated due to chance (the "winners curse" effect). Also, the use of different clinical definitions compared to the original reports resulting in enrichment of cases with different clinical subtypes makes replication difficult. In addition, interactions with other factors such as age, sex and urban/rural residency may have an impact on replication. To investigate the ability of the present study to detect the previously reported associations, we estimated the power for the allele-based test in the present investigation. Given calculated or published ORs and the sample sizes used in the present study, the power was calculated at significance levels 0.05 and 0.001. The results are shown in Table 2 where most SNPs show high power to detect an association. The expected number of significant *P*-values is calculated as the sum of the power estimates with standard deviation $= (\sum power_i(1-power_i))^{1/2}$. The expected number varies between 16.3 and 22.3 with standard deviations between 1.0 and 1.8. Since the observed number of significant *P*-values varies between 0 and 2 (Table 1), the expected numbers exceed the observed by many standard deviations, i.e. if the published ORs would have been true a number of significant results would have been expected. However, it is not an uncommon observation that early association studies report highly inflated ORs. Although the observed results are not surprising, the present investigation is the first systematic study of this aspect in AR.

If the originally reported significant ORs are due to a "winners curse" effect, the power in our analysis may be insufficient. If this is true, an effect could perhaps still be traced via a correlation of effects between investigations. Spearman correlation coefficients were therefore calculated from the ORs for allelic effects for the different sets of data. Comparing data from the SP with published data from the other European populations, a non-significant result was obtained with a correlation coefficient of 0.08 ($P=0.84$). In the corresponding comparison between data obtained from the CP and published data from other Asian populations the correlation coefficient was higher but still non-significant ($R=0.33$ and $P=0.19$). Finally, the concordance between SP and CP was calculated. Also this comparison gave a low and non-significant correlation coefficient ($R=0.03$ and $P=0.87$).

A third strategy to investigate potential associations would be to test for identical trends among SNPs. This was done by calculating the number of concordant SNPs, i.e. SNPs for which both ORs were either larger than 1 or less than 1, as well as the number of discordant SNPs, i.e. SNPs where one OR was less than 1 and the other was larger than 1. In the comparison between the Swedish and Singapore results, 23 SNPs were concordant and 20 were

Table 1. Observed and expected numbers of *P*-values for the different association tests in the Swedish population (n = 1061) and the Singapore Chinese population (n = 1528).

P-value range		Swedish population					Singapore Chinese population				
		Allele	**Genotype**	**Birch**	**Timothy**	**Total**	**Allele**	**Genotype**	***B. tropicalis***	***D. pteronyssinus***	**Total**
1.0–0.1	Obs/Exp	45/44	45/44	42/43	42/43	174/174	41/41	39/41	43/41	41/41	166/162
	Q-values	0.88–0.99	0.59–0.74	0.73–0.97	0.50–0.80	0.50–0.99	0.88–0.97	0.53–0.77	0.76–0.90	0.42–0.97	0.42–0.97
0.1–0.05	Obs/Exp	3/2.5	2/2.5	4/2.4	4/2.4	13/9.8	2/2.3	4/2.3	1/2.3	1/2.3	7/9.2
	Q-values	0.88–0.93	0.59	0.73	0.45–0.49	0.45–0.93	0.88	0.46	0.76	0.42	0.42–0.88
0.05–0.01	Obs/Exp	0/2.0	0/2.0	1/1.9	1/1.9	2/7.8	2/1.8	2/1.8	0/1.8	2/1.8	6/7.2
	Q-values	–	–	0.73	0.45	0.45–0.73	0.60	0.46	–	0.15–0.19	0.15–0.60
0.01–0.001	Obs/Exp	1/0.44	1/0.44	1/0.43	1/0.43	4/1.7	0/0.40	0/0.40	2/0.40	1/0.40	3/1.6
	Q-values	0.28	0.085	0.23	0.12	0.085–0.28	–	–	0.11–0.13	0.14	0.11–0.14
0.001	Obs/Exp	0/0.05	1/0.050	0/0.050	0/0.050	1/0.20	0/0.040	0/0.040	0/0.040	0/0.040	0/0.16
	Q-values	–	0.033	–	–	–	–	–	–	–	–

Obs/Exp = Observed number of *P*-values/Expected number of *P*-values in the absence of effect.
Q-values = Observed *Q*-values calculated according to Storey JD (2002) A direct approach to false discovery rates. J R Stat Soc Series B Stat Methodol 64:479–498.

Table 2. Power estimates in present investigation given odds ratios extracted or calculated from published data.

Gene	SNP ID	Polymorphism	Population	Population size (case; control)	OR†	Power (SP)‡		Power (CP)‡		Reference*
						0.05	0.001	0.05	0.001	
IL28RA	rs7525481	g.32349 G>A	Korean	267; 559	0.74	0.72	0.20	0.98	0.76	[10]
FCGR2A	rs1801274	R131R	Turkish	180; 234	1.93	1.00	1.00	1.00	1.00	[11]
CD55 (DAF)	rs10746463		Japanese	684; 346	0.73	0.86	0.40	–	–	[12]
CCR3	rs4987053	51T/C	Japanese	151; 157	7.75	1.00	1.00	1.00	1.00	[13]
IL2	rs2069762	−330T/G	German	318; 322	1.29	0.72	0.22	0.91	0.49	[14]
IL13	rs1800925	C-1112T	Spanish	146; 50	0.16	1.00	1.00	1.00	1.00	[15]
IL13	rs20541	R130Q	Spanish	146; 50	1.52	0.97	0.73	1.00	0.98	[15]
HAVCR2	rs1036199	4259G>T	Korean	201; 319	1.54	0.98	0.75	0.16	0.00	[16]
CCL26	rs2302009	2497T>G	Korean	178; 281	2.87	1.00	1.00	1.00	1.00	[17]
CCL24	rs2302004	179T>C	Korean	178; 281	1.10	0.19	0.01	0.22	0.02	[17]
IL33	rs1929992		Japanese	170; 100	1.41	0.95	0.63	1.00	0.90	[18]
GATA3	rs1269486		Han Chinese	109; 112	0.35	1.00	1.00	1.00	0.97	[19]
MS4A2	rs569108	Glu237Gly	Japanese	233; 100	1.47	0.17	0.01	0.99	0.81	[20]
IL18	rs187238	−137G>C	Swiss	1105; 2953	1.12	0.20	0.01	0.17	0.01	[21]
IL18	rs187238	−137C	German	25; 80	2.72*	1.00	1.00	1.00	1.00	[22]
RNASE3	rs2233860		Korean	440; 478	1.36	0.78	0.30	0.87	0.41	[23]
IL4R	rs1805010	Ile50Val	Japanese	145; 206	0.62	1.00	0.96	1.00	1.00	[24]
IL4R	rs1805011	Glu375Ala	Japanese	145; 206	0.35	1.00	1.00	1.00	1.00	[24]
NOD2	rs5743266		German	488; 978	0.82*	0.43	0.06	0.08	0.00	[25]
NOD2	rs2066842		German	488; 978	0.80*	0.49	0.08	0.08	0.00	[25]
NOD2	rs2066844	C2104T	German	154; 1765	1.73*	0.53	0.13	–	–	[26]
NOD2	rs2066845	G2722C	German	154; 1765	3.16*	0.87	0.46	–	–	[26]
CCL5	rs2280788	−28C/G	Korean	151; 278	1.58	0.43	0.08	0.98	0.78	[27]
CCL5	rs2107538	−403G/A	Korean	151; 278	1.42	0.85	0.41	1.00	0.89	[27]
EPX	rs2240815	3979A/G	Czech	294; 319	1.28	0.76	0.27	0.85	0.39	[28]
FOXJ1	rs3192453	g.3375G>C	Korean	295; 418	0.62	0.78	0.25	0.98	0.78	[29]
FOXJ1	rs880213	g. −460C>T	Korean	295; 418	0.64	0.89	0.43	0.95	0.64	[29]
ADAM33	rs2787094		Chinese Han	128; 151	4.01	1.00	1.00	1.00	1.00	[30]
ADAM33	rs2280089	12540C/T	Japanese	95; 95	0.32	1.00	1.00	1.00	1.00	[31]
ADAM33	rs2280089	12540C/T	Chinese Han	128; 151	1.91	1.00	0.98	1.00	0.99	[30]
ADAM33	rs2280090	12462C/T	Japanese	95; 95	0.28	1.00	1.00	1.00	1.00	[31]
ADAM33	rs2280090	12462C/T	Chinese Han	128; 151	0.40	1.00	0.99	1.00	1.00	[30]
ADAM33	rs511898	7575G/A	Japanese	95; 95	0.60	1.00	0.96	1.00	1.00	[31]

†Odds ratios (OR) as reported in reference (*) or calculated for minor allele given published data.
‡Power calculations at different levels of significance in the Swedish (SP) and the Singapore Chinese (CP) population. The significance level 0.001 corresponds approximately to the Bonferroni correction level.

discordant, which of course is not significantly different from equal proportions. Thus, even at this basic level no sign of effects of the investigated SNPs could be detected.

Several GWAS have been performed to identify genetic variants for asthma and related phenotypes whereas only one study has been performed aiming specifically for AR [4]. In the latter no associations were detected at a genome-wide significance level, and only two at a suggestive significance level. A genome-wide meta-analysis based on self-reported phenotyping identified few genetic variants associated with AR in spite of analyzing 2.2 million SNPs in close to 4000 AR cases and 9000 controls [5]. Only one locus reached genome-wide significance and six suggestive loci were identified. When this data set was used in a candidate gene approach analyzing 164 genes only one locus was identified as suggestive for the AR phenotype [5]. Comparing these two GWAS there were no significant association signals in common, and the ORs identified for the significant SNPs were in the size ranges 0.6–1.4 and 1.1–1.3, respectively, in the two studies [4,5]. This is in contrast to the previously reported associations listed in Table S1 and S2 where many show much stronger effects (OR = 0.16–7.8). In addition, none of these associations are detected in the GWAS described above.

In conclusion, the overall pattern of *P*- and *Q*-values indicates that very few, if any, of the 49 investigated SNPs are significantly associated with AR in our populations. If associations do exist they must have much lower effect sizes than reported. This is in agreement with the results of the GWAS where reported effect sizes are fairly modest. The results above do not exclude that certain cases may represent true associations. Due to the necessary compensation for the multiple testing involved, the larger the number of SNPs that are included in a study, the harder it is to detect true associations. The obvious candidates are of course the SNPs with low *P*-values mentioned above. In these cases, the likelihood of an association is strengthened if the ORs in CP, SP and the original publication are concordant. This is not the case for the SNPs in *CCL24*, *FOXJ1* and *IL33*. The strongest case using this criterion would be rs20541 in *IL13* where there is complete concordance in the direction of the ORs between both populations and the original result. Thus, even though this SNP did not yield the lowest *P*-value, it is potentially the best candidate for future investigations. There are a number of other reasons for the lack of replication, such as the use of different clinical definitions or that different studies may be enriched in cases with different clinical subtypes. This indicates that future GWAS or candidate gene studies favorably would use much larger population sizes and more careful phenotyping using strictly defined guidelines than what has been used in the past. In addition, alternative strategies for the identification of AR-associated genes, such as exome sequencing, may be more successful strategies.

Materials and Methods

Ethics Statement

This study was approved by the Ethics Committee of the Medical Faculty, Lund University and the Institutional Review Board of National University of Singapore and written informed consent was obtained from all subjects. This study is also in compliance with the Helsinki declaration.

Study Populations and Phenotype Definitions

The Swedish study population was recruited at Malmö University hospital (Malmö, Sweden) between the years 2003 and 2009 and consists of unrelated subjects from the general population. It is comprised of 360 AR-cases (169 females, 191 males, mean age 33 years) and 720 controls (294 females, 426 males, mean age 43 years) with no atopy and allergic symptomology. All cases were patients at the allergy clinic and were diagnosed with symptomatic birch and/or timothy grass pollen induced intermittent AR. Both cases and controls were of Caucasian origin, with both parents born in Sweden. In the Swedish population skin prick tests (SPT) [32] were performed with a standard panel of 11 common airborne allergens (ALK-Abelló, Hørsholm, Denmark). This study population has previously been analyzed in several AR studies [33,34,35].

The Singapore Chinese population was collected in Singapore over multiple volunteer recruitment drives and consists of unrelated subjects. In the Singapore Chinese population SPT was using a panel consisting of common allergens in Singapore such as *Dermatophagoides pteronyssinus* and *Blomia tropicalis*. The population used in this study consists of 1024 AR cases (549 females, 475 males, mean age 22 years) with symptomatic dust mite induced AR and 605 controls (449 females, 156 males, mean age 22 years) with no atopy and allergic symptomology. This study population has previously been analyzed in several AR studies [4,35,36,37,38].

Diagnostic procedures for the study populations included personal interview of medical history and SPT or Phadiatop tests and were performed using standard panels of common airborne allergens. SPT were performed on the volar side of the forearm with saline buffer as negative and histamine chloride (10 mg/ml) as positive controls. A wheal reaction diameter of ≥3 mm was considered a positive SPT response. SPT was only performed if the AR cases had not taken any anti-allergic drugs for at least 3 days prior to the test. Atopy is defined as a positive SPT reaction to either one of allergens tested. AR is thus diagnosed based on the presence of atopic status and typical AR symptoms as defined by the Allergic Rhinitis Impact on Asthma (ARIA) guidelines i.e., two or more AR symptoms (nasal congestion, rhinorrhea, nasal itching, sneezing) persisting for four or more days per week during the past year [1,39]. Conversely, the non-allergic controls are defined by having no atopy and no typical AR symptoms.

Literature Mining and SNP Selection

PubMed (www.ncbi.nlm.nih.gov/pubmed/) was used to search for reports on AR associations using the search terms: (rhinitis OR hay fever) AND (association OR "case control") AND (polymorphism OR SNP OR mutation) AND English [language]. Studies that only reported skin prick test scores, associations with severity or related phenotypes such as IgE levels, but not allergic rhinitis *per se* were not considered in this study. The first literature search was conducted 2010-03-16 and served as a base for selection of 49 randomly chosen SNPs previously reported to be associated with AR ($P<0.05$). A second literature search was made 2012-06-26, using the same search terms as described above, to make an up-to-date list containing all previously associated SNPs with AR (Table S1 and S2).

Genotyping of Candidate Polymorphisms

Genomic DNA was extracted from blood collected in EDTA using QIAamp DNA Blood Maxi or Mini kits (Qiagen, Hilden, Germany) and DNA concentrations determined by fluorometry using PicoGreen (Molecular Probes, Eugene, OR, USA). Genotypes were determined using the Sequenom MassARRAY MALDI-TOF system. The system analyzes allele-specific primer extension products using mass-spectrometry. Assay design was made using the MassARRAY Assay Design ver. 2.0 software (Sequenom Inc, San Diego, CA, USA). Primers were obtained from Metabion GmbH, Germany and all reactions were run under the same conditions except for the primer annealing temperature of the primary PCR. PCR reactions were performed in a total volume of 6 µl containing 2.5 ng of template DNA, 1.25X HotStar Taq PCR buffer, 0.15 units of HotStar Taq polymerase, 3.5 mM $MgCl_2$, 0.5 mM dNTPs and 100 nM of each primer. Amplifications were performed using GeneAmp 9700 machines with dual-384 heads as follows: 95°C for 15 min, 45 cycles of 95°C for 20 s, 56°C, 60°C or 64°C for 30 s, 72°C for 60 s and finally 72°C for 3 min. Dephosphorylation of unincorporated dNTPs was achieved using shrimp alkaline phosphatase. Concentrations of individual hME primer pairs were adjusted to even out peak heights in the mass spectrum. The extension reactions were then made by mixing the adjusted MassEXTEND primer mix (containing approximately 1 µM of each primer) with hME EXTEND mix containing buffer and 50 µM of each d/ddNTP mix and 1.25 units of Thermo Sequenase. PCR amplification of hME reactions was performed as follows: 94°C for 2 min and 99 cycles of 94°C for 5 s, 52°C for 5 s and 72°C for 5 s. The samples were then manually desalted by using 6 mg of Clean Resin and a dimple plate and subsequently transferred to a 384-well SpectroCHIP using a nanodispenser.

Analyzing 49 SNPs, the total genotyping rate in the Swedish population was 99.4% in 352 (168 female, 184 male) cases and 709 (291 female, 418 male) controls after removal of low-quality DNA samples. In the Chinese population, the total genotyping rate after removal of low-quality data was 99.7% in 948 (514 female, 434 male) cases and 580 (440 female, 140 male) controls. Only 45 SNPs were polymorphic in the Singapore Chinese population.

Statistical Analysis

Statistical analyses were made using R statistical software [40] and the genetics package [41]. Genotype frequencies were calculated and tested for Hardy-Weinberg equilibrium in both cases and controls. Allele and genotype frequencies were then investigated for association with AR using a χ^2-homogeneity test. ORs and 95% confidence intervals were estimated by using the most common allele as the referent and are reported for each minor allele. The Kruskal-Wallis rank sum test was used for analysis of associations between genotypes and SPT-scores. The score is defined as the size of the wheel reaction in relation to histamine. In order to compensate for the effect of multiple testing, *Q*-values was calculated using the software QVALUE (ver.1.0) [42]. One of the assumptions underlying the calculation of the *Q*-values is that the *P*-values will be uniformly distributed under the null hypothesis. We have calculated the number of expected *P*-values in the different ranges, with a higher resolution for the lower values.

Power calculations were made through simulations for the association tests of allele effects. The calculations were made separately for the Swedish and Singapore populations. For each SNP we simulated a data set with the actual numbers of cases and controls of the respective population, using the published or calculated ORs (given published data) and the allele frequencies observed in our populations. A total of 10 000 runs were made in each case. For these, a full data set was simulated and the χ^2-value was calculated. The number of times the test quantity exceeded the critical values for 0.05 and 0.001 was subsequently scored.

Supporting Information

Table S1 Genes and SNPs reported to be associated with allergic rhinitis in case-control studies.

Table S2 Genes and SNPs reported to be associated with allergic rhinitis in family-based studies.

Table S3 Minor allele frequencies (MAF) and P-values for Hardy-Weinberg (HW), association and skin prick test in the Singapore Chinese population.

Table S4 Observed odds ratios (OR) and 95% confidence intervalls (CI) in the Singapore Chinese population.

Table S5 Minor allele frequencies (MAF) and P-values for Hardy-Weinberg (HW), association and skin prick test in the Swedish population.

Table S6 Observed odds ratios (OR) and 95% confidence intervalls (CI) in the Swedish population.

Author Contributions

Conceived and designed the experiments: DN CH LOC. Analyzed the data: DN TS CFT AKA. Wrote the paper: DN CH TS LOC. Performed recruitment of subjects and clinical examinations of patients: LOC DYW. Critically revised the manuscript and approved the final form of the manuscript: LOC DN AKA CH CFT TS DYW.

References

1. Bousquet J, Khaltaev N, Cruz AA, Denburg J, Fokkens WJ, et al. (2008) Allergic rhinitis and its impact on asthma (ARIA) 2008 update (in collaboration with the World Health Organization, GA(2)LEN and AllerGen). Allergy 63 Suppl 86: 8–160.
2. Rasanen M, Laitinen T, Kaprio J, Koskenvuo M, Laitinen LA (1998) Hay fever–a Finnish nationwide study of adolescent twins and their parents. Allergy 53: 885–890.
3. van Beijsterveldt CE, Boomsma DI (2007) Genetics of parentally reported asthma, eczema and rhinitis in 5-yr-old twins. Eur Respir J 29: 516–521.
4. Andiappan AK, Wang dY, Anantharaman R, Parate PN, Suri BK, et al. (2011) Genome-wide association study for atopy and allergic rhinitis in a Singapore Chinese population. PLoS One 6: e19719.
5. Ramasamy A, Curjuric I, Coin LJ, Kumar A, McArdle WL, et al. (2011) A genome-wide meta-analysis of genetic variants associated with allergic rhinitis and grass sensitization and their interaction with birth order. J Allergy Clin Immunol 128: 996–1005.
6. Tung JY, Do CB, Hinds DA, Kiefer AK, Macpherson JM, et al. (2011) Efficient replication of over 180 genetic associations with self-reported medical data. PLoS One 6: e23473.
7. Klein RJ, Halldén C, Gupta A, Savage CJ, Dahlin A, et al. (2011) Evaluation of multiple risk-associated single nucleotide polymorphisms versus prostate-specific antigen at baseline to predict prostate cancer in unscreened men. Eur Urol 61: 471–477.
8. Rogers AJ, Raby BA, Lasky-Su JA, Murphy A, Lazarus R, et al. (2009) Assessing the reproducibility of asthma candidate gene associations, using genome-wide data. Am J Respir Crit Care Med 179: 1084–1090.
9. Murk W, Walsh K, Hsu LI, Zhao L, Bracken MB, et al. (2011) Attempted replication of 50 reported asthma risk genes identifies a SNP in RAD50 as associated with childhood atopic asthma. Hum Hered 71: 97–105.
10. Chae SC, Park YR, Li CS, Lee JH, Yang YS, et al. (2006) Analysis of the variations in IL-28RA gene and their association with allergic rhinitis. Exp Mol Med 38: 302–309.
11. Gulen F, Tanac R, Altinoz S, Berdeli A, Zeyrek D, et al. (2007) The Fc gammaRIIa polymorphism in Turkish children with asthma bronchial and allergic rhinitis. Clin Biochem 40: 392–396.
12. Kawai T, Takeshita S, Imoto Y, Matsumoto Y, Sakashita M, et al. (2009) Associations between decay-accelerating factor polymorphisms and allergic respiratory diseases. Clin Exp Allergy 39: 1508–1514.
13. Nakamura H, Higashikawa F, Nobukuni Y, Miyagawa K, Endo T, et al. (2007) Genotypes and haplotypes of CCR2 and CCR3 genes in Japanese cedar pollinosis. Int Arch Allergy Immunol 142: 329–334.
14. Nieters A, Linseisen J, Becker N (2004) Association of polymorphisms in Th1, Th2 cytokine genes with hayfever and atopy in a subsample of EPIC-Heidelberg. Clin Exp Allergy 34: 346–353.
15. Llanes E, Quiralte J, Lopez E, Sastre B, Chacartegui M, et al. (2009) Analysis of polymorphisms in olive pollen allergy: IL13, IL4RA, IL5 and ADRB2 genes. Int Arch Allergy Immunol 148: 228–238.
16. Chae SC, Park YR, Lee YC, Lee JH, Chung HT (2004) The association of TIM-3 gene polymorphism with atopic disease in Korean population. Hum Immunol 65: 1427–1431.
17. Chae SC, Park YR, Oh GJ, Lee JH, Chung HT (2005) The suggestive association of eotaxin-2 and eotaxin-3 gene polymorphisms in Korean population with allergic rhinitis. Immunogenetics 56: 760–764.
18. Sakashita M, Yoshimoto T, Hirota T, Harada M, Okubo K, et al. (2008) Association of serum interleukin-33 level and the interleukin-33 genetic variant with Japanese cedar pollinosis. Clin Exp Allergy 38: 1875–1881.
19. Zhang L, Wang X, Han D, Duan H, Zhao Y (2009) Association of single nucleotide polymorphisms in GATA-3 with allergic rhinitis. Acta Otolaryngol 129: 190–194.
20. Nagata H, Mutoh H, Kumahara K, Arimoto Y, Tomemori T, et al. (2001) Association between nasal allergy and a coding variant of the Fc epsilon RI beta gene Glu237Gly in a Japanese population. Hum Genet 109: 262–266.
21. Imboden M, Nieters A, Bircher AJ, Brutsche M, Becker N, et al. (2006) Cytokine gene polymorphisms and atopic disease in two European cohorts. (ECRHS-Basel and SAPALDIA). Clin Mol Allergy 4: 1–9.
22. Kruse S, Kuehr J, Moseler M, Kopp MV, Kurz T, et al. (2003) Polymorphisms in the IL 18 gene are associated with specific sensitization to common allergens and allergic rhinitis. J Allergy Clin Immunol 111: 117–122.
23. Kang I, An XH, Oh YK, Lee SH, Jung HM, et al. (2009) Identification of polymorphisms in the RNase3 gene and the association with allergic rhinitis. Eur Arch Otorhinolaryngol 267: 391–395.
24. Nakamura H, Miyagawa K, Ogino K, Endo T, Imai T, et al. (2003) High contribution contrast between the genes of eosinophil peroxidase and IL-4 receptor alpha-chain in Japanese cedar pollinosis. J Allergy Clin Immunol 112: 1127–1131.

25. Weidinger S, Klopp N, Rummler L, Wagenpfeil S, Baurecht HJ, et al. (2005) Association of CARD15 polymorphisms with atopy-related traits in a population-based cohort of Caucasian adults. Clin Exp Allergy 35: 866–872.
26. Kabesch M, Peters W, Carr D, Leupold W, Weiland SK, et al. (2003) Association between polymorphisms in caspase recruitment domain containing protein 15 and allergy in two German populations. J Allergy Clin Immunol 111: 813–817.
27. Kim JJ, Lee JH, Jang CH, Kim YS, Chae SC, et al. (2004) Chemokine RANTES promoter polymorphisms in allergic rhinitis. Laryngoscope 114: 666–669.
28. Hrdlickova B, Izakovicova-Holla L (2009) Association of single nucleotide polymorphisms in the eosinophil peroxidase gene with allergic rhinitis in the Czech population. Int Arch Allergy Immunol 150: 184–191.
29. Li CS, Chae SC, Lee JH, Zhang Q, Chung HT (2006) Identification of single nucleotide polymorphisms in FOXJ1 and their association with allergic rhinitis. J Hum Genet 51: 292–297.
30. Su D, Zhang X, Sui H, Lu F, Jin L, et al. (2008) Association of ADAM33 gene polymorphisms with adult allergic asthma and rhinitis in a Chinese Han population. BMC Med Genet 9: 82.
31. Cheng L, Enomoto T, Hirota T, Shimizu M, Takahashi N, et al. (2004) Polymorphisms in ADAM33 are associated with allergic rhinitis due to Japanese cedar pollen. Clin Exp Allergy 34: 1192–1201.
32. Bousquet J, Heinzerling L, Bachert C, Papadopoulos NG, Bousquet PJ, et al. (2011) Practical guide to skin prick tests in allergy to aeroallergens. Allergy 67: 18–24.
33. Bryborn M, Halldén C, Säll T, Adner M, Cardell LO (2008) Comprehensive evaluation of genetic variation in S100A7 suggests an association with the occurrence of allergic rhinitis. Respir Res 9: 29.
34. Bryborn M, Halldén C, Säll T, Cardell LO (2010) CLC - a novel susceptibility gene for allergic rhinitis? Allergy 65: 220–228.
35. Nilsson D, Andiappan AK, Halldén C, Yun WD, Säll T, et al. (2012) Toll-like receptor gene polymorphisms are associated with allergic rhinitis: a case control study. BMC Med Genet 13: 66.
36. Andiappan AK, Anantharaman R, Nilkanth PP, Wang dY, Chew FT (2010) Evaluating the transferability of Hapmap SNPs to a Singapore Chinese population. BMC Genet 11: 36.
37. Andiappan AK, Parate PN, Anantharaman R, Suri BK, Wang dY, et al. (2011) Genetic variation in BDNF is associated with allergic asthma and allergic rhinitis in an ethnic Chinese population in Singapore. Cytokine 56: 218–223.
38. Andiappan AK, Yeo WS, Parate PN, Anantharaman R, Suri BK, et al. (2011) Variation in Uteroglobin-Related Protein 1 (UGRP1) gene is associated with allergic rhinitis in Singapore Chinese. BMC Med Genet 12: 39.
39. Bousquet J, Van Cauwenberge P, Khaltaev N, Group AW, Organization WH (2001) Allergic rhinitis and its impact on asthma. J Allergy Clin Immunol 108: S147–334.
40. R Development Core Team (2009) R: A language and environment for statistical computing. Vienna, Austria: R Foundation for Statistical Computing.
41. Warnes G, Gorjanc G, Leisch F, Man M (2008) Genetics: Population Genetics.
42. Storey JD (2002) A direct approach to false discovery rates. J R Stat Soc Series B Stat Methodol 64: 479–498.

3

ASXL1 but Not *TET2 Mutations* Adversely Impact Overall Survival of Patients Suffering Systemic Mastocytosis with Associated Clonal Hematologic Non-Mast-Cell Diseases

Gandhi Damaj[1,2,3*], Magalie Joris[1], Olivia Chandesris[2,4], Katia Hanssens[5], Erinn Soucie[5], Danielle Canioni[6], Brigitte Kolb[7], Isabelle Durieu[8], Emanuel Gyan[9], Cristina Livideanu[10], Stephane Chèze[11], Momar Diouf[12], Reda Garidi[13], Sophie Georgin-Lavialle[14], Vahid Asnafi[15], Ludovic Lhermitte[15], Christian Lavigne[16], David Launay[17], Michel Arock[18,19], Olivier Lortholary[20], Patrice Dubreuil[5¶], Olivier Hermine[2,3,4¶]

1 Service d'Hématologie, Centre Hospitalier Universitaire, Hôpital Sud; Amiens, France, **2** Centre de Référence des Mastocytoses, Faculté de Médecine et AP-HP Necker-Enfants Malades, Paris, France, **3** CNRS UMR 8147 and Institut Imagine, AP-HP, Hôpital Necker-Enfants Malades, Paris, France, **4** Service d'Hématologie Adulte, Université Paris Descartes, Paris Sorbonne Cité, Faculté de Médecine et AP-HP Necker-Enfants Malades, Paris, France, **5** Inserm, U1068, CRCM, (Signaling, Hematopoiesis and Mechanism of Oncogenesis); Institut Paoli-Calmettes,Marseille; Aix-Marseille Univ; CNRS, UMR7258, Marseille, France, **6** Service d'Anatomo-pathologie, Université Paris Descartes, Paris Sorbonne Cité, Faculté de Médecine et AP-HP Necker-Enfants Malades, Paris, France, **7** Service d'Hématologie, Centre Hospitalier Universitaire, Reims, France, **8** Service de médecine interne, Groupe Hospitalier Sud. Hospices Civils, Lyon, France, **9** Service d'Hématologie et thérapie cellulaire, CIC INSERMU202, Centre Hospitalier Universitaire, Tours, France, **10** Département de Dermatologie, Centre Hospitalier Universitaire, Toulouse, France, **11** Service d'Hématologie, Centre Hospitalier Universitaire, Caen, France, **12** Département de bio-statistiques et de Recherche clinique, Centre Hospitalier Universitaire, Amiens, France, **13** Service d'Hématologie, Centre Hospitalier, St Quentin, France, **14** Service de Médecine Interne, Hôpital Tenon, Assistance Publique-Hôpitaux, Université Pierre et Marie Curie, Paris, France, **15** Laboratoire d'hématologie Biologique et UMR CNRS 8147, Université Paris Descartes, Paris Sorbonne Cité, Faculté de Médecine et Assistance Publique-Hôpitaux de Paris (AP-HP) Necker-Enfants Malades, Paris, France, **16** Service d'Hématologie, Centre Hospitalier Universitaire, Angers, France, **17** Service de Médecine Interne, CHRU, Lille, France, **18** CNRS UMR 8113, Laboratoire de Biologie et Pharmacologie Appliquée, Ecole Normale Supérieure, Cachan, France, **19** Laboratoire Central d'Hématologie, Groupe Hospitalier Pitié-Salpetrière, Paris, France, **20** Service de Médecine Interne et de Maladie Infectieuses, Université Paris Descartes, Paris Sorbonne Cité, Faculté de Médecine et AP-HP Necker-Enfants Malades, Paris, France

Abstract

Systemic mastocytosis with associated hematologic clonal non-mast cell disease (SM-AHNMD) is a rare and heterogeneous subtype of SM and few studies on this specific entity have been reported. Sixty two patients with Systemic mastocytosis with associated hematologic clonal non-mast cell disease (SM-AHNMD) were presented. Myeloid AHNMD was the most frequent (82%) cases. This subset of patients were older, had more cutaneous lesions, splenomegaly, liver enlargement, ascites; lower bone mineral density and hemoglobin levels and higher tryptase level than lymphoid AHNMD. Defects in *KIT*, *TET2*, *ASXL1* and *CBL* were positive in 87%, 27%, 14%, and 11% of cases respectively. The overall survival of patients with SM-AHNMD was 85.2 months. Within the myeloid group, SM-MPN fared better than SM-MDS or SM-AML (p = 0.044,). In univariate analysis, the presence of C-findings, the AHNMD subtypes (SM-MDS/CMML/AML *versus* SM-MPN/hypereosinophilia) (p = 0.044), Neutropenia (p = 0.015), high monocyte level (p = 0.015) and the presence of *ASXL1* mutation had detrimental effects on OS (p = 0.007). In multivariate analysis and penalized Cox model, only the presence of *ASXL1* mutation remained an independent prognostic factor that negatively affected OS (p = 0.035). SM-AHNMD is heterogeneous with variable prognosis according to the type of the AHNMD. ASXL1 is mutated in a subset of myeloid AHNMD and adversely impact on OS.

Editor: Ivan Cruz Moura, Institut national de la santé et de la recherche médicale (INSERM), France

Funding: The authors have no funding or support to report.

Competing Interests: The authors have declared that no competing interests exist.

* E-mail: damaj.gandhi@chu-amiens.fr

¶ These authors contributed equally to this work.

Introduction

Mastocytosis is a heterogeneous group of disorders characterized by abnormal growth and accumulation of mast cells (MCs) in one or more organ systems. Indolent forms of mastocytosis are the most frequent followed by systemic mastocytosis (SM) with associated clonal hematologic non-MC lineage disease (SM-AHNMD) which constitutes a sub-category of aggressive SM [1–3].

Although most of these patients display *KIT* mutations, little is known about the clinical and prognostic relevance of other gene defects in SM-AHNMD. Only studies with a small number of SM cases, including few cases of SM-AHNMD, have been reported in 23 and 8 patients respectively [4,5]. The overall prognosis for this disease is poor as compared to indolent SM patients. Furthermore, the subtype of the AHNMD has a prognostic value [6]. For example, patients with associated AML or MDS have a worse prognosis compared to patients with SM-MPN [6]. Nevertheless, some SM-AHNMD patients have a chronic course that seems to embrace the course of the associated hematologic disease.

The prognostic value of gene mutations has not been evaluated in large studies. In one study, reporting on 42 patients with SM, *TET2* mutations were not found to alter the prognosis of the disease [4], whereas two other studies showed that the presence of *TET2* mutations conferred a poor prognosis to patients with aggressive SM [5,7].

In the present study, we report on 62 patients with SM-AHNMD with the following aims: 1/ To describe the clinical and laboratory characteristics of myeloid and lymphoid AHNMD patients; 2/ To evaluate the occurrence of genetic mutations such as *KIT* D816V and *JAK2* V617F as well as *TET-2, ASXL1, and CBL*; 3/ To evaluate a possible impact of these genetic mutations on the clinical and laboratory characteristics of SM-AHNMD patients as well as on their prognosis.

Patients and Methods

This retrospective study was approved by the Institutional Review Board of Necker Enfants-Malades Hospital, and was carried out according to the Helsinki Declaration. Written Informed consent was obtained from adult patients or parents or next of kin for teenage patients at the first or second hematology clinic appointment. Patients aged 16 years or more, diagnosed with SM-AHNMD according to the WHO criteria [1] for mastocytosis and other hematologic neoplasms were eligible. Mutations analyses were centrally performed for all patients (KH, ES, PD). Mutations analyses were done on bone marrow samples and/or skin biopsy as previously described using a highly sensitive technique for *KIT* D816V [8], *JAK-2* [9] and *TET-2* [10]. *ASLX1* mutations status was detected in blood and/or marrow as already described [11].

Overall survival (OS) was defined as the time between diagnosis of AHNMD and the date of death or last follow-up. Survival distributions were estimated using the Kaplan-Meier method. Univariate and multivariate Cox proportional hazards model were used to assess prognostic factors of OS and to compute hazard ratios (HRs) and their 95% confidence interval (95% CI). Variables tested in the univariate model were those listed in table 1. Variables eligible for the multivariate Cox model were those having a p-value<0.15 in univariate Cox model because most of the variables significant at 10% other than ASXL1 were highly correlated with each other; thus limiting multicollinearity in the multivariate model. Proportional hazard assumption was tested using Schoenfeld residuals test. P values were two sided and values <0.05 were considered significant. Due to the low proportion of event in our study, a complementary analysis using a penalized ridge Cox model [12] was applied with a shrinkage parameter equal to 3. The SAS software version 9.2® (SAS Institute, Cary, NC) was used for all analysis.

Results and Discussion

Sixty-two SM-AHNMD patients were analyzed. Myeloid AHNMD were the most frequent type of AHNMD encountered (82% of the patients) (table S1). MDS was the leading myeloid disease (29%) of patients, followed by CMML (16%) and MPN (16%) including essential thrombocytopenia (n = 4), primary myelofibrosis (n = 2) and polycythemia (n = 1). MDS/MPNs were present in 8% along with PDGFRα negative hypereosinophilia (8%). AML was associated with true SM in only 5% of cases. Lymphoid AHNMD were rare and constituted only 17% of cases. They were represented mainly by non-Hodgkin's lymphoma (6 patients; 8%) and monoclonal gammapathy of undetermined significance (MGUS) (4 patients; 5%).

Patients' characteristics are detailed in Table 1. Briefly, patients with myeloid AHNMD were older (p = 0.032), had less cutaneous lesions (p = 0.038), splenomegaly (p = 0.003), ascites (p = 0.046) and less bone mineral density (p = 0.045). They had significantly lower hemoglobin level (p = 0.029), higher monocyte counts (p = 0.028), and tryptase (p = 0.046) and LDH (p = 0.020) levels than lymphoid AHNMD. AHNMD was diagnosed concomitantly with SM in 39(67%) patients. For the other patients, the median time from the diagnosis of SM to the diagnosis of the AHNMD was 110 (3–370) months. Of note, in one patient, the diagnosis of polycythemia vera was diagnosed 18 months before the diagnosis of SM was made.

KIT mutations were the most frequent alteration, found in 87% of the patients. *TET2* mutation was positive in 12 (27%) cases, only in the myeloid AHNMD group (SM-MDS = 5, SM-CMM = 6; SM-AML = 1). *TET2* positive patients tended to be older (p = 0.08), with more hepatomegaly (p = 0.03), splenomegaly (p = 0.003), ascites p = 0.04), low bone mineral density (p = 0.02). The same patients had lower hemoglobin level (p = 0.01), and had lower platelet counts (p = 0.009) than those negative for *TET2* mutation (table 1). The presence of *TET2* mutation correlated with the presence of *KIT* D816V mutations (p = 0.03) but not with that of *ASXL1* mutations (p = 0.45).

Six (14%) patients (SM-MDS = 3, SM-CMML = 1, SM-AML = 1, SM-PMF = 1) were found positive for *ASXL1* mutations. Patients with lymphoid AHNMD all tested negative for *ASLX1*. Again, *ASXL1* positive patients were not different from *ASXL1* negative patients regarding the main clinical and biological characteristics. *CBL* mutations were found positive in 3 (11%) patients (ET = 1, CMML = 1, MDS/MPN = 1) and *JAK2* Val617Phe mutation in 3 (6%) patients (MDS = 1; ET = 1; PMF = 1).

For the whole group of patients, the median OS time was 85.2 months (58.8–111.7) (Figure S1A). The OS was not statistically different between the lymphoid AHNMD and the myeloid AHNMD groups (median OS: 85.2 *vs* 60months respectively; p = 0.928). However, within the myeloid group, SM-MPN fared better than SM-MDS or SM-AML (median OS: not reached *vs* 79.6 months respectively; p = 0.044,) (data not shown). While median survival time for SM-MPN/SM-hypereosinophilia was not reached, it was of 91.8 (13.2–170.4) months for SM-MDS, of 79.6 (0.1–159.5) months for SM-CMML, of 39.9 (8.5–71.4) months for SM-AML and of 60 (58.8–111.7) months for SM-lymphoproliferative diseases (Figure S1B).

In univariate analysis, the presence of C-findings as defined by the WHO criteria (cytopenia, organomegaly with organ dysfunction, malabsorption, weight loss, hypoalbuminemia) [HR = 3.12; (1.11–8.77); p = 0.030], the AHNMD subtypes (SM-MDS/CMML/AML *vs* SM-MPN/hypereosinophilia) (median OS: 79.66 months *vs* not reached; p = 0.044), Neutropenia [HR = 1.10; (1.02–1.20); p = 0.015], high monocytes level [HR = 1.31; (1.02–1.20); p = 0.015] and the presence of *ASXL1* mutations [HR = 4.91; (1.53–15.71); p = 0.007] had detrimental effects on overall survival.

In multivariate analysis, as well as, after using penalized Cox regression model [12], only the presence of *ASXL1* mutation remained an independent prognostic factor that negatively affected OS [HR = 5.75; 95%CI (1.09–30.25); p = 0.035] (Figure 1).

Table 1. Demographic, clinical and biological characteristics of patients with myeloid and lymphoid SM-AHNMD patients at inclusion.

	Total n = 62 (%)	**Myeloid AHNMD n = 51 (%)**	**Lymphoid AHNMD n = 11 (%)**	*P*
Age (years); median (range)	64 (16–84)	67 (16–84)	53 (23–74)	*0.032*
Sex; n (%)				*1.0*
Female	23 (37)	19 (37)	4 (36)	
Male	39 (63)	32 (63)	7 (64)	
CM subtypes; n (%)				*0.038*
UP	23 (38)	16 (33)	7 (64)	
TEMP	9 (15)	8 (16)	1 (9)	
DCM	7 (12)	6 (12)	1 (9)	
No lesions	21 (35)	19 (39)	2 (18)	
[1]C-findings; n (%)				*0.045*
Yes	35 (56)	32 (63)	3 (27)	
No	27 (44)	19 (27)	8 (73)	
C-findings excluding cytopenia; n (%)				*1.0*
Yes	16 (26)	13 (25)	3 (27)	
No	46 (74)	38 (75)	8 (73)	
[2]Mast cell activating symptoms				*0.394*
Yes	51 (82)	43 (84)	8 (73)	
No	11 (18)	8 (12)	3 (27)	
Pruritus				*0.167*
Yes	23 (38)	17 (33)	6 (60)	
No	38 (62)	34 (67)	4 (40)	
Pollakiuria; n (%)				*0.142*
Yes	8 (13)	5 (9)	3 (27)	
No	54 (87)	46 (91)	8 (73)	
Neuropsychological symptoms; n (%)				*0.685*
Yes	13 (21)	10 (18)	3 (27)	
No	48 (79)	41 (72)	8 (73)	
Digestive symptoms; n (%)				*1.0*
Yes	30 (61)	26 (60)	4 (67)	
No	19 (39)	17 (40)	2 (33)	
Hepatomegaly; n (%)				*0.149*
Yes	27 (49)	25 (52)	2 (22)	
No	30 (51)	23 (48)	7 (78)	
Splenomegaly; n (%)				*0.003*
Yes	38 (68)	36 (76)	2 (22)	
No	18 (32)	11 (24)	7 (78)	
Ascites; n (%)				*0.046*
Yes	17 (30)	17 (35)	0	
No	40 (70)	31 (65)	9 (82)	
Lymph nodes enlargement; n (%)				*1.0*
Yes	21 (37)	18 (37)	3 (33)	
No	36 (63)	30 (63)	6 (67)	
BMD; n (%)				*0.045*
Normal	29 (52)	27 (56)	2 (25)	
Osteoporosis	14 (25)	9 (19)	5 (63)	
Osteopenia	13 (23)	12 (25)	1 (12)	
Hemoglobin, (mean; range, g/dl)	11.6 (7.7–16.9)	11.4 (7.7–16.9)	12.9 (11.1–13.5)	0.029

Table 1. Cont.

	Total n = 62 (%)	Myeloid AHNMD n = 51 (%)	Lymphoid AHNMD n = 11 (%)	*P*
Neutrophils (mean; range,10^9/l)	4.2 (0.1–24.3)	4.2 (0.1–24.3)	4.0 (1.5–8.08)	0.547
Eosinophils (mean; range,10^9/l)	0.59 (0–6.4)	0.6 (0.0–6.4)	0.2 (0.0–2.4)	0.160
Basophils (mean; range,10^9/l)	0.0 (0–0.5)	0.0 (0–0.5)	0.0 (0–0.05)	0.399
Monocytes (mean; range,10^9/l)	0.7 (0.08–6.96)	1.2 (0.2–6.96)	0.5 (0.08–0.8)	0.028
Lymphocyte (mean; range,10^9/l)	1.6 (0.1–5.20)	1.6 (0.1–5.20)	2.2 (1.1–2.9)	0.149
Platelets (mean; range,10^9/l)	181 (10–1036)	133 (10–1036)	250 (170–466)	0.126
Tryptase (ng/ml)	137 (10–697)	169 (10–697)	50 (19.4–204)	0.046
LDH (mean; range,UI/l)	292 (126–737)	302 (141–737)	213 (126–329)	0.020
KIT genotype; n (%)				0.674
D816 positive	53 (85)	44 (86)	8 (75)	
Non D816V	1 (2)	1 (2)	0	
WT	8 (13)	6 (12)	2 (25)	
TET2 mutations; n (%)				0.163
Yes	12 (27)	12 (32)	0	
No	32 (73)	25 (68)	7	
ASXL1 mutations; n (%)				0.567
Yes	6 (14)	6 (17)	0	
No	37 (86)	30 (83)	7	
JAK2 mutations; n (%)				0.567
Yes	3 (13)	3 (7.5)	0	
No	44 (87)	37 (92.5)	7	
CBL mutations; n (%)				0.778
Yes	3 (11.5)	3 (12.5)		
No	23 (88.5)	21 (87.5)	0	

[1]C-findings according to WHO classification.
[2]including fatigue, headache, flushes, fever, hypotension, choc, syncope, WHO; world health organization, CM; cutaneous mastocytosis, AHNMD; associated clonal hematologic non-mast cell lineage disease, UP; urticaria pigmentosa, TEMP; telengietasia eruptive macularis persistans, DCM; diffuse cutaneous mastocytosis, BMD; bone mineral density.

This study is, to the best of our knowledge, the second largest study which reports [6,13–15] on SM-AHNMD. *KIT*, *TET2*, *ASXL1*, *JAK2*, and *CBL* were found mutated in 87%, 27%, 14%, 14%, and 11% of the patients respectively.

In this series dedicated to SM-AHNMD subtypes myeloid AHNMD was the most frequent associated disease (82%) where MDS, CMML and MPN represented 29%, 16% and 16% of AHNMD respectively. The median age at the onset of the disease was higher in the myeloid AHNMD than in the lymphoid one, and higher than the median age of mastocytosis patients without AHNMD as already reported [16].

Patients with SM-myeloid AHNMD had more splenomegaly, ascites, low bone density, lower hemoglobin and higher tryptase levels than SM-lymphoid AHNMD patients. However, there was no difference in OS between the 2 groups and this might be explained by the heterogeneity of the subcategories of AHNMD and their prognosis within the myeloid and lymphoid groups.

KIT D816V, *JAK2* and *C-CBL* mutations were found in 85%,13% and 11.5% of the patients as already reported [5,6].

We found *TET2* mutations in 27% of SM-AHNMD patients. This frequency is higher than the incidence encountered in patients with MPN [17] and lower than previously reported in SM-AHNMD in two series of 23 and 8 patients respectively [5,18].

TET2 mutated patients tended to be older with more C-findings than patients with wild type *TET2*. However, these findings did not translate into poor prognosis in contrast to the negative prognostic value in cytogenetically normal AML [19], MPNs or mastocytosis patients [20].

Recently, *ASXL1* mutations have been analyzed in only 8 SM patients and found mutated in 2(25%) patients [5]. In our cohort, we found an intermediate frequency of *ASXL1* mutations (14%). They are of prognostic value and shown to adversely affect the OS of patients with SM-AHNMD independently from other clinically utilized prognosticators. *ASXL1* mutations retained also its independent negative impact in the group of patients with SM-MDS/AML (Figure S1C).

As such, mutations in *ASXL1* appear to be novel biomarkers of adverse overall survival in patients with SM-myeloid AHNMD as it has been reported with other myeloid malignancies such as MDS, CMML and subgroups of AML [21–23].

In conclusion

ASXL1 mutations in SM-AHNMD adversely impact on OS. More studies comparing individual subcategories of SM-AHNMD to their hematological non MCs counterpart without SM are needed.

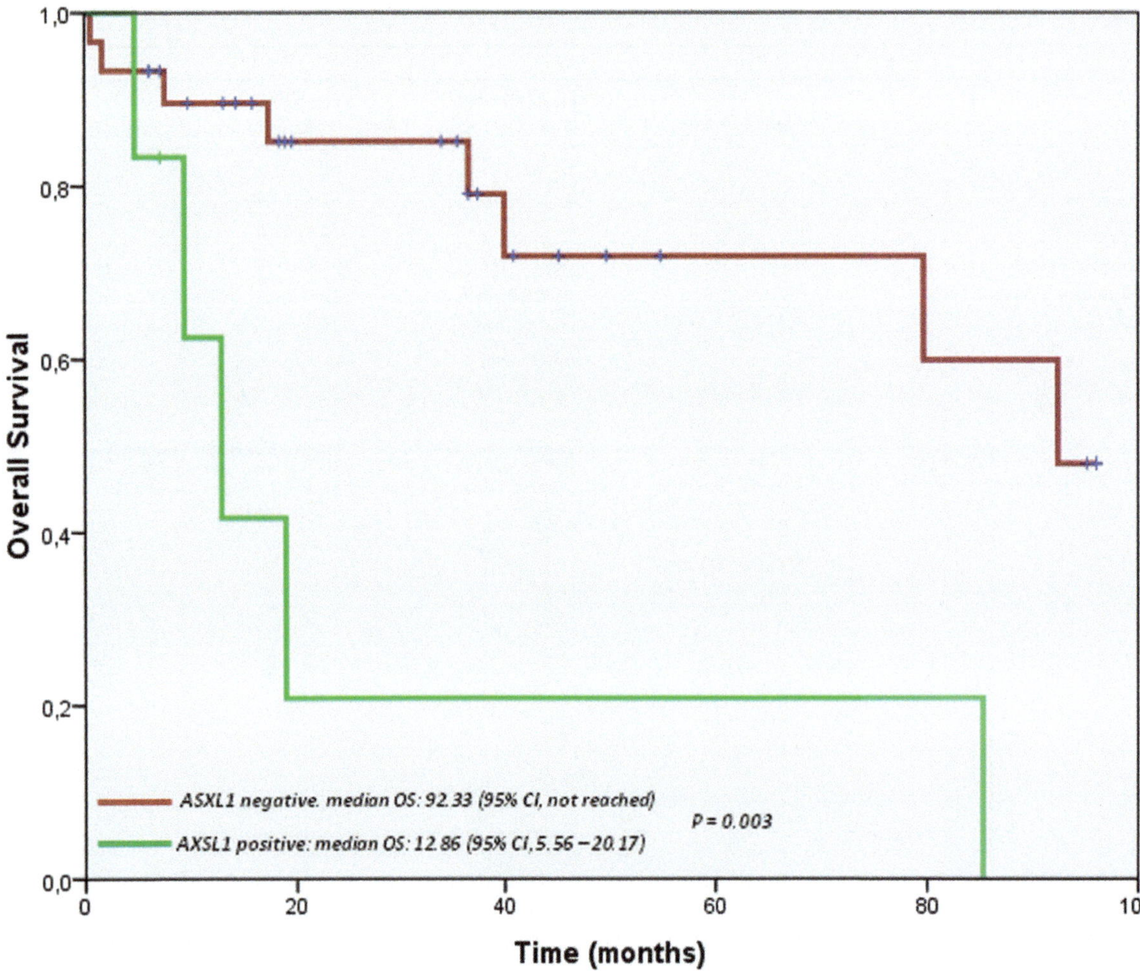

Figure 1. Overall Survival according to *AXSL1* mutations.

Supporting Information

Table S1 Patient's characteristics.

Figure S1 Overall survival (OS) of the whole group (S1A); OS according to the subtype of the AHNMD (S1B); OS of SM-MDS according to ASXL1 mutations (S1C).

Acknowledgments

We would like to thank Isabelle Hirsch and Cedric Baude for technical help and data management

Author Contributions

Conceived and designed the experiments: GD OH. Analyzed the data: GD MD. Wrote the paper: GD. Approved the manuscript: GD MJ OC KH ES DC BK ID EG CL SC MD RG SGL VA LL CL DL MA OL PD OH. Enrollment of patients: GD MJ OC KH ES DC BK ID EG CL SC MD RG SGL VA LL CL DL MA OL PD OH.

References

1. Horny AC, Metcalfe DD, et al. (2008) Mastocytosis. In: Swerdlow S, Campo E, Lee Harris N. WHO Classification of Tumours of Haematopoietic and Lymphoid Tissues. In: Press I, ed. WHO Classification of Tumours of Haematopoietic and Lymphoid Tissues. Lyon:53–63.
2. Valent P, Horny HP, Escribano L, Longley BJ, Li CY, et al. (2001) Diagnostic criteria and classification of mastocytosis: a consensus proposal. Leuk Res 25:603–25.
3. Horny HP, Valent P. (2001) Diagnosis of mastocytosis: general histopathological aspects, morphological criteria, and immunohistochemical findings. Leuk Res 25:543–51.
4. Tefferi A, Levine RL, Lim KH, Abdel-Wahab O, Lasho TL, et al. (2009) Frequent TET2 mutations in systemic mastocytosis: clinical, KITD816V and FIP1L1-PDGFRA correlates. Leukemia 23:900–4.
5. Traina F, Visconte V, Jankowska AM, Makishima H, O'Keefe CL, et al. (2012) Single nucleotide polymorphism array lesions, TET2, DNMT3A, ASXL1 and CBL mutations are present in systemic mastocytosis. PLoS One 7:e43090.
6. Pardanani A, Lim KH, Lasho TL, Finke C, McClure RF, et al. (2009) Prognostically relevant breakdown of 123 patients with systemic mastocytosis associated with other myeloid malignancies. Blood 114:3769–72.
7. Soucie E HK, Mercher T, Georgin-Lavialle S, Damaj G, Chandesris MO, et al.(2012) In Aggressive Forms of Mastocytosis, TET2 Loss Cooperates with c-KITD816V to Transform Mast Cells. Blood 120: 4846–9.

8. Lanternier F, Cohen-Akenine A, Palmerini F, Feger F, Yang Y, et al. (2008) Phenotypic and genotypic characteristics of mastocytosis according to the age of onset. PLoS One Apr 9:e1906.
9. Delhommeau F, Dupont S, Tonetti C, Masse A, Godin I, et al.(2007) Evidence that the JAK2 G1849T (V617F) mutation occurs in a lymphomyeloid progenitor in polycythemia vera and idiopathic myelofibrosis. Blood 109:71–7.
10. Delhommeau F, Dupont S, Della Valle V, James C, Trannoy S, et al. (2009) Mutation in TET2 in myeloid cancers. N Engl J Med 360:2289–301.
11. Gelsi-Boyer V, Trouplin V, Adelaide J, Bonansea J, Cervera N, et al. (2009) Mutations of polycomb-associated gene ASXL1 in myelodysplastic syndromes and chronic myelomonocytic leukaemia. Br J Haematol 145:788–800.
12. Ambler G, Seaman S, Omar RZ. (2011) An evaluation of penalised survival methods for developing prognostic models with rare events. Stat Med 31:1150–61.
13. Travis WD, Li CY, Bergstralh EJ, Yam LT, Swee RG. (1988) Systemic mast cell disease. Analysis of 58 cases and literature review. Medicine (Baltimore) 67:345–68.
14. Horny HP, Sotlar K, Sperr WR, Valent P. (2004) Systemic mastocytosis with associated clonal haematological non-mast cell lineage diseases: a histopathological challenge. J Clin Pathol 57:604–8.
15. Sotlar K, Colak S, Bache A, Berezowska S, Krokowski M, et al. (2010) Variable presence of KITD816V in clonal haematological non-mast cell lineage diseases associated with systemic mastocytosis (SM-AHNMD). J Pathol 220:586–95.
16. Hermine O, Lortholary O, Leventhal PS, Catteau A, Soppelsa F, et al. (2008) Case-control cohort study of patients' perceptions of disability in mastocytosis. PLoS One 3:e2266.
17. Shih AH, Abdel-Wahab O, Patel JP, Levine RL. (2012) The role of mutations in epigenetic regulators in myeloid malignancies. Nat Rev Cancer 12:599–612.
18. Tefferi A, Lim KH, Abdel-Wahab O, Lasho TL, Patel J, et al. (2009) Detection of mutant TET2 in myeloid malignancies other than myeloproliferative neoplasms: CMML, MDS, MDS/MPN and AML. Leukemia 23:1343–5.
19. Metzeler KH, Maharry K, Radmacher MD, Mrozek K, Margeson D, et al. (2011) TET2 mutations improve the new European LeukemiaNet risk classification of acute myeloid leukemia: a Cancer and Leukemia Group B study. J Clin Oncol 2011; 29:1373–81.
20. Tefferi A, Pardanani A, Lim KH, Abdel-Wahab O, Lasho TL, et al. (2009) TET2 mutations and their clinical correlates in polycythemia vera, essential thrombocythemia and myelofibrosis. Leukemia 23:905–11.
21. Thol F, Friesen I, Damm F, Yun H, Weissinger EM, et al. (2011) Prognostic significance of ASXL1 mutations in patients with myelodysplastic syndromes. J Clin Oncol 29:2499–506.
22. Patel JP, Gonen M, Figueroa ME, Fernandez H, Sun Z, et al. (2012) Prognostic relevance of integrated genetic profiling in acute myeloid leukemia. N Engl J Med 366:1079–89.
23. Gelsi-Boyer V, Brecqueville M, Devillier R, Murati A, Mozziconacci MJ, et al. (2012) Mutations in ASXL1 are associated with poor prognosis across the spectrum of malignant myeloid diseases. J Hematol Oncol 5:12.

4

Association Study on *ADAM33* Polymorphisms in Mite-Sensitized Persistent Allergic Rhinitis in a Chinese Population

Ruo-Xi Chen[1], Wen-Min Lu[1], Lu-Ping Zhu[1¤a], Mei-Ping Lu[1], Mei-Lin Wang[2], Yun-Li Wang[1¤b], Xin-Yuan Chen[1], Xin-Jie Zhu[1], Min Yin[1,3], Zheng-Dong Zhang[2], Lei Cheng[1,3]*

1 Department of Otorhinolaryngology, The First Affiliated Hospital, Nanjing Medical University, Nanjing, China, **2** Department of Molecular and Genetic Toxicology, School of Public Health, Nanjing Medical University, Nanjing, China, **3** International Centre for Allergy Research, Nanjing Medical University, Nanjing, China

Abstract

Background: The *ADAM33* gene has been identified as a potentially important asthma candidate gene and polymorphisms in this gene have been shown to be associated with asthma and seasonal allergic rhinitis.

Objective: To assess whether the *ADAM33* polymorphisms are associated with persistent allergic rhinitis (PER) due to house dust mites in a Chinese population.

Methods: In a hospital-based case-control study of 515 patients with mite-sensitized PER and 495 healthy controls, we genotyped seven single nucleotide polymorphisms (SNPs) in *ADAM33*. Serum levels of eosinophil cationic protein, total IgE and allergen-specific IgE against *Dermatophagoides pteronyssinus* and *Dermatophagoides farinae* were measured by the ImmunoCAP assays.

Results: In the single-locus analysis, three polymorphisms, rs3918392 (F1), rs528557 (S2) and rs2787093, were significantly associated with mite-sensitized PER. SNP S2 was associated with significantly increased risk both of asthmatic and nonasthmatic mite-sensitized PER. In the combined genotypes analysis, individuals with 2–4 risk alleles had a significantly higher risk of mite-sensitized PER (adjusted OR = 1.99, 95% CI = 1.50–2.62) than those with 0–1 risk alleles. Haplotype-based association analysis revealed that the ACAGCCT haplotype might have potential to protect against mite-sensitized PER (adjusted OR = 0.67; 95% CI = 0.49–0.90).

Conclusions: Polymorphisms in the *ADAM33* gene may contribute to susceptibility of mite-sensitized PER in this Chinese population.

Editor: Giuseppe Novelli, Tor Vergata University of Rome, Italy

Funding: This study was supported by the Priority Academic Program Development of Jiangsu Higher Education Institutions (PAPD 2010–2013), the Health Promotion Project (XK200719, RC2007065 and RC2011071) of Jiangsu Province, and the Scientific Research Foundation for the Returned Overseas Chinese Scholars (SRF for ROCS 2008-890), Ministry of Education, the People's Republic of China. The funders had no role in study design, data collection and analysis, decision to publish, or preparation of the manuscript.

Competing Interests: The authors have declared that no competing interests exist.

* E-mail: jspent@126.com

¤a Current address: Department of Otorhinolaryngology, The Second Affiliated Hospital, Nanjing Medical University, Nanjing, China
¤b Current address: Department of Otorhinolaryngology, Nanjing Tongren Hospital, Medical School of Southeast University, Nanjing, China

These authors contributed equally to this work.

Introduction

Allergic rhinitis (AR) is defined as a nasal disorder induced by immunoglobulin E (IgE)-mediated immune response and characterized by nasal symptoms including rhinorrhoea, sneezing, nasal obstruction, and itching [1]. It is one of the most common atopic diseases throughout the world. In China, the prevalence of AR ranges from 8.7% to 24.1% [2]. Meanwhile, epidemiologic studies have consistently shown that rhinitis and asthma often coexist in one patient [3,4,5]. AR and asthma, respectively affecting upper and lower airway, where mucosa present similarities and complement in function, both manifest atopy symptoms and likely share a common genetic background [6], suggesting the concept of 'one airway, one disease' [7].

AR and asthma are both multi-factorial diseases with genetic as well as environmental factors influencing disease progression. A gene encoding a disintegrin and metalloprotease (ADAM) 33 located on chromosome 20p13 was identified by positional cloning as a putative candidate gene for the development of asthma and bronchial hyperresponsiveness (BHR) [8]. Selective expression of ADAM33 in lung mesenchymocytes suggests that alterations in its activity may underlie abnormalities in the function of airway smooth muscle cells and fibroblasts linked to BHR and airway remolding [9]. One possible explain is that ADAM33 may serve as

Table 1. Primers and probes for genotypes screening by TaqMan allelic discrimination.

NCBI rs No.	Base change	Primers*	Probes*
rs3918392	A>G	F: CTCAACCCACGAGATCTTTCG	G allele: FAM-CCTGGAAAGGAGCCT-MGB
		R: GGTCATGCCCGCTTTGTT	A allele: HEX-CCTGGAAAGGAACC-MGB
rs528557	C>G	F: CTTCCTGCTGGCCATGCT	G allele: FAM-TGCTCCCAGGGGC-MGB
		R: CCTGGGAGTCGGTAGCAACA	C allele: HEX-TGCTCCCAGGCGC-MGB
rs2280091	A>G	F: CCCAAAGATGGCCCACACA	C allele: FAM-CACCCCACGGAGTT-MGB
		R: GGCATGAGCCCTTCCCTTCT	T allele: HEX- ACCCCATGGAGTTGG-MGB
rs2280090	A>G	F: CCCAAAGATGGCCCACACA	C allele: FAM-TGGACAGCCCTGGC-MGB
		R: GGCATGAGCCCTTCCCTTCT	T allele: HEX-TGGACAGTCCTGGC-MGB
rs3918400	C>T	F: GCAGGCAGCTTGGAAGTTTC	T allele: FAM-AGTGGAGCTTTGACC-MGB
		R: TCTAATGTGGCTCTGGGTTCCT	C allele: HEX-TGGAGCTTCGACCC-MGB
rs2787094	C>G	F: TGGCCAGAAGCTAGTGGTCCT	C allele: FAM-CTCCCCTGCAGCCT-MGB
		R: CAGGAAGGAAGGTCCCCAAA	G allele: HEX-CTCCCCTGGAGCCT-MGB
rs2787093	C>T	F: GTGGGGTGGTGGCTGATG	A allele: FAM-AGCCTAGATGGCAGC-MGB
		R: AAAGAGGGTGTTCAAACTAGGCAA	G allele: HEX-CCGAGCCTAGGTGG-MGB

*The alleles were arrayed as the location of the primers or probes from 5′to 3′.

a cell surface 'sheddase' to release growth factors such as transforming growth factor (TGF)-β and modify cell-surface receptor expression to induce the proliferation of airway mesenchymocyte [10].

Significant associations between single nucleotide polymorphisms (SNPs) of the *ADAM33* gene and asthma in ethnically diverse populations have been reported [8,11,12,13,14,15,16, 17,18,19]; however, little attention was given to rhinitis. Six SNPs (F+1, L−1, S2, T1, T2 and T+1) in *ADAM33* were reported to have significant association in seasonal allergic rhinitis (SAR) induced by Japanese cedar pollen [20], while three SNPs (T1, T+1 and V4) were reported to be associated with AR or concomitant AR and Asthma in a Chinese population [12,21]. Recently, a

Table 2. Distribution of selected variables among cases and controls.

Variables	Cases (n=515)		Controls (n=495)		P
	N	%	N	%	
Age (years), mean ± SD	19.68±12.6		20.10±12.61		0.597*
Sex					
Male	342	66.4	299	60.4	0.086*
Female	173	33.6	196	39.6	
Serum total IgE (kU/L), median (IQR)	265.0 (120.2–573.0)		26.8 (11.1–52.2)		<0.001†
Eosinophil cationic protein (μg/L), median (IQR)	14.3 (5.6–30.1)		4.8 (3.1–7.5)		<0.001†
Duration of rhinitis (years), mean ± SD	6.62±5.87				
Total nasal symptoms (VAS score), mean ± SD	5.23±2.41				
Concomitant asthma‡					
Yes	130	30.1			
No	304	70.0			
Family history of allergic diseases‡					
Yes	306	70.2			
No	130	29.8			
Specific IgE (kU_A/L), median (IQR)					
Dermatophagoides pteronyssinus	27.4 (5.0–69.4)				
Dermatophagoides farinae	23.1 (5.0–63.3)				

*Derived from two-sided χ^2 test for comparison of discrete variables and unpaired Student's t-test for continuous variables.
†Selective variables were transformed into logarithmic model before unpaired Student's t-test between cases and controls.
‡Some information of concomitant asthma or family history of allergic diseases was not available in cases.
IQR, interquartile range; VAS, visual analogue scales.

Table 3. Primary information of seven genotyped SNPs in the *ADAM33* gene.

SNP No.	NCBI rs No.	Chromosome position*	SNP name in ref. [8]	Location	Base change	MAF Database†	MAF Case	MAF Control	P for HWE‡	Genotyped (%)
1	rs3918392	3655219	F1	exon	A>G	0.067	0.119	0.077	0.175	98.6
2	rs528557	3651742	S2	exon	C>G	0.250	0.266	0.206	0.916	98.3
3	rs2280091	3650234	T1	exon	A>G	0.078	0.093	0.072	0.782	96.6
4	rs2280090	3650205	T2	exon	G>A	0.100	0.109	0.102	0.332	98.1
5	rs3918400	3649463	V2	3'-UTR	C>T	0.159	0.188	0.163	0.300	99.1
6	rs2787094	3649161	V4	3'-UTR	C>G	0.410	0.563	0.547	0.251	99.1
7	rs2787093	3648462		3'near gene	T>C	0.233	0.282	0.226	0.145	98.0

*SNP position in NCBI dbSNP (http://www.ncbi.nlm.nih.gov/snp).
†MAF for CHB from the HapMap databases (http://www.hapmap.org) or NCBI dbSNP (http://www.ncbi.nlm.nih.gov/snp).
‡HWE *P* value in the control group.
SNP, single nucleotide polymorphism; MAF, minor allele frequencies; HWE, Hardy-Weinberg equilibrium; CHB: Han Chinese in Beijing, China.

study showed that haplotypes of ADAM33 polymorphisms exhibited significant association with AR among Jordanians [22].

To confirm the association between *ADAM33* polymorphisms and AR induced by house dust mites (HDM), and to examine the association with clinical phenotypes including rhinitis severity, concomitant asthma, and serum total IgE levels, we genotyped and analyzed seven SNPs of the *ADAM33* gene in a Chinese population.

Materials and Methods

Subjects

The 515 unrelated individuals (342 males and 173 females) with persistent allergic rhinitis (PER) were aged from 3 to 66 years with a mean age of 19.68±12.6 years. The 495 unrelated healthy controls (299 males and 196 females) were aged from 3 to 65 years with a mean age of 20.10±12.61 years. All the cases and controls were recruited from Jiangsu and Anhui provinces, eastern China. All patients were enrolled in the First Affiliated Hospital of Nanjing Medical University (Nanjing, China) from May 2008 to January 2013. PER was diagnosed according to the guidelines of Allergic Rhinitis and its Impact on Asthma (ARIA) 2008 update [1]. A questionnaire was used to obtain information of disease condition and status, including history, family history, symptoms and concomitant diseases from each PER case. In this study, control subjects were recruited from the hospital who seeking health care or doing routine health examinations, and were frequency matched with the cases by age (±5 years) and sex. Individuals selected for controls must meet all the following criteria: (i) no symptoms or history of rhinitis or other nasal diseases; (ii) no symptoms or history of asthma or other atopic disorders; (iii) have negative allergen-specific IgE in serum (Phadiatop<0.35 kU_A/L); (iv) absence of first-degree relatives with a history of AR or other allergic diseases. Subjects of all only Han Chinese were included in this study and the participation rate was approximately 95%. The research protocol was approved by the ethical review board of Nanjing Medical University, and written informed consent was obtained from all participants.

Clinical Parameters

A visual analogue scales (VAS) ranging from 0 (not at all bothersome) to 10 cm (extremely bothersome) was used to assess the severity of total nasal symptoms (VAS score) as well as individual symptoms including rhinorrhoea, sneezing, nasal obstruction, and nose and eye itching. Patients with VAS score ≤5 were diagnosed as mild rhinitis and those with VAS score >5 as moderate/severe [23].

About 5 mL venous blood samples were obtained from each participant for *in vitro* allergy testing. The serum total IgE, specific IgE, and eosinophil cationic protein (ECP) levels were measured with ImmunoCAP100 assays (Phadia, Uppsala, Sweden), according to the manufacturer's standard procedures. Total IgE and ECP were determined in all subjects. Specific IgE antibodies to common inhalant allergens including *Dermatophagoides pteronyssinus* (*Der p*; d1), *Dermatophagoides farinae* (*Der f*; d2), cat dander (e1), dog dander (e5), *Blatella germanica* (i6), *Alternaria alternata* (m6), *Ambrosia elatior* (w1), and *Artemisia vulgaris* (w6) were determined in patients with PER.

SNP Selection and Genotyping

Seven SNPs in the *ADAM33* gene, including rs3918392 (F1), rs528557 (S2), rs2280091 (T1), rs2280090 (T2), rs3918400 (V2) rs2787094 (V4), and rs2787093 (located in 3′ near gene), were selected by using genotype data obtained from unrelated Han

Table 4. Genotype and allele frequencies in *ADAM33* polymorphisms among cases and controls.

SNP No.	NCBI rs No.	Genotypes	Cases		Controls		Crude OR	Adjusted OR	$P^{\dagger}$
			N	%	N	%	(95% CI)	(95% CI)*	
1	rs3918392		$n=507$		$n=489$				
		AA	405	79.9	419	85.7	1.00 (reference)	1.00 (reference)	**0.006**
		AG	83	16.4	65	13.3	1.32 (0.93–1.88)	1.34 (0.94–1.91)	
		GG	19	3.8	5	1.0	**3.93 (1.45–10.63)**	**4.03 (1.49–10.93)**	
		AG/GG	102	20.1	70	14.3	**1.51 (1.08–2.10)**	**1.53 (1.09–2.14)**	**0.015**
		G allele‡	0.119		0.077				**0.001**
2	rs528557		$n=508$		$n=485$				
		CC	288	56.7	306	63.1	1.00 (reference)	1.00 (reference)	**0.002**
		CG	170	33.5	158	32.6	1.14 (0.87–1.50)	1.15 (0.88–1.51)	
		GG	50	9.8	21	4.3	**2.53 (1.48–4.32)**	**2.56 (1.50–4.38)**	
		CG/GG	220	43.3	179	36.9	**1.31 (1.01–1.68)**	**1.32 (1.02–1.70)**	**0.040**
		G allele‡	0.266		0.206				**0.002**
3	rs2280091		$n=508$		$n=468$				
		AA	416	81.9	403	86.1	1.00 (reference)	1.00 (reference)	0.190
		AG	90	17.7	63	13.5	1.38 (0.98–1.96)	1.38 (0.97–1.96)	
		GG	2	3.9	2	4.3	0.97 (0.14–6.91)	0.91 (0.13–6.49)	
		AG/GG	91	17.9	64	13.7	1.38 (0.97–1.95)	1.37 (0.97–1.94)	0.073
		G allele	0.093		0.072				0.093
4	rs2280090		$n=505$		$n=486$				
		GG	406	80.4	394	81.1	1.00 (reference)	1.00 (reference)	0.685
		GA	88	17.4	85	17.5	1.01 (0.72–1.40)	1.00 (0.72–1.40)	
		AA	11	2.2	7	1.4	1.53 (0.59–3.97)	1.57 (0.60–4.10)	
		GA/AA	99	19.6	92	18.9	1.04 (0.76–1.43)	1.05 (0.76–1.43)	0.788
		A allele	0.109		0.102				0.609
5	rs3918400		$n=508$		$n=493$				
		CC	337	66.3	342	69.4	1.00 (reference)	1.00 (reference)	0.175
		CT	151	29.7	141	28.6	1.09 (0.83–1.43)	1.07 (0.81–1.40)	
		TT	20	3.9	10	2	2.03 (0.94–4.40)	2.07 (0.95–4.50)	
		CT/TT	171	33.7	151	30.6	1.15 (0.88–1.50)	1.13 (0.87–1.48)	0.305
		T allele	0.188		0.163				0.147
6	rs2787094		$n=508$		$n=493$				
		CC	87	17.1	95	19.3	1.00 (reference)	1.00 (reference)	0.674
		CG	270	53.2	257	52.1	1.15 (0.82–1.61)	1.14 (0.81–1.60)	
		GG	151	29.7	141	28.6	1.17 (0.81–1.69)	1.18 (0.81–1.71)	

Table 4. Cont.

SNP No.	NCBI rs No.	Genotypes	Cases		Controls		Crude OR	Adjusted OR	$P^{†}$
			N	%	N	%	(95% CI)	(95% CI)*	
		CG/GG	421	82.9	398	80.7	1.16 (0.84–1.59)	1.15 (0.84–1.59)	0.379
		G allele	0.563		0.547				0.462
7	rs2787093		n = 506		n = 483				
		TT	259	51.2	284	58.8	1.00 (reference)	1.00 (reference)	**0.011**
		CT	209	41.3	180	37.3	1.27 (0.98–1.65)	1.29 (0.99–1.67)	
		CC	38	7.5	19	3.9	**2.19 (1.23–3.90)**	**2.24 (1.26–4.00)**	
		CT/CC	247	48.8	199	41.2	**1.36 (1.06–1.75)**	**1.38 (1.07–1.78)**	**0.016**
		C allele‡	0.282		0.226				**0.004**

*Adjusted for age and sex in logistic regression model.
†Two-sided χ^2 test for the distributions of genotype and allele frequencies.
‡Assumed risk alleles.
SNP, single nucleotide polymorphism; OR, odds ratio; CI, confidence interval.

Chinese in Beijing (CHB) individuals in the HapMap (HapMap Data Rel 28 Phase II+III, August 10, on NCBI B36 assembly, dbSNP b126) and based on previously published studies [8,12,20,21] identifying putative risk alleles. Genotyping was performed with the TaqMan SNP Genotyping Assay using the 384-well ABI 7900HT Real-Time PCR System (Applied Biosystems, Foster City, CA, USA). More than 15% of the samples were randomly selected for confirmation, and the results were 100% concordant. The primers and TaqMan probes are shown in Table 1.

Statistical Analysis

Differences in the distributions of demographic characteristics, selected variables, and frequencies of *ADAM33* genotypes between the cases and controls were evaluated using Student's *t*-test (for continuous variables) or the Chi-square test (for categorical variables). Serum levels of total IgE and ECP were transformed into logarithmic model for normalize the distribution. Percentiles were calculated based on all available subjects with existing total IgE measurements (n = 973) and logarithmic total IgE 90th percentile (999.9 kU/L) was used as dependent variable (above/below the 90th percentile) with two categories denoted as 'high' and 'low' total IgE levels, respectively [24]. Hardy-Weinberg equilibrium (HWE) of the genotype distribution among control groups was tested by a goodness-of-fit Chi-square test. Chi-square test and one-way ANOVA were used to assess the difference between the *ADAM33* polymorphisms and clinical phenotypes. The crude and adjusted odds ratios (ORs) and 95% confidence intervals (CIs) were obtained to assess the association between the *ADAM33* polymorphisms and risk of mite-sensitized PER using unconditional univariate and multivariate logistic regression models. The multivariate adjustment included age and sex. The combined genotypes were further stratified by subgroups of age, sex, asthma, history, VAS score, total IgE and HDM-specific IgE levels. The computation of linkage disequilibrium (LD) between SNPs was estimated using the normalized measure of allelic association D' and r^2, and the characterization of these patterns was determined using Haploview 4.0 software [25]. EM algorithm (SAS 9.1.3 PROC HAPLOTYPE) was used to infer haplotype frequencies based on the observed *ADAM33* genotypes. All of the statistical analyses were carried out with SAS software version 9.1.3 (SAS Institute, Cary, NC, USA), unless indicated otherwise. *P*-value <0.05 was considered statistically significant.

Results

Characteristics of the Study Subjects

The frequency distributions of selected characteristics of the PER cases and healthy controls are presented in Table 2. The cases and controls appeared to be well matched on age ($P = 0.579$) and sex ($P = 0.086$). Apparently, serum levels of ECP (14.3 [5.6–30.1] μg/L) and total IgE (256.0 [120.2–573.0] kU/L) in cases were significantly higher ($P<0.001$) than those in controls (4.8 [3.1–7.5] μg/L and 26.8 [11.1–52.2] kU/L, respectively). In patients with PER, the serum level of allergen-specific IgE against *Der p* and *Der f* was 27.4 (5.0–69.4) kU_A/L and 23.1 (5.0–63.3) kU_A/L, respectively. Of the patients, 277 (53.8%) cases were mild and 270 (52.4%) were moderate/severe according to VAS score, and 130 (30.1%) cases reported to have concomitant asthma and 306 (70.2%) cases had family history of allergic diseases. These variables were further adjusted in the multivariate logistic regression analysis for any residual confounding effect.

Table 5. Genotype frequencies of *ADAM33* polymorphisms in dominant model in PER patients with and without asthma.

SNP No.	NCBI rs No.	Case with asthma *vs.* control		Case without asthma *vs.* control	
		Adjusted OR (95% CI)*	$P^{\dagger}$	Adjusted OR (95% CI)*	$P^{\dagger}$
1	rs3918392	1.28 (0.83–2.00)	0.258	**1.70 (1.19–2.42)**	**0.003**
2	rs528557	**1.54 (1.11–2.14)**	**0.011**	**1.32 (1.01–1.74)**	**0.048**
3	rs2280091	**1.71 (1.12–2.61)**	**0.013**	1.35 (0.93–1.95)	0.118
4	rs2280090	1.24 (0.83–1.85)	0.297	1.06 (0.75–1.49)	0.748
5	rs3918400	1.00 (0.70–1.42)	1.000	1.12 (0.84–1.50)	0.426
6	rs2787094	1.48 (0.94–2.23)	0.090	1.04 (0.74–1.47)	0.818
7	rs2787093	1.24 (0.89–1.72)	0.208	**1.39 (1.06–1.83)**	**0.018**

Dominant model: MW+MM/WW; MW: heterozygotes; MM: mutation homozygotes; WW: wild homozygotes.
*Adjusted for age and sex in logistic regression model.
†Two-sided χ^2 test for the distributions of genotype frequencies.
PER, persistent allergic rhinitis; SNP, single nucleotide polymorphism; OR, odds ratio; CI, confidence interval.

Individual SNP Association Analysis

The primary information and allele frequencies observed are listed in Table 3. All genotype distributions of control subjects were consistent with those expected from the HWE (all $P>0.05$). As shown in Table 4, the individual SNP analyses revealed that the genotype frequencies of three SNPs (SNP F1, S2, and rs2787093) were significantly different between the cases and controls ($P=0.006$ for F1, $P=0.002$ for S2, and $P=0.011$ for rs2787093). The homozygous genotype GG of SNP F1 was associated with a significantly increased risk of mite-sensitized PER compared with the wild-type genotype CC (adjusted OR = 4.03, 95% CI = 1.49–10.93). Similar associations were also found in SNP S2 and rs2787093 (adjusted OR = 2.56, 95% CI = 1.50–4.38 for S2 and 2.24, 1.26–4.00 for rs2787093, respectively). We also found that the dominant models (MW+MM/WW) of SNP F1 (AG+GG/AA), S2 (CG+GG/CC) and rs2787093 (CT+TT/CC) showing significant associations with mite-sensitized PER (adjusted OR = 1.53, 95% CI = 1.09–2.14 for F1; 1.32, 1.02–1.70 for S2 and 1.38, 1.07–1.78 for rs2787093).

Association and Stratification Analysis between the Individual SNP and AR-related Phenotypes

As shown in Table 5, significantly increased risk of mite-sensitized PER with asthma were found for SNP S2 (OR = 1.54, 95% CI = 1.11–2.14) and T1 (OR = 1.71, 95% CI = 1.12–2.61) under the dominant models. Comparing nonasthmatic PER patients with controls, we also found that the dominant models of F1 (OR = 1.70, 95% CI = 1.19–2.42), S2 (OR = 1.32, 95% CI = 1.01–1.74) and rs2787093 (OR = 1.39, 95% CI = 1.06–1.83) had a significantly higher risk of mite-sensitized PER than those with wild-type genotypes.

Given the significant difference between cases and controls, the correlations between serum total IgE levels and individual locus in cases and controls were evaluated separately. No significant association was shown between total IgE levels and genotypes of each SNP in controls (all $P>0.05$). No significant difference was observed in total IgE levels among individuals with different genotypes of seven SNPs (all $P>0.05$). We also evaluated the association between other AR-related phenotypes and different genotypes of individual SNP; however, no statistical evidence was found for interactions between the different genotypes and the

Table 6. Distributions of the *ADAM33* combined genotypes among cases and controls.

No. variant (risk) alleles of the combined alleles*	Cases ($n=481$)		Controls ($n=443$)		$P^{\dagger}$
	N	%	N	%	
0	117	23.5	135	28.9	**<0.0001**
1	186	37.4	218	46.6	
2	125	25.5	92	19.7	
3	57	11.5	21	4.5	
4	12	2.4	2	0.4	
Dichotomized groups					
0–1	303	61.0	353	75.4	**<0.0001**
2–4	194	39.0	115	24.6	

*The number represents the numbers of risk genotypes.
†Two-sided χ^2 test for the distributions of combined genotype frequencies.

Table 7. Association and stratification analyses between the *ADAM33* combined genotypes and risk of PER.

Variables	Subcategory	N (case/control)	Combined genotypes (case/control)*				Adjusted OR (95% CI)†
			0–1		2–4		
			N	%	N	%	
Total		497/468	303/353	61.0/75.4	194/115	39.0/24.6	**1.99 (1.50–2.62)**
Age (years)							
	<18	288/230	180/171	62.5/74.4	108/59	37.5/25.7	**1.72 (1.16–2.54)**
	≥18	209/238	123/182	58.9/76.5	86/56	41.2/23.5	**2.30 (1.53–3.46)**
Sex							
	Male	329/292	207/221	62.9/75.7	122/71	37.1/24.3	**1.87 (1.32–2.66)**
	Female	168/176	96/132	57.1/75.0	72/44	42.9/25.0	**2.29 (1.44–3.64)**
Concomitant asthma							
	No	294/468	188/353	63.9/75.4	106/115	36.1/24.6	1.00 (reference)
	Yes	126/468	78/353	61.9/75.4	48/115	38.1/24.6	0.92 (0.59–1.42)
Family history of allergic diseases							
	No	293/468	188/353	64.2/75.4	105/115	35.8/24.6	1.00 (reference)
	Yes	129/468	79/353	61.2/75.4	50/115	38.8/24.6	0.87 (0.56–1.36)
VAS score							
	≤5	277/468	162/353	58.5/75.4	115/115	41.5/24.6	1.00 (reference)
	>5	220/468	141/353	64.1/75.4	79/115	35.9/24.6	1.34 (0.92–1.94)
Total IgE ‡							
	Lower level	403/468	237/353	58.8/75.4	166/115	41.2/24.6	1.00 (reference)
	Higher level	94/468	66/353	70.2/75.4	28/115	29.8/24.6	1.14 (0.72–1.82)

*The number represents the numbers of risk genotypes.
†Adjusted for age and sex in logistic regression model.
‡Lower level: below the 90th percentile of logarithmic total IgE; Higher level: above the 90th percentile of logarithmic total IgE.
PER, persistent allergic rhinitis; VAS, visual analogue scale; OR, odds ratio; CI, confidence interval.

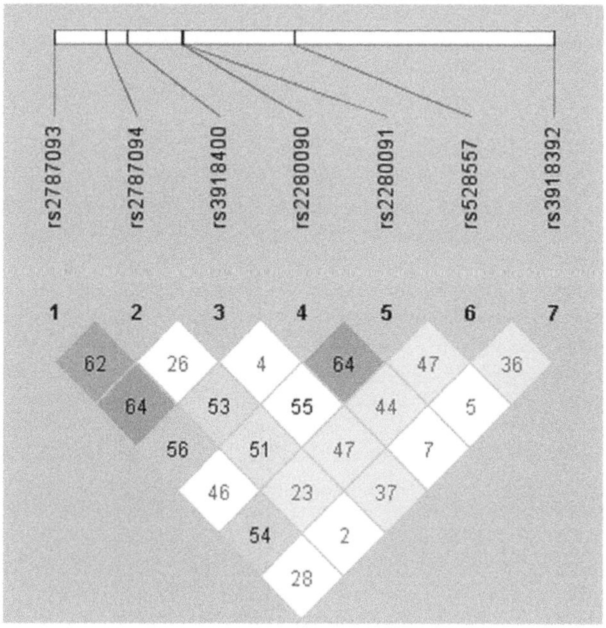

Figure 1. Linkage disequilibrium of seven SNPs in the *ADAM33* gene. Linkage disequilibrium (LD) of 7 SNPs was determined using the solid spine of LD option of Haploview 4.1. *D'* values are displayed in the squares. Empty red squares have a pairwise *D'* of 1.00. Red squares indicate high pairwise LD, gradually coloring down to white squares of low pairwise LD.

variables (i.e., rhinitis severity, serum specific IgE and ECP levels) (all $P>0.05$; data not shown).

Distribution of the ADAM33 Combined Genotypes among Cases and Controls

In Table 4, the frequencies in *ADAM33* SNP F1 G (0.119 *vs.* 0.077), SNP S2 G (0.266 *vs.* 0.206), and rs2787093 C (0.282 *vs.* 0.226) alleles among the cases were significantly higher than those among the controls. Considering potential interactions of these three SNPs on the risk of mite-sensitized PER, we combined these three SNPs based on the numbers of variant (risk) alleles (SNP F1 G, S2 G and rs2787093 C).

As shown in Table 6, the combined genotypes with 0–1 variant (risk) alleles were more common (28.9% and 46.6%, respectively) and those with 2–4 variant (risk) alleles were less common (19.7%, 4.5% and 0.4%, respectively) among the controls than among the cases (23.5%, 37.4%, 25.5%, 11.5%, and 2.4%, respectively). In our study, no individual carried the combined genotypes with 5 or 6 variant (risk) alleles, presumably due to the LD. When these combined genotypes were dichotomized into two groups (i.e., zero to one *vs.* two to four risk alleles), their distributions differed significantly between the cases and controls ($P<0.0001$).

Association and Stratification Analysis between the ADAM33 Combined Genotypes and AR-related Phenotypes

As shown in Table 7, we found that the individuals with 2–4 variant (risk) alleles had a significantly higher risk of mite-sensitized PER (adjusted OR = 1.99, 95% CI = 1.50–2.62) than those with 0–1 risk genotypes. Further stratification analysis showed that this increased risk was pronounced among subgroups of both age <18 years (adjusted OR = 1.72, 95% CI = 1.16–2.54) and age ≥18 years (adjusted OR = 2.30, 95% CI = 1.53–3.46). This increased risk was also pronounced among both male (adjusted OR = 1.87, 95% CI = 1.32–2.66) and female (adjusted OR = 2.29, 95% CI = 1.44–3.64) groups. However, no statistical evidence was observed for interactions between the combined genotypes and the variables (i.e., concomitant asthma, family history of allergic diseases, VAS score, and total IgE) (all $P>0.05$).

Association and Stratification Analysis between the Haplotypes and Risk of AR

The LD between each pair of SNPs in *ADAM33* is presented in Fig. 1. Haplotype analysis including 7 SNPs was performed, there were >100 possible haplotypes derived from the known genotypes. Haplotypes with a frequency <0.01 in both the cases and controls were pooled into a single group, and the remaining 9 haplotypes were analyzed. As shown in Table 8, the frequency of ACAGCCT haplotype in controls was significantly higher than that in cases

Table 8. Associations between risk of PER and frequencies of inferred haplotypes on the basis of the observed genotypes among cases and controls.

Haplotypes*	Haplotype frequencies		$P^†$	Adjusted OR (95% CI)[‡]
	Cases	Controls		
A-C-A-G-C-G-T	0.291	0.312	0.3161	1.00 (reference)
A-C-A-G-C-C-C	0.209	0.191	0.3305	1.17 (0.90–1.52)
A-C-A-G-C-C-T	0.102	0.162	**0.0001**	**0.67 (0.49–0.90)**
A-G-A-G-T-G-T	0.054	0.059	0.6011	0.99 (0.65–1.49)
A-C-A-G-C-G-C	0.025	0.019	0.4246	1.35 (0.72–2.55)
A-G-G-A-C-G-T	0.035	0.037	0.8596	1.02 (0.62–1.70)
A-G-A-G-C-G-T	0.033	0.017	**0.0284**	**2.03 (1.09–3.79)**
A-G-A-G-C-C-T	0.027	0.024	0.6621	1.21 (0.67–2.18)
A-C-A-G-T-G-T	0.016	0.017	0.7647	0.95 (0.46–1.96)

*The alleles of haplotypes were arrayed as the location of the SNPs in *ADAM33* from 5′to 3′.
[†]Two-sided χ^2 test for each haplotype *vs.* all others combined in cases and controls.
[‡]Adjusted for age and sex in logistic regression model.
PER, persistent allergic rhinitis; OR, odds ratio; CI, confidence interval.

($P=0.0001$, adjusted OR = 0.67, 95%CI = 0.49–0.90) compared with the common haplotype ACAGCGT, and the association was also statistically significant after Bonferroni's correction ($P=0.001$), suggesting that ACAGCCT haplotype may have potential to protect against mite-sensitized PER. We also found AGAGCGT haplotype carrying the S2 G allele was associated with a significantly increased risk of mite-sensitized PER (adjusted OR = 2.03, 95% CI = 1.09–3.79), compared with the common haplotype ACAGCGT. However, the significance did not remain after the Bonferroni's correction ($P=0.256$).

Discussion

ADAM33 is a member of the ADAM protein family of zinc-dependent metalloproteinase superfamily [26]. We selected seven SNPs in the *ADAM33* gene and conducted an association study in a Han Chinese Han population. The results showed that three polymorphisms (SNP F1, S2 and rs2787093) were significantly associated with mite-sensitized PER and nonasthmatic mite-sensitized PER. Moreover, associations of SNPs (S2 and T1) with asthmatic mite-sensitized PER were observed in the study.

The normal structure of mucosa in nasal cavity is similar to that of bronchial mucosa, which characteristically manifests pseudo-stratified ciliated columnar epithelium [27]. Also, they both share the commonness of immunological process. Allergens and inflammation factors absorbed in nasal mucosa can influence lower part of airway and inflammatory infiltration of mucosa is resembled both in AR and asthma. Viewing as a whole, hyperresponsiveness present in upper airway contribute to AR and in lower airway represent asthma. ADAM33 protein has been proposed to contribute to the remodeling process present in asthma and BHR [8]. ADAM33 mRNA was seen in asthmatic subepithelial fibroblasts and smooth muscle [28] and was significantly higher in the epithelium, submucosal cells and airway smooth muscle in severe bronchial asthma [29,30,31]. Thus, we proposed that ADAM33 may also be implicated in the progression of PER and upper airway remodeling process.

ADAMs were originally identified as membrane-anchored proteins on the cell surface that mediate adhesion and proteolysis, and play pivotal roles in cell-to-cell interactions, cell signaling and the remodeling of extracellular matrix components [32]. ADAMs include matrix metalloproteinases (MMPs), specifically regulated by tissue inhibitors of metalloproteinases (TIMPs) during tissue remodeling. ADAM33 may release growth factors (such as EGF, TGF-β and IGF) and modify cell-surface receptor expression to stimulate the proliferation of airway mesenchymocytes in response to injury. Besides, ADAM33 might act as a dominant negative regulator, fusagen or an enhancer of a mesenchymal cell migration in the progress of airway remodeling [33,34].

As indicated above, SNPs located in functional domain of the *ADAM33* gene may contribute to transcription and expression of ADAM33 mRNA and protein, and finally influence the function of ADAM33 in the pathogenesis of AR. For instance, F1 (Thr178Ala, in exon 6) may influence the gene expression and the composition and structure of protein. S2 is a polymorphism located in exon encoding the transmembrane domain, which is predicted to influence anchoring ADAM33 protein to the cell membrane. Although S2 encodes the synonymous exon (Gly717Gly) which does not change amino acid sequence or missense, it may alter the mRNA folding, mRNA stability and translation [35]. Further studies are warranted to reveal the influence of S2 variation to ADAM33 function. Additionally, the intracellular domain of *ADAM33* is relatively short in comparison with its nearest homologues but it is very rich in prolines and has a putative SH3 binding site (PsWPLDP) where T2 is located and may affect function [9]. T1 is in the intracellular domain that may affect bi-directional signaling. V2 and V4 located in 3′UTR and rs2787093 located in 3′near gene may affect the mRNA transcription.

Our result of the association of S2 and F1 polymorphisms in *ADAM33* with mite-sensitized PER had been previously confirmed in SAR due to Japanese cedar pollen [20]. However, the significant association of other SNPs (T1 and T2) with cedar pollinosis was observed in the Japanese patients, but not in our patients with mite-sensitized PER. The S2 polymorphism in *ADAM33* had also been reported to be associated with asthma in many case-control studies of diverse population, including Japanese [14], British [36], and Irish [13], but not American [16], Germany [37], Brazilian [38], and Colombians [24]. Several reasons can explain the variety results of association of S2 with Asthma. Firstly, it is important to consider the genetic diversity of the populations reflected in differences in the occurrence of polymorphisms and their allelic frequencies. The minor allele frequency (MAF) of S2 in Chinese may be similar to that of Japanese (MAF = 0.250 in CHB+JBT show in Table 3), yet different from that in European (MAF = 0.091 showed in the HapMap) or other populations. Secondly, environmental influence is also a crucial factor in the progression of allergic diseases. Numerous environmental exposures such as allergen, air pollution, smoking, diet, pet keeping, microbial exposure, moisture and dampness, and chemicals at the workplace have been related to the new onset of asthma [39]. Thereby, the gene effect may differ from various populations respect to their environmental exposure. Further studies should focus on the gene-environment interaction of AR and asthma to uncover the mechanism of onset and progression of the diseases.

Three SNPs (T1, T+1 and V4), which have no association with mite-sensitized PER in our study, had been previously reported to be significantly associated with AR in population of northern China [12]. The controversial results may due to its small sample size (135 cases and 151 controls) that did not have enough statistical power to reveal any significant ORs and the environmental differences between northern and eastern part of China. Also, several studies have reported no significant difference in variant genotype distributions of SNPs in the *ADAM33* gene between the asthmatics and controls [37,40,41,42,43]. More studies of larger sample size are necessary for further confirming the association between the *ADAM33* polymorphisms and AR in diverse populations.

In the analysis of the association of individual SNP with AR-related clinical phenotypes, we found that two SNPs (S2 and T1) were significantly associated with concomitant asthma in PER patients, supporting the previous findings about the relation between *ADAM33* polymorphisms and asthma. The association between *ADAM33* polymorphisms and asthma has been reported in American (T1, T2 and T+1) [8], British (S2) [15], Japanese (S2, T1 and T2) [14], and Chinese (S2, T1, T2, and V4) [12] population. Moreover, recently several meta-analysis showed that polymorphisms in the *ADAM33* gene are risk factors for asthma in the Asian (T1, V4, F+1, T2, and T+1) [44,45] and European (S2) [46] population. However, a genome-wide association studies (GWAS) of Spanish individuals revealed that among 19 selected tag SNPs of *ADAM33*, only one SNP (rs2787095) was associated with asthma [17]. No evidence of *ADAM33* polymorphisms associated with either serum total IgE or allergen-specific IgE level was found in our study. It suggests that airway remodeling function due to activity of ADAM33 protein may not accompany with the increase of IgE production. Lack of association between

ADAM33 polymorphisms and serum total IgE levels was also reported in Japanese patients with cedar pollinosis [20] and in German and Australian Caucasian populations [19], yet was contradicted by the data from asthmatics of Dutch (S2), US white (T1 and T2) and US hispantic (T1 and T2) [16], and Colombian (T1 and T2) [24] population, suggesting an existence of race and ethnic difference.

As shown in Table 7, we found that the combined genotypes with 2–4 risk alleles were associated with a higher risk of mite-sensitized PER among subgroups of adult subjects (≥18 years old). The difference of nasal structure and development of immune system between children and adults contribute to the dissimilarity of allergic symptoms between them. Moreover, prenatal factors and early life exposures, coupled with genetically determined susceptibility from parents, have a major impact on the natural history of childhood allergy [47,48]. According to our results, we suggested that compared with children, adults might be more susceptible to the genetic effect caused by *ADAM33*, and the effect caused by *ADAM33*, such as airway remolding. Thus, besides the discrepancy of exposure environment, pediatric allergy may differ from adult allergy in effect of genetic variation. However, lack of the analysis in the interaction of environment and genetic polymorphism may cause this finding due to chance.

In addition, we also were looking for a dose-response effect as one might expect that gene variants associated with increased airway remodeling, as suggested by Jongepier *et al.* [49], to be likewise increased in more severe AR. Actually, we did not found such relation of *ADAM33* polymorphism and rhinitis severity in patients with mite-sensitized PER. Coherent with the negative results of individual SNP with IgE, no evidence of an increased risk of PER associated with elevated serum total or specific IgE was found in combined genotypes. Nevertheless, since our sample size might not be large enough and the selected bias could not be excluded completely, the finding might be due to chance and should be interpreted with caution.

As multiple SNPs may act in combination to increase the risk of AR, we further analyzed the *ADAM33* haplotype structure and frequencies, and identified a haplotype (ACAGCCT), carrying wild-type alleles of each polymorphism, that might account for susceptibility to protect against mite-sensitized PER. Although the significance for AGAGCGT haplotype did not remain after the Bonferroni's correction, consistent with our genotype analysis, AGAGCGT haplotype carrying S2 G allele was pronounced a borderline significantly increased risk of mite-sensitized PER.

In conclusion, our data suggested that *ADAM33* polymorphisms might play an important role in the pathogenesis of mite-sensitized PER in this Chinese population. However, functional studies are needed to elucidate the role of *ADAM33* polymorphisms in the molecular mechanisms underlying nasal allergy, and more detailed environmental exposure data are needed to confirm the effect of gene-environment interaction on mite-sensitized PER.

Author Contributions

Conceived and designed the experiments: R-XC L-PZ LC. Performed the experiments: R-XC W-ML L-PZ M-PL X-YC X-JZ. Analyzed the data: R-XC M-LW MY Z-DZ. Contributed reagents/materials/analysis tools: Z-DZ LC Y-LW. Wrote the paper: R-XC W-ML LC.

References

1. Bousquet J, Khaltaev N, Cruz AA, Denburg J, Fokkens WJ, et al. (2008) Allergic Rhinitis and its Impact on Asthma (ARIA) 2008 update (in collaboration with the World Health Organization, GA^{2}LEN and AllerGen). Allergy 63 Suppl 86: 8–160.
2. Zhang L, Han D, Huang D, Wu Y, Dong Z, et al. (2009) Prevalence of self-reported allergic rhinitis in eleven major cities in china. Int Arch Allergy Immunol 149: 47–57.
3. Leynaert B, Neukirch F, Demoly P, Bousquet J (2000) Epidemiologic evidence for asthma and rhinitis comorbidity. J Allergy Clin Immunol 106: S201–205.
4. Linneberg A, Henrik Nielsen N, Frolund L, Madsen F, Dirksen A, et al. (2002) The link between allergic rhinitis and allergic asthma: a prospective population-based study. The Copenhagen Allergy Study. Allergy 57: 1048–1052.
5. Bugiani M, Carosso A, Migliore E, Piccioni P, Corsico A, et al. (2005) Allergic rhinitis and asthma comorbidity in a survey of young adults in Italy. Allergy 60: 165–170.
6. Barnes KC (2000) Evidence for common genetic elements in allergic disease. J Allergy Clin Immunol 106: S192–200.
7. Grossman J (1997) One airway, one disease. Chest 111: 11S–16S.
8. Van Eerdewegh P, Little RD, Dupuis J, Del Mastro RG, Falls K, et al. (2002) Association of the ADAM33 gene with asthma and bronchial hyperresponsiveness. Nature 418: 426–430.
9. Cakebread JA, Haitchi HM, Holloway JW, Powell RM, Keith T, et al. (2004) The role of ADAM33 in the pathogenesis of asthma. Springer Semin Immunopathol 25: 361–375.
10. Holgate ST, Davies DE, Powell RM, Holloway JW (2006) ADAM33: a newly identified protease involved in airway remodelling. Pulm Pharmacol Ther 19: 3–11.
11. Bijanzadeh M, Ramachandra NB, Mahesh PA, Mysore RS, Kumar P, et al. (2010) Association of IL-4 and ADAM33 gene polymorphisms with asthma in an Indian population. Lung 188: 415–422.
12. Su D, Zhang X, Sui H, Lu F, Jin L, et al. (2008) Association of ADAM33 gene polymorphisms with adult allergic asthma and rhinitis in a Chinese Han population. BMC Med Genet 9: 82.
13. Reijmerink NE, Kerkhof M, Koppelman GH, Gerritsen J, de Jongste JC, et al. (2009) Smoke exposure interacts with ADAM33 polymorphisms in the development of lung function and hyperresponsiveness. Allergy 64: 898–904.
14. Hirota T, Hasegawa K, Obara K, Matsuda A, Akahoshi M, et al. (2006) Association between ADAM33 polymorphisms and adult asthma in the Japanese population. Clin Exp Allergy 36: 884–891.
15. Blakey J, Halapi E, Bjornsdottir US, Wheatley A, Kristinsson S, et al. (2005) Contribution of ADAM33 polymorphisms to the population risk of asthma. Thorax 60: 274–276.
16. Howard TD, Postma DS, Jongepier H, Moore WC, Koppelman GH, et al. (2003) Association of a disintegrin and metalloprotease 33 (ADAM33) gene with asthma in ethnically diverse populations. J Allergy Clin Immunol 112: 717–722.
17. Pino-Yanes M, Corrales A, Cumplido J, Poza P, Sanchez-Machin I, et al. (2013) Assessing the validity of asthma associations for eight candidate genes and age at diagnosis effects. PLoS One 8: e73157.
18. Xue W, Han W, Zhou ZS (2013) ADAM33 polymorphisms are associated with asthma and a distinctive palm dermatoglyphic pattern. Mol Med Rep 8: 1795–1800.
19. Godava M, Kopriva F, Bohmova J, Vodicka R, Dusek L, et al. (2012) Association of STAT6 and ADAM33 single nucleotide polymorphisms with asthma bronchiale and IgE level and its possible epigenetic background. Biomed Pap Med Fac Univ Palacky Olomouc Czech Repub 156: 236–247.
20. Cheng L, Enomoto T, Hirota T, Shimizu M, Takahashi N, et al. (2004) Polymorphisms in ADAM33 are associated with allergic rhinitis due to Japanese cedar pollen. Clin Exp Allergy 34: 1192–1201.
21. Zhang X, Su D, Sui H, Jin L, Lu F, et al. (2009) Association of ADAM33 gene polymorphisms with adult concomitant allergic rhinitis and asthma in Chinese Han population. Mol Biol Rep 36: 1505–1509.
22. Zihlif M, Mahafza T, Obeidat NM, Froukh T, Shaban M, et al. (2013) Frequency of genetic polymorphisms of ADAM33 and their association with allergic rhinitis among Jordanians. Gene 531: 462–466.
23. Bousquet PJ, Combescure C, Neukirch F, Klossek JM (2007) Visual analog scales can assess the severity of rhinitis graded according to ARIA guidelines. Allergy 62: 367–372.
24. Vergara CI, Acevedo N, Jimenez S, Martinez B, Mercado D, et al. (2010) A Six-SNP haplotype of ADAM33 is associated with asthma in a population of Cartagena, Colombia. Int Arch Allergy Immunol 152: 32–40.
25. Barrett JC, Fry B, Maller J, Daly MJ (2005) Haploview: analysis and visualization of LD and haplotype maps. Bioinformatics 21: 263–265.
26. Yoshinaka T, Nishii K, Yamada K, Sawada H, Nishiwaki E, et al. (2002) Identification and characterization of novel mouse and human ADAM33s with potential metalloprotease activity. Gene 282: 227–236.
27. Harkema JR, Carey SA, Wagner JG (2006) The nose revisited: a brief review of the comparative structure, function, and toxicologic pathology of the nasal epithelium. Toxicol Pathol 34: 252–269.
28. Umland SP, Garlisi CG, Shah H, Wan Y, Zou J, et al. (2003) Human ADAM33 messenger RNA expression profile and post-transcriptional regulation. Am J Respir Cell Mol Biol 29: 571–582.
29. Ito I, Laporte JD, Fiset PO, Asai K, Yamauchi Y, et al. (2007) Downregulation of a disintegrin and metalloproteinase 33 by IFN-gamma in human airway smooth muscle cells. J Allergy Clin Immunol 119: 89–97.

30. Foley SC, Mogas AK, Olivenstein R, Fiset PO, Chakir J, et al. (2007) Increased expression of ADAM33 and ADAM8 with disease progression in asthma. J Allergy Clin Immunol 119: 863–871.
31. Tripathi P, Awasthi S, Husain N, Prasad R, Mishra V (2013) Increased expression of ADAM33 protein in asthmatic patients as compared to non-asthmatic controls. Indian J Med Res 137: 507–514.
32. Primakoff P, Myles DG (2000) The ADAM gene family: surface proteins with adhesion and protease activity. Trends Genet 16: 83–87.
33. Holloway JW, Davies DE, Powell R, Haitchi HM, Keith TP, et al. (2004) The discovery and role of ADAM33, a new candidate gene for asthma. Expert Rev Mol Med 6: 1–12.
34. Holgate ST (2010) ADAM metallopeptidase domain 33 (ADAM33): identification and role in airways disease. Drug News Perspect 23: 381–387.
35. Duan J, Wainwright MS, Comeron JM, Saitou N, Sanders AR, et al. (2003) Synonymous mutations in the human dopamine receptor D2 (DRD2) affect mRNA stability and synthesis of the receptor. Hum Mol Genet 12: 205–216.
36. Blakey JD, Sayers I, Ring SM, Strachan DP, Hall IP (2009) Positionally cloned asthma susceptibility gene polymorphisms and disease risk in the British 1958 Birth Cohort. Thorax 64: 381–387.
37. Schedel M, Depner M, Schoen C, Weiland SK, Vogelberg C, et al. (2006) The role of polymorphisms in ADAM33, a disintegrin and metalloprotease 33, in childhood asthma and lung function in two German populations. Respir Res 7: 91.
38. de Faria IC, de Faria EJ, Toro AA, Ribeiro JD, Bertuzzo CS (2008) Association of TGF-beta1, CD14, IL-4, IL-4R and ADAM33 gene polymorphisms with asthma severity in children and adolescents. J Pediatr (Rio J) 84: 203–210.
39. von Mutius E (2009) Gene-environment interactions in asthma. J Allergy Clin Immunol 123: 3–11; quiz 12–13.
40. Kedda MA, Duffy DL, Bradley B, O'Hehir RE, Thompson PJ (2006) ADAM33 haplotypes are associated with asthma in a large Australian population. European journal of human genetics : EJHG 14: 1027–1036.
41. Lee JH, Park HS, Park SW, Jang AS, Uh ST, et al. (2004) ADAM33 polymorphism: association with bronchial hyper-responsiveness in Korean asthmatics. Clin Exp Allergy 34: 860–865.
42. Wang P, Liu QJ, Li JS, Li HC, Wei CH, et al. (2006) Lack of association between ADAM33 gene and asthma in a Chinese population. Int J Immunogenet 33: 303–306.
43. Lind DL, Choudhry S, Ung N, Ziv E, Avila PC, et al. (2003) ADAM33 is not associated with asthma in Puerto Rican or Mexican populations. Am J Respir Crit Care Med 168: 1312–1316.
44. Lee YH, Song GG (2012) Association between ADAM33 T1 polymorphism and susceptibility to asthma in Asians. Inflamm Res 61: 1355–1362.
45. Liang S, Wei X, Gong C, Wei J, Chen Z, et al. (2013) A disintegrin and metalloprotease 33 (ADAM33) gene polymorphisms and the risk of asthma: a meta-analysis. Hum Immunol 74: 648–657.
46. Song GG, Kim JH, Lee YH (2013) Association between ADAM33 S2 and ST+4 polymorphisms and susceptibility to asthma: a meta-analysis. Gene 524: 72–78.
47. Gelfand EW (2009) Pediatric asthma: a different disease. Proc Am Thorac Soc 6: 278–282.
48. Szefler SJ (2011) Advances in pediatric asthma in 2010: addressing the major issues. J Allergy Clin Immunol 127: 102–115.
49. Jongepier H, Boezen HM, Dijkstra A, Howard TD, Vonk JM, et al. (2004) Polymorphisms of the ADAM33 gene are associated with accelerated lung function decline in asthma. Clin Exp Allergy 34: 757–760.

5

Inverse Immunological Responses Induced by Allergic Rhinitis and Head and Neck Squamous Cell Carcinoma

Camilla Rydberg Millrud[1], Terese Hylander[1], Susanna Kumlien Georen[1], Åsa Kågedal[1], Ola Winqvist[2], Lars Olaf Cardell[1]*

1 Division of ENT diseases, Department of Clinical Science, Intervention and Technology, Karolinska Institutet, Karolinska University Hospital, Stockholm, Sweden, 2 Department of Medicine, Translational Immunology Unit, Karolinska Institutet, Stockholm, Sweden

Abstract

Several epidemiological studies have investigated the relation between allergy and cancer with contradicting conclusions, and reports on immunological differences are scarce. By focusing on inflammation, the present study was designed to compare the immune response induced by allergic rhinitis (AR) and head and neck squamous cell carcinoma (HNSCC). Blood and serum was obtained from patients with symptomatic seasonal AR, and newly detected HNSCC, as well as healthy controls. Peripheral blood mononuclear cells (PBMC) and polymorphonuclear leukocytes (PMN) were isolated and cultured with or without the toll-like receptor ligands, Pam_3CSK_4, LPS, R837, and CpG. Cellular activation and cytokine release were assessed with ELISA, Luminex Multiplex Immunoassay, flow cytometry, and real-time RT-PCR. Sera from HNSCC patients showed elevated levels of innate immune cytokines, and exhibited a response profile consistent with an increased innate immune reaction. In contrast, sera and stimulated PBMC from AR patients displayed increased concentrations of T cell related cytokines, consistent with an adaptive immune response. The presented data demonstrate that AR and HNSCC induce two distinct immunological processes, indicating an inverse association between the immunological responses seen in patients with allergy and cancer of the upper airway.

Editor: Luo Zhang, Beijing Instiiute of Otolaryngology, China

Funding: Funding was obtained from the Swedish Medical Research Council, Karolinska Institutet and the Karolinska University Hospital. This study was also supported by grants from the Swedish Cancer Society, IMTAC. The funders had no role in study design, data Collection and analysis, decision to published, or preparation of the manuscript.

Competing Interests: The authors have declared that no competing interests exist.

* E-mail: lars-olaf.cardell@ki.se

Introduction

The existence of a possible association between allergic airway inflammation and cancer has been debated over the past several years. Because reports on immunological differences are scarce, the discussion has almost entirely been based on information derived from epidemiological studies with diverse outcomes [1,2,3,4,5].

Allergic inflammation is a lymphocyte mediated disease with a T helper (Th)2 dominated phenotype [6]. The adaptive immune system, especially T cells, is important in cancer [7]. Patients with head and neck squamous cell carcinoma (HNSCC) have been demonstrated to have a shift towards the pro-tumorigenic Th2 response that inhibits the anti-tumor activity of the Th1 reaction [8,9]. The innate immune system is interposed as a bridge between the external environment and the adaptive system [10]. Pattern-recognition receptors (PRRs), especially toll-like receptors (TLRs), are known to have an important role in this interplay [11]. The present study focus on differences in the immunological reactions seen during ongoing allergic rhinitis (AR) and early stages of still untreated HNSCC, with focus on effects induced by external TLR stimulation. The HNSCC investigated were found foremost in the oral and nasopharyngeal regions, and the allergic individuals were sampled during pollen season. Cells were stimulated with the TLR agonists Pam_3CSK_4 (TLR1/2), LPS (TLR4), R837 (TLR7) and CpG (TLR9). Subsequently, the cell activation was analyzed for CD11b which is involved in leukocyte recruitment, the interleukin-2 (IL-2) receptor CD25 presented on activated T cells, CD69 a very early activation marker, and CD98 an early marker for T cell activation. In addition, the cytokine profile was investigated, and IL-6 and IL-8, secreted by activated innate immune cells, were analyzed.

Materials and Methods

Ethics Statement

This study was approved by the Ethics Committees of Karolinska Institutet and Lund University, and a written consent was obtained from all participants.

Patients

The study included 13 patients (8 females and 5 males) with symptomatic, pollen-induced AR and 10 patients (3 females and 7 males) newly diagnosed with HNSCC prior to initiation of treatment, along with 18 healthy controls (15 females and 4 males). The median age of the allergic patients was 42 years (range 25–77), HNSCC patients 67 years (range 51–80), and controls 52.5 years (range 26–69). Allergic individuals that exhibited a positive skin prick test towards birch and/or grass were sampled during pollen season, when their disease was the most active. At the time of sampling, the patients had to fill in a symptom score to verify that they had an ongoing allergic reaction. They also had to avoid allergy medications a week before blood samples were collected. The HNSCC patients were sampled in connection with the detection of their disease, prior to initiation of treatment. None of the cancer patients were on immune modulating medication, and they had no previous history of malignant disease. The control individuals were healthy volunteers without medication. The tumor (T) and lymph node (N) classification of the cancer patients at the time of inclusion are shown in Table 1. The study included cancer patients with the following tumor localization: 7 oral, 2 nasopharyngeal, and 1 glottic.

Cell Line

The human pharyngeal squamous cell carcinoma cell line FaDu (HTB-43; ATCC; Manassa, VA) was cultured in minimum essential medium (MEM) with Earl's salts and 2 mM L-glutamine (GIBCO, Grand Island, NY), and supplemented with 10% FBS (PAN Biotech, Aidenbach, Germany), and 100 U/ml penicillin and 100 μg/ml streptomycin (GIBCO). Cells were cultured in tissue culture flasks at 37°C in a humidified 5% CO_2 air atmosphere.

Cell Separation

Freshly drawn blood was diluted 1:1 with PBS and centrifuged using Ficoll-Paque (Amersham Bioscience, Uppsala, Sweden). The interphase containing peripheral blood mononuclear cells (PBMC) was collected and washed in PBS before resuspended in complete medium, consisting of RPMI-1640 supplemented with 0.3 g/l L-glutamine (Sigma Aldrich, St. Louis, MO), 100 U/ml penicillin and 100 μg/ml streptomycin (GIBCO), and 10% autologous plasma, to a concentration of 1×10^6 cells/ml. The polymorphonuclear leukocytes (PMN) rich pellet was recovered and treated with ammonium chloride erythrocyte lysis solution (0.8% NH_4Cl, 10 mM $KHCO_3$, and 0.1 mM EDTA) for 15 min on ice. The cell suspension was centrifuged at 400 g, washed in PBS, and resuspended in complete medium to a density of 4×10^6 cells/ml.

Cell Culture

Both PBMC and PMN were treated with 1 μg/ml Pam_3CSK_4, 1 μg/ml LPS, 5 μg/ml R837 (Invivogen, San Diego, CA, USA), 0.3 μM CpG (sequence 5′-tcgtcgttttgtcgttttgtcgtt-3′; DNA technology, Aarhus, Denmark), or with vehicle (as the control). PBMC was cultured for 24 or 72 h, and PMN for 4 or 24 h at 37°C in a humidified air atmosphere with 5% CO_2. Thereafter, the supernatants were analyzed with ELISA, Luminex Multiplex Immunoassay, and the cells with flow cytometry. PMN obtained from healthy individuals was also cultured in the presence or absence of culture medium supernatants from FaDu, and stimulated with or without 1 μg/ml LPS for 4 h at 37°C in a humidified air atmosphere with 5% CO_2. Subsequently, the supernatant were analyzed for cytokine secretion with ELISA.

Table 1. Clinical tumor (T) and lymph node (N) classification of the head and neck squamous cell carcinoma (HNSCC) patients.

N stage		**0**	**1**	**2**	**3**	***Total***
T stage	**1**	1	1	1	0	*3*
	2	2	0	1	0	*3*
	3	1	0	3	0	*4*
	4	0	0	0	0	*0*
Total		*4*	*1*	*5*	*0*	*10*

Elisa and Luminex Multiplex Immunoassay

The levels of IL-6 (Limit of detection (LOD): 2 pg/ml) and IL-8 (2 pg/ml) in cell culture supernatants from PMN were analyzed with ELISA plates from eBioscience (San Diego, CA, USA). In addition, levels of 17 cytokines were measured in supernatants from PBMC using Bio-Plex Pro Human Cytokine 17-plex Assay from Bio-Rad Laboratories (Herculeas, CA, USA) according to the manufacturer's instructions. The following cytokines were measured: IL-1β (0.6 pg/ml), IL-2 (1.6 pg/ml), IL-4 (0.7 pg/ml), IL-5 (0.6 pg/ml), IL-6 (2.6 pg/ml), IL-7 (1.1 pg/ml), IL-8 (1.0 pg/ml), IL-10 (0.3 pg/ml), IL-12p70 (3.5 pg/ml), IL-13 (0.7 pg/ml), IL-17 (3.3 pg/ml), granulocyte-colony stimulating factor (G-CSF; 1.7 pg/ml), granulocyte monocyte-colony stimulating factor (GM-CSF; 2.2 pg/ml), interferon (IFN)-γ (6.4 pg/ml), monocyte chemotactic protein (MCP)-1 (1.1 pg/ml), macrophage inflammatory protein (MIP)-1β (2.4 pg/ml), and TNF-α (6.0 pg/ml). The cytokine levels were measured by the Bio-Plex 200 system (Bio-Rad).

Antibodies

The following antibodies (Abs) were purchased from BD Bioscience (San Jose, CA, USA): CD4-APC (clone: RPA-T4), CD11b-APC (ICRF44), CD16-FITC (3G8), CD25-FITC (M-A251), CD62L-PE (DREG-56), CD69-APC-Cy7 (FN50), and CD98-FITC (UM7F8).

Flow Cytometry

Flow cytometry analyses were performed on a Beckman Coulter FC500 (Marseille, France) or a BD LSRFortessa flow cytometer (BD Bioscience). Events in the range 50 000–100 000 were collected depending on the occurrence of the investigated leukocyte population. Data was analyzed using the FlowJo software (Tree Star Inc., Ashland, OR, USA). To ensure flow cytometric standardization, the voltage settings were updated daily using FlowSet calibration beads. All Abs were titrated before use. For staining, cells were incubated with Abs for 20 min, washed and resuspended in PBS prior to analysis.

Real-Time RT-PCR

PBMC was lysed in RLT buffer (Qiagen, Hilden, Germany) supplemented with 1% 2-mercaptoethanol and stored in −80° until use. RNA was extracted using the RNeasy Mini Kit (Qiagen) according to manufacturer's instruction. The RNA quality and quantity was determined by spectrophotometry, based on the A_{260}/A_{280} ratio (1.7–2.1 in all samples). Reverse transcription of RNA into cDNA was carried out using the Omniscript Reverse Transcriptase Kit (Qiagen) and Oligo(dT) primer (DNA Technology) in a Mastercycler personal PCR machine (Eppendorf AG, Hamburg, Germany). Real-time PCR was performed in a Stratagen Mx3000P (Agilent Technologies Inc., Santa Clara, CA) using Brilliant II SYBR® Green QPCR Master Mix (Agilent Technology) to detect COX-1 (PTGS1; Hs00924808_ml) and COX-2 (PTGS2; Hs00153133_ml). The thermal cycler was programmed as followed: initial set up for 10 min at 95°C, 45 cycles of denaturation at 95°C for 15 s each and thereafter annealing/extension at 60°C for 1 min. The gene expression was assessed using the comparative threshold cycle (C_t) method [12].

Statistics

Statistical analyses were performed using GraphPad Prism 5 (GraphPad Software, San Diego, CA, USA), and data are presented as mean ± standard error of the mean (SEM). *n* is equal to the number of independent donors, and a *p*-value of ≤0.05 were considered statistically significant. The nonparametric Mann-Whitney test was used to determine the statistical difference between the groups, and for paired data the nonparametric Wilcoxon signed rank test was used.

Results

Distinct Serum Cytokine Profiles in Patients with Allergy and Head and Neck Cancer

Cytokine levels in serum samples from healthy controls, AR patients, and HNSCC patients were analyzed with Luminex Multiplex Immunoassay. Cytokines involved in innate inflammation, IL-1β, IL-17, MCP-1, MIP-1β, and G-CSF, all showed a suggestive tendency to be increased in HNSCC patients as compared to AR patients. GM-CSF was the only exception. However, the concentration of IL-1β and IL-17 were close to the LOD value 0.6 pg/ml for IL-1β, and 3.3 pg/ml for IL-17 (Figure 1A). In addition, IL-7 was increased, and IL-6 was slightly elevated in sera from HNSCC patients compared to healthy controls (Figure 1D). As expected, sera from allergic individuals displayed an increased level of the Th2 cytokines IL-5 and IL-13 compared to sera from healthy controls and HNSCC patients (Figure 1B). Only very low levels close to detection limit of IL-4 were found (Figure 1B). In addition, sera from AR patients displayed a significant decrease in the serum levels of the innate cytokine IL-1β compared to sera from healthy controls (Figure 1A). More surprisingly, the serum levels of the Th1 cytokines IL-12, IFN-γ, and TNF-α were increased in AR patients compared to sera from healthy controls and patients with HNSCC patients (Figure 1C).

PMN from Head and Neck Cancer Patients Respond with Increased Activation after TLR Stimuli

To determine the differences in leukocyte functionality between patients with AR, HNSCC, and healthy controls, PMN were isolated and stimulated with or without TLR ligands (Pam_3CSK_4, LPS, R837, and CpG) for 4 and 24 h, and subsequently analyzed with ELISA and flow cytometry. PMN obtained from HNSCC patients displayed an increased basal secretion of IL-8, and exhibited a higher IL-8 response to the different TLR ligands compare to the response of PMN from AR patients and healthy controls after 4 h (Figure 2A). When investigating the 24 h time point, the IL-8 production was equal in the supernatant from AR and HNSCC patients when compared to the control. In contrast, the IL-6 release remained the same in all three groups (Figure 2A and Figure S1A). When studying the expression of cell surface markers, we found significantly increased expression levels (mean fluorescent intensity; MFI) of CD11b and the early activation marker CD69 on stimulated PMN isolated from the HNSCC patients compared to PMN from AR patients and healthy controls (Figure 2B). The increased expression levels of CD11b was found on foremost LPS stimulated PMN after both 4 and 24 h, whereas the elevated level of CD69 was observed for all types of stimuli except CpG after 4 h of stimulation (Figure 2B and Figure S1B, C).

To investigate whether it is the tumor that dictates the activation pattern of PMN, PMN from healthy donors were cultured in supernatants from the HNSCC cell line FaDu with or without LPS for 4 h, using IL-8 and IL-6 secretion as read outs. Since the FaDu supernatants contained a basal level of IL-8 and IL-6, the concentration of these cytokines in the media alone was subtracted from PMN cultured samples. The IL-8 levels were decreased in LPS stimulated cells in FaDu supernatant. The unstimulated PMN controls cultured in the presence of FaDu supernatants were found to have a decreased level of IL-6 expression compared to the FaDu medium alone and the unstimulated PMN in complete RPMI medium. LPS stimulated cells cultured in FaDu supernatants were also found to release a lower amount of IL-6 compared to LPS treated PMN in complete RPMI medium (Figure 2C).

Decreased Activation Of PBMC from Head and Neck Cancer Patients after TLR Stimuli

Further, the functionality of PBMC from healthy controls, AR individuals and HNSCC patients was determined. PBMC were isolated, stimulated with or without Pam_3CSK_4, LPS R837, or CpG for 24 and 72 h. Cytokine profiles were analyzed with Luminex Multiplex Immunoassay, and T cell activation was monitored by flow cytometry. Four representative cytokines are displayed in Figure 3 and the other 13 cytokines can be found in Figure S2. PBMC obtained from the cancer patients showed a decreased IL-1β secretion after 24 h of LPS stimulation compared to PBMC from the AR individuals. Low levels of IL-5, IL-7 and IL-12 were also released from PBMC isolated from HNSCC patients, whereas PBMC from AR patients showed high concentrations of these cytokines (Figure 3A). No differences in cytokine levels were observed between 24 and 72 h. The HNSCC patients also displayed a decreased Th cell activation as observed by a reduction in MFI of CD25 and CD98 after both 24 (Figure 3B) and 72 h (Figure S3A, B). However, a high percentage of CD98-positive Th cells were also found in the cancer patients (Figure S3B). Finally, real-time RT-PCR was used to determine the expression of COX-1 and COX-2 mRNA in PBMC obtained from healthy individuals, AR patients and HNSCC patients. PBMC isolated from cancer patients were found to display a lower expression of COX-2 compared to PBMC from healthy controls (Figure 3C).

Discussion

This study demonstrates that allergy and cancer induce two distinct immunological reactions. The tumorigenic immune response is dominated by an innate immune reaction, and by suppressed T cells, whereas the allergic reaction is characterized by an adaptive response with enhanced activation of T cells.

The innate and neutrophil dominated inflammation seen among the HNSCC patients is characterized by a strong PMN activation, and a suggestive tendency of high serum levels of IL-1β, IL-17, MCP-1, MIP-1β, and G-CSF. These findings are well in line with previous studies reporting altered peripheral PMN activation in HNSCC [13,14]. The presented data show that PMN isolated from patients with HNSCC have an increased basal secretion of IL-8 that was confirmed to be mediated by the tumor. This highlights that the tumor cells and its release of mediators modulate the activation process of PMN. The suppressed release of IL-8 from LPS stimulated PMN from healthy donors cultured in FaDu supernatants indicates that the tumor cells release mediators that inhibit the TLR4 signaling pathway for IL-8 secretion. These inhibitory substances seem to be effective locally in the tumor without reaching the circulation, since PMN isolated from the blood of patients with HNSCC displayed an increased IL-8 release after TLR stimulation. This is in concert with previous observations of tumor cells expressing and releasing mediators that

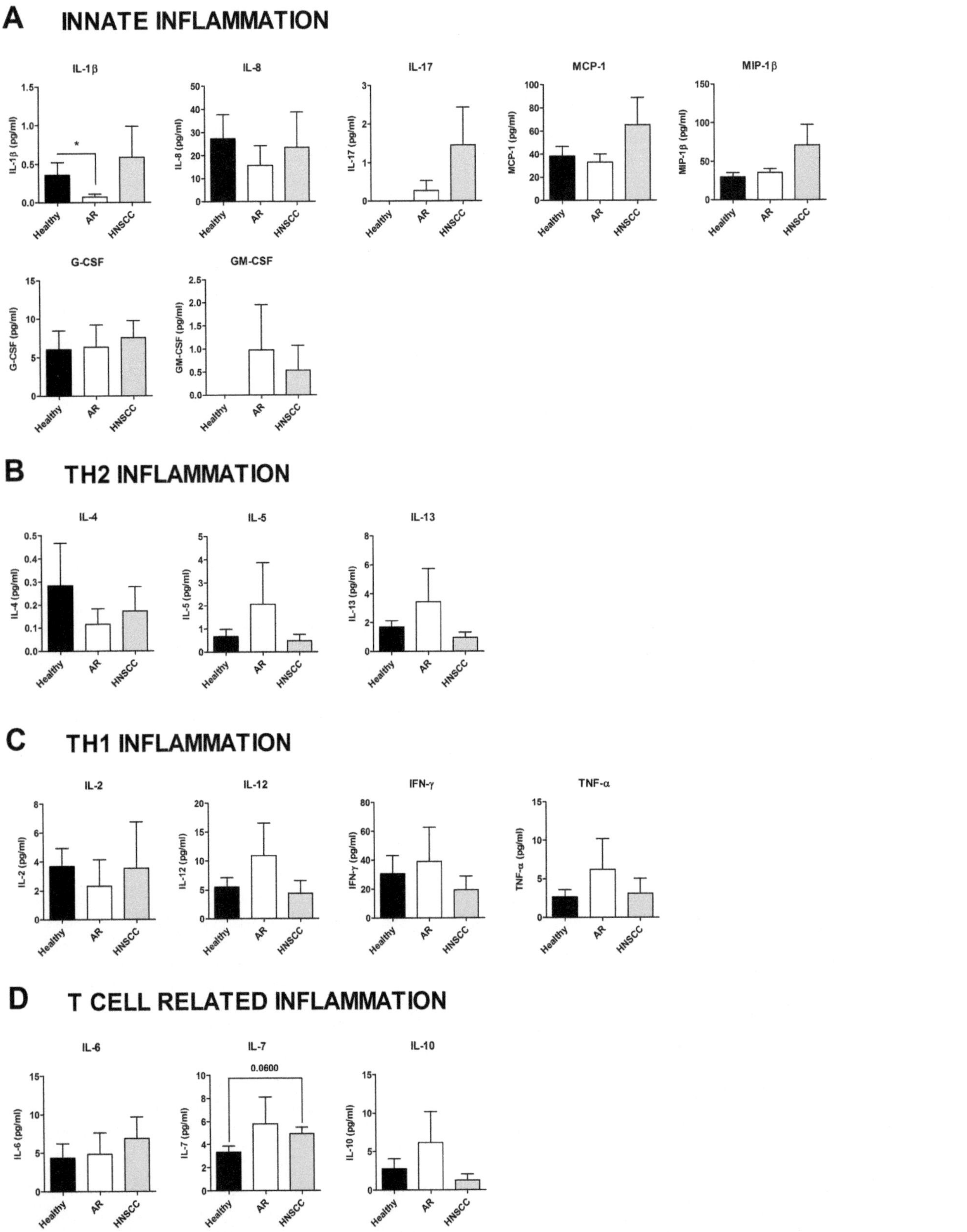

Figure 1. Cytokine concentrations in serum. Sera were collected from healthy controls (n = 10), patients with an ongoing seasonal allergic rhinitis (AR; n = 13) and patients with head and neck squamous cell carcinoma (HNSCC; n = 8), and analyzed for cytokine levels with Luminex Multiplex Immunoassay. *$p \leq 0.05$.

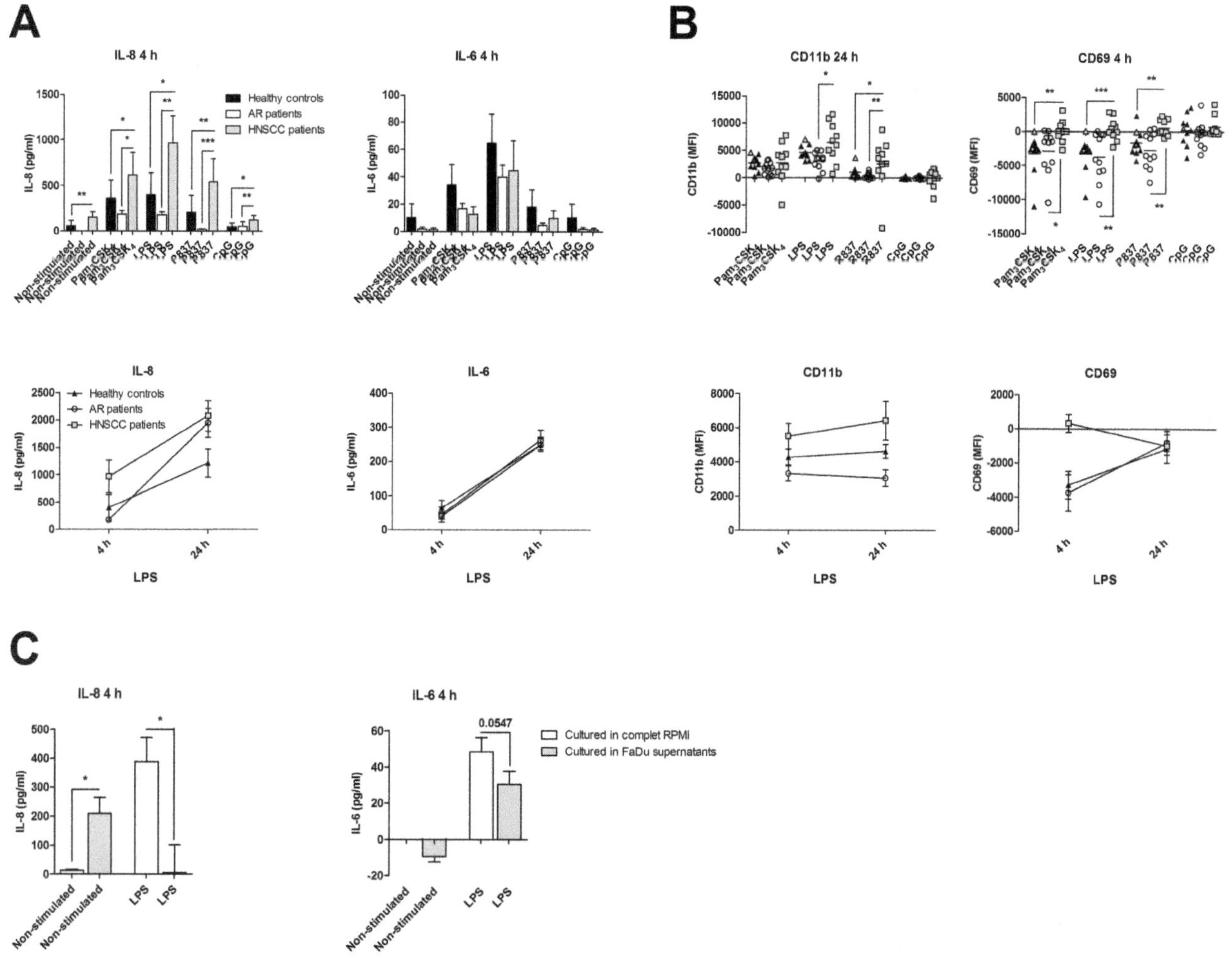

Figure 2. Increased activation of polymorphonuclear leukocytes (PMN) in patients with head and neck squamous cell carcinoma (HNSCC). Blood was obtained from healthy controls (n = 10), patients with an ongoing seasonal allergic rhinitis (AR; n = 11) and patients with HNSCC (ELISA n = 9; FACS n = 10). PMN were isolated and cultured in the presence or absence of Pam_3CSK_4 (1 µg/ml), LPS (1 µg/ml), R837 (5 µg/ml) or CpG (0.3 µM) for 4 and 24 h. (**A**) The cell free supernatants were then analyzed for IL-6 and IL-8 with ELISA, (**B**) and the CD16 positive cells were investigated for the expression of CD11b and CD69 using flow cytometry. The results are presented as the non-stimulated value minus the TLR stimulated values. Grey colored samples were analyzed on a BD LSRFortessa, whereas the rest of the samples were investigated on a Beckman Coulter Navios flow cytometer. (**C**) PMN from healthy individuals (n = 9) were incubated with or without culture medium supernatant from the HNSCC cell line FaDu, and stimulated with or without 1 µg/ml LPS for 4 h, and analyzed for IL-6 and IL-8 secretion with ELISA. The basal cytokine levels in the media were subtracted from the concentrations present in the PMN cultures. MFI = mean fluorescence intensity; $^*p \leq 0.05$; $^{**}p \leq 0.01$; $^{***}p \leq 0.001$.

modulate the immune system in its favor [15]. IL-6 is known to facilitate the proliferation and differentiation of T cells [16,17]. The failure to induce IL-6 secretion in tumor derived PMN, and the suppressed IL-6 release from LPS stimulated PMN from healthy controls cultured in supernatants from FaDu cancer cells may therefore be a tumor induced immune evasive mechanism to attenuate the effective anti-tumoral T cell responses. This assumption is partially supported by the reduced response of T cells from HNSCC patients, and the low expression of COX mRNA levels in PBMC. The high number of CD98-positive Th cells indicates that these cells have the ability to detect unfamiliar substances. However, the low CD98 expression might indicate a deficiency in the clonal T cell expansion [18], and that the suppressed and anergic state render them incapable of eliciting a response. This might explain the increased number of activated T cells previously reported [19]. An altered T cell function has been described among HNSCC patients [20,21]. The increased frequency of regulatory T cells in patients with HNSCC, and their suppressive function on effector T cells [22,23] further verifies that T cells in HNSCC are generally suppressed.

In addition to its important role in the adaptive immunity, CD98 have been shown to be expressed by solid tumors where it promotes transformation, tumor growth and progression [18,24,25]. Center and Ginsberg conclude that the benefits of the adaptive immunity come with a price, in this case increased susceptibility to invasive cancer [18].

The high cytokine secretion by PBMC from allergic patients, the indicative tendency of increased levels of T cells related cytokines, and the suggestive reduced serum concentration of IL-1β in AR patients acknowledge the awareness of allergy as a lymphocyte mediated immune disease with relatively low innate immune reactivity detected. The findings of both Th1 and Th2 cytokines in PBMC supernatants and suggestive in sera supports recent notions that allergy is a more complex immunological

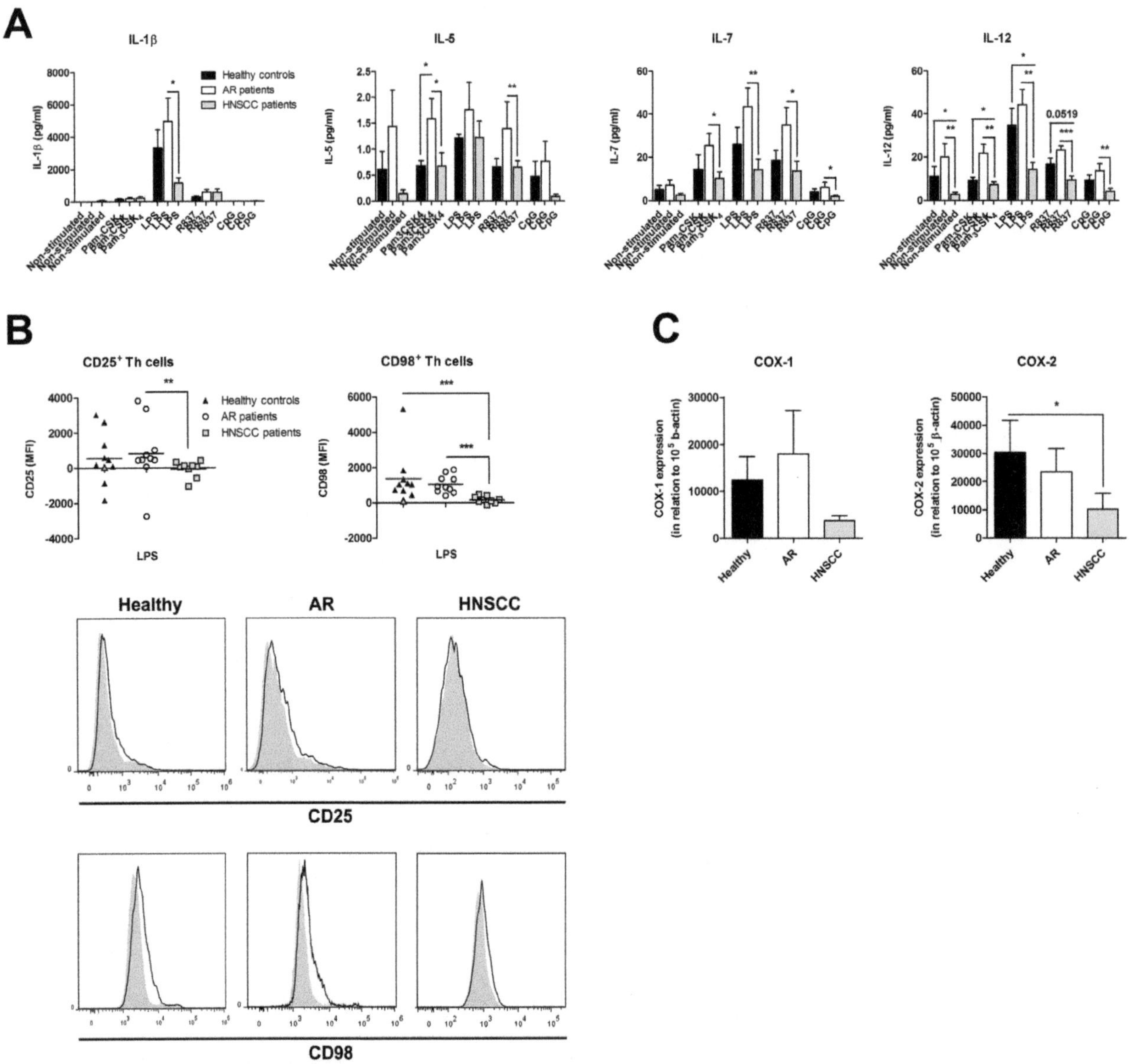

Figure 3. Decreased peripheral blood mononuclear cells (PBMC) activation in patients with head and neck squamous cell carcinoma (HNSCC). PBMC were isolated from blood collected from healthy controls (n = 10), patients with an ongoing seasonal allergic rhinitis (AR; n = 11) and patients with HNSCC (n = 9), and cultured with or without Pam_3CSK_4 (1 µg/ml), LPS (1 µg/ml), R837 (5 µg/ml) or CpG (0.3 µM) for 24 h. (**A**) Thereafter, the supernatants were analyzed for the secreted cytokine profile with Luminex Multiplex Immunoassay, 4 out of 17 investigated cytokines are shown, (**B**) and the cells were examined for the expression of CD25 and CD98 on CD4 positive T helper (Th) cells with flow cytometry. The results are presented as the non-stimulated value minus the TLR stimulated values. Grey colored samples were analyzed on a BD LSRFortessa, whereas the rest of the samples were investigated on a Beckman Coulter Navios flow cytometer. One representative histogram from the healthy controls, AR patients and HNSCC patients is displayed. The open histograms represent LPS stimulated cells, and the light grey histograms are denoting the non-stimulated samples. (**C**) RNA was extracted from peripheral PBMC, isolated from healthy individuals (n = 8), AR patients (n = 10), and HNSCC patients (n = 7), made into cDNA, and thereafter analyzed for COX-1 and COX-2 mRNA expression with real-time PCR. Data are given in relation to the housekeeping gene β-actin, $100\,000 \times 2^{-\Delta Ct}$, and presented as mean ± SEM. MFI = mean fluorescence intensity; *$p \leq 0.05$; **$p \leq 0.01$; ***$p \leq 0.001$.

disease than merely an imbalance between Th1 and Th2 activity [26].

T cells and the adaptive branch of the immune system play an important role in the defense against malignantly transformed cells, and enhanced lymphocyte activity can prevent cancer development [27,28]. In contrast, cancer patients exhibit increased number of regulatory T cells causing a general suppression of the immune reaction. The reversed phenomenon is seen in allergic patients with a more depressed function of their regulatory T cells [29,30] that may facilitate a more active adaptive immune response. In regard of this, we can only speculate whether the increased adaptive response in the AR patients might have an increased ability to raise a tumor specific immune response against malignantly transformed cells, thus providing protection against development of HNSCC.

To summarize, the presented results reflect the principal inflammatory mechanisms involved in allergy and head and neck cancer. The differences in the inflammatory response between AR and HNSCC are distinct despite the somewhat widespread distribution of the tumors and disease progression. The occurrence of two distinct immunological processes, in combination with results from previous epidemiological studies, suggests an inverse association between the immunological responses in patients with allergy and HNSCC.

Supporting Information

Figure S1 Increased activation of polymorphonuclear leukocytes (PMN) in patients with head and neck squamous cell carcinoma (HNSCC). Blood was obtained from healthy controls (n = 10), patients with an ongoing seasonal allergic rhinitis (AR; n = 11) and patients with HNSCC (ELISA n = 9; FACS n = 10). PMN was isolated and cultured in the presence or absence of Pam_3CSK_4 (1 µg/ml), LPS (1 µg/ml), R837 (5 µg/ml) or CpG (0.3 µm) for 4 and 24 h. **(A)** The cell free supernatants were then analyzed for IL-6 and IL-8 with ELISA, and the CD16 positive cells were investigated for the expression of **(B)** CD11b and **(C)** CD69 with flow cytometry. The flow cytometry results are presented as the non-stimulated value minus the TLR stimulated values. Grey colored samples were analyzed on a BD LSRFortessa, whereas the rest of the samples were investigated on a Beckman Coulter Navios flow cytometer. MFI = mean fluorescence intensity; $*p \leq 0.05$; $**p \leq 0.01$; $***p \leq 0.001$.

Figure S2 Increased cytokine secretion by peripheral blood mononuclear cells (PBMC) from patients with allergic rhinitis (AR). PBMC was isolated from blood collected from healthy controls (n = 9), patients with an ongoing seasonal AR (n = 11) and patients with head and neck squamous cell carcinoma (HNSCC; n = 9), and cultured in the presence or absence of Pam_3CSK_4 (1 µg/ml), LPS (1 µg/ml), R837 (5 µg/ml) or CpG (0.3 µm) for 24 h. Thereafter, the supernatants were analyzed for the secreted cytokine profile with Luminex Multiplex Immunoassay. MFI = mean fluorescence intensity; $*p \leq 0.05$; $**p \leq 0.01$; $***p \leq 0.001$.

Figure S3 Increased T helper (Th) cell activation in patients with allergic rhinitis (AR). Peripheral blood mononuclear cells (PBMC) were isolated from blood obtained from healthy controls (24 h and 72 h n = 10), patients with an ongoing seasonal AR (24 h n = 10, 72 h n = 11) and patients with head and neck squamous cell carcinoma (HNSCC; 24 h n = 9, 72 h n = 10), and incubated with or without Pam_3CSK_4 (1 µg/ml), LPS (1 µg/ml), R837 (5 µg/ml) or CpG (0.3 µm) for 24 and 72 h. Subsequently, the cells were examined for the expression of **(A)** CD25 and **(B)** CD98 on CD4 positive Th cells with flow cytometry. The results are presented as the non-stimulated value minus the TLR stimulated values. Grey colored samples were analyzed on a BD LSRFortessa, whereas the rest of the samples were investigated on a Beckman Coulter Navios flow cytometer. MFI = mean fluorescence intensity; $*p \leq 0.05$; $**p \leq 0.01$; $***p \leq 0.001$.

Acknowledgments

The authors would like to acknowledge Eva Johansson and Annette Ingemansson at the flow cytometry lab for helpful assistance. We would also like to express our gratitude to Ann Reutherborg, Josefine P Riikonen, and Anna-Karin Bastos, and Carina Israelsson for collecting blood samples, and to Ingegerd Larsson for helpful technical assistance during the course of this study.

Author Contributions

Conceived and designed the experiments: CRM TH LOC. Performed the experiments: CRM TH SKG. Analyzed the data: CRM TH SKG ÅK OW LOC. Contributed reagents/materials/analysis tools: ÅK OW. Wrote the paper: CRM LOC. Supervised the whole project: LOC.

References

1. Santillan AA, Camargo CA,Jr, Colditz GA (2003) A meta-analysis of asthma and risk of lung cancer (United States). Cancer Causes Control 14: 327–334.
2. Boffetta P, Ye W, Boman G, Nyren (2002) Lung cancer risk in a population-based cohort of patients hospitalized for asthma in Sweden. Eur Respir J 19: 127–133.
3. Turner MC, Chen Y, Krewski D, Ghadirian P, Thun MJ, et al. (2005) Cancer mortality among US men and women with asthma and hay fever. Am J Epidemiol 162: 212–221.
4. Holly EA, Eberle CA, Bracci PM (2003) Prior history of allergies and pancreatic cancer in the San Francisco Bay area. Am J Epidemiol 158: 432–441.
5. Turner MC, Chen Y, Krewski D, Ghadirian P (2006) An overview of the association between allergy and cancer. Int J Cancer 118: 3124–3132.
6. Wisniewski JA, Borish L (2011) Novel cytokines and cytokine-producing T cells in allergic disorders. Allergy Asthma Proc 32: 83–94.
7. Coussens LM, Zitvogel L, Palucka AK (2013) Neutralizing tumor-promoting chronic inflammation: a magic bullet? Science 339: 286–291.
8. Lathers DM, Achille NJ, Young MR (2003) Incomplete Th2 skewing of cytokines in plasma of patients with squamous cell carcinoma of the head and neck. Hum Immunol 64: 1160–1166.
9. Lathers DM, Young MR (2004) Increased aberrance of cytokine expression in plasma of patients with more advanced squamous cell carcinoma of the head and neck. Cytokine 25: 220–228.
10. Minnicozzi M, Sawyer RT, Fenton MJ (2011) Innate immunity in allergic disease. Immunol Rev 242: 106–127.
11. Takeuchi O, Akira S (2010) Pattern recognition receptors and inflammation. Cell 140: 805–820.
12. Fransson M, Adner M, Erjefalt J, Jansson L, Uddman R, et al. (2005) Up-regulation of Toll-like receptors 2, 3 and 4 in allergic rhinitis. Respir Res 6: 100.
13. Trellakis S, Farjah H, Bruderek K, Dumitru CA, Hoffmann TK, et al. (2011) Peripheral blood neutrophil granulocytes from patients with head and neck squamous cell carcinoma functionally differ from their counterparts in healthy donors. Int J Immunopathol Pharmacol 24: 683–693.
14. Jablonska E, Puzewska W, Grabowska Z, Jablonski J, Talarek L (2005) VEGF, IL-18 and NO production by neutrophils and their serum levels in patients with oral cavity cancer. Cytokine 30: 93–99.
15. Coussens LM, Werb Z (2002) Inflammation and cancer. Nature 420: 860–867.
16. Teague TK, Marrack P, Kappler JW, Vella AT (1997) IL-6 rescues resting mouse T cells from apoptosis. J Immunol 158: 5791–5796.
17. Rincon M, Anguita J, Nakamura T, Fikrig E, Flavell RA (1997) Interleukin (IL)-6 directs the differentiation of IL-4-producing CD4+ T cells. J Exp Med 185: 461–469.
18. Cantor JM, Ginsberg MH (2012) CD98 at the crossroads of adaptive immunity and cancer. J Cell Sci 125: 1373–1382.
19. Millrud CR, Mansson Kvarnhammar A, Uddman R, Bjornsson S, Riesbeck K, et al. (2012) The activation pattern of blood leukocytes in head and neck squamous cell carcinoma is correlated to survival. PLoS One 7: e51120.
20. Heimdal JH, Aarstad HJ, Aakvaag A, Olofsson J (1997) In vitro T-lymphocyte function in head and neck cancer patients. Eur Arch Otorhinolaryngol 254: 318–322.
21. Kuss I, Donnenberg AD, Gooding W, Whiteside TL (2003) Effector CD8+CD45RO-CD27-T cells have signalling defects in patients with squamous cell carcinoma of the head and neck. Br J Cancer 88: 223–230.
22. Schaefer C, Kim GG, Albers A, Hoermann K, Myers EN, et al. (2005) Characteristics of CD4+CD25+ regulatory T cells in the peripheral circulation of patients with head and neck cancer. Br J Cancer 92: 913–920.
23. Schott AK, Pries R, Wollenberg B (2010) Permanent up-regulation of regulatory T-lymphocytes in patients with head and neck cancer. Int J Mol Med 26: 67–75.
24. Hara K, Kudoh H, Enomoto T, Hashimoto Y, Masuko T (1999) Malignant transformation of NIH3T3 cells by overexpression of early lymphocyte activation antigen CD98. Biochem Biophys Res Commun 262: 720–725.
25. Henderson NC, Collis EA, Mackinnon AC, Simpson KJ, Haslett C, et al. (2004) CD98hc (SLC3A2) interaction with beta 1 integrins is required for transformation. J Biol Chem 279: 54731–54741.

26. Woodfolk JA (2006) Cytokines as a therapeutic target for allergic diseases: a complex picture. Curr Pharm Des 12: 2349–2363.
27. Jensen-Jarolim E, Achatz G, Turner MC, Karagiannis S, Legrand F, et al. (2008) AllergoOncology: the role of IgE-mediated allergy in cancer. Allergy 63: 1255–1266.
28. Gould HJ, Mackay GA, Karagiannis SN, O'Toole CM, Marsh PJ, et al. (1999) Comparison of IgE and IgG antibody-dependent cytotoxicity in vitro and in a SCID mouse xenograft model of ovarian carcinoma. Eur J Immunol 29: 3527–3537.
29. Ling EM, Smith T, Nguyen XD, Pridgeon C, Dallman M, et al. (2004) Relation of CD4+CD25+ regulatory T-cell suppression of allergen-driven T-cell activation to atopic status and expression of allergic disease. Lancet 363: 608–615.
30. Grindebacke H, Wing K, Andersson AC, Suri-Payer E, Rak S, et al. (2004) Defective suppression of Th2 cytokines by CD4CD25 regulatory T cells in birch allergics during birch pollen season. Clin Exp Allergy 34: 1364–1372.

Citrus Allergy from Pollen to Clinical Symptoms

Rosa Anna Iorio[1], Stefano Del Duca[1]*, Elisabetta Calamelli[2], Chiara Pula[2], Magda Lodolini[3], Fortuna Scamardella[3], Andrea Pession[2], Giampaolo Ricci[2]

1 Department of Biological, Earth and Environmental Sciences, University of Bologna, Bologna, Italy, 2 Department of Pediatric Allergology of the Women's, Children's and Adolescents' Health Gozzadini Children's Hospital Sant'Orsola-Malpighi, University of Bologna, Bologna, Italy, 3 Laboratory Analysis Unit. Maggiore Hospital, Bologna, Italy

Abstract

Allergy to citrus fruits is often associated with pollinosis and sensitization to other plants due to a phenomenon of cross-reactivity. The aims of the present study were to highlight the cross-reactivity among citrus and the major allergenic pollens/fruits, throughout clinical and molecular investigations, and to evaluate the sensitization frequency to citrus fruits in a population of children and adults with pollinosis. We found a relevant percentage of sensitisation (39%) to citrus fruits in the patients recruited and in all of them the IgE-mediated mechanism has been confirmed by the positive response to the prick-to-prick test. RT-PCR experiments showed the expression of Cit s 1, Cit s 3 and a profilin isoform, already described in apple, also in *Citrus clementine* pollen. Data of multiple sequence alignments demonstrated that *Citrus* allergens shared high percentage identity values with other clinically relevant species (i.e. *Triticum aestivum, Malus domestica*), confirming the possible cross-allergenicity citrus/grasses and citrus/apple. Finally, a novelty of the present work has been the expression of two phospholipaseA2 isoforms (PLA2 α and β) in *Citrus* as well as in *Triticum* pollens; being PLA2 able to generate pro-inflammatory factors, this enzyme could participate in the activation of the allergenic inflammatory cascade.

Editor: Phillip A. Stumbles, Murdoch University, Australia

Funding: This work was supported by the Programma Operativo Regionale (POR FESR 2007-2013) of Regione Calabria "My Darling Clementine": un prodotto salutistico nuovo e innovativo dalle clementine e dal limone di Calabria". The funders had no role in study design, data collection and analysis, decision to publish, or preparation of the manuscript.

Competing Interests: The authors have declared that no competing interests exist.

* E-mail: stefano.delduca@unibo.it

Introduction

The regular consumption of fruit and vegetables is generally encouraged also by the European Community as the basis of a daily diet healthy and able to improve human health and prevent some diseases: there are many data that confirm the direct correlation between the consumption of fresh fruit and the reduction in the incidence of cardio-vascular disease, asthma, diabetes and cancer [1,2]. The benefit derives not only from their nutritional properties in terms of vitamins, minerals and fibres, but also from the "non-nutritional" component, such as the high content in secondary metabolites (phenols, flavonoids, carotenoids) that play an important antioxidant role.

Unfortunately, about 1/5 of the population in Western countries suffer from respiratory allergies [3]. Recent epidemiological studies estimate that food allergies are increasing and affecting millions of people (1–2% of world population), as to consider them as the epidemic of the XXI century [4]. Nearly 4% of the US populations are afflicted with food allergies, a prevalence much higher than appreciated in the past. In addition, the frequency of food hypersensitivities is greater in the first few years of life, affecting about 6% of infants less than 3 years of age and decreasing over the first decade [5].

For food allergies there is still no effective treatment and, consequently, up to now the only therapy is still the avoidance of fruits that cause allergy [6] and, considering that a regular consumption of fruits is reported to enhance human health and prevent various diseases, it is easy to understand that allergy can significantly affect the quality of life of allergic patients in a profoundly negative way [7]. The problem is compounded by the fact that food allergy may also arise as a result of cross-pollen allergy [8].

Oranges (*Citrus sinensis*) are largely consumed worldwide and commonly included in the population's diet in many countries, both as fresh fruit or derived beverages (juices) and foods (jams) [9,10]. This fact has probably led to point to orange among the main allergenic plant food in a public perception survey of food allergies [11]. Although in the daily clinical practice orange allergy is obviously rarely observed in Central Europe, some early studies suggested oranges being an important allergenic food, as for other foods and pollens such as kiwi, strawberry, peach, banana, grasses (www.foodallergyitalia.org) [12]. However, allergy to oranges or other citrus fruits has been scarcely investigated [10]; when present, it is often associated with pollinosis and sensitization to other plants [10] due to a phenomenon of cross-reactivity, whereby the pollen would be the cause of a sensitization by the respiratory way that could predispose to allergy towards foods that contain homologous proteins to those in sensitizing pollen. In an English study on 67 asthmatic children which compared a multiple food specific IgE antibodies (sIgE) test to parental perception of food allergy, oranges resulted implicated in the 15% of patients [13]. Another study reported a frequency of 17% of adverse food reactions after eating oranges in a population of 100 adults suffering from oral allergy syndrome (OAS) as common manifestations of allergy to oranges [14]. Previous studies indicated mild local reactions and described subjects affected from orange-dependent exercise-induced anaphylaxis after eating oranges [12].

The three major orange allergens that have been recently identified and characterized are Cit s 1, a germin-like protein (GLP) [14,15], Cit s 2, a profilin [9,10] and Cit s 3, a new member of the lipid transfer protein pan-allergen family (LTP) [9]. Cit s 1 is a glycoprotein of 24 kDa recognized by patients' sera IgE recently described by Ibáñez et al. [15] and Pignataro et al. in lemon fruit flavedo [16]; its biological activity in fruit need to be clarified, but it is considered one of the major orange allergen [12] displaying an high *in vitro* reactivity with its glycans constituting the major IgE epitopes [9]. Moreover, the protein could be present in different isoforms ranging from 20 to 120 kDa [16]. Cit s 2 represents the other major allergen according to its *in vitro* and *in vivo* reactivity in patients with allergy to this fruit [10]. Its biological activity is associated to the structural organization of actin filament; in particular it is believed to be involved in the transition between G- and F-actin, playing a very important role for pollen germination and indeed for plant fertilization [17]; its reactivity with patient-s'sera is associated to plan pollen allergy [18]. Cit s 3 behaves as a minor allergen (approximately 35% prevalence) [9], contrary to the fact that LTPs are considered in general the major fruit allergen in the Mediterranean area [12]. Cit s 3 is present in pulp, but in lower amount comparing to flavedo, so the moderate IgE reactivity observed might be explained by the low nsLTP concentration in the orange pulp [19]. LTP role in plant is believed to be related to the defence mechanisms and in the control of pathogen attack responses. Moreover, a role in transporting lipid molecules to the outer layers of plant organs, in embryogenesis and in abiotic stress response has been also proposed [20]. The multiple function of LTPs is also supported by the presence of isoforms showing moderate levels of amino acid sequence identity and different gene expression patterns [21].

Ahrazem et al. [19] sought to identify and isolated citrus fruit LTPs and to explore their relevance in orange allergy in 27 patients with OAS after orange ingestion and with positive skin-prick test (SPT) as well as prick-to-prick test (PPT) responses and sIgE levels to orange. This study showed that members of the LTP allergen family are involved in orange's allergy, displaying positive *in vivo* and *in vitro* tests in 30–50% of the subjects studied. Furthermore, both orange and lemon allergens showed cross-reactivity with the major peach LTP allergen Pru p 3: the recombinant orange isoform (rCit s 3) presented 67% sequence identity with rPru p 3 [19].

Crespo et al. [12] documented a statistically significant correlation between the presence of IgE mediated sensitization to the two orange major allergens, Cit s 1 and Cit s 2 and the positive response to Skin-Prick test (SPT) respectively to olive and cypress (Cit s 1) and to platanus (Cit s 2) in 56 patients with self-reported adverse reactions to oranges.

The purposes of the present study were to i) deeply investigate the cross-reactivity among citrus and the major allergenic pollens and fruits, either under clinical and molecular points of view, and to ii) evaluate the frequency of sensitization and/or allergy to citrus fruits (oranges, lemons and clementines) in a population of children and young adults with pollinosis (allergic hay fever and/or asthma) recruited for this monocentric observational study.

The cross-reactivity aspect has focused on the analysis of i) the sIgE levels in patients serum in order to determine the major citrus allergens levels by the use of the recombinant molecules Pru p 3 (LTP protein homolog to Cit s 3), r Phl p 12 (profilin homolog to Cit s 2) and MuxF3-CCD, marker of sensitization for Cross-reactive carbohydrate determinants (CCD) and of ii) allergens expression (Cit s 1, Cit s 2, Cit s 3) in *Citrus clementine* pollen, in order to assess its potential allergenicity and cross-reactivity with other pollens, especially *Triticum aestivum*, whose allergens sequences are conserved in the *poaceae* family. The three important citrus allergens reported above were also analyzed in citrus pollen because of the possible cross-reactivity between pollen and fruits, as documented for apple [22]. *Citrus clementine* pollen can be potentially important from the allergenic point of view because present in some foods as marmalade and honey and for farmers cultivating citrus fields.

The research for sensitizing agents in pollen continued with the evaluation of the expression of two isoforms of secretory phospholipase (PLA2 α and β), key enzymes in the synthesis of pro-inflammatory eicosanoids that may have a key role in raising sensitization and allergic reaction [23,24].

Materials and Methods

Chemicals and Antibodies

All chemicals (unless otherwise indicated) were obtained from Sigma-Aldrich (Milan, Italy).

Plant material

Mature pollen of clementine (*Citrus clementine* Hort. Ex Tan. cv. Comune) was collected from flowers kindly donated by Professor S. Mazzucca, University of Calabria (Dipartimento di Ecologia), and pollen of *Triticum aestivum* (wheat) was kindly donated by Azienda Agricola Rondinini (Faenza, Ra). Handling and storage were performed as reported by Bagni et al. [25], stored at $-20°C$ with NaOH pellets to maintain it dry.

Fruits of oranges, clementines and lemons have been provided by Azienda Agricola "San Mauro" di Minisci Edmondo (Corigliano Calabro, Cosenza) within the project "My Darling Clementine": un prodotto salutistico nuovo e innovativo dalle clementine e dal limone di Calabria" (POR FESR 2007–2013).

In vitro germination

Pollen was hydrated at 20°C-100% rHu for 1 h and allowed to germinate (1 mg/mL in germination medium: 15% sucrose, 324 µM boric acid, 2% agar) 13 h (overnight, o/n) into glass Petri dishes at 20°C-100% rHu.

Total RNA isolation and cDNA synthesis

Total RNA was extracted from 30 mg of frozen ungerminated (UGP) and germinated (GP) *Citrus c.* and *Triticum a.* pollens following the basic protocol for phenol/SDS method [26] with minor modifications as published by Paris et al. [27]. The purity and concentration of the extracted RNAs were evaluated by measuring the absorbance at 260 and 280 nm wavelengths using a NanoDrop Spectrophotometer ND-1000 (EuroClone S.p.A., Italy). RNA was considered pure if the A260/280 ratio was grater than 1.8 and A260/230 ratio higher than 2. First-strand cDNA was synthesized following the instruction from Stratagene (Agilent Technologies, USA), starting from 1 µg DNA-free RNA, and 2 µl was used for the semi-quantitative PCR analyses.

Primer design

Specific primer pairs (Table 1 and Table 2) were designed on the basis of the sequences obtained from National Center for Biotechnology Information (NCBI) Reference Sequence database (http://www.ncbi.nlm.nih.gov) with the software Primer3 version 0.4.0 (http://frodo.wi.mit.edu/primer3) and further tested with the software PrimerSelect® v8.0-MegAlign for the formation of primer homo and heterodimers. As endogenous control the EF1-α gene of *Citrus sinensis* (GenBank ID AY498567) and the UBQ10 (GenBank ID CB322134.1) genes were used.

Table 1. Primer sequences and amplicon characteristics for *Citrus sinensis* genes used in semi-quantitative and qRT-PCR.

Gene	GeneBank accension number	Sequence 5′-3′	Product size (bp)	Ta (°C)	qRT-PCR Efficiency *	R^2*
UB10	CB322134.1	GATCCCACCAGACCAGCAA	105	60	1,953	1
		ACCAAATGAAGGGTTGATTCCTT				
EF1	AY498567.1	ATTGACAAGCGTGTGATTGAGC	132	60	1,948	0,999
		TCCACAAGGCAATATCAATGGTA				
Cit s 1	UniProt P84159	CATTCCAGTTGGACCCAAAG	191	60	1,961	1
		CAGTCAGCCTGGAGAGAGGT				
Cit s 2	AJ865015.1	CTTTCCTGCGTTTAGGCTTG	189	60	n.d.	n.d.
		AGGGCCTGATTGGTCTTCTT				
Cit s 3	AJ783335.1	CCCTATACCTGTGCCATGCT	199	60	1,902	1
		GCAGTCAGTGGAGATGCTGA				
PLA2 α	GU075396	GCCATAGCCCATGTTTTCAT	184	60	1,89	1
		CACTGTACAGCAGCCCACAG				
PLA2 β	GU075398	GTATCTCTGCAAGCGCACTG	180	60	1,961	1
		TGCCATGTCCATACCCTGTA				

*The qRT-PCR efficiency and correlations; R^2 were determined with LinRegPCR software.

Allergen gene expression analysis by semi-quantitative PCR

The PCR reactions were performed in a 15 µl reaction containing 2 µl cDNA, 0.1 µM specific primers (Table 1 and Table 2), 1.5 mM MgCl2, 100 µM dNTPs, 0.5 Unit Taq DNA Polymerase (Fermentas, M-Medical, Italy) and 1X reaction buffer. The reaction included an initial 5 min denaturation step at 94°C, followed by 40 PCR cycles at 94°C 30 s, the optimised annealing temperature for 45 s and 1 min at 72°C.

The number of amplification cycles was chosen to be in the exponential phase of amplification. The amplicons were visualised with a transilluminator (Vilber Lournet, Genenco) at 302 nm after electrophoresis in 2% (w/v) agarose gels in TAE 1X Buffer, containing 0.5 µg/ml ethidium bromide, and photographed (Nikon E5400 Coolpix). The experiment was repeated twice.

Real-time PCR (qRT-PCR) analysis

The transcript levels were determined by real-time quantitative RT-PCR (qRT-PCR) using a StepOnePlus™ Real Time PCR System (Applied Biosystems, USA) and the Power SYBR Green PCR Master Mix (Applied Biosystems, USA) as recommended by the manufacturer. PCR reactions were carried out in 96-well plates (10 µl per well) in a buffer containing SYBR Green (including Taq polymerase, dNTPs, SYBR Green dye) and 200 nM of each primer (forward and reverse, Table 1). After denaturing at 95°C for 10 min, a two-step amplification occurred: 15 s of denaturation at 95°C and 1 min of annealing/extension at 60°C, with a total of 40 cycles. The melting curves were analyzed at 60°C-95°C after 40 cycles to ensure that the resulting fluorescence originated from a single PCR product did not represent primer-dimers formed during the PCR or a nonspecific product. Each qRT-PCR analysis was performed in triplicate. Negative controls without cDNA were routinely included.

qRT-PCR results were analyzed with the sequence detection software SDS version 1.1 (Applied Biosystems, USA). The SYBR green fluorescent signal was standardized to a passive reference dye (ROX) included in the PCR master mix. Direct detection of the PCR product was measured by monitoring the increase in

Table 2. Primer sequences and amplicon characteristics of *Triticum aestivum* (wheat) and *Malus domestica* (apple) cross-allergens.

Gene	GeneBank accension number	Sequence 5′-3′	Product size (bp)	Ta (°C)
Tri a 12	X89827.1	CCTTGCACCAACTGGTCTTT	162	60
		CCAGGAGTCATGGGTTCATC		
Tri a 14	AJ784902.1	GGCGTCAAGAACCTCCATAA	177	60
		GCTGCAGTCGATGTTGAGAC		
Mal d 3.02	AY572532.1	TGGCCAGGTGAGCTCCAA	247	60
		TGGTGGAGGTGCTGATCTTG		
Mal d 4.02	AY792613.1	GTGTTACTTGTCAAGAAGAGCACAA	126	58
		GCTCAATGAGATAATCCGCA		
PLA 2.23	EEF48118.1	TGGGAAGTATTGTGGGCTTT	259	52
		AGCAACTAAAGCAGCCTCCA		

fluorescence caused by the binding of SYBR green dye to double-stranded DNA.

To estimate the expression variation levels of the eight candidate genes, geNorm software package for Microsoft Excel (http://medgen.ugent.be/*jvdesomp/genorm/) [28] was applied to analyze the data obtained from the samples of citrus pollen [29]. The PCR efficiency was calculated for each gene with LinRegPCR program [30] from raw fluorescence data taken from the Applied Biosystems detection system. Results from the LinRegPCR software were imported into Microsoft Excel, transformed to relative quantities using the comparative Ct (ΔΔCt) method, and taken into account the different amplification efficiencies for the different genes (just replace value 2 with the actual efficiency of the gene (e.g. 1.95 for 95%) in the formula of ΔCt [31]. Data have been normalized to the geometric mean of two housekeeping genes (EF-1 and UBQ 10), chosen according to the geNorm software.

Multiple sequence alignments

The multiple sequence alignments of the sensitizing factors annotated in the UniProtKB database (http://www.ebi.ac.uk/uniprot/) has been performed through ClustalΩ tool (http://www.ebi.ac.uk/Tools/msa/clustalo/) to find sequence homology among *Citrus sinensis* and *Triticum aestivum, Phleum pratense, Cynodon dactylon, Betula pendula, Artemisia vulgaris, Parietaria judaica, Malus domestica, Corylus avellana, Olea europaea, Arachis hypogaea.*

Study population for clinical trials

This monocentric observational study enrolled all caucasian children and young adults affected from pollinosis [allergic rhino-conjunctivitis (RC) and/or asthma] consecutively referred to the Allergologic Center of the Paediatric Department of Bologna University (Northern Italy) from December 2011 to May 2012.

The criteria for study inclusion were:

- aged between 4 and 22 years;
- diagnosis of allergic RC and/or asthma with or without sensitization/allergy to oranges;
- Written informed consent from all patients (or from parents for patients younger than 18 years old).

The criteria for study exclusion were:

- Children with height or weight less than 3rd centile;
- Patient affected from systemic disease (different from allergy or asthma) including: gastro-esophageal reflux disease under medical treatment, epilepsy, severe neurological or neurodevelopmental disorders, tuberculosis, previous thoracic surgery, major congenital malformations, heart diseases (with the exception of atrial sept defect without hemodynamic significance and ventricular sept defect), primary or secondary immunodeficiencies.

Allergometric assays

In each patient, the presence of symptoms of food allergy and/or OAS to oranges and other citrus fruits was investigated. Skin-Prick test (SPT) with commercial extracts (Lofarma, Milano) of pollens (grass, composites, parietaria) were performed as well as prick-by-prick test (PPT) with fresh fruit pulp of oranges, lemons and clementines. A SPT result was considered positive when elicited a wheal at least greater than half of histamine control.

In the patients with a positive PPT with citrus fruits pulp, the levels of specific IgE were determined to a panel of the main pollens (*Phleum p., Parietaria j., Olea e., Betula v., Corylus a.*), recombinant allergens (rPhl p 1, rPhl p 12, rBet v 2, rPru p 3), fruit extracts (orange, apple, peanut, wheat) and MuxF3-CCD, a marker of sensitization for cross-reactive carbohydrate determinants (CCD) (ImmunoCAP 1000 FEIA, ThermoFisher-Sweden). In addition, the choice of determining the sIgE levels for rPhl p 12 and rPru p 3 has been made on the base of the high degree of homology with orange profilin Cit s 2 (almost 75%) [32] and orange LTP Cit s 3 (almost 67%) [18] respectively. Levels of sIgE greater than 0.35 kU/L were considered positive.

Data and Statistics

The values reported are expressed as mean ± SD; they have been calculated on the basis of the data obtained from three independent experiments run separately and each sample was undertaken in triplicate (total nine replicates for each determination). Differences between sample sets were determined by the Student's *t*-test with 95% confidence limits. When indicated statistical analysis was performed using GraphPad Prism (version 5.03 Windows GraphPad Software Inc., La Jolla, CA, USA).

Ethic Statement

The research was conducted according to the principles expressed in the Declaration of Helsinki, and approved by Ethic Committee of Bologna University, S. Orsola-Malpighi Hospital (protocol name: OrangeAllergy; number: 108/2011/U/Oss.). Written informed consent was obtained from all the parents or guardians of the minors involved in the study.

Results

Clinical results

We have recruited 72 children and young adults (50 males, 69% and 22 females, 31%) with mean age of 12,3 years (range 6–22 years) and clinical history of pollinosis, who presented a positive reactions to SPT with grass pollen extract.

Forty-seven patients (65%) had symptoms of allergic RC, 25 (35%) presented both RC and asthma. Nine patients (12%) referred systemic symptoms after ingesting the following foods (alone or in combination): 6 to nuts (2 to hazelnut, 1 to peanut, 1 to walnut, and 2 to a not specified nut), 2 to citrus fruits (1 to orange and 1 to clementine), 1 to kiwi, 1 to apple, 1 to tomato, 1 to egg, 1 to fish and 1 to milk. Four patients (6%) presented symptoms of OAS to the following plant-derived foods (alone or in combination): 2 to kiwi, 2 to melon, 1 to orange, 1 to strawberry and 1 to peanut. Overall three out of patients (4%) showed symptoms after ingestion of citrus fruits (2 systemic food allergy – 1 to orange and 1 to clementine – and 1 OAS to orange). The patient with systemic orange allergy showed a severe reaction with urticaria and vomiting immediately after ingestion of orange, otherwise the other patient with systemic citrus allergy presented abdominal pain and diarrhea after the assumption of a clementine. The case of OAS due to citrus fruits was elicited by the contact with an orange. The clinical features and allergological assays of the three patients with documented citrus fruits allergy are reported in Table 3.

PPT with the pulp of fresh orange, lemon and clementine resulted positive in 28 patients (39%): 24 (33%) to orange (mean wheal diameter = 2.8 mm, range: 2–7 mm), 16 (22%) to lemon (mean wheal diameter = 2.8 mm, range: 2–6 mm) and 12 (17%) to clementine (mean wheal diameter = 2,9 mm, range 2–6 mm).

Fourteen out of the 28 patients with a positive PPT performed with fresh citrus fruit accepted to perform blood test: the mean values of sIgE against orange and the main pollens and plant

Table 3. Clinical features of the three patients with citrus fruit allergy.

PATIENT DATA	Patient	**1**	**2**	**3**
	Sex	F	M	M
	Age yrs	20	20	12
	Respiratory disease (A/RC)	A, RC	A, RC	RC
	Symptoms with citrus fruits	Urticaria Vomiting (Orange)	OAS (Orange)	Abdominal pain Diarrhoea (clementine)
	Food Allergy/ OAS to other foods	apple, nuts, tomato	kiwy, melon, strawberry	kiwy
PRICK-TO-PRICK WITH FRUIT PULP *Mean wheal diameter (mm)*	*Orange*	7	4	0
	Clementine	6	3	3
	Lemon	6	0	0
SPECIFIC IGE (KU/L)	*Orange*	39.2	<0.10	4.3
	Wheat	14.3	<0.10	6.5
	Apple	45.7	<0.10	24.4
	Peanut	47.8	<0.10	13.1
	Phleum p.	87.8	14.3	83.9
	Olea e.	56.8	0.8	33.3
	Betula v.	>100	<0.10	57.3
	Corylus a.	92.7	0.4	59
	r Phl p 1	41	15.1	71.2
	r Phl p 12	34.2	0.31	4
	r Bet v 2	47	<0.10	7.1
	r Pru p 3	19.7	<0.10	16.6
	MuxF3-CCD	1.23	<0.10	0.74

Patient data, results of prick-to-prick (PPT) with fresh citrus fruit pulp and specific IgE (sIgE) against the main pollens, (*Phleum p., Olea e., Betula v., Corylus a.*), fruit extracts (orange, apple, peanut, wheat), recombinant allergens (rPhl p 1, rPhl p 12, rBet v 2, rPru p 3) and MuxF3-CCD.
A: Asthma; OAS: oral allergy syndrome; RC: rhino-conjunctivitis; yrs: years.

derived foods are reported in Table 4; the geometric mean value of sIgE for orange was 3.5 kU/L (range: 0.85–39,2 kU/L). A direct correlation seems to exist between the high level of sIgE for the rPhl p12 and rPru p 3, homolog to the two orange allergens Cit s 2 and Cit s 3 respectively, and the generalized clinical symptoms (vomiting and urticaria, abdominal pain and diarrhoea) as reported in Table 3 for the patient 1 (sIgE = 34.2 and 19.7 for rPhl p 12 and rPur p 3 respectively) and patient 3 (sIgE = 4 and 16.6 for rPhl p 12 and rPur p 3 respectively).

Expression analysis of sensitizing factors in citrus pollen

The gene expression analysis were conducted in order to study which allergens and other sensitizing factors were actually expressed even in the pollen, after the recently identification and characterization of the three major orange allergens in fruits [9,10,12,15,16]: transcripts for Germin-like proteins (GLP, Cit s 1), profilins (Cit s 2), non specific Lipid Transfer Proteins (nsLTP, Cit s 3) and two isoforms of secretory phospholipase A2 (PLA2 α and PLA2 β) were tested in ungerminated (UGP) and germinated (GP) pollen of *Citrus clementine* (Cit UGP and Cit GP) and *Triticum aestivum* (Tri UGP and Tri GP) through either semi-quantitative RT-PCR (Figure 1A) and qRT-PCR (Figure 1D). The evaluation of the expression profile of the *Cit s* 1–3 allergens by semi-quantitative RT-PCR (Figure 1A) allowed to verify the presence of Cit s 1 (GLP) and Cit s 3 (nsLTP) transcripts even in the citrus pollen with a different pattern of expression than those observed in the literature for the orange fruits [12]: for the citrus pollen the two major allergens are the Cit s 1 and Cit s 3, whereas the expression of Cit s 2 is not detectable according to the experimental conditions described in Material and Methods section. The densitometry analysis (Figure 1B) performed on the semi-quantitative RT-PCR shown in Figure 1A, confirmed differences in the expression profile between Cit UGP and Cit GP: Cit s 1 and Cit s 3 are both expressed almost with the same intensity in UGP, whereas in GP Cit s 1 showed an higher expression signal (about 2.5 fold) when compared to Cit s 3 ($1{,}55\pm0{,}08$ Cit s 1 *vs* $0{,}58\pm0{,}05$ Cit s 3); as concerning PLA2 isoforms, both enzymes were expressed more in Cit GP ($1{,}3\pm0{,}03$ PLA2 α *vs* $1{,}25\pm0{,}03$ PLA2 β) compared to Cit UGP ($1\pm0{,}03$ PLA2 α *vs* $1{,}16\pm0{,}03$ PLA2 β).

Since clinical data reported in literature [12] often shown that allergic patients to citrus fruits also manifest sensitization to grass pollens, expression analysis of *Cit s* 1–3 and grass specific allergens has been assessed to confirm cross-reactivity between pollens; among grass allergens have been chosen those from *Triticum aestivum* (wheat) pollen (Figure 1A and Figure 1B): Tri a 12.0103 (GenBank ID X89827.1), a profilin, and Tri a 14.0101 (GenBank ID AJ784902), a nsLTP. They represented conserved allergens among the most allergenic species of the *poaceae* family (i.e. *Triticum aestivum, Cynodon dactylon* and *Phelum pratense*) as shown by the

Table 4. Pollinosis patients' clinical features.

ALLERGENS	n of positive/14 (≥ 0.35 kU/L)	g mean sIgE (kU/L)°	range (kU/L)°
Orange	9	3.5	0.85–39.2
Phleum p.	14	52.0	1.5–>100
Betula v.	13	8.2	0.4–>100
Corylus a.	14	7.0	0.4–92.7
Olea e.	13	7.5	0.8–70.8
Parietaria j.	13	5.2	0.36–43.2
r Phl p 1	12	49.2	15.1–>100
r Phl p 12	11	2	0.35–34.2
r Bet v 2	4	9.6	2.38–47
r Pru p 3	5	4.83	1.07–19.7
MuxF3-CCD	5	1.14	0.42–6.43
CITRUS FRUITS	**N of positive PPT (%)**[§]		**PPT** Mean wheal diameter mm (range) [§]
Orange	**24/72 (33)**		2.8 (2–7)
Lemon	**16/72 (22)**		2.8 (2–6)
Clementine	**12/72 (17)**		(2–6)

Levels of specific IgE (sIgE) against the main pollens (*Phleum p., Parietaria j., Olea e., Betula v., Corylus a.*), fruit extracts (orange, apple, peanut, wheat), recombinant allergens (rPhl p 1, rPhl p 12, rBet v 2, rPru p 3) and MuxF3-CCD in children and young adults with pollinosis. The geometric mean values of sIgE were calculated on the 14 out of the 28 patients with a positive reaction to prick-to-prick (PPT) with fresh citrus fruit pulp who accepted to perform blood test.
g mean: geometric mean; N: number; sIgE: specific IgE; PPT: prick-to-prick test.
§Calculated on the 72 patients enrolled in the study.
° Calculated on the 14 patients who perform blood test.

multiple sequence alignments performed with ClustalΩ for profilin proteins, that shared identity values in the range between 76–82% (Figure 2A); on the contrary only isoforms for *Triticum a.* nsLTP proteins were annotated in the UniProtKB database, while sequences for *Cynodon d.* and *Phelum p.* were not yet present. Since one of the aims of the present study was to investigate on molecules involved in the cross-allergenicity citrus *vs* grass pollens, we have chosen that of *Triticum aestivum* as model.

The expression profiles performed through semi-quantitative RT-PCR (Figure 1A) and the densitometry analysis reported in Figure 1B showed that wheat allergens were remarkably expressed in *Triticum a.* pollen, with significantly differences between Tri UGP and Tri GP: GP showed the highest expression levels of both allergens with Tri a 12 more expressed than Tri a 14; the difference between Tri a 12 and Tri a 14 is higher in Tri UGP, where Tri a 12 showed an almost double fold expression level than Tri a 14. Moreover, we observed a faint signal for Cit s 1 and Cit s 2 allergens and PLA2 α enzyme also in wheat pollen grain (Figure 1A), with Cit s 1 expressed only in Tri GP and Cit s 2 and PLA2 α in both Tri UGP and Tri GP, emphasizing the cross-sensitization between citrus and grass pollens. Finally, it should be noted as the Tri a 14 is also expressed in *Citrus c.* pollen, both Cit UGP and Cit GP, emphasizing the pan-allergenic nature of nsLTPs.

Unexpectedly, the presence of allergens with common sequence has been observed also between *Citrus c.* and *Malus domestica* pollens. Among all the apple allergen sequences tested (known to be present also in apple fruits), it has been obtained signal for two specific allergen isoforms (Mal d 3.02, an nsLTP and Mal d 4.02, a profilin) and for potential sensitizing factors, PLA2 (isoform 23): in fact, these three pairs of primers were able to generate transcripts in *Citrus c.* both Cit UGP and Cit GP (Figure 1C) with different expression profile as Mal d 3.02 and PLA 2.23 showed an higher signal in UGP when compared to GP. These data were confirmed by the multiple sequence alignments for *Citrus c.* and *Malus d.* proteins, which shared values of 69% identity Mal d 3 *vs* Cit s 3, 90% identity Mal d 4 *vs* Cit s 2 and 77% identity PLA 2.23 *vs* PLA2 β.

To confirm previous results and to obtained quantitative data about allergens expression, the qRT-PCR methodology was followed and data are shown in Figure 1D. The technique of qRT-PCR combined with the use of highly specific primers designed for each allergen allowed to test in a precise, accurate and sensitive manner the gene expression at the level of messenger RNA. The selection of the optimal reference target has been performed by geNorm software [28]: in this experimental situation the optimal number of housekeeping genes was 2, represented by EF1 and UBQ10 (geNorm V <0.15 when comparing a normalization factor based on the 2 or 3 most stable targets). As shown in Figure 1D, Cit s 2 was not detected even after 40 cycles; Cit s 1 was higher expressed in Cit GP when compared to Cit UGP (2,03±0,02 in Cit GP *vs* 1,53±0,1 in Cit UGP), whereas Cit s 3 expression was higher in Cit UGP (2,24±0,1) than in Cit GP (1,08±0,14), being also the allergen with the highest level detected in *Citrus c.* pollen. As described before and confirmed also by qRT-PCR for Cit GP, Cit s 1 showed an expression signal double higher than Cit s 3. The two isoforms of PLA2 (PLA2 α and PLA2 β), were differentially expressed in Cit UGP and Cit GP with a stronger signal for PLA2 β in respect to PLA2 α, showing the same trend reported for the densitometry analysis (Figure 1B): an higher signal in Cit GP (1,61±0,34 PLA2 α *vs* 1,81±0,18 PLA2 β) when compared to Cit UGP (1,14±0,18 PLA2 α *vs* 1,65±0,15 PLA2 β) for both PLA enzyme isoforms.

According to the World Health Organization (WHO), two proteins can be considered cross-allergens if they share 35% identity on 80 residues and have an exact match of 6–8 residues

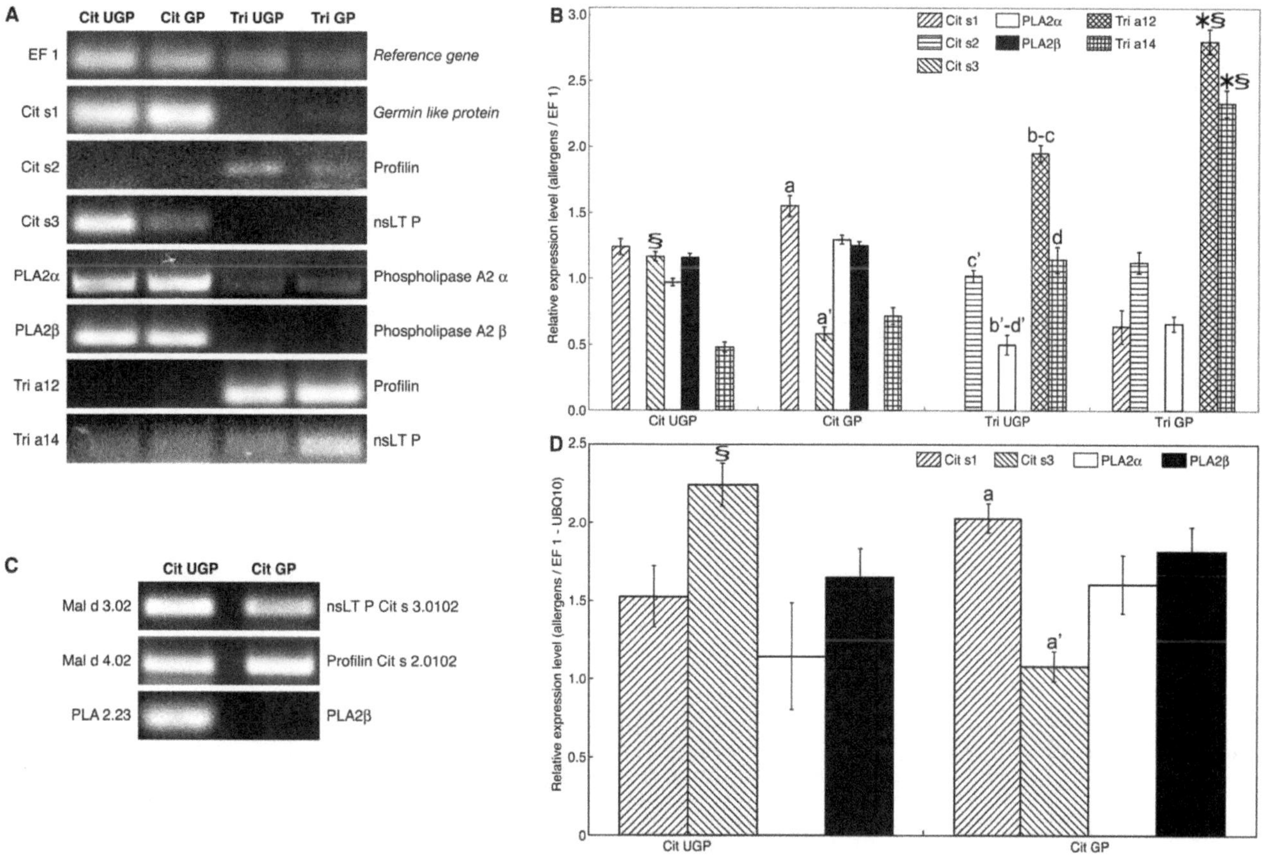

Figure 1. Allergens and phospholipase expression analysis in *Citrus clementine* and *Triticum aestivum* pollens. The cDNAs obtained from mRNA of *Citrus c.* (Cit) and *Triticum a.* (Tri) pollens ungerminated (UGP) and germinated (GP) have been tested for the different allergens (Cit s 1, Cit s 2, Cit s 3, Tri a 12 and Tri a 14) and phospholipase isoforms (PLA2 α and PLA2 β) through semi-quantitative RT-PCR after 40 cycles. EF-1 expression was used as reference gene (**A**). Lanes: *Citrus clementine* pollen ungerminated: Cit UGP; *Citrus clementine* pollen germinated: Cit GP; *Triticum aestivum* pollen ungerminated: Tri UGP; *Triticum aestivum* pollen germinated: Tri GP. Densitometries of the PCR bands revealed through semi-quantitative RT-PCR (**B**). Data are expressed as allergen/reference gene ratio ± SD. EF-1 expression was used as reference gene. The cDNAs of *Citrus clementine* UGP and GP have been tested for two different apple allergens (Mal d 3.02 and Mal d 4.02), and one isoform of apple secretory phospholipase (PLA 2.23) through semi-quantitative RT-PCR after 40 cycles (**C**). Logarithmic histogram (LOG10) of the expression levels of the different allergens (Cit s 1, Cit s 2, Cit s 3) and phospholipase isoforms (PLA2 α and PLA2 β) obtained through qRT-PCR in samples of *Citrus c.* pollen (Cit UGP and Cit GP) after 40 cycles of reaction (**D**). Data were calculated on the basis of the quantitative-comparative Ct (ΔΔCt) method normalized to the geometric mean of two housekeeping genes (EF-1 and UBQ 10), chosen according to the geNorm software. Values are the mean (n = 9) ± SD. Different letters (a–a', b–b', c–c', d–d') indicate means that are significantly different in allergens pairwise comparison (between bars marked by the same letter, i.e. a and a', b and b' etc.); * Statistical significance compared different allergens in the same sample (Tri GP); § Statistical significance compared the same allergen among the different samples ($p \leq 0.05$ with the Student's *t*-test [two-tailed distribution, two-sample equal variance]).

on a single peptide (http://www.codexalimenatarius.net) [32]. On these basis and according to the data reported both in literature [12,33,34] and in the clinical results section about cross-allergenicity, we performed a bioinformatics approach based on the ClustalΩ multiple sequence alignments to find sequence homologies among the three main allergens in *Citrus sinensis* (Cit s 1, Cit s 2 and Cit s 3) and the same class of proteins, that may be present in the well known allergenic plant species considered in the clinical trials (i.e. *Triticum aestivum, Phleum pratense, Cynodon dactylon, Betula pendula, Artemisia vulgaris, Parietaria judaica, Malus domestica, Corylus avellana, Olea europaea, Arachis hypogaea*). As reported in Figure 2B, profilin proteins were the most conserved and with the highest identity percentage values (70–90%); on the contrary, nsLTP sequence identity values were lower in the range between 23% Cit s 3 *vs Parietaria judaica* to 69% Cit s 3 *vs Malus domestica*; as regards GLP, the identity values didn't exceed the percentages of 35% to consider them cross-allergens (it was in the range 12–32%).

Discussion

Pollen allergens studies and sensitization patients' analysis to plant allergens describe a picture in which allergies to citrus fruit and cross-allergies with other pollen/fruit proteins could play an important role in the insurgence of sensitization and/or allergy reactions.

The allergy to citrus fruits is not clinically relevant as other foods and pollens (www.foodallergyitalia.org), even if some early studies suggested oranges being an important allergenic food [9,10,12,35]. This is possibly due to the fact that a very high percentage of sensitization to citrus is not accompanied by clinical reactivity to these fruit, because only one third of self-reported reactions were confirmed by oral provocations [12]; it is also evident that clinical orange allergy exists and confirmed by challenge tests [10,15].

As in literature few data are reported about allergy to citrus fruits, above all in paediatric population, the aim of this study was to investigate this topic in a population of children and young

A

Poaceae **PROFILIN**	Identity (%) PROF_WHEAT	PROF_PHLPR	PROF_CYNDA
PROF_WHEAT	89 - 98	76 - 80	77 - 79
PROF_PHLPR	76 - 80	96 - 99	82
PROF_CYNDA	77 - 79	82	100

B

GLP	Identity (%)	PROFILIN	Identity (%)	nsLTP	Identity (%)
GLP_CITSI	100	PROF_CITSI	100	NLTP_CITSI	100
GER_WHEAT	20 - 32	PROF_WHEAT	75 - 76	NLTP_WHEAT	36 - 47
GLP_BETPN	12 - 18	PROF_PHLPR	70 - 73	NLTP_ARTVU	43 - 54
		PROF_CYNDA	78	NLTP_PARJU	23 - 27
		PROF_ARTVU	71 - 72	NLTP_OLEEU	55
		PROF_BETPN	74 - 75	NLTP_ARAHY	61
		PROF_PARJU	74	NLTP_MALDO	69
		PROF_OLEEU	79 - 80	NLTP_CORAV	59
		PROF_ARAHY	73 - 78		
		PROF_MALDO	75 - 91		
		PROF_CORAV	76 - 81		

Figure 2. ClustalΩ multiple sequence alignments of allergen sequences annotated in UniProtKB database. Identity degree values expressed as multiple sequence alignment percentages of *Triticum aestivum* (PROF_WHEAT, Uniprot ID P49232-34, B6EF35), *Phleum pratense* (PROF_PHLPR, Uniprot ID P35079, O24650, O24282) and *Cynodon dactylon* (PROF_CYNDA, Uniprot ID O04725) profilin proteins (**A**). Identity percentages obtained from *Citrus sinensis* Cit s 1 (GLP), Cit s 2 (PROFILIN) and Cit s 3 (nsLTP) multiple sequence alignments (**B**). First column: *Citrus sinensis* GLP (GLP_CITSI, Uniprot ID P84159) with those for *Triticum aestivum* (GER_WHEAT, Uniprot ID P15290, B9VR55, C3UZE8, P26759, Q9SM34, Q9LD27, Q70PK0) and *Betula pendula* (GLP_BETPN, Uniprot ID P85352-54, P85336). Second column: *Citrus sinensis* PROFILIN (PROF_CITSI, Uniprot ID P84177) with those of *Triticum aestivum* (PROF_WHEAT, Uniprot ID P49232-34, B6EF35), *Phleum pratense* (PROF_PHLPR, Uniprot ID P35079, O24650, O24282), *Cynodon dactylon* (PROF_CYNDA, Uniprot ID O04725), *Artemisia vulgaris* (PROF_ARTVU, Uniprot ID Q8H2C8-9), *Betula pendula* (PROF_BETPN, Uniprot ID A4K9Z8, P25816), *Parietaria judaica* (PROF_PARJU, Uniprot ID Q9XG85, Q9T0M8), *Olea europaea* (PROF_OLEEU, Uniprot ID O24169-71), *Arachis hypogaea* (PROF_ARAHY, Uniprot ID Q9SQI9, Q5XXQ5, D3K177), *Malus domestica* (PROF_MALDO, Uniprot ID Q9XF40-42), *Corylus avellana* (PROF_CORAV, Uniprot ID A4KA40-45, Q9AXH4-5). Third column: *Citrus sinensis* nsLTP (NLTP_CITSI, Uniprot ID Q8L5S8, Q6EV47) with those of *Triticum aestivum* (NLTP_WHEAT, Uniprot ID Q5NE27-31, Q2PCB0, Q2PCB7-8, Q2PCD1-2, Q84N29), *Artemisia vulgaris* (NLTP_ARTVU, Uniprot ID P0C088, C4MGH0-2, C4MGG9), *Parietaria judaica* (NLTP_PARJU, Uniprot ID P43217, P55958, O04403-4, Q40905), *Olea europaea* (NLTP_OLEEU, Uniprot ID B2BGS3), *Arachis hypogaea* (NLTP_ARAHY, Uniprot ID B6CEX8, B6CG41), *Malus domestica* (NLTP_MALDO, Uniprot ID Q5GLH0, Q9M5X7, Q5J026), *Corylus avellana* (NLTP_CORAV, Uniprot ID Q9ATH2). Data are presented as range of percentage identity values as it has been considered all the allergen isoforms annotated and reviewed in UniProtKB database.

adults with pollinosis. Interestingly, we found a relevant percentage of sensitisation (39%) to citrus fruits in the population of pollen allergic patients recruited. Moreover, three out of the 72 pollen allergic patients (4%) presented adverse reactions after the ingestion of orange (2 patients) and clementine (1 patient) and in all of them the IgE- mediated mechanism has been confirmed by the positive response to the PPT with the fresh citrus fruit pulp. In a previous study, Kumar et al. [36] described a lower percentage (9.2%) of citrus fruit sensitization in 216 Indian children and adults affected from asthma. Asero et al. [37] reported that out of 200 children and adults with pollen allergy, 7 (3.5%) presented adverse reactions to a citrus fruit (orange, tangerine) with a similar percentage obtained also for the present study. Moreover, the present data reported that 2 out of 3 citrus allergic patients presented systemic reactions (urticaria, gastrointestinal symptoms) and 1 patient OAS after the ingestion of citrus fruits. The 2 patients with the generalized clinical symptoms showed high level of sIgE for the rPhl p12 and rPru p 3, homolog to the two orange allergens Cit s 2 and Cit s 3 respectively, emphasizing a direct correlation between sensitization/specific antibodies levels and the allergenic symptomatology. In particular, profilin are mainly involved in local symptoms (i.e. OAS) [15] contrary to systemic symptomatology mainly due to a sensitization towards nsLTPs, as highlighted by our clinical data.

The other patient with OAS has clear skin sensitization but not significant positivity to profilins and nsLTPs: probably other allergenic molecules are implied for such symptoms.

As suggested from previous works [38,39], patients allergic to pollen may present different kinds of symptoms after eating several plant foods due to the cross-reactivity of pollen allergen specific IgE that reacts with homologous plant food proteins. Examples for such cross-reactive allergens are profilins as Phl p 12 or Bet v 2, which are recognised by IgE from 10% to 20% of pollen-allergic patients [40] and cause IgE cross-reactivity among botanically unrelated pollen and between pollen and food [41,42]. In a previous study [15] about the evaluation of different pattern of allergen recognition in 6 orange allergic children, all the patients with isolated OAS presented sensitization to a profilin (Bet v 2), and the 2 patients with systemic reactions (general discomfort, urticaria) were Bet v 2 negative. In contrast, in the present study the patients recruited with generalized symptoms were all Bet v 2 positive and the one with OAS resulted Bet v 2 negative.

Moreover all patients who presented a positive PPT reactions to citrus fruit, included the three patients with citrus fruit allergy, presented a positive response to SPT with grass pollen extract and/or the presence of sIgE against *Phleum p.*, which belongs as *Triticum a.* to *poaceae* family. The presence of cross-reactivity between grass and citrus pollen has been described even by El-Qutob Lòpez et al. [43], who reported a case of systemic reaction (urticaria and angioedema) after ingestion of orange blossom pollen in a woman sensitized to several pollens included the grass one. In conclusion the present clinical data confirm a relevant prevalence of citrus fruit sensitization and show that orange and clementine allergy is not a so rare condition in pollen sensitized patients.

The molecular characterization of citrus pollen and cross-allergenicity was aimed to verify whether some important citrus allergen genes (Cit s 1, Cit s 2 and Cit s 3), known to be expressed in the fruit and to provoke allergic reactions after ingestion [12] were also expressed in pollen.

In the international allergen database (http://www.allergen.org/index.php) a single GLP, a single profilin and two nsLTPs were listed as allergens in sweet orange (*Citrus sinensis*). We demonstrated the expression of these allergens also in *Citrus clementine* pollen and in particular, Cit s 1 and Cit s 3 represent the two allergens commonly expressed in fruit and pollen, whereas Cit s 2 is present in citrus fruit and not detectable in citrus pollen. Hyun and Kim [44] reported the genomic identification of putative members of *Citrus c.* allergens, five different isoforms of nsLTP (Cit c 3) and three different isoforms of profilin (Cit c 2) annotated on Phytozome (http://www.phytozome.net/) and the Citrus Genome Database (http://www.citrusgenomedb.org/); the molecular data presented in this study demonstrated the presence of a GLP also in clementine pollen.

About profilin, when the RT-PCR was performed with the primers for a profilin isoform of *Malus domestica* fruit, the *Citrus c.* pollen showed a clear band either in Cit UGP and Cit GP; however, this result was not obtained when the RT-PCR was assessed with primers specific for the *Citrus sinensis* profilin. The data could mean that the isoform of *Citrus sinensis* annotated in UniProtKB database is not present in clementine pollen. Interestingly, the Cit s 2 isoform present in citrus fruit is also present in *Triticum a.* pollen, supporting the hypothesis of a cross-sensitization between *poaceae* pollen and citrus fruits. On the other hand, the Tri a 14, the nsLTP specific of *Triticum a.* is present in citrus pollen both Cit UGP and Cit GP, emphasizing the pan-allergenic nature of nsLTPs. As *Triticum a.* profilin and nsLTP protein sequences are annotated in UniProtKB database, we verified their homology sequences among the well known species of *poaceae* family considered allergenic (i.e. *Phleum pratense* and *Cynodon dactylon*) to assessed the degree of sequences identity and the possible cross-allergenicity between citrus and grass pollens. From the bioinformatics data, we showed that profilin were the most conserved proteins and with the highest identity percentage values, whereas nsLTP sequence identity values were lower; on the contrary, GLP cannot be considered involved in the cross-allergenicity, being the identity values lower than 35%.

Interestingly, we demonstrated both through clinical data and molecular approaches that *Citrus c.* and *Malus d.* specific allergen isoforms (Mal d 3.02, an nsLTP and Mal d 4.02, a profilin) shared high percentage identity values, confirming the possible cross-allergenicity citrus/apple.

The presence of phospholipase A2 (PLA2) in pollen of *Arabidopsis thaliana* has been reported only recently [45]; although the proven involvement of plant PLA2s in many biological functions, including i.e. senescence, wounding and stress responses, relatively little is known about plant PLA2s, and their genes essentially remain uncharacterized. In *Arabidopsis t.* three of four PLA2 paralogs (PLA2 β, γ and δ) have been characterized and found to be expressed in pollen, localized to the endoplasmic reticulum and/or Golgi, and playing critical roles in pollen development and tube growth.

A novelty of the present work is the finding of the PLA2 α and β in *Citrus c.* pollen, either UGP and GP, as in fruits, as well as the presence of PLA2 α also in *Triticum a.*; being PLA2 able to generate pro-inflammatory factors as eicosanoid substances, this enzyme could represent a key factor in the inflammatory response to allergens possibly activating the inflammatory cascade. From the apple genome database (http://genomics.research.iasma.it), we found that the apple PLA2.23 is conserved also in Cit UGP as shown by the semi-quantitative RT-PCR; the sequence alignments of PLA2.23 with PLA2 β from citrus fruit showed that the two sequences are very conserved [identities = 116/150 (77%), positives = 129/150 (86%)].

In conclusion, according to the molecular analysis performed in this work, Cit s 1 and Cit s 3, but also profilin, even if a different isoform from that expressed in orange fruit, and two isoforms of PLA2 enzyme (PLA2 α and PLA2 β) were identified as important allergens and sensitizing factors in *Citrus c.* pollen UGP and GP. As consequence, data obtained support the evidences that cross-sensitization among citrus and other plant homolog allergens, could play an important role in inflammatory response to citrus proteins and emphasize that citrus allergy can be considered a relevant food related allergy in pollen sensitizing patients.

Finally, we can hypothesize that allergy to oranges can occur mainly through local symptoms (i.e OAS and erythema) unlike other food allergy, such as apple or peach, characterized with more generalized symptoms such as vomiting, diarrhea and abdominal pain. The clinical data presented support the hypothesis that a sensitization towards nsLTPs mainly cause a systemic symptomatology and the relevant high percentages (39%) of children and young adults sensitized to citrus fruits recruited for our monocentric observational study suggest that there is a risk to develop an allergenic symptomatology in the future.

Acknowledgments

We thank the project "My Darling Clementine": un prodotto salutistico nuovo e innovativo dalle clementine e dal limone di Calabria"(POR FESR 2007-2013)", Prof. Mazzucca who kindly donated pollen of *Citrus clementine* and Mr. Rondinini for the pollen of *Triticum aestivum*.

We thank Mr. N. Mele for the image elaboration.

Author Contributions

Conceived and designed the experiments: SDD GR AP. Performed the experiments: RI CP EC ML FS. Analyzed the data: SDD RI GR AP. Contributed reagents/materials/analysis tools: SDD GR AP. Wrote the paper: SDD RI GR CP EC. Designed the pollen molecular investigation: SDD. Designed the clinical investigation: GR AP. Performed the molecular biology experiments: RI. Performed the clinical observational studies: CP EC. Performed the immunological tests of sera against Phl p12: ML FS.

References

1. Knekt P, Isotupa S, Rissanen H, Heliövaara M, Järvinen R, et al. (2000) Quercetin intake and the incidence of cerebrovascular disease. Eur J Clin Nutr 54: 415–417.
2. Le Marchand L, Murphy SP, Hankin JH, Wilkens LR, Kolonel LN (2000) Intake of flavonoids and lung cancer. J Natl Cancer Inst 92: 154–160.
3. D'Amato G, Cecchi L, D'Amato M, Liccardi G (2010) Urban air pollution and climate change as environmental risk factors of respiratory allergy: an update. J Investig Allergol Clin Immunol 20: 95–102.
4. Sampson HA (1999) Food allergy. Part 1: Immunopathogenesis and clinical disorders. J Allergy Clin Immun 103: 717–728.
5. Sampson HA (2004) Update on food allergy. J Allergy Clin Immun 113: 805–819.
6. Bolhaar ST, van de Weg WE, van Ree R, Gonzalez-Mancebo E, Zuidmee L, et al. (2005) In vivo assessment with prick-to-prick testing and double-blind, placebo-controlled food challenge of allergenicity of apple cultivars. J Allergy Clin Immun 116: 1080–1086.
7. Mills EN, Mackie AR, Burney P, Beyer K, Frewer L, et al. (2007) The prevalence, cost and basis of food allergy across Europe. Allergy 62: 717–722.
8. Marzban G, Puehringer H, Dey R, Brynda S, Ma Y, et al. (2005) Localisation and distribution of the major allergens in apple fruits. Plant Sci 169: 387–394.
9. Ahrazem O, Ibàñez MD, Lòpez-Torrejòn G, Sánchez-Monge R, Sastre J, et al. (2006) Orange Germin-Like Glycoprotein Cit s 1: An Equivocal Allergen. Int Arch Allergy Immunol 139: 96–103.
10. Lòpez-Torrejòn G, Ibàñez MD, Ahrazem O, Sánchez-Monge R, Sastre J, et al. (2005) Isolation, cloning and allergenic reactivity of natural profilin Cit s 2, a major orange allergen. Allergy 60: 1424–1429.
11. Sloan AE, Powers ME (1986) A perspective on popular perceptions of adverse reactions to food. J Allergy Clin Immun 78: 127–132.
12. Crespo JF, Retzek M, Foetish K, Sierra Maestro E, Cid-Sanchez AB, et al. (2006) Germin-like protein Cit s 1 and profilin Cit s 2 are major allergen in orange (*Citrus sinensis*) fruits. Mol Nutr Food Res 50: 282–290.
13. Adler BR, Assadullahi T, Warner JA, Warner JO (1991) Evaluation of a multiple food specific IgE antibody test compared to parental perception, allergy skin tests and RAST. Clin Exp Allergy 21: 683–688.
14. Ortolani C, Ispano M, Pastorello EA, Ansaloni R, Magri GC (1989) Comparison of results of skin prick tests (with fresh foods and commercial food extracts) and RAST in 100 patients with oral allergy syndrome. J Allergy Clin Immunl 83: 683–690.
15. Ibañez MD, Sastre J, Martinez SAN Ireneo M, Laso MT, et al. (2004) Differents patterns of allergen recognition in children allergic to orange. J Allergy Clin Immun 113: 175–177.
16. Pignataro V, Canton C, Spadafora A, Mazzuca S (2010) Proteome from lemon fruit flavedo reveals that this tissue produces high amounts of the Cit s1 germin-like isoforms. J Agric Food Chem 58: 7239–7244.
17. Krishnan K, Moens PDJ (2009) Structure and functions of profilins. Biophys Rev 1: 71–81.
18. Enrique E, Alonso R, Bartolome B, San Miguel-Moncin M, Bartra J, et al. (2004) IgE reactivity to profilin in Platanus acerifolia pollen-sensitized subjects with plant-derived food allergy J Investig Allergol Clin Immunol 14: 335 – 342.
19. Ahrazem O, Ibanez MD, Lopez-Torrejon G, Sanchez- Monge R, Sastre J, et al. (2005) Lipid transfer proteins and allergy to oranges. Int Arch Allergy Immunol 137: 201–210.
20. Kader JC (1996) Lipid-transfer proteins in plants. Annu Rev Plant Physiol Plant Mol Biol 47: 627–654.
21. Botton A, Begheldo M, Rasori A, Bonghi C, Tonutti P (2002) Differential expression of two lipid transfer protein genes in reproductive organs of peach (Prunus persica L. Batsch). Plant Sci 163: 993–1000.
22. Iorio RA, Di Sandro A, Paris R, Pagliarani G, Tartarini S, et al. (2012) Simulated environmental criticalities affect transglutaminase of *Malus* and *Corylus* pollens having different allergenic potential. Amino Acids 42: 1007–1024.
23. Behrendt H, Kasche A, Ebner von Eschenbach C, Risse U, Huss-Marp J, et al. (2001) Secretion of proinflammatory eicosanoid-like substances precedes allergen release from pollen grains in the initiation of allergic sensitization. Int Arch Allergy Immunol 124: 121–125.
24. Gunawan H, Takai T, Kamijo S, Wang XL, Ikeda S, et al. (2008) Characterization of proteases, proteins, and eicosanoid-like substances in soluble extracts from allergenic pollen grains. Int Arch Allergy Immunol 147: 276–288.
25. Bagni N, Adamo P, Serafini-Fracassini D, Villanueva VR (1981) RNA, proteins and polyamines during tube growth in germinating apple pollen. Plant Physiol 68: 727–730.
26. Wilkins TA, Smart LB (1996) Isolation of RNA from plant tissue – A laboratory guide to RNA: isolation, analysis, and synthesis. In: Krieg PA, editor. New York: Wiley-Liss. 21–42.
27. Paris R, Cova V, Pagliarani G, Tartarini S, Komjanc M, et al. (2009) Expression profiling in *HcrVf2*-transformed apple plants in response to *Venturia inaequalis*. Tree Genetics & Genomes 5: 81–91.
28. Vandesompele J, De Preter K, Pattyn F, Poppe B, Van Roy N, et al. (2002) Accurate normalization of real-time quantitative RT-PCR by geometric averaging of multiple internal control genes. Genome Biol 3: RESEARCH0034.
29. Yan J, Yuan F, Long G, Qin L, Deng Z (2012) Selection of reference genes for quantitative real-time PCR analysis in citrus. Mol Biol Rep 39: 1831–1838.
30. Ramakers C, Ruijter JM, Deprez RH, Moorman AF (2003) Assumption-free analysis of quantitative real-time polymerase chain reaction (PCR) data. Neurosci Lett 339: 62–66.
31. Livak KJ, Schmittgen TD (2001) Analysis of relative gene expression data using real-time quantitative PCR and the 2-ΔΔCT method. Methods 25: 402–408.
32. Garcia BE, Lizaso MT (2011) Cross-reactivity Syndromes in Food Allergy. J Investig Allergol Clin Immunol 21: 162–170.
33. Eriksson NE, Werner S, Foucard T, Möller C, Berg T, et al. (2003) Self-reported hypersensitivity to exotic fruit in birch pollen-allergic patients. Allergol Int 52: 199–206.
34. Glaspole IN, de Leon MP, Rolland JM, O'Hehir R (2007) Anaphylaxis to lemon soap: citrus seed and peanut allergen cross-reactivity. Ann Allergy Asthma Immunol 98: 286–289.
35. Ebo DG, Ahrazem O, Lopez-Torrejon G, Bridts CH, Salcedo G, et al. (2007) Anaphylaxis from mandarin (Citrus reticulata): identification of potential responsible allergens. Int Arch Allergy Immunol 144: 39–41.
36. Kumar R, Singh BP, Srivastava P, Sridhara S, Arora N, et al. (2006) Relevance of serum IgE estimation in allergic bronchial asthma with special reference to food allergy. Asian Pac J Allergy Immunol 24: 191–199.
37. Asero R, Monsalve R, Barber D (2008) Profilin sensitization detected in the office by skin prick test: a study of prevalence and clinical relevance of profilin as a plant food allergen. Clin Exp Allergy 38: 1033–1037.
38. Ricci G, Righetti F, Menna G, Bellini F, Miniaci A, et al. (2005) Relationship between Bet v 1 and Bet v 2 specific IgE and food allergy in children with grass pollen respiratory allergy. Mol Immunol 42: 1251–1257.
39. Bohle B (2007) The impact of pollen-related food allergens on pollen allergy. Allergy 63: 3–10.
40. Radauer C, Hoffmann-Sommergruber K (2004) Profilins. Plant food allergens. In: Mills ENC, Shewry PR, editors. Oxford: Blackwell Publishing. 105–124.
41. Mari A (2001) Multiple pollen sensitization: a molecular approach to the diagnosis. Int Arch Allergy Immunol 125: 57–65.
42. van Ree R, Voitenko V, van Leeuwen WA, Aalberse RC (1992) Profilin is a cross-reactive allergen in pollen and vegetable foods. Int Arch Allergy Immunol 98: 97–104.
43. El-Qutob López D, Morales Rubio C, Cervera Aznar R, Pelaez Hernández A (2006) Allergic reaction after ingestion of orange blossom pollen. J Investig Allergol Clin Immunol 16: 140–141.
44. Hyun KT, Kim J (2011) Genomic identification of putative allergen genes in woodland strawberry (*Fragaria vesca*) and mandarin orange (*Citrus clementina*). Plant Omics J 4: 428–434.
45. Kim HJ, Ok SH, Bahn SC, Jang J, Oh SA, et al. (2011) Endoplasmic Reticulum– and Golgi-Localized Phospholipase A2 Plays Critical Roles in Arabidopsis Pollen Development and Germination. The Plant Cell 23: 94–110.

7

In silico Identification of IgE-Binding Epitopes of Osmotin Protein

Prerna Sharma[1], Shailendra Nath Gaur[2], Naveen Arora[1]*

1 Allergy and Immunology Section, CSIR-Institute of Genomics and Integrative Biology, Delhi, India, 2 Department of Respiratory Medicine, Vallabhbhai Patel Chest Institute, University of Delhi, Delhi, India

Abstract

The identification of B-cell epitopes is an important step to study the antigen- antibody interactions for diagnosis and therapy. The present study aimed to identify B- cell epitopes of osmotin using bioinformatic tools and further modify these regions to study the allergenic property. B-cell epitopes were predicted based on amino acid physicochemical properties. Three single point mutations M1, M2, and M3 and a multiple point mutant (M123) were selected to disrupt the IgE binding. These mutants were cloned, expressed and proteins purified to homogeneity. The IgE binding of the purified proteins was evaluated by ELISA and ELISA inhibition with patients' sera. Three regions of osmotin M1 (57–70 aa), M2 (72–85 aa) and M3 (147–165 aa) were identified as potential antibody recognition sites using *in silico* tools. The sequence similarity search of the predicted epitopes of osmotin using Structural Database of Allergenic proteins (SDAP) showed similarity with known allergens from tomato, kiwifruit, bell pepper, apple, mountain cedar and cypress. Mutants M1, M2 and M3 showed up to 72%, 60% and 76% reduction, respectively in IgE binding whereas M123 showed up to 90% reduction with patients' sera. The immunoblot of M123 mutant showed 40% reduction in spot density as compared to osmotin. All mutants showed decreased inhibition potency with M123 exhibiting lowest potency of 32% with osmotin positive pooled patients' sera. The three B- cell epitopes of osmotin predicted by *in silico* method correlated with the experimental approach. The mutant M123 showed a reduction of 90% in IgE binding. The present method may be employed for prediction of B- cell epitopes of allergenic proteins.

Editor: Christian Schönbach, Kyushu Institute of Technology, Japan

Funding: The work covered in this manuscript was funded by the Council for Scientific and Industrial Reasearch (CSIR). The URL for the funder's website is "http://rdpp.csir.res.in/csir_acsir/Home. aspx". The funders had no role in study design, data collection and analysis, decision to publish, or preparation of the manuscript.

Competing Interests: The authors have declared that no competing interests exist.

* E-mail: naveen@igib.res.in

Introduction

The prevalence of food allergy is increasing worldwide and as many as 8% of children and 2% of adults are affected in western countries [1]. Primary treatment of food allergy is strict avoidance of the diets containing food allergens. Recently new strategies have been designed to reduce allergic reactions [2]. Specific immunotherapy is not used to treat food allergies because of the risk of severe side effects, including anaphylactic shock [3]. Several studies have shown the development of hypoallergenic molecules with reduced or no allergenic potential, which may be useful for specific immunotherapy [4], [5].

The knowledge of the B-cell epitopes can be applied in diagnosis, therapy or development of effective vaccines for immunotherapy [6]. In case of food allergens, digestion/heating may lead to loss of the structure of the protein thereby rendering the conformational epitopes inactive. Thus sequential epitopes play an important role for diagnosis of food allergy. Moreover, it is difficult to study the conformational epitopes of allergens as considerable efforts are required for validation [7]. Epitopes can be identified by many methods but computational tools provide a promising and rapid alternative [8]. These epitopes may be modified to reduce allergenicity of an allergen. These variants can be produced by disruption of IgE binding epitopes either by chemical modification [5] or genetic engineering [9]. The key requirement is to identify IgE-binding epitopes on food allergens. The recombinant allergens have similar structure and immunologic properties as that of native counterparts, hence these can be modified to reduce the allergenicity while maintaining important immunologic properties [10]. Earlier studies on recombinant food allergens have demonstrated reduced allergenicity of shrimp [4], peanut allergen [11], apple [12], olive [13], etc.

Osmotin is a stress-responsive multifunctional protein from tobacco (*Nicotiana tabacum*). It accumulates in cells on osmotic stress adaptation and provides osmotolerance to plants [14]. It belongs to pathogenesis related-5 (PR-5) protein family and exhibits antifungal activity as it permeabilizes the plasma membrane and dissipates the membrane pH gradient of the fungal species [15]. These two properties of osmotin have been exploited for developing transgenic crops such as tobacco [16], strawberry [17], wheat [18], cotton [19], tomato [20], and mulberry [21]. In our previous study we had identified osmotin as a potential allergen using bioinformatic and immunobiochemical methods [22]. In the present study we identified sequential epitopes of osmotin by *in silico* approach. The potential IgE binding residues in these epitopes were mutated to reduce allergenicity of osmotin.

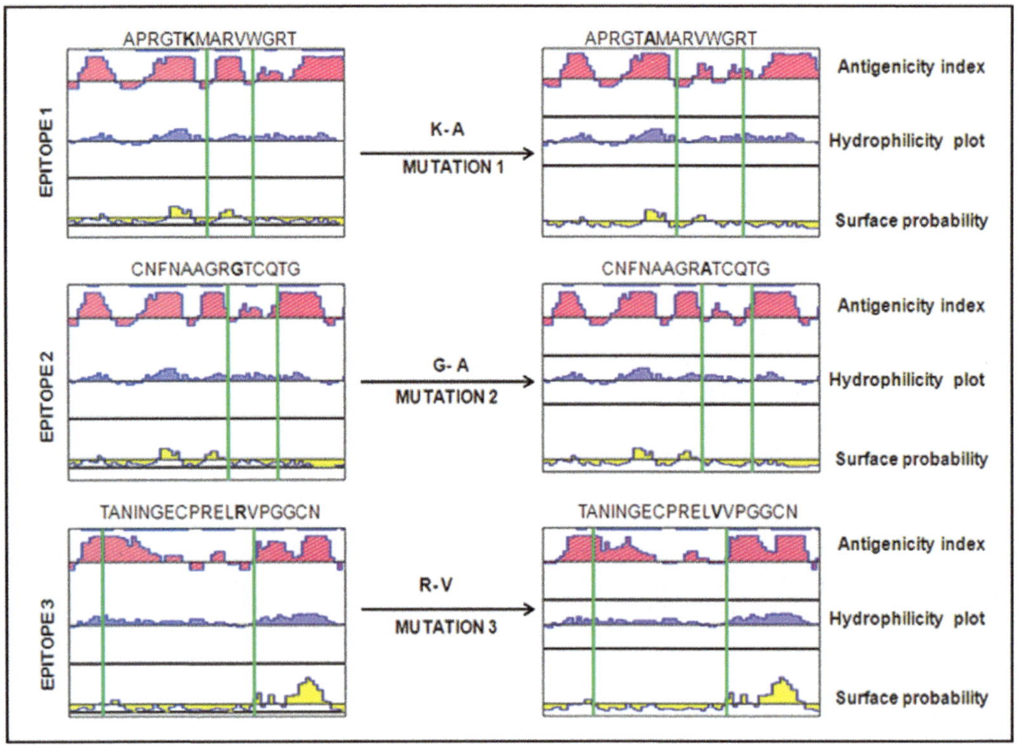

Figure 1. Comparative analysis of antigenic index of osmotin epitopes and its mutants by DNAstar protean system. The region between vertical lines show the three regions mutated by site directed mutagenesis. Mutation in epitope regions shows reduction in antigenic index in DNAstar program.

Materials and Methods

Ethics statement

The study protocol was approved by human ethics committee of the Institute of Genomics and Integrative Biology, Delhi. Informed written consent was obtained from the patients and healthy subjects that participated in the study. The study did not involve any minors/children.

B-cell epitope prediction

B-cell epitopes are classified as either continuous or discontinuous. A number of algorithms have been developed for predicting the continuous B-cell epitopes based on physico-chemical properties like hydrophilicity (Parker method), flexibility (Karplus and Schulz method), accessibility (Emini method) and turns (Pellequer method) [23]. The prediction methods of the linear or continuous epitopes have improved over the years. The linear B- cell epitopes were predicted by different servers namely, BcePred (based on a combination of physico-chemical properties), BepiPred 1.0b (based on hydorophilicity scale with a Hidden Markov Model), ABCpred (uses artificial neural networks), and BCPred (uses support vector machine) [23]. DNASTAR Lasergene version 7.2. (DNASTAR Inc., Madison, WI, USA) was also used which uses amino acid propensity scales of Hopp -Woods (hydrophilicity), Emini (Surface probability), Jameson-Wolf (antigenic index) and Karplus-Schulz (flexibility). The epitopes identified frequently by most of the tools were selected.

Site directed mutagenesis of osmotin

Osmotin was mutated at three residues to generate three single point mutants M1, M2 and M3. A fourth mutant M123 with all three point mutations was also generated. Mutagenesis was performed using oligonucleotide primers and mutation-specific oligonucleotide primers accommodating each mutation. Internal amino acid substitution in osmotin was performed by a three step PCR reaction. The first two steps of PCR reaction was carried out with an internal mutant primer and one of the flanking primers. Final products of these two steps were purified from agarose gel, mixed and amplified using flanking primers. The fourth mutant with all three point mutations was generated step wise using mutant M2 as template. The mutation 1 was generated using forward primer 5′ATCAATGCGCCACGATTTACTAAAAAG3′ and reverse primer 5′CATTTTAGTAAATCGTGGCGCATTG3′, mutant 2 was generated using forward primer 5′ATGCTGCTGGTAGGTTTACGTGCCAA3′ and reverse primer 5′TTTGGCACGTAAA CCTACCAGCAGCA3′, mutant 3 using forward primer 5′ACGGCTAATATATTCGGCGAATGTCC3′ and reverse primer 5′GGACATTCGCCGAATATATTAGCCGTAC3′ and the flanking primers 5′GAATTGAATTCGATGGGCAACTTGAGATCTTCTTTTG3′with *EcoR I* site and 5′GCTCGAG CTCCTTAGCCACTTCATCACTTCCAG 3′ with *Xho I* site. The PCR products were digested with *EcoRI* and *XhoI* enzymes, subcloned in pET22b+ vector and sequenced to confirm the mutations. Constructs containing the mutations in the epitopes were used for the expression of fully modified recombinant osmotin protein mutants.

Expression and purification of mutants

The constructs of M1, M2, M3 and M123 mutant sequences in pET22b+ vector were transformed into BL-21 *Escherichia coli* cells. The cells were grown till 0.6 O.D., induced with 1 mM isopropyl-beta-D-thiogalactopyranoside for 3 h, harvested and the pellet was suspended in binding buffer containing 50 mM NaH_2PO_4, 300 mM NaCl, 10 mM imidazole (pH 8.0), sonicated and centrifuged. The supernatant was incubated for 2 h with 2 ml Ni-NTA equilibrated with binding buffer. The column was washed with buffer containing 20 mM imidazole, 300 mM NaCl and 50 Mm NaH_2PO_4 (pH 8.0) and bound proteins were eluted using buffer containing 250 mM imidazole, 300 mM NaCl and 50 mM NaH_2PO_4. The purified mutant proteins were resolved on 12% SDS-PAGE, transferred to nitrocellulose membrane and probed with osmotin positive patients' pooled sera. Densitometry of the immunoblot was performed by Gene Tools software from SynGene (Synoptics Ltd, Cambridge, UK).

Circular dichroism (CD) spectroscopy

Osmotin protein and its mutant M123 were dialyzed against 10 mM KH_2PO_4/K_2HPO_4 buffer (pH 7.4). Circular dichroism spectroscopy was performed on a J-815 S spectropolarimeter (Jasco) with constant nitrogen flushing at 25°C. Wavelength was analysed with a step width of 0.2 nm and a band width of 1 nm. The spectral range was 200–240 nm at a scan speed of 50 nm/min. The final spectra were corrected by subtracting the corresponding baseline spectrum obtained under identical conditions. Average of three scans was taken and the mean residue molar ellipticity was calculated.

Sera collection

The patients of allergic rhinitis and asthma aged 15–50 years were skin prick tested with various aeroallergens and food extracts to detect sensitization. The guidelines of the American Thoracic Society were followed for diagnosis of asthma [24]. The patients having any two of the symptoms, viz. sneezing, rhinorrhea, nasal blockage, postnasal drip, etc. for most of the time since the last two years were diagnosed as rhinitis. Blood samples were collected from patients showing marked positive skin reactions to different food extracts and healthy subjects at the outpatient department, V.P. Chest Institute, Delhi, a referral chest hospital.

Specific IgE estimation

Specific IgE binding for the mutants and osmotin protein was determined by ELISA. Briefly the proteins were incubated in carbonate buffer overnight at 4°C in a microtitre plate (Nunc, Roskilde, Denmark). After washing with PBS– Tween 20 (0.05%), the nonspecific sites were blocked with 3% defatted milk for 3 h at 37°C. The plate was washed again and incubated with 100 µl diluted (1:10 v/v) sera of food allergic patients which were positive to osmotin, overnight at 4°C. Normal human sera (n = 4) were used as negative control. The plate was washed and incubated with antihuman IgE-horse radish peroxidase (1:1000 v/v, Sigma) for 3 h at 37°C. The plate was washed with PBS- Tween 20 and followed by PBS and colour was developed with orthophenylene diamine in citrate – phosphate buffer, pH 5.0. The reaction was stopped after 30 min by adding 5 N H_2SO_4 and the absorbance was read at 492 nm.

ELISA inhibition

ELISA inhibition with the mutants was performed to determine the allergenic potency and relative ability of the mutants for IgE binding. The microtitre plate was coated with purified osmotin protein and blocked with 3% defatted milk. Further it was incubated with pre- incubated mixture of 1:10 v/v osmotin positive pooled patients' sera (n = 5) and graded amounts of

Table 1. Peptide similarity search of the three predicted epitopes of osmotin with known allergens in SDAP database.

S. No.	Predicted osmotin Epitopes	Allergen	*PD* Sequence Similarity Index	Matching region
1	APRGTKMARVWGRT	Lyc e NP24	0.39	**APRGTKMAR**i**WGRT**
		Cap a 1	2.01	**AP**p**GTKMAR**i**WGRT**
		Cap a 1w	3.47	**AP**p**GT**a**MAR**i**WGRT**
		Act c 2	7.31	pgag**TK**g**ARVW**p**RT**
2	CNFNAAGRGTCQTG	Lyc e NP24	0.00	**CNFNAAGRGTCQTG**
		Act c 2	2.92	**CNF**dg**AGRG**k**CQTG**
		Jun a 3	3.26	**C**t**F**d**A**s**G**k**G**s**CQTG**
		Cap a 1	3.39	**CNF**dg**AGRG**w**CQTG**
		Cup s 3.0101	4.34	**C**t**F**d**A**s**G**g**G**s**C**rs**G**
		Cup a 3	4.34	**C**t**F**d**A**s**G**k**G**s**C**rs**G**
		Mus a 4.0101	4.49	CSFDGSGRGRCQTG
		Mal d 2	7.08	**C**std**AAG**kft**C**e**T**a
3	TANINGECPRELRVPGGCN	Lyc e NP24	1.21	**TANINGECPR**a**L**k**VPGGCN**
		Cap a 1w	2.42	**TANINGECP**gs**LRVPGGCN**
		Act c 2	2.46	**TA**d**ING**q**CP**n**ELR**a**PGGCN**
		Cap a 1	3.24	v**ANINGECP**gs**LRVPGGCN**
		Mus a 4.0101	5.07	aad**ING**q**CP**ga**L**ka**PGGCN**
		Cup a 3	5.73	kad**IN**av**CP**s**EL**k**V**d**GGCN**
		Jun a 3	5.79	kad**IN**av**CP**s**EL**k**V**d**GGCN**

The table shows similarity of the predicted B- cell epitopes of osmotin with peptides of known allergens with a PD value less than 8.5 in SDAP database. Matching amino acids are depicted in bold and upper case. Unmatched amino acids in lower case.

osmotin and each of the purified mutants i.e. 0.1, 1, 10, 100 and 1000 ng as inhibitor. Sera of non-allergic subjects were used as control. The remaining steps were the same as followed for ELISA. Inhibition was presented as percentage decrease in absorbance of sample with inhibitor to that of sample without inhibitor and allergenic potency was defined by establishing the concentration of protein required for 50% inhibition.

Statistical analysis

Statistical analysis of results was done by using GraphPad Prism and GraphPad Instat software (GraphPad Software, San Diego, CA, USA). The statistically significant difference was determined using one way ANOVA followed by Bonferroni comparison test between osmotin and the mutant M123 challenged mice groups. The p value <0.05 was considered as significant.

Results

Mapping of IgE-binding epitopes

IgE binding regions were identified by sequence based tools which fall in common regions of the sequence map. Three stretches of amino acids 57–70, 72–85 and 147–165 recognized by at least four tools were predicted as B- cell epitopes. Residues 60 (Gly → Phe), 80 (Gly → Phe) and 151(Asn → Phe) in each epitope were selected for substitution mutation. These epitopes on mutation using *in silico* approach showed reduction in the antigenic index in DNAstar program (Fig. 1). In Structural Database of Allergenic Proteins (SDAP; 737 sequences; http://fermi.utmb.edu/SDAP/), these epitopes showed similarity with tomato allergen Lyc (NP24), kiwi fruit allergen (Act c 2), cypress allergen (Cup s 3.0102), bell pepper allergen (Cap a 1), apple allergen (Mal d 2) and mountain cedar allergen (Jun a 3) with a *PD* (property distance) value of less than 8.5 (Table 1).

Expression and purification of the mutants

Four osmotin mutants M1, M2, M3 and M123 proteins were expressed in *E. coli* and purified as His-tag proteins. The yield obtained of these proteins were 2.5 mg/L, 2 mg/L, 2 mg/L, 3 mg/L of the culture. The protein expression in the culture after induction at 1h, 2 h and 3 h with IPTG was visualized by SDS-PAGE (Fig. 2). The purified recombinant proteins were resolved on SDS-PAGE (Fig. 3a) and reacted with osmotin positive pooled patients' sera on immunoblot (Fig. 3b). The intensity of spots on the blot was measured by densitometric scan and osmotin was set as a reference point. The mutant M123 showed 40% reduction in the spot density followed by M1, M3 and M2 as compared to osmotin (Figure 3c).

Circular dichroism analysis of purified recombinant osmotin and mutant M123

Figure 4 shows the comparison of the osmotin protein and M123 mutant by circular dichroism analysis. The far-UV spectra showed similar characteristics. Minima were obtained at 208 nm, 218 nm and 222 nm. It shows the presence of both α- helices and β- sheets in the secondary structure of the osmotin protein. The CD spectrum of the M123 mutant was similar to osmotin indicating that the mutant has probably adopted the same folded state.

IgE binding of the mutants with osmotin positive patients' sera

IgE-binding of the four mutants was compared with that of osmotin by ELISA. The mutants showed a reduction in specific

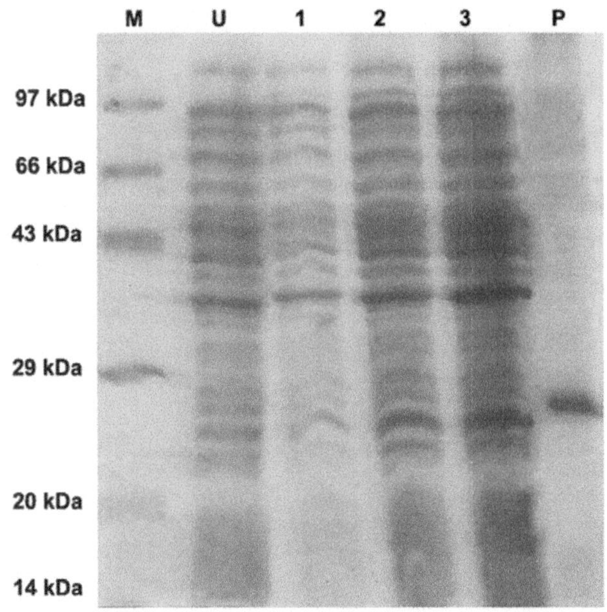

Figure 2. SDS-PAGE analysis of protein expression in culture. The uninduced and induced stages of expression of osmotin protein was resolved on 12% gel and stained with Coomassie brilliant blue. Lane M was loaded with Molecular weight marker. Lane U uninduced protein expression. Lane 1, 2, 3 shows expression after induction for 1 h, 2 h, 3 h respectively and lane P represents purified protein.

IgE binding between 25%–72% (M1), 22%–60% (M2), 43%–76% (M3) and 50%–90% (M123) as compared to osmotin (Fig. 5). All the mutants showed significant reduction in IgE binding as compared to osmotin ($p<0.001$) with mutant M123 having maximum reduction.

Potency of osmotin mutants

IgE-binding and immunoblot of the mutants were further substantiated by ELISA inhibition assay. Pooled osmotin positive patients' sera preincubated with different amounts of the four mutants were added to ELISA plate coated with osmotin. Here, wild-type osmotin gave 66% inhibition at 1000 ng of protein. In contrast, all mutants showed decreased ability to inhibit IgE binding. M1, M2, M3 and M123 reached a maximum inhibition of 39%, 53%, 43% and 32% respectively at 1000 ng/ml inhibitor concentrations. Osmotin required 4 ng of protein to reach the EC_{50}. Only M2 showed the inhibition with an EC_{50} of 500 ng whereas the other mutants did not reach the EC_{50} value (Fig. 6).

Discussion

The knowledge of epitopes is a prerequisite for understanding mechanism of antigen antibody interactions. Various methods like X-ray crystallography, enzymatic fragmentation, synthetic overlapping peptides, site-directed mutagenesis and phage display may be used to determine B- cell epitopes. However, these approaches are time consuming, exhaustive and require many experiments. Hence, we used computational methods to predict the location of B- cell epitopes. Earlier studies have shown the use of bioinformatic approach to predict eptiopes which correlated well with the experimental approach [8], [25]. In the present study, three IgE binding regions of osmotin were identified and validated by *in vitro* experiments. Further, residues in these regions were mutated to study the allergenic properties.

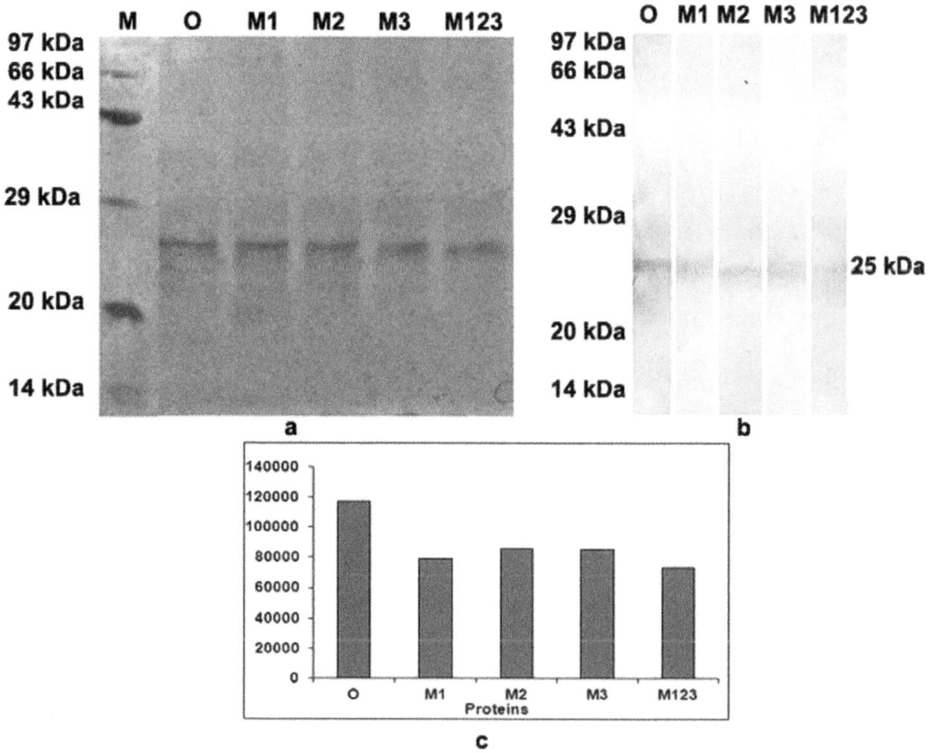

Figure 3. SDS-PAGE profile of purified osmotin and the three mutants. (a) The proteins were resolved on 12% gel and stained with Coomassie brilliant blue. (b) SDS-PAGE resolved protein was transferred on to nitrocellulose membrane and probed with osmotin positive patients' pooled sera. Lane M was loaded with Molecular weight marker. Lanes O, M1, M2, M3, M123 were loaded with osmotin and the mutants respectively. (c) Graph showing densitometric scan of spots of the blot.

Linear epitopes are more relevant as compared to conformational epitopes for food allergens as these allergens are encountered by the immune system only after they are subjected to digestion/heating [26]. Further it is difficult to validate computationally predicted epitopes except by cocrystallographic approach [7]. Conformational epitopes are preferred in case of globular allergens such as aeroallergens or food allergens involved in oral allergy syndrome [27]. It has been demonstrated that many food allergens like Ara h 1, Ara h 2, Ara h 3 [28], shrimp allergen Pen a 1 [29], hen's egg ovomucoid [30] and milk allergen [31] have linear epitopes that binds to IgE. Many algorithms have been developed to predict linear epitopes on a protein sequence based on propensity values of amino acid properties of hydrophilicity, antigenicity, segmental mobility, flexibility and accessibility [27]. In our study, we selected three linear epitopes commonly recognized by most of the sequence based tools. The three epitopes predicted comprise approximately 50% hydrophobic residues and 25% charged residues. The SDAP sequence similarity search of the predicted epitopes of osmotin showed similarity with known allergens which are members of the PR-5

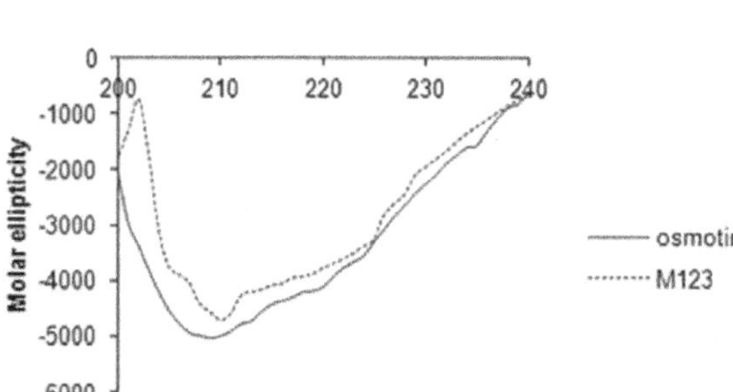

Figure 4. Circular dichroism analysis. Far-UV CD analysis of purified osmotin protein and M123 mutant. Results are expressed as mean residue ellipticity (y-axis) at a given wavelength (x-axis).

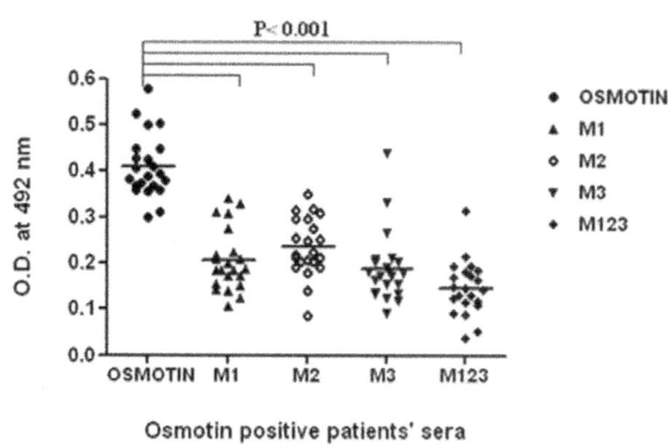

Figure 5. IgE affinity of osmotin, M1, M2, M3, M123 with food allergic patients' sera (n = 22). Specific IgE values against the respective proteins in patients' sera by ELISA. Specific IgE values ≥3 times of control were taken as cutoff for the positive results. (—) median value. Statistical difference in IgE binding among osmotin and the mutants is $p<0.001$ was considered statistically significant.

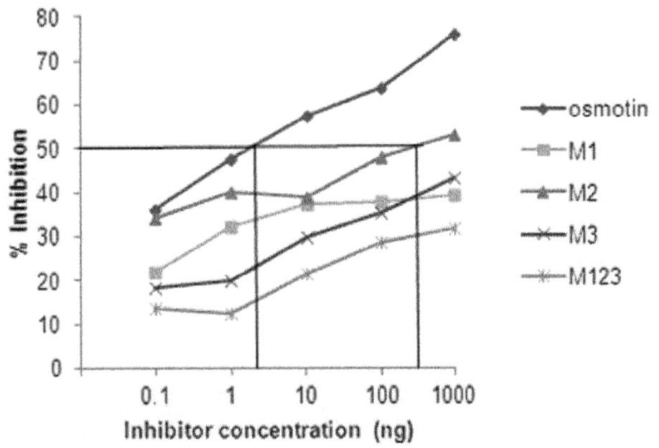

Figure 6. IgE reactivity of osmotin, M1, M2, M3 and M123. For IgE inhibition, osmotin positive patients' pooled sera were incubated with 0.1–1000 ng of osmotin protein and mutants as inhibitor. The assay was carried out with purified osmotin protein coated on microtitre plate. Competition of IgE binding to osmotin on the solid phase was quantified by ELISA. The (EC_{50}) value for Osmotin is 4 ng and for M2 is 500 ng.

protein family. Maleki et al., 2011 reported that peptides with a *PD* value similarity (<8.5) to known IgE epitopes could contribute to IgE binding and cross-reactivity [32]. This indicates that osmotin may share cross reactive epitopes with other similar proteins. In our earlier study osmotin showed IgE binding with sera of tomato and apple allergic patients confirming the predicted epitopes [22].

In the present study, three single point mutants (M1, M2 and M3) and a triple point mutant, M123 was subcloned and protein purified to homogeneity. These were developed by mutating a single residue in each of the three IgE binding predicted areas. Previous study has shown that single point allergen mutants do not lead to significant changes in protein structure but reduces allergenicity [33]. Mutational analysis of Pen a 1 showed that at least three substitutions per epitope were necessary to abolish the IgE Ab reactivity in >99% of the mutated epitopes [4]. In our study, all the mutants of osmotin showed reduction in IgE binding with patients' sera. The pattern of IgE binding of the mutants was not similar among all the patients suggesting the contribution was not same for all the mutations. However, the triple mutant of osmotin showed maximum reduction of up to 90% in the IgE binding as compared to osmotin. The reduction in IgE binding may be attributed to the phenylalanine substitution that is non reactive and tend to bury in hydrophobic cores of the protein molecule [34].

The *Brassica* pollen allergen Bra r 1 showed 74% and 94% inhibition of IgE binding with two patients' sera respectively at the highest inhibitor concentration. The double mutant of Bra r 1 showed 13% and 19% inhibition indicating reduced affinity of the IgE antibodies [35]. Peach allergen, Pru p 3 mutated at single position showed no change in IgE binding pattern whereas the triple mutant showed a 5 times reduction in IgE binding and inhibition potency [36]. Allergic response is elicited due to the multiple epitopes on an allergen, therefore multiple mutations are required to inhibit IgE binding completely. In the present study, triple mutant M123 of osmotin showed up to 90% reduction as compared to osmotin whereas single point mutants showed reduction of up to 76% in IgE binding. The circular dichroism spectra of the recombinant osmotin and M123 mutant showed that the secondary structure was not affected by three substitutions.

The potential of introduced foreign or engineered proteins in genetically modified crops to cause allergy has been of concern worldwide [37]. Many food allergens have been modified to generate the hypoallergenic mutants that showed reduced IgE binding. Osmotin has been shown as a potential allergen using *in silico* and *in vitro* studies [22]. It is still being used for developing transgenic crops owing to its properties of osmotic stress tolerance and antifungal activity. Therefore, genetically modified foods containing osmotin may not get clearance from regulatory bodies. Osmotin with no IgE binding having biological activity may be employed in developing genetically modified crops.

Specific immunotherapy against allergic disorders requires frequent injections of allergen extract to slowly build up the maintenance dose [38]. Allergen specific immunotherapy with purified protein has shown potential but may cause anaphylactic reactions. This can be prevented by modifying the IgE binding epitopes of the protein. In the present study IgE binding linear epitopes of osmotin were modified to have a hypoallergenic. These mutant proteins will have potential for immunotherapy.

In conclusion, three B- cell epitopes of osmotin were predicted by *in silico* method that correlated well with the experimental approach. Osmotin mutant M123 showed a reduction of 90% in IgE binding. The present method may be employed for prediction of B- cell epitopes of allergenic proteins.

Acknowledgments

The authors thank Prof. K.C. Bansal, Indian Agricultural Research Institute, New Delhi, for providing the osmotin gene.

Author Contributions

Conceived and designed the experiments: NA PS. Performed the experiments: PS SNG NA. Analyzed the data: PS NA. Contributed reagents/materials/analysis tools: PS SNG NA. Wrote the paper: PS SNG NA.

References

1. Cianferoni A, Spergel JM (2009) Food allergy: review, classification and diagnosis. Allergol Int 58: 457–466.
2. Vrtala S (2008) From allergen genes to new forms of allergy diagnosis and treatment. Allergy 63: 299–309.
3. Nelson HS, Lahr J, Rule R, Bock A, Leung D (1997) Treatment of anaphylactic sensitivity to peanuts by immunotherapy with injections of aqueous peanut extract. J Allergy Clin Immunol 99: 744–751.
4. Reese G, Viebranz J, Leong-Kee SM, Plante M, Lauer I, et al. (2005) Reduced Allergenic Potency of VR9-1, a Mutant of the Major Shrimp Allergen Pen a 1 (Tropomyosin). J Immunol 175: 8354–8364.
5. Toda M, Reese G, Gadermaier G, Schulten V, Lauer I, et al. (2011) Protein unfolding strongly modulates the allergenicity and immunogenicity of Pru p 3, the major peach allergen. J Allergy Clin Immunol 128: 1022–1030.
6. Xiao Y, Lu Y, Chen YH (2001) Epitope-vaccine as a new strategy against HIV-1 mutation. Immunol Lett 77: 3–6.
7. Wang HW, Lin YC, Pai TW, Chang HT (2011) Prediction of B-cell linear epitopes with a combination of support vector machine classification and amino acid propensity identification. J Biomed Biotechnol 2011: 432830.
8. Nair S, Kukreja N, Singh BP, Arora N (2011) Identification of B cell epitopes of alcohol dehydrogenase allergen of *Curvularia lunata*. PLoS One 6: e20020.
9. Thalhamer T, Dobias H, Stepanoska T, Pröll M, Stutz H, et al. (2010) Designing hypoallergenic derivatives for allergy treatment by means of in silico mutation and screening. J Allergy Clin Immunol 125: 926–934.
10. Valenta R, Niederberger V (2007) Recombinant allergens for immunotherapy. J Allergy Clin Immunol 119: 826–830.
11. King N, Helm R, Stanley JS, Vieths S, Luttkopf D, et al. (2005) Allergenic characteristics of a modified peanut allergen. Mol Nutr Food Res 49: 963–971.

12. Bolhaar ST, Zuidmeer L, Ma Y, Ferreira F, Bruijnzeel-Koomen CA, et al. (2005) A mutant of the major apple allergen, Mal d 1 demonstrating hypo-allergenicity in the target organ by double-blind placebo-controlled food challenge. Clin Exp Allergy 35: 1638–1644.
13. Marazuela EG, Rodríguez R, Barber D, Villalba M, Batanero E (2007) Hypoallergenic mutants of Ole e 1, the major olive pollen allergen, as candidates for allergy vaccines. Clin Exp Allergy 37: 251–260.
14. Cornelissen BJC, Hooft van Huijsduijnen RA, Bol JFA (1986) Tobacco mosaic virus-induced tobacco protein is homologous to the sweet-tasting protein thaumatin. Nature 321: 531–532.
15. Abad LR, D'Urzo MP, Liu D, Narasimhan ML, Reuveni M, et al. (1996) Antifungal activity of tobacco osmotin has specificity and involves plasma membrane permeabilization. Plant Sci 118: 11–23.
16. Barthakur S, Babu V, Bansal KC (2001) Overexpression of osmotin induces proline accumulation and confers tolerance to osmotic stress in transgenic tobacco. J Plant Biochem Biotechnol 10: 31–37.
17. Hussaini AM, Abdin MZ (2008) Overexpression of tobacco osmotin geneleads to salt stress tolerance in strawberry (*Fragaria* X *ananassa* Duch.) plants. Indian J Biotechnol 7: 465–471.
18. Noori SAS, Sokhansanj A (2008) Wheat plants containing an osmotin gene show enhanced ability to produce roots at high NaCl concentration. Russ J Plant Physiol 55: 256–258.
19. Parkhi V, Kumar V, Sunilkumar G, Campbell LM, Singh NK, et al. (2009) Expression of apoplastically secreted tobacco osmotin in cotton confers drought tolerance. Mol Breed 23: 625–639.
20. Goel D, Singh AK, Yadav V, Babbar SB, Bansal KC (2010) Overexpression of osmotin gene confers tolerance to salt and drought stresses in transgenic tomato (*Solanum lycopersicum* L.). Protoplasma 245: 133–141.
21. Das M, Chauhan H, Chhibbar A, Rizwanul Haq QM, Khurana P (2011) High-efficiency transformation and selective tolerance against biotic and abiotic stress in mulberry, *Morus indica* cv. K2, by constitutive and inducible expression of tobacco osmotin. Transgenic Res 20: 231–246.
22. Sharma P, Singh AK, Singh BP, Gaur SN, Arora N (2011) Allergenicity assessment of osmotin, a pathogenesis-related protein, used for transgenic crops. J Agric Food Chem 59: 9990–9995.
23. El-Manzalawy Y, Honavar V (2010) Recent advances in B-cell epitope prediction methods. Immunome Res 6 Suppl 2: S2.
24. American Thoracic Society (1991) Lung function testing: selection of reference values and interpretative strategies. Am Rev Respir Dis 144: 1202–1218.
25. Sharma V, Singh BP, Gaur SN, Pasha S, Arora N (2009) Bioinformatics and immunologic investigation on B and T cell epitopes of Cur l 3, a major allergen of *Curvularia lunata*. J Proteome Res 8: 2650–2655.
26. Bannon GA (2004) What makes a food protein an allergen? Curr Allergy Asthma Rep 4: 43–46.
27. Pomes A (2010) Relevant B cell epitopes in allergic disease. Int Arch Allergy Immunol 152: 1–11.
28. Sicherer SH, Sampson HA (2007) Peanut allergy: emerging concepts and approaches for an apparent epidemic. J Allergy Clin Immunol 120: 491–503.
29. Ayuso R, Lehrer SB, Reese G (2002) Identification of continuous, allergenic regions of the major shrimp allergen Pen a 1 (tropomyosin). Int Arch Allergy Immunol 127: 27–37.
30. Jarvinen KM, Beyer K, Vila L, Bardina L, Mishoe M, et al. (2007) Specificity of IgE antibodies to sequential epitopes of hen's egg ovomucoid as a marker for persistence of egg allergy. Allergy 62: 758–765.
31. Busse PJ, Järvinen KM, Vila L Beyer K, Sampson HA (2002) Identification of sequential IgE-binding epitopes on bovine alpha (s2)-casein in cow's milk allergic patients. Int Arch Allergy Immunol 129: 93–96.
32. Maleki SJ, Teuber SS, Cheng H, Chen D, Comstock SS, et al. (2011) Computationally predicted IgE epitopes of walnut allergens contribute to cross-reactivity with peanuts. Allergy 66: 1522–1529.
33. Chan SL, Ong TC, Gao YF, Tiong YS, Wang de Y, et al. (2008) Nuclear magnetic resonance structure and IgE epitopes of Blo t 5, a major dust mite allergen. J Immunol 181: 2586–2596.
34. Betts MJ, Russell RB (2003) Amino acid properties and consequences of subsitutions. In: Barnes MR, Gray IC, Editors. Bioinformatics for Geneticists. Wiley Chichester UK. pp. 289–316.
35. Okada T, Swoboda I, Bhalla PL, Toriyama K, Singh MB (1998) Engineering of hypoallergenic mutants of the *Brassica* pollen allergen, Bra r 1, for immunotherapy. FEBS Lett 434: 255–260.
36. García-Casado G, Pacios LF, Díaz-Perales A, Sánchez-Monge R, Lombardero M, et al. (2003) Identification of IgE-binding epitopes of the major peach allergen Pru p 3. J Allergy Clin Immunol 112: 599–605.
37. Herman EM (2003) Genetically modified soybeans and food allergies. J Exp Bot 54: 1317–1319.
38. Srivastava D, Arora N, Singh BP (2009) Current immunological approaches for management of allergic rhinitis and bronchial asthma. Inflamm Res 58: 523–36.

Peripheral Erythrocytes Decrease upon Specific Respiratory Challenge with Grass Pollen Allergen in Sensitized Mice and in Human Subjects

Galateja Jordakieva[1,2]✉, Julia Wallmann[1]✉, René Schmutz[3], Patrick Lemell[3], Michael Wegmann[4], Thomas Nittke[1], Martina Mittlböck[5], Heinz Fehrenbach[4], Jasminka Godnic-Cvar[2], René Zieglmayer[3], Erika Jensen-Jarolim[1,6]*

1 Comparative Medicine, Messerli Research Institute of the University of Veterinary Medicine Vienna, Medical University of Vienna & University of Vienna, Vienna, Austria, **2** Institute of Occupational Medicine, Department of Internal Medicine II, Medical University of Vienna, Vienna, Austria, **3** Vienna Challenge Chamber (VCC), Vienna, Austria, **4** Priority Area Asthma & Allergy, Leibniz Center for Medicine and Biosciences, Research Center Borstel, Airway Research Center North, Member of the German Center for Lung Research, Borstel, Germany, **5** Section for Clinical Biometrics, Center for Medical Statistics, Informatics, and Intelligent Systems, Medical University of Vienna, Vienna, Austria, **6** Institute of Pathophysiology and Allergy Research, Center of Pathophysiology Infectiology and Immunology, Medical University of Vienna, Vienna, Austria

Abstract

Background and Aims: Specific hyper-responsiveness towards an allergen and non-specific airway hyperreactivity both impair quality of life in patients with respiratory allergic diseases. We aimed to investigate cellular responses following specific and non-specific airway challenges locally and systemically in i) sensitized BALB/c mice challenged with grass pollen allergen Phl p 5, and in ii) grass pollen sensitized allergic rhinitis subjects undergoing specific airway challenge in the Vienna Challenge Chamber (VCC).

Methods and Results: BALB/c mice (n = 20) were intraperitoneally immunized with grass pollen allergen Phl p 5 and afterwards aerosol challenged with either the specific allergen Phl p 5 (n = 10) or the non-specific antigen ovalbumin (OVA) (n = 10). A protocol for inducing allergic asthma as well as allergic rhinitis, according to the united airway concept, was used. Both groups of exposed mice showed significantly reduced physical activity after airway challenge. Specific airway challenge further resulted in goblet cell hyperplasia, enhanced mucous secretion, intrapulmonary leukocyte infiltration and lymphoid follicle formation, associated with significant expression of IL-4, IL-5 and IL-13 in splenocytes and also partially in lung tissue. Concerning circulating blood cell dynamics, we observed a significant drop of erythrocyte counts, hemoglobin and hematocrit levels in both mouse groups, challenged with allergen or OVA. A significant decrease in circulating erythrocytes and hematocrit levels after airway challenges with grass pollen allergen was also found in grass pollen sensitized human rhinitis subjects (n = 42) at the VCC. The effects on peripheral leukocyte counts in mice and humans however were opposed, possibly due to the different primary inflammation sites.

Conclusion: Our data revealed that, besides significant leukocyte dynamics, particularly erythrocytes are involved in acute hypersensitivity reactions to respiratory allergens. A rapid recruitment of erythrocytes to the lungs to compensate for hypoxia is a possible explanation for these findings.

Editor: Bernhard Ryffel, French National Centre for Scientific Research, France

Funding: This work was supported by an SFB project F4606-B19 of the Austrian Science Fund and partially by the German Research Foundation (Cluster of Excellence EXC306). Further support was contributed by the Vienna Science and Technology Fund (project LS07-058). The funders had no role in study design, data collection and analysis, decision to publish, or preparation of the manuscript.

Competing Interests: The authors have declared that no competing interests exist.

* E-mail: erika.jensen-jarolim@meduniwien.ac.at

✉ These authors contributed equally to this work.

Introduction

The prevalence of allergy mediated medical conditions is increasing worldwide and currently affecting approximately a fifth of the world population. [1] Especially allergic airway diseases are associated with significant quality of life limitations in affected patients. [2] Although less limiting than bronchial asthma, allergic rhinitis has been described as a global health concern causing major illness and disability worldwide. [3] Allergic rhinitis and allergic asthma are often found in the same patients and considered manifestations of the same inflammatory disease emphasized in different parts of the airways [2,3].

Allergic asthma is defined as a chronic inflammatory disorder of the lower airways and is characterized by airway inflammation, persistent airway hyperresponsiveness (AHR) and intermittent acute, reversible airways obstruction. [4] Typically, the IgE-mediated, immediate obstruction is followed by a late phase reaction triggered by the release of inflammatory mediators like leukotrienes and cytokines (i.e. IL-4) from cells recruited to the lungs. This results in respiratory and, consequently, physical deficits of affected patients for a considerable time after an asthma attack. Additionally, in the absence of allergen, even exposure to unrelated antigens may trigger shortness of breath and wheezing, again limiting lung function and thus, seriously affecting the patients' quality of life. Pallor is an additional well known clinical sign of severe asthma and has recently been described to occur in 10% of emergency cases [5].

Although mouse models of respiratory allergies exhibit some limitations compared to the human disease, they have provided important information about the conditions necessary for allergen sensitization. The common basis for the induction of Th2-type airway inflammation in mice is systemic sensitization followed by aerosol or intranasal challenges with the allergen. [6] Using this protocol renders an phenotype in mice mirroring the united airway concept in human patients, characterized by eosinophilic nasal and bronchial inflammation, increased Th2-type cytokines and antibody levels, mucus hyper-secretion and airway hyper-responsiveness. [7] However, the expression of each of these parameters can vary within the disease, with other sensitization protocols used [8,9].

With respect to the profound impairment of capability in allergic airway diseases, we aimed to analyze peripheral blood cell dynamics during specific and non-specific aerosol allergen challenge in this study. For this purpose, data from BALB/c mice sensitized to Phl p 5 followed by aerosol challenges with allergen or non-specific control antigen was compared to data from grass pollen sensitized human rhinitis subjects who underwent airway challenge with specific allergen in the Vienna Challenge Chamber.

Methods

Mouse Study

Immunization of mice. BALB/c mice (female; 6–10 weeks) were purchased from Charles River Laboratories (Sulzfeld, Germany GmbH) and treated according to European Community rules of animal care [10] with the permission of the Austrian Ministry of Science (BMWF-66.012/0015-CIGT/2007); study approval was granted by the Ethics Commission of the Medical University of Vienna. BALB/c mice ($n = 20$) were immunized intraperitoneally (i.p.) with rPhl p 5a (10 μ g/100 μ l PBS) on days 0 and 21. Ten days later, mice ($n = 10$) were aerosol challenged with nebulized rPhl p 5a or OVA (protein and plasmid kindly provided by Prof. Arnd Petersen, Research Institute Borstel, Germany) (0.25 mg rPhl p 5a/100 ml PBS/challenge or Ovalbumin from chicken egg white 1%/100 mL PBS/challenge) with an ultrasonic nebulizer (Kendall, Aerodyne X, MTE Medizintechnik, Oldendorf, Germany) for 60 min twice daily with a four hours interval, on two consecutive days (day 31 and 32). Control groups were sensitized either with rPhl p 5a ($n = 5$) or PBS ($n = 5$) on days 0 and 21 and aerosol challenged 10 days later with PBS. One mouse group ($n = 5$) remained naïve. Measurements were performed on day 31 before, immediately after (day 32) and 48 hours after aerosol challenges (day 34) (Fig. S2A).

Assessment of activity. Activity was evaluated using Infra-Red Actimeter frames equipped with infrared beam and detector units (Bioseb, France). Activity measurements were performed on day 31 before aerosol challenges, on day 32 and on day 34 (Fig. S2A).

Arterial blood analysis and differential blood cell counts in mice. Arterial blood samples from the tails of mice were taken and measured by a radiometer ABL800 FLEX (Wiener Neudorf, Austria). Differential blood cell counts were performed simultaneously with an Abbott Cell Dyn CD 3500 CS Analyzer, Vienna, Austria.

Measurements on naïve mice were performed on day 0 and immediately after sensitized mice were aerosol challenged with either Phl p 5 or OVA on day 31. Beside red blood cells (RBC) and white blood cells (WBC), hemoglobin (HGB) and hematocrit (HCT) were assessed by differential blood cell counts.

Histopathology. On day 35, mice were anesthetized (200 μ l 2% Rompun (Bayer, Leverkusen, Germany) and 5 ml Ketanest S (5 mg/ml); 600 μ l per mouse)) before fixation procedures were initiated. Lungs were fixed by intratracheal instillation performed with 4% paraformaldehyde in 0.1 M Sörensen's phosphate buffer (12.0 mM NaH2PO4, 69.0 mM Na2HPO4) (pH 7.4), as described. [11] Lungs were embedded into paraffin as described earlier. [12] Systematic uniform random samples (SURS) of lung tissue were analyzed according to standard methods. Paraffin sections of 2 μ m in thickness were stained with periodic-acid-Schiff (PAS) for airway epithelial mucus. The surface area of mucus-secreting goblet cells (*Sgc*) per total surface area of airway epithelial basal membrane (*Sep*) and the volume of PAS-stained epithelial mucus (*Vmuc*) per *Sep* were determined using a computer-assisted Olympus BX61 microscope equipped with the newCAST stereology tool box (Visiopharm, Hoersholm, Denmark) according to following formulas:

$$Sgc/Sep = \sum Igc \Big/ \sum Iep$$

$$Vmuc/Sep = LP \times \sum Pmuc/2 \times \sum Iep$$

$\sum Igc$ = sum of intersections of test-lines with goblet cells

$\sum Iep$ = sum of all intersections of test-lines with epithelial basal membrane

$\sum Pmuc$ = sum of all test-points hitting stored mucus

LP = test-line length per test-point at final magnification (490×).

The volume of lymphoid follicles (*Vfol*) per total surface area of airway epithelial basal membrane (*Sep*) was determined according to the formula:

$$Vfol/Sep = LP \times \sum Pfol \Big/ 2 \times \sum Iep$$

$\sum Iep$ = sum of all intersections of test-lines with epithelial basal membrane

$\sum Pfol$ = sum of all test-points hitting mucus

LP = test-line length per test-point at final magnification (490×).

Eosinophilic infiltration. Paraffin sections of 2 μ m in thickness were stained with Congo Red as previously reported [13] for the assessment of airway wall infiltration with eosinophilic granulocytes. The degree of infiltration within each field of view collected according to SURS, was ascribed to one of the three scores; (A) no (B) one or (C) two or more eosinophils in the airway wall.

RNA isolation and quantitative reverse transcriptase polymerase chain reaction (qRT-PCR). Total RNA was extracted using the Trizol Reagent from Invitrogen (Invitrogen, Lofer, Austria) according to the manufacturer's instructions. RNA was quantified by measuring the absorption at 260/280 nm using a NanoDrop spectrophotometer (Nanodrop Technologies Montchanin, DE, USA). 3 µ g of total RNA from each sample were reverse transcribed in a total volume of 20 µl using the high capacity cDNA reverse transcription kit (Applied Biosystems, Vienna, Austria), according to the manufacturer's instructions. 2 µ l of cDNA were used for amplification by qRT-PCR which was performed with POWER SYBR®Green PCR Master Mix on an ABI StepOnePlus Realtime PCR System (Applied Biosystems, Vienna, Austria). IL-4, IL-5 and IL-13 mRNA levels were quantified by the comparative ΔΔCT method using the SDS software (Applied Biosystems, Foster City, CA, USA).

For each of the samples, relative expression was normalized to the housekeeping gene Hypoxanthine-phophoribosyl-transferase (HPRT). Pooled cDNA of naïve tissue was used as a calibrator and set the value 1; the relative expression levels of the other samples were compared hereto. Each sample was applied in duplicates. Following qRT-PCR program was used: 50°C for 2 min, 94°C for 2 min, followed by 40 cycles of 94°C for 15 s and 60°C for 30 s. Primers were designed using Primer Express (Applied Biosystems) and were located on different exons to prevent amplification of potentially contaminating genomic DNA.

Following primer sequences were used:

IL-4: fwd primer: ccatgcttgaagaagaactctagtgt
rev primer: attcatggtgcagcttatcgatg

IL-5: fwd primer: gaggcttcctgtccctatcataa
rev primer: tacccccacggacagtttga

IL-13: fwd primer: ccatctacaggacccagaggat
rev primer: gggaggctggagaccgtagt

Human Study

Study subjects. Forty-two white subjects (n = 42, age 30±7.4, 88% male) (Tab. 1) with medical history of recurrent allergic airway symptoms were included. The subjects were divided in two groups differing in total duration of airway challenge and time points of baseline blood sampling. In *group 1* (n = 26) blood sampling was performed on the day before and immediately after allergen challenge in accordance with our mouse model. The total duration of continuous allergen exposure was 4 hours in this group. In *group 2* (n = 16) blood sampling was performed immediately before and after 2 hours of continuous allergen challenge. (Fig. S2B+C) Follow-up blood samples were collected approximately 1–3 weeks after allergen challenge to evaluate a return to baseline values.

All subjects reported rhinitis symptoms (not attributed to infections and/or nasal abnormalities) manifesting for at least one year preceding the study; additionally few subjects reported occasional asthmatic symptoms. Sensitization to grass pollen allergen (Dac g, Phl p) was assessed by positive serologic and clinical examination (RAST [radioallergosorbent test] class 4±1.2, skin prick test 10±2.6 mm). Subjects had discontinued eventual immunomodulating medication prior to airway challenge (antihistamines: 72 hours; glucocorticosteroids: nasal 24 hours, bronchial 1 week, oral 12 weeks; other drugs potentially inducing enzymatic activity: 7 to 14 days). The study was approved by the ethics committee of the "Österreichische Arbeitsgemeinschaft für Klinische Pharmakologie" and performed between November 2010 and April 2011 after obtaining written informed consent of each subject.

Table 1. Demographic and clinical characteristics of study subjects.

	Group 1	*Group 2*	**Total**
N	26	16	**42**
Sex (male)	26 (100%)	11 (69%)	**37 (88%)**
Age (years)	30±7.5	29±7.5	**30±7.4**
SPT	10±2.6	9.6±2.6	**9.8±2.6**
IgE RAST class	4±1.2	4±1.2	**4±1.2**
FEV1 baseline	4.229±0.7	3.730±0.8	**4.039±0.8**
FEV1 after challenge	4.190±0.7	3.675±0.8	**3.994±0.7**

Data are mean±standard deviation, SPT = Skin-Prick-Test, RAST = Radioallergosorbent Test, FEV1 = forced expiratory volume in 1 second.

Inclusion criteria.

- Age 18–50 years.
- Healthy individuals (medical history, physical examination and routine laboratory without pathological findings), except for allergic rhinitis and intermittent or mild asthma [14] not requiring treatment and associated with normal baseline lung function (FEV1≥80%).
- Manifest allergic symptoms, positive skin prick test (≥4 mm) and elevated specific IgE (RAST class ≥2) results for grass pollen within the last 12 months preceding the study.

Exclusion criteria.

- Planned or ongoing pregnancy during the study as well as breastfeeding.
- Nasal abnormalities (septum perforation, polyps, malformations, frequent epistaxis).
- Cold symptoms or acute infections of the upper respiratory tract within 3 weeks.
- Active respiratory tract disease, other than mild asthma not requiring treatment.
- Cigarette smoking within 6 months prior to study.
- Ongoing immunotherapy and/or immunomodulating medication.
- Known severe illness (e.g. heart disease) or malignancy.
- Alcohol and/or other drug abuse.
- Insufficient language abilities or compliance.
- Psychological disorders causing mental or legal incapacitation.

Materials and Methods

A mixture of >93% pure pollen allergen (Allergon, Thermo Fisher Scientific) containing equal parts of pollen derived from Phleum pratense (phl p), Dactylis glomerata (Dac g), Lolium perenne (Lol p) and Anthoxanthum odoratum (Ant o) was used for airway challenge. The pollen were provided by the manufacturer with microbiological and chemical quality analysis certificates and dry stored at +2 to +10°C in their original containers. During airway challenge the pollen allergen mix was canalized into a feeding system (regulatory apparatus with vacuum outlet) connected to the air supply of the enclosed challenge chamber every five minutes. The allergen concentration in the challenge chamber was measured by persistent visual checking (Light

Microscope, Olympus) of adhesive coated slides that were exposed to a constant air flow of 9–10 l/min (approximately equal to human nasal inspiratory flow) for five minutes inside a modified pollen trap (Burkard Co Ltd., Rickmansworth, England). The records were then saved to an Excel® spreadsheet every 5 min throughout the duration of a provocation session and used as basis for calculation of average, standard deviation, minimum and maximum value for the entire provocation session. Inside the challenge chamber climatic conditions were kept constant throughout each trial by a complex external air conditioning system combined with a processing plant for the supply and exhaustion of air. Temperature (24°C), humidity (40%), CO2 (%), air velocity (m/s) and air flow (m^3/h or l/min) were monitored via several sensors (Alhborn) within the challenge chamber.

The subjects were exposed to the allergen for 4 h (*group 1*) or 2 h (*group 2*) in the provocation chamber. (Fig. S2B+C) Air concentration was kept at about ~1500 pollen/m^3 constantly (approximate air pollen concentration on a midsummer day). Every 15 min the study participants' reported presence or absence of allergic symptoms, every 30 min the volume of air flow through the nose was measured by active anterior rhinomanometry, permitting indirect conclusions about the extent of swelling in the nasal mucosa and every 60 min spirometry was performed to assess changes in lung function (FEV1, FVC) for safety reasons.

Differential Blood Cell Counts in Humans

Peripheral venous blood was sampled in ethylenediamine tetraacetic acid (EDTA) tubes at two time-points: on the day before (*group 1*) as in the mouse model or immediately before (*group 2*) and immediately after allergen challenge (both groups); a third blood sample (follow-up) was collected between 6 and 21 days after the allergen challenge sessions. EDTA blood samples were stored at +2°C to +10°C and analyzed within 2 days at an ISO 9001-certified laboratory (Labors Mühl-Speiser, Vienna, Austria) performing total and differential blood cell counts.

Statistical Analysis

Continuous variables with a normal distribution are expressed as mean ± standard deviation (SD) or as median (minimum, maximum) if assumption of normal distribution was violated. Statistical comparisons between groups were made either by unpaired t-tests if data were normally distributed within groups or by Wilcoxon rank-sum test otherwise. Differences in before and after (paired) measurements are tested by paired t-test, if the differences were approximately normally distributed and by Wilcoxon's signed rank test otherwise. All tests are based on a two-sided significance level of 0.05. The statistical software SPSS® (version 17.0 for Windows) was used for all statistical calculations.

Results

Mouse Model

Airway challenge with specific allergen and nonspecific antigen results in a significant reduction of motor activity in sensitized mice. The physical activity of mice was recorded before and after aerosolizations by counting the rearings (Z-axis movements) using an infrared beam at three different time-points; before, immediately after challenge and 48 hours later. Regardless of the allergen/antigen used for provocation of the airways, physical activity was drastically reduced in both mouse groups (Fig. 1), mirroring the clinical impairment in human patients. At the 48 hour time point, activity continued to be significantly reduced, irrespective of the agent used for challenge.

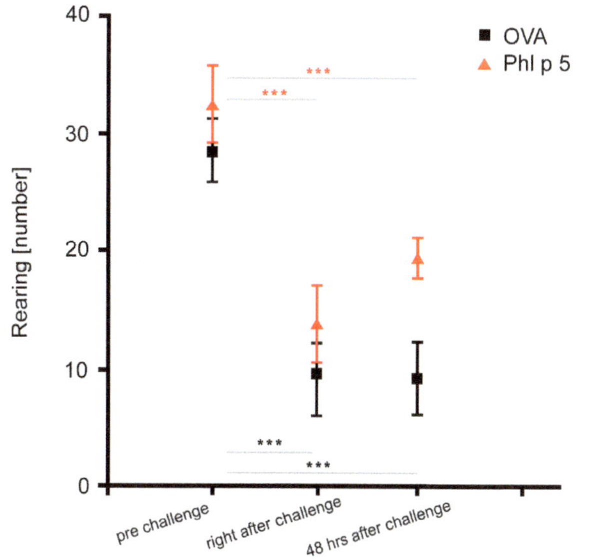

Figure 1. Physical activity after airway challenge. Rearing of Phl p 5-allergic in allergen (red squares) or nonspecific antigen (black points) challenged mice. Data are mean ± SD and n=5 mice/group. ***, p<0.001.

Peripheral erythrocyte parameters and leucocyte numbers after specific allergen aerosol challenges in sensitized mice. After aerosol challenge we observed significant decreases of peripheral red blood cell counts (RBC), hemoglobin (HGB) and hematocrit (HCT) compared to baseline values, suggestive of increased redistribution and dynamics of erythrocytes upon challenge with a specific allergen, and less with an irrelevant antigen (Fig. 2, A–C).

White blood cell counts (WBC) decreased in arterial blood of mice hypersensitive to Phl p 5, in the allergen-aerosol exposed group but remained almost unchanged in the group nebulized with control antigen OVA (Fig. 2D).

Allergen-specific, but less non-specific respiratory challenge, is associated with lymphoid airway inflammation. Systematic uniform random samples (SURS) were collected from the entire lung and analyzed for goblet cell metaplasia, mucus production, lymphoid follicles and infiltration of the airways with eosinophils 64 hours after aerosol challenge (Fig. 3 and 4). In contrast to mice challenged with the allergen Phl p 5, mice immunized with Phl p 5 but challenged with OVA hardly exhibited any goblet cell metaplasia (Fig. 3A) or mucus production (Fig. 3B and C–E). Moreover, total volume of lymphoid follicles found peribronchially together with qualitative microscopic observations indicated that more and larger lymphoid follicles were present after mice were challenged with the specific allergen compared to OVA (Fig. 4A and C–E). Peripheral counts of lymphocytes were not affected (data not shown). Determining the percentage of airway walls containing eosinophils in the fields of view (FOVs) showed that eosinophilic infiltration was significantly increased in both, OVA and Phl p 5 challenged allergic mouse groups compared to naïve controls (Fig. 4B).

Phlp 5 sensitized mice aerosolized with the specific allergen exhibited higher Th2 cytokine mRNA production in lung tissue and splenocytes. As a measure for systemic immune deviation, expression of Th2 associated cytokines of spleen cells was investigated and compared to local effects in lungs. The spleens and the left lung of each mouse were isolated 64 hours

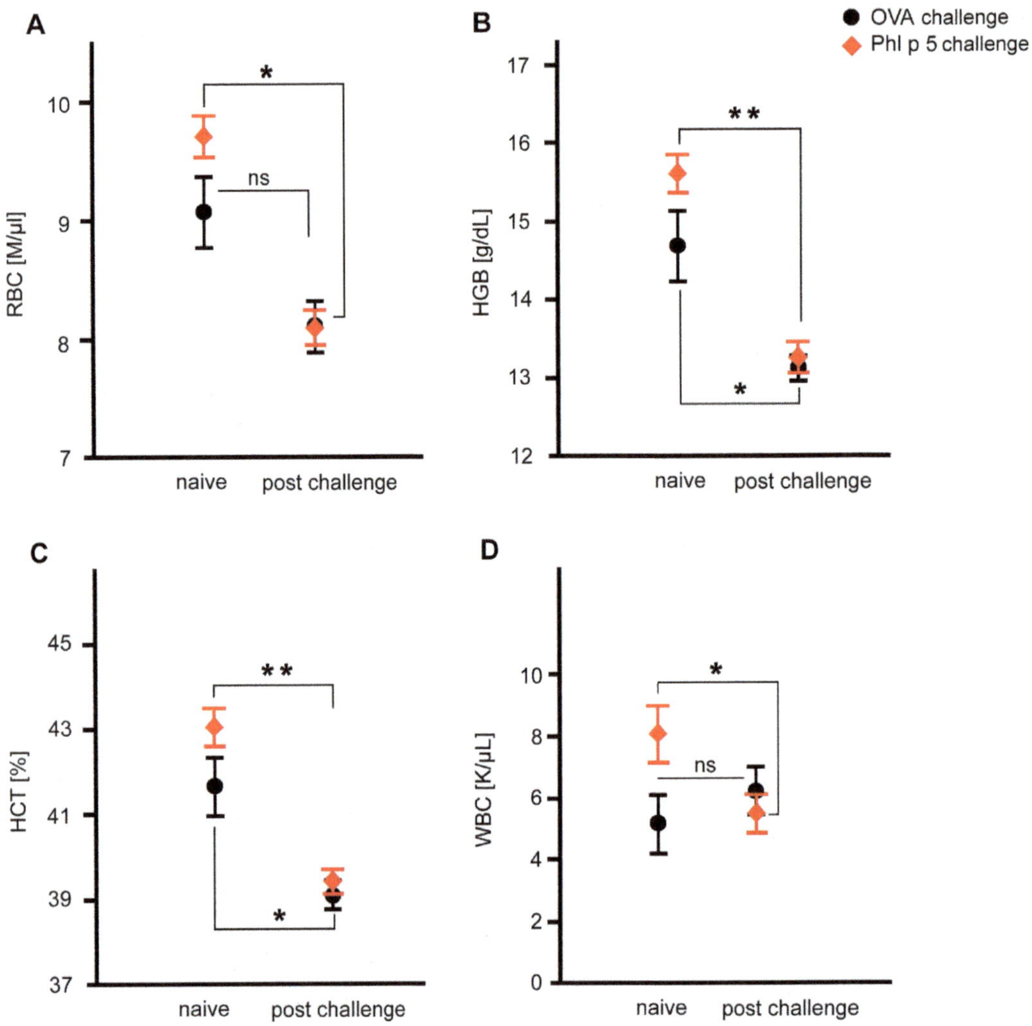

Figure 2. Specific and nonspecific airway provocation of allergic mice: impact on blood cells. (**A**) RBC, (**B**) HGB and (**C**) HCT levels of naïve, non-sensitized versus sensitized and Phl p 5 nebulized (red squares) and OVA challenged mice (black points) after airway challenge. Data are mean ± SD and n = 5 mice/group. *, $p<0.05$, **, $p<0.01$ and n.s. means not significant. (**D**) White blood cell counts (WBC) from naïve versus sensitized and Phl p 5 challenged (red squares) or OVA aerosolized mice (black points).

after the last treatment. Relative expression of IL-4, IL-5 and IL-13 mRNA levels was quantified by qRT-PCR.

Aerosol challenges of Phl p 5-sensitized mice with OVA did neither elevate Th2 cytokine mRNA in spleens nor in lungs, as compared to naïve animals. As expected, challenges with the specific allergen Phl p 5 induced Th2 cytokine mRNA production in lungs and even more significantly in spleens (Fig. S1). These data indicate that significant transcription of IL-4, IL-5 and IL-13 is initiated as a consequence of specific allergen challenge and that it is a systemic event.

Human Subjects

Peripheral erythrocyte numbers and hemoglobin decrease after specific allergen challenge in grass-pollen sensitized rhinitis subjects. Analogous to our findings in mice, the overall RBC counts were significantly decreased in sensitized subjects immediately after allergen airway challenge compared to baseline values ($p<0.01$); similarly HGB levels were reduced ($p<0.05$). These findings were significant in subjects exposed to grass pollen allergens for 4 h (*group 1*), however were not found in the smaller subject group exposed to allergen for 2 h only (*group 2*). The changes in HCT, MCV (mean corpuscular volume), MCH (mean corpuscular hemoglobin) or MCHC (mean corpuscular hemoglobin concentration) after allergen challenge did not reach statistical significance in any group (Tab. 2). In the follow-up blood samples no significant differences in RBC count, HGB or HCT were noted when compared to the respective baseline values before allergen challenge.

Segmented neutrophils increase after allergen challenge in sensitized human subjects. In contrast to the described outcomes in aerosol-challenged mice we found significantly elevated peripheral leukocyte numbers immediately after allergen challenge in the grass-pollen sensitized human subjects ($p<0.001$) independent of the allergen exposure duration (4 h or 2 h; in *group 1* or *group 2*) (Fig. S3A). As depicted in Fig. S3B the most outstandingly increased leukocyte subset was that of segmented neutrophils ($p<0.001$ in both groups). In subjects who underwent 4 h of continuous allergen challenge absolute basophil numbers ($p<0.05$) were also significantly increased compared to baseline (pre-challenge) values. Overall post-challenge eosinophil numbers

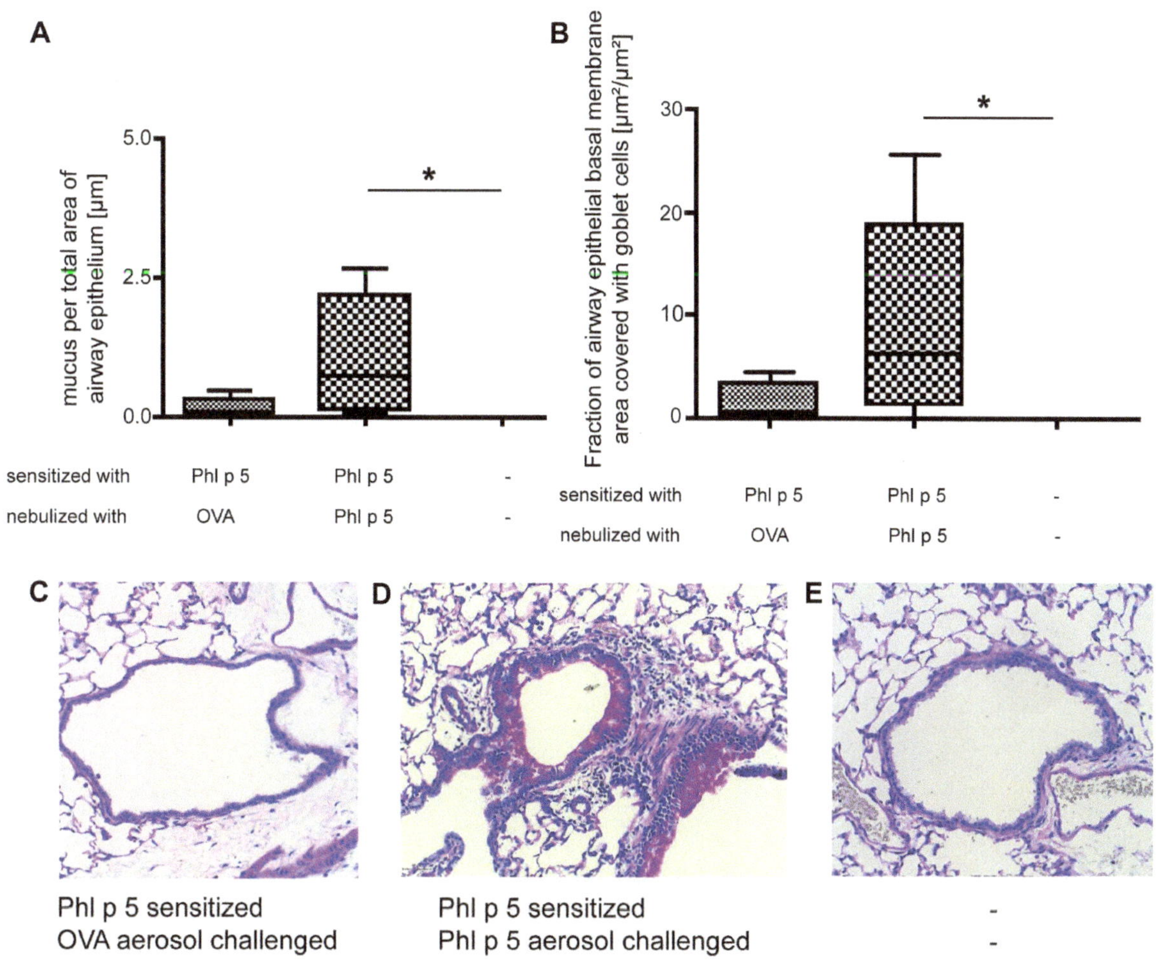

Figure 3. Goblet cell metaplasia, mucus production, lymphoid follicles and infiltration of airways with eosinophils after aerosol challenge. (**A**) Volume of epithelial mucus, (**B**) fraction of epithelial basal membrane covered by goblet cells. Representative lung histology from (**C**) Phl p 5 sensitized and OVA challenged (**D**), Phl p 5 sensitized and Phl p 5 challenged (**E**) naïve mice. Data are presented by boxplots (median, quartiles, minimum and maximum) and n = 5 mice/group. *, $p<0.05$.

did not significantly differ from baseline values; also no clear trend was found for lymphocyte dynamics in the subgroup analysis. (Tab. 2) In the follow-up blood samples no significant dynamics were found in the leukocyte subsets, when compared to baseline values before allergen challenge, except for a shift in relative basophil ratio ($p<0.05$, data not shown) without significant changes in total basophil numbers.

Thrombocyte numbers increased after allergen exposure in both groups; however a statistical significance was only found in subjects after 2 h of continuous allergen challenge ($p<0.01$). In the follow-up blood samples, thrombocyte counts did not differ significantly from the respective baseline values.

Discussion

In the present study we evaluated the local and systemic effects of specific allergen and non-specific antigen challenges in sensitized mice compared to data gained from airway challenges in human allergic rhinitis subjects at the Vienna Challenge Chamber. After allergen-specific as well as non-specific airway challenge in our study motor activity in mice immediately decreased and remained low until more than 48 hours after challenge which corresponds to sustained physical impairment in asthmatic patients [15] and allergic rhinitis patients [16].

In mouse models the degree of overall airway inflammation, depends on the experimental protocol used. [6] Here [17] immunization and aerosol challenges with Phl p 5 as the specific allergen rendered modest induction of mucus production, lymphoid follicle formation and eosinophilic infiltration in the proximal parts of the airways. Nebulization with the irrelevant antigen rendered milder inflammation and smaller lymphoid infiltration.

The levels of different Th2-associated cytokines and mRNA increased upon allergen challenge (S1) from splenocytes and lung tissues indicating systemic and local immune bias. The Th2-type lung inflammation was less pronounced upon non-specific aerosol challenge. IL-4 and IL-13 not only play a pivotal role in the production of IgE antibodies, but also contribute to narrowing of the airways. IL-4 also causes epithelial cells to swell and increases the contractibility of airway smooth muscle cells, thereby playing an essential role in AHR. [18,19] IL-13 supports goblet cell metaplasia and mucus production. [20] Counter-regulation of Th2 cytokines also has therapeutic implications in allergic rhinitis. [21] IL-5 is primarily engaged in the recruitment of eosinophils, which

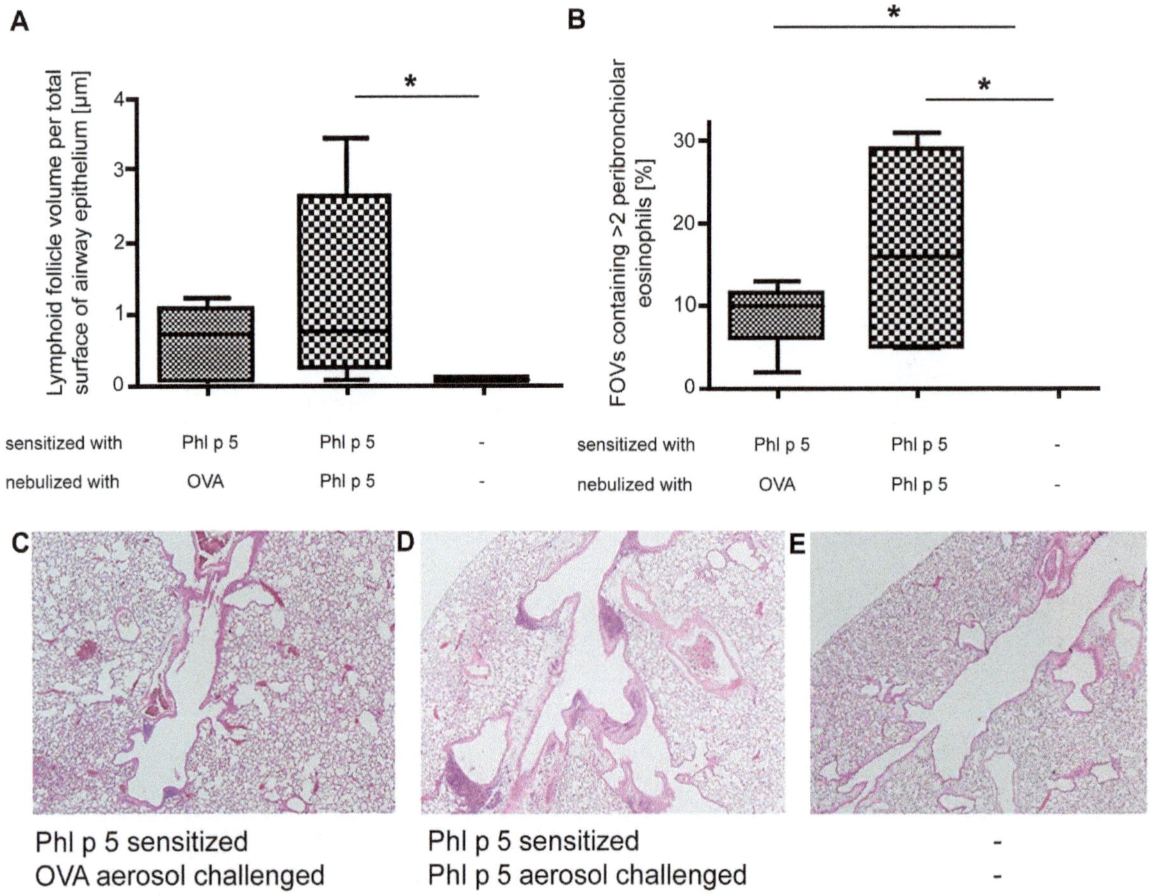

Figure 4. Aerosol allergen challenge specifically attracts leukocytes to lungs. (**A**) Volume of lymphoid follicles V/S (fol, epi) per total surface area of airway epithelial basal membrane [µm] (**B**) and percentage of airway walls containing eosinophils in fields of view (FOVs). Lung histology representatives with respect to lymphoid follicles from Phl p 5 sensitized and (**C**) OVA challenged or (**D**) Phl p 5 challenged and (**E**) naïve mice. Data are presented by boxplots (median, quartiles, minimum and maximum) and n = 5 mice/group. *, $p<0.05$, **, $p<0.01$ and n.s. means not significant.

negatively correlate with nasal airflow in asthma and rhinitis patients. [7] In our study, eosinophilic infiltration of the airways occurred to a comparable extent in both, specifically and non-specifically challenged sensitized mouse groups.

In mice, we observed a substantial decrease of red blood cell count, hemoglobin and hematocrit levels immediately following specific airway allergen challenge, with twofold significance upon specific provocation with Phl p 5.

We addressed the relevance of these phenomena in human grass pollen-sensitized rhinitis subjects undergoing respiratory airway challenge in the Vienna Challenge Chamber. [22–24] Like in the mouse study a significant decrease in erythrocyte and hemoglobin levels in the peripheral blood of the subjects was found after inhalative allergen challenge over 4 hours. The drop in circulating erythrocytes may to some extent be attributed to minor interstitial bleedings previously described as micro-epistaxis; [25] however taking the analogous results from our mouse model into consideration, we assume a compensatory re-distribution of erythrocytes to the respective site of inflammation for oxygen loading. Since erythrocytes may induce hypoxic lung inflammation, [26] the changes in erythrocyte counts upon allergen-challenge may also indicate a participation of the lungs in early wheezing, compatible with the United Airways concept. [27] No reports on effects of allergic asthma or rhinitis on red blood cell counts have been made so far, except sporadic evidence suggesting that human asthmatics may experience a decrease of hematocrit during recovery from acute episodes. [28] Our findings that acute allergic airway episodes are associated with in a significant fall of peripheral erythrocyte counts explain the facial pallor of the patients [29] and may contribute to the perception of respiratory discomfort [30].

The drop of leukocytes upon allergen challenge in the mouse study is in accordance with a previous observation in anaphylaxis, [31] but opposed the results from the human allergic subjects in our study, where peripheral leukocyte counts significantly increased after allergen challenge. A subset analysis showed that human segmented neutrophils and to some extent basophils accounted for the total leukocyte elevation, without relevant changes in less matured neutrophils or eosinophils. Neutrophils are known to have a crucial function in the allergy-mediated inflammatory response, for instance by release of proteases, [19,20] myeloperoxidase (MPO) or elastase. [32–35] Neutrophils were elevated in blood and sputum after specific bronchial challenge in asthmatics; recently a rise in leukocytes in the delayed asthmatic response was observed proposing the monitoring of peripheral blood cell counts as a useful supplementary parameter to bronchial allergen challenge. [36,37] In intermittent allergic rhinitis neutrophils are elevated in nasal lavage fluid within an hour after local allergen exposure and correlate with rhinitis symptoms. [38] Although conducted in allergic rhinitis rather than

Table 2. Changes in number of peripheral blood cells before and after airway challenge with grass-pollen mix in subjects with allergic rhinitis, after 4 h (*group 1*) or 2 h (*group 2*) of allergen exposure; follow-up data shows the respective blood cell counts 6–21 days after airway allergen challenge.

	All subjects (n = 42)			**Subgroups**			
				Group 1 **(n = 26)**		*Group 2* **(n = 16)**	
Allergen challenge status	*baseline*	*after*	*follow-up*	*baseline*	*after*	*baseline*	*after*
Red blood cells (RBC) × 10^{12}/l	5 (4.1, 5.7)	**4.95 (4.1, 5.7)****	*5,01 (4.2, 5.6)*	5.08 (4.54, 5.57)	**5 (4.46, 5.4)****	4.8 (4.1, 5.7)	4.85 (4.1, 5.7)
HGB *g/dl*	15 (13.2, 16.4)	**14.7 (13.3, 16.4)***	*15 (12.8, 16.7)*	15.1(14.0, 16.1)	**14.65 (13.7, 16.4)****	14.65 (13.2, 16.4)	14.7 (13.3, 16)
HCT %	44 (39, 49)	44 (39, 49)	*44 (39, 49)*	45 (42, 49)	43 (41, 49)	44 (39, 49)	44 (39, 48)
MCV *femtoliters/cell*	89 (82, 95)	89.5 (82, 98)	*89 (82, 98)*	89 (82, 95)	90 (82, 95)	88.5 (82, 95)	88.5 (82, 98)
MCH *picograms/cell*	30 (27, 33)	30 (27, 33)	***30 (27, 33)**[a]***	30 (27, 32)	30 (27, 32)	30 (27, 33)	29.5 (27, 33)
MCHC *g/dl*	34 (32, 36)	33 (32, 35)	*34 (32, 35)*	34 (32, 35)	33 (32, 35)	34 (32, 36)	34 (32, 35)
Leukocytes (WBC) × 10^9/l	6.4 (3.9, 10.4)	**7.4 (4.3, 11.4)*****	*6.33 (2.7, 12.7)*	6.74 (3.91, 9.26)	**7.8 (4.49, 10.89)*****	5.45 (3.9, 10.4)	**6.4 (4.3, 11.4)****
Segmented neutrophils × 10^9/l	3.05 (1.95, 7.1)	**4.37 (1.9, 7.69)*****	*3.29 (0.9, 8.9)*	3.12 (1.95, 5.88)	**4.58 (1.92, 7.69)*****	2.7 (2, 7.1)	**3.4 (1.9, 7.1)****
Band neutrophils × 10^9/l	0.1 (0, 0.3)	0.1 (0, 0.3)	*0.1 (0, 0.3)*	0.1 (0.1, 0.3)	**0.1 (0.1, 0.2)***	0.1 (0, 0.2)	0.1 (0, 0.3)
Eosinophils × 10^9/l	0.22 (0.08, 0.65)	0.2 (0.05, 0.6)	*0.27 (0.08, 0.66)*	0.23 (0.1, 0.53)	0.19 (0.05, 0.5)	0.21 (0.08, 0.65)	0.25 (0.1, 0.6)
Basophils × 10^9/l	0.04 (0.01, 0.15)	**0.06 (0.02, 0.12)***	*0.06 (0.02, 0.13)*	0.05 (0.03, 0.15)	0.06 (0.02, 0.12)	0.04 (0.01, 0.07)	**0.06 (0.02, 0.07)****
Monocytes × 10^9/l	0.32 (0.2, 0.66)	0.37 (0.1, 0.68)	*0.39 (0.19, 0.58)*	0.34 (0.20, 0.66)	0.38 (0.24, 0.68)	0.3 (0.2, 0.5)	0.3 (0.1, 0.5)
Lymphocytes × 10^9/l	2.06 (1.1, 3.58)	2.05 (1.2, 3.3)	*1.94 (0.91, 3.14)*	2.22 (1.22. 3.58)	**1.98(1.31, 2.86)***	1.85 (1.1, 2.6)	**2.15 (1.2, 3.3)***
Thrombocytes × 10^9/l	239 (153, 418)	**246 (159, 452)****	*235 (170, 409)*	232.5 (153, 341)	239 (159, 346)	269 (160, 418)	**275 (170, 452)****

Data are median (minimum, maximum); *$p<0.05$, **$p<0.01$, ***$p<0.001$ compared to baseline values;
[a]Significantly more intra-individual decreases than increases from baseline.

in bronchial asthma subjects, we also report a significant elevation of absolute and relative peripheral neutrophil numbers after allergen challenge. This reflects a first-line innate immune system response and supports the assumption that allergic rhinitis, like asthma, is a systemic condition [3,39].

Taken together, we report significant peripheral blood cell dynamics as a non-classical parameter in acute allergic airways disease; in line with published data we confirm that white blood cells counts, specifically segmented neutrophils, significantly rise upon specific respiratory allergen challenge in human allergic rhinitis subjects. However, we consider the decrease in erythrocytes upon allergen challenge in sensitized mice as well as in human subjects as the most significant and novel result of our study. This finding may explain the profound systemic impairment of patients upon to specific and non-specific antigen inhalation.

Supporting Information

Figure S1 Nebulization of allergic mice with the allergen increases local and systemic Th2 mRNA cytokine levels. **(A)** IL-4, **(B)** IL-5 and **(C)** IL-13 mRNA levels from spleens (left) and lungs (right) of challenged mice. Naïve organs served as negative controls. Data are presented by boxplots (median, quartiles, minimum and maximum) and n = 5 mice/group. *, $p<0.05$.

Figure S2 Schematic protocol flow chart for allergen challenge in grass pollen-sensitized allergic rhinitis subjects, compared to the mouse model (A), and blood sampling after 4 h (*group 1*) (B) or 2 h (*group 2*) (C) of continuous allergen exposure.

Figure S3 Changes in peripheral blood cell counts in subjects after allergen challenge. **(A)** White blood cells count and especially **(B)** total segmented neutrophils are significantly elevated after airway challenge. Data are represented by boxplots (median and quartiles) and n = 42. ***, $p<0.001$ respectively.

Acknowledgments

We would like to thank Franziska Ganzert and Erika Bajna for their excellent technical assistance.

Author Contributions

Conceived and designed the experiments: EJJ. Performed the experiments: JW TN MW PL RS RZ. Analyzed the data: GJ JW MM HF EJJ. Contributed reagents/materials/analysis tools: HF JGC RZ EJJ. Wrote the paper: GJ JW EJJ.

References

1. Pawankar R, Bunnag C, Khaltaev N, Bousquet J (2012) Allergic Rhinitis and Its Impact on Asthma in Asia Pacific and the ARIA Update 2008. World Allergy Organ J 5: S212–217.
2. Bousquet J, Schunemann HJ, Samolinski B, Demoly P, Baena-Cagnani CE, et al. (2012) Allergic Rhinitis and its Impact on Asthma (ARIA): achievements in 10 years and future needs. J Allergy Clin Immunol 130: 1049–1062.
3. Bousquet J, Khaltaev N, Cruz AA, Denburg J, Fokkens WJ, et al. (2008) Allergic Rhinitis and its Impact on Asthma (ARIA) 2008 update (in collaboration with the World Health Organization, GA(2)LEN and AllerGen). Allergy 63 Suppl 86: 8–160.
4. Bousquet J, Jeffery PK, Busse WW, Johnson M, Vignola AM (2000) Asthma. From bronchoconstriction to airways inflammation and remodeling. Am J Respir Crit Care Med 161: 1720–1745.
5. Bazaraa HM, El Houchi S, Rady HI (2012) Profile of patients visiting the pediatric emergency service in an Egyptian university hospital. Pediatr Emerg Care 28: 148–152.
6. McCusker CT (2004) Use of mouse models of allergic rhinitis to study the upper and lower airway link. Curr Opin Allergy Clin Immunol 4: 11–16.
7. Yukselen A, Kendirli SG, Yilmaz M, Altintas DU, Karakoc GB (2012) Correlation between nasal eosinophils and nasal airflows in children with asthma and/or rhinitis monosensitised to house dust mites. Allergol Immunopathol (Madr).
8. Epstein MM (2006) Are mouse models of allergic asthma useful for testing novel therapeutics? Exp Toxicol Pathol 57 Suppl 2: 41–44.
9. Wallmann J, Epstein MM, Singh P, Brunner R, Szalai K, et al. (2010) Mimotope vaccination for therapy of allergic asthma: anti-inflammatory effects in a mouse model. Clin Exp Allergy 40: 650–658.
10. Waldegrave W (1986) Directive CEE. J Officiel Communautés. 1–28.
11. Forkert PG (1995) CYP2E1 is preferentially expressed in Clara cells of murine lung: localization by in situ hybridization and immunohistochemical methods. Am J Respir Cell Mol Biol 12: 589–596.
12. Wegmann M, Fehrenbach H, Fehrenbach A, Held T, Schramm C, et al. (2005) Involvement of distal airways in a chronic model of experimental asthma. Clin Exp Allergy 35: 1263–1271.
13. Pali-Scholl I, Yildirim AO, Ackermann U, Knauer T, Becker C, et al. (2008) Anti-acids lead to immunological and morphological changes in the intestine of BALB/c mice similar to human food allergy. Exp Toxicol Pathol 60: 337–345.
14. Global Initiative for Asthma (GINA) NH, Lung and Blood Institute (NHLBI) Bethesda (MD); (2006) Global strategy for asthma management and prevention.
15. Everhart RS, Smyth JM, Santuzzi AM, Fiese BH (2010) Validation of the Asthma Quality of Life Questionnaire with momentary assessments of symptoms and functional limitations in patient daily life. Respir Care 55: 427–432.
16. Canonica GW, Bousquet J, Mullol J, Scadding GK, Virchow JC (2007) A survey of the burden of allergic rhinitis in Europe. Allergy 62 Suppl 85: 17–25.
17. Mojtabavi N, Dekan G, Stingl G, Epstein MM (2002) Long-lived Th2 memory in experimental allergic asthma. J Immunol 169: 4788–4796.
18. Corry DB, Folkesson HG, Warnock ML, Erle DJ, Matthay MA, et al. (1996) Interleukin 4, but not interleukin 5 or eosinophils, is required in a murine model of acute airway hyperreactivity. J Exp Med 183: 109–117.
19. Galli SJ, Tsai M, Piliponsky AM (2008) The development of allergic inflammation. Nature 454: 445–454.
20. Mitchell J, Dimov V, Townley RG (2010) IL-13 and the IL-13 receptor as therapeutic targets for asthma and allergic disease. Curr Opin Investig Drugs 11: 527–534.
21. Erin EM, Zacharasiewicz AS, Nicholson GC, Tan AJ, Higgins LA, et al. (2005) Topical corticosteroid inhibits interleukin-4, -5 and -13 in nasal secretions following allergen challenge. Clin Exp Allergy 35: 1608–1614.
22. Zieglmayer PU (2013) Are results of environmental exposure units transferable to real-life exposure? Curr Opin Allergy Clin Immunol.
23. Horak F, Zieglmayer P, Zieglmayer R, Lemell P, Devillier P, et al. (2009) Early onset of action of a 5-grass-pollen 300-IR sublingual immunotherapy tablet evaluated in an allergen challenge chamber. J Allergy Clin Immunol 124: 471–477, 477 e471.
24. Horak F, Jager S, Berger U (1992) Onset and duration of the effects of three antihistamines in current use–astemizole, loratadine and terfenadine forte–studied during prolonged, controlled allergen challenges in volunteers. J Int Med Res 20: 422–434.
25. Park YJ, Repka-Ramirez MS, Naranch K, Velarde A, Clauw D, et al. (2002) Nasal lavage concentrations of free hemoglobin as a marker of microepistaxis during nasal provocation testing. Allergy 57: 329–335.
26. Kiefmann R, Rifkind JM, Nagababu E, Bhattacharya J (2008) Red blood cells induce hypoxic lung inflammation. Blood 111: 5205–5214.
27. Compalati E, Ridolo E, Passalacqua G, Braido F, Villa E, et al. (2010) The link between allergic rhinitis and asthma: the united airways disease. Expert Rev Clin Immunol 6: 413–423.
28. Gopalan AV, Govindan UT, Govindaraj M (1983) Asthma and chronic bronchitis: contrasting changes in body weight and hematocrit values during recovery from acute episodes. J Asthma 20: 53–55.
29. Przybilla B, Ring J, Enders F, Winkelmann H (1991) Stigmata of atopic constitution in patients with atopic eczema or atopic respiratory disease. Acta Derm Venereol 71: 407–410.
30. Scano G, Stendardi L (2006) Dyspnea and asthma. Curr Opin Pulm Med 12: 18–22.
31. Krishnamurthy D, Starkl P, Szalai K, Roth-Walter F, Diesner SC, et al. (2012) Monitoring neutrophils and platelets during casein-induced anaphylaxis in an experimental BALB/c mouse model. Clin Exp Allergy 42: 1119–1128.
32. Monteseirin J (2009) Neutrophils and asthma. J Investig Allergol Clin Immunol 19: 340–354.
33. Takeyama K, Agusti C, Ueki I, Lausier J, Cardell LO, et al. (1998) Neutrophil-dependent goblet cell degranulation: role of membrane-bound elastase and adhesion molecules. Am J Physiol 275: L294–302.
34. Nadel JA, Takeyama K, Agusti C (1999) Role of neutrophil elastase in hypersecretion in asthma. Eur Respir J 13: 190–196.
35. Westin U, Lundberg E, Wihl JA, Ohlsson K (1999) The effect of immediate-hypersensitivity reactions on the level of SLPI, granulocyte elastase, alpha1-antitrypsin, and albumin in nasal secretions, by the method of unilateral antigen challenge. Allergy 54: 857–864.
36. Pelikan Z (2011) Delayed asthmatic response to bronchial challenge with allergen-mediators, eicosanoids, eosinophil and neutrophil constituents in the blood and urine. Respiration 82: 225–236.
37. Pelikan Z (2012) Cellular Profiles in Peripheral Blood Accompanying Particular Asthmatic Response Types. International Journal of Clinical Medicine 3: 485–497.
38. Fransson M, Benson M, Wennergren G, Cardell LO (2004) A role for neutrophils in intermittent allergic rhinitis. Acta Otolaryngol 124: 616–620.
39. Togias A (2004) Systemic effects of local allergic disease. J Allergy Clin Immunol 113: S8–14.

9

Comparative Effectiveness of Homoeopathic vs. Conventional Therapy in Usual Care of Atopic Eczema in Children: Long-Term Medical and Economic Outcomes

Stephanie Roll[1]*, Thomas Reinhold[1], Daniel Pach[1], Benno Brinkhaus[1], Katja Icke[1], Doris Staab[2], Tanja Jäckel[1], Karl Wegscheider[3], Stefan N. Willich[1], Claudia M. Witt[1,4]

1 Institute for Social Medicine, Epidemiology, and Health Economics, Charité University Medical Centre, Berlin, Germany, **2** Department of Paediatric Pulmonology and Immunology, Charité University Medical Centre, Berlin, Germany, **3** Department of Medical Biometry and Epidemiology, University Medical Centre, Hamburg-Eppendorf, Germany, **4** Centre for Integrative Medicine, University of Maryland School of Medicine, Baltimore, Maryland, United States of America

Abstract

Background: One in five children visiting a homeopathic physician suffers from atopic eczema.

Objectives: We aimed to examine the long-term effectiveness, safety and costs of homoeopathic vs. conventional treatment in usual medical care of children with atopic eczema.

Methods: In this prospective multi-centre comparative observational non-randomized rater-blinded study, 135 children (48 homoeopathy, 87 conventional) with mild to moderate atopic eczema were included by their respective physicians. Depending on the specialisation of the physician, the primary treatment was either standard conventional treatment or individualized homeopathy as delivered in routine medical care. The main outcome was the SCORAD (SCORing Atopic Dermatitis) at 36 months by a blinded rater. Further outcomes included quality of life, conventional medicine consumption, safety and disease related costs at six, 12 and 36 months after baseline. A multilevel ANCOVA was used, with physician as random effect and the following fixed effects: age, gender, baseline value, severity score, social class and parents' expectation.

Results: The adjusted mean SCORAD showed no significant differences between the groups at 36 months (13.7 95% CI [7.9–19.5] vs. 14.9 [10.4–19.4], $p = 0.741$). The SCORAD response rates at 36 months were similar in both groups (33% response: homoeopathic 63.9% vs. conventional 64.5%, $p = 0.94$; 50% response: 52.0% vs. 52.3%, $p = 0.974$). Total costs were higher in the homoeopathic versus the conventional group (months 31–36 200.54 Euro [132.33–268.76] vs. 68.86 Euro [9.13–128.58], $p = 0.005$).

Conclusions: Taking patient preferences into account, while being unable to rule out residual confounding, in this long-term observational study, the effects of homoeopathic treatment were not superior to conventional treatment for children with mild to moderate atopic eczema, but involved higher costs.

Editor: Monica da Silva Nunes, Universidade Federal do Acre (Federal University of Acre), Brazil

Funding: Funding source: Robert Bosch Foundation (grant number 12.5.1060.0083.1). The funders had no role in study design, data collection and analysis, decision to publish, or preparation of the manuscript.

Competing Interests: The authors have declared that no competing interests exist.

* E-mail: stephanie.roll@charite.de

Introduction

Comparative Effectiveness Research (CER) is a growing field in health care research; it has considerable potential to inform stakeholders on decision-making. Different definitions for CER have been published. In this paper we use the working definition as established by the Institute of Medicine (IOM) Committee, which defines CER as "the generation and synthesis of evidence that compares the benefits and harms of alternative methods to prevent, diagnose, treat, and monitor a clinical condition or to improve the delivery of care". The purpose of CER is to assist consumers, clinicians, purchasers, and policy makers to make informed decisions that will improve health care at both the individual and population levels [1]. CER is especially valuable for disorders that are most common and most costly to society, have the highest morbidity rates and have a great degree of variation in the treatment of the disorder [2].

Atopic eczema is a chronic inflammatory skin disease associated with pruritus, which occurs predominantly in children [3,4]. Atopic eczema, as well as other atopic diseases, has become even more prevalent in Western industrialized countries in recent years, affecting around 7 to 8% children aged 6 to 7 and 13 to 14 with current eczema symptoms, and up to 22 to 25% worldwide [4]. The nationwide population-based German Health Interview and Examination Survey for Children and Adolescents (KIGGS) found a life-time prevalence of 13% and a point prevalence of 7% for atopic eczema in children and adolescents [5].

Atopic eczema can impose great burden on both the child's and their parents' overall wellbeing and has relevant economic impact on both the individual and to society [6,7] with estimated annual costs of 1.1 to 3.6 Billion Euro [8,9] in Germany alone.

Complementary medicine is increasingly asked for in the treatment of atopic eczema, as well as other allergic conditions [10–12]. Homoeopathy, for example, is widely used in Germany for treating atopic eczema, although official guidelines do not recommend it. Data from a cohort study showed that one in five children who sought a homoeopathic medical doctor suffer from atopic eczema [13]. However, very little data on the efficacy or effectiveness of homoeopathy for eczema is available. A meta-analysis on homeopathy included nine dermatological studies, none of which looked specifically at atopic eczema [14]. A small randomized, placebo-controlled trial could not show a superior effect of individualized homeopathic treatment over placebo [15]. In addition, most trials focus on the short-term effects, however this yields little insight into the longer treatment options for this chronic condition.

A comparative effectiveness research study (ADEV study) was performed to examine the effectiveness, safety and cost of homoeopathic vs. conventional treatment in usual care of children with atopic eczema taking patient preferences into account [16].

Children were included and followed between January 2005 and October 2009. The primary endpoint of the study was a symptom score after six months (SCORAD; SCORing-Atopic-Dermatitis). Those results (including a follow-up after 12-months) have already been published [16]. After six and 12 months homoeopathic treatment was not superior to conventional treatment and higher costs were observed in the homoeopathic compared to the conventional group.

Information on the long-term effects is of great interest, especially for chronic conditions. Thus, the aim of the present analysis was to describe the effectiveness and the costs involved in the long-term follow-up after 36 months.

Materials and Methods

Study Design and Participants

Children were recruited from January 2005 to June 2006 in Berlin, Germany for this non-randomized prospective multicentre open comparative observational study. Data was collected up until October 2009 for the long-term follow-up, allowing a total observation period of 36 months per patient. Children and their parents were recruited at either homoeopathic or conventional doctors' practices and had already made their own choice of therapy. Thus, the parents' preference towards treatment of atopic eczema generated the groups to be compared. The recruitment of homoeopathic doctors was through the association of homoeopathic doctors in Berlin, while doctors for conventional treatment (paediatricians or dermatologists) were chosen from address lists or by recommendation. Further methods of this study have been described in detail previously [16]. Inclusion and exclusion criteria, intervention details and outcome measures are summarized in Fig. 1. The study was compliant with Good Epidemiological Practice (GEP) and applicable data-protection laws. Oral and written informed consent was obtained from the parent accompanying the child after verbal information about the study was provided by the physician. The signed consent form was sent to the central study center, and a copy was kept at the physician's office. The study and the consent procedure were approved by the Ethics Committee of the Charité-Universitätsmedizin Berlin, Germany.

Study Procedures

At baseline, a conventional case history, screening and recruitment took place at the physicians' practice before the patients were enrolled in the study. Patients were then asked to complete a questionnaire on socio-demographic characteristics, outcome measures, and adverse events. The main outcome was the SCORAD (SCORing-Atopic-Dermatitis) score, which includes the rating of the extent and intensity of AD, as well as subjective items on pruritus and sleeplessness. To reduce bias, the SCORAD was centrally assessed by two specially trained staff members who were blinded of the treatment group. Patients were asked to respect the blinding of the rater. Each patient was assigned to one rater only for the whole study period to ensure intra-rater stability. After the central rating had taken place, patients could visit their respective physician and start with either the homoeopathic case history taking and the subsequent individualised treatment or the conventional treatment. The children's physicians documented the treatment over a 12 months period. To reflect usual care, patients visited their physician whenever needed. At each visit, data was obtained by filling out questionnaires and ratings. For the final three-year follow-up, all patients that had attended at least one of the prior follow-up visits (at six or 12 months) were invited. After 36 months no follow-up data was retrieved from the physicians.

Economic Analysis

The cost-comparison analysis was made from a societal perspective and was performed from a diagnosis specific view (only costs with direct relation to atopic eczema were considered). We summarized costs for 12 months before study onset (months −12 to months 0), and for the following 6 month periods after study onset: 1–6 months, 7–12 months and 31–36 months, where available. Data on resource consumption such as hospital stays, use of medication and days on sick leave were obtained from the patient questionnaires and diaries. Costs of days spent in hospitals were based on the appropriate dermatological German DRGs. The cost of medication was based on consumed units and package prices. If this data was not available, daily defined dosage [17] was multiplied by the number of days of intake. Outpatient visits were valued by multiplying the number of visits and the mean contact-costs depending on the physician's profession (data provided by the Association of German Statutory Health Insurance Physicians). For the follow-up between months 31 and 36, the costs were discounted by 3% per year. For the first 12 months of the study, the costs incurred due to visits to the ADEV-study physician were directly extracted from the doctors' documentation. For the long-term follow-up for the months 31 to 36, no physicians' documentation was available. The mean cost values from the respective treatment group at months 7–12 were used for those patients who documented that they still visited their study physician. As a post-hoc sensitivity analysis we calculated the costs for these visits in months 31 to 36 for the treatment group to be 40% of the costs at months 7–12, as there is evidence for a reduction in costs in homoeopathic treatments over time [18].The cost for patients who had no further contact with their ADEV-study physician was valued at 0€.

Indirect costs were calculated by adopting the human capital approach. In cases of disease-related absence from work, the indirect costs were measured according to the parents' income level.

Inclusion criteria

- children (aged 1-14 years) with atopic eczema
- disease duration at least 6 months
- fulfilling 3 out of 4 Williams' criteria [30, 31]
- Three Item Severity (TIS) Score: 2-7 (mild/moderate symptoms [32])

Exclusion criteria

- other dermal disease, or severe medical or psychological disease
- oral or intravenous corticosteroids during the last 3 months
- psychotherapy, allergy desensitization, or additional complementary therapy during the last 3 months

Treatments

Homoeopathic group

- classical homoeopathy defined as a homoeopathic case history taking and a prescription of a single remedy according to the simile law
- emollient creams were recommended
- corticosteroids were reserved for rescue medication only

Conventional group

- routine treatment according to German guidelines

Outcomes

Main outcome

- SCORAD (SCORing Atopic Dermatitis; evaluated outcome measure for atopic eczema [33-35])

Other outcomes

- self-rated skin condition, pruritus, sleep disturbance, general well being (by visual analogue scale (VAS) from 0 to 100)
- parents' quality of life [36, 37]
- childrens' quality of life (CDLQI: Children Dermatology Life Quality Index; validated for age 3 to 16) [38]
- use of conventional medicine
- response rates
- safety measures
- disease related costs

Figure 1. Description of inclusion and exclusion criteria, treatments and outcome measures.

Statistics

Statistical analyses were based on the intention-to-treat (ITT) principle, including all patients with baseline values who received treatment and with assessed outcome using multilevel models (analysis of covariance (ANCOVA) or generalized estimating equations (GEE)). In these models, physicians were considered random effect and fixed effects were: baseline value (continuous), Three item severity (TIS) Score (continuous), social class (high, average, low), parents' expectation of a good outcome (high, low), children's age (continuous) and gender (male/female). Results are presented as adjusted mean or proportion with a standard error (SE) and/or 95% confidence interval (CI). All tests were exploratory and two-sided with a level of significance of 5%. Adverse events and intake of corticosteroids of different potency groups [19] were analyzed descriptively by frequencies, percentages and by Chi-squared or Fisher's exact test (if feasible). As a sensitivity analysis, analysis was additionally performed with replacing missing outcome data by the last observation carried forward (LOCF) method.

As a post-hoc analysis on a subset of patients with SCORAD data available for all time points, a repeated measures ANCOVA for differences to baseline of SCORAD values was used to test if changes over time were different for the two groups (time by group effect).

The nonparametric bootstrapping method was used to generate a picture of variability around the arithmetic mean for the cost-effectiveness analyses. The original sample was bootstrapped 1000 times in order to obtain 1000 means for costs and effect differences. Each bootstrap sample was adjusted for confounding variables as previously described.

For detailed description and sample size calculation, see the previously published article [16]. Statistical analyses were performed according to a predefined statistical analysis plan using PASW Statistics 18.0 (SPSS Chicago, IL) and SAS for Windows, version 9.2 (SAS Institute, Cary, NC, USA).

Results

Population

135 children were included into the study and analyzed in the primary analysis after 6 months (mean age 4.01±2.97 (SD), 48% girls, conventional group n = 87, homeopathic group n = 48, Table 1). Children were recruited by 26 physicians experienced in the treatment of atopic eczema in children (10 homoeopaths and 16 conventional doctors). For details on the doctors'

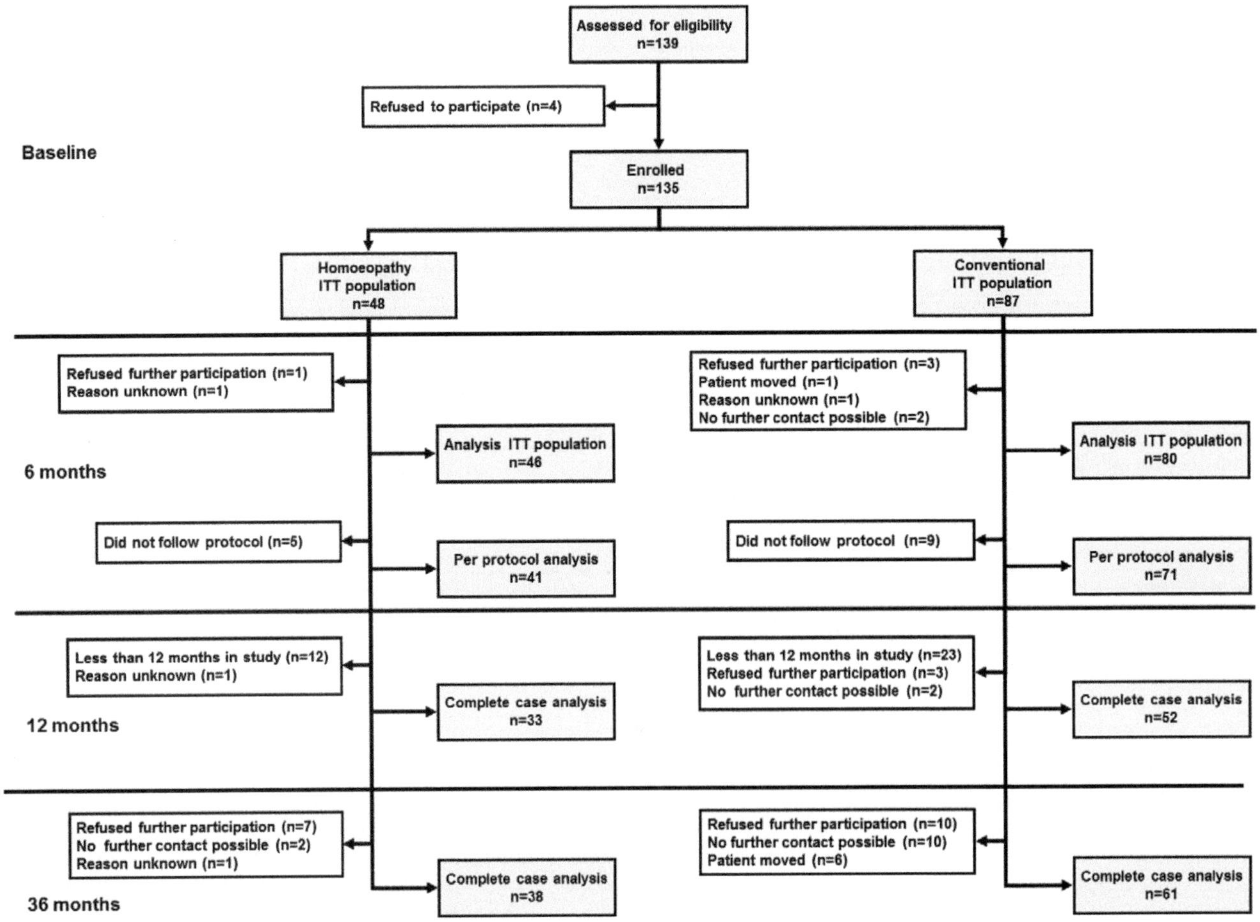

Figure 2. Trial flow chart (ITT: intention to treat).

specialisations please see the previously published article [16]. After 36 months, data from 99 participants (38 in the homeopathic and 61 in the conventional group) were available (Fig. 2). Reasons for missing follow-up data included refusal of further participation, relocation, or not contactable.

Patient preferences resulted in the following baseline differences: patients in the homeopathic group showed more severe SCORAD scores and a trend to a longer symptom duration, while the TIS score was higher in the conventional group. On average, the parents of the homoeopathic group were older, had a higher income level and were better educated, i.e. had a higher social status than the parents of the conventional group (Table 1). In addition, higher baseline costs in the homoeopathic group were seen. These differences in baseline characteristics were similar for the patients who were still available to be assessed at 36 months.

Outcome Parameters

After 36 months the primary outcome parameter SCORAD showed no significant differences between groups: homeopathy group 13.68±2.91 (adjusted mean±SE) 95% CI [7.88–19.48] vs. conventional group 14.90±2.25 [10.41–19.40], $p = 0.741$) (Table 2, Fig. 3). When replacing missing SCORAD values at 36 months by LOCF as a sensitivity analysis, results remained similar (homeopathy group 13.29±2.51 [8.30–18.28] vs. conventional group 15.24±1.92 [11.43–19.05], $p = 0.541$). Neither the SCORAD at six or 12 months [29] nor the SCORAD subscales showed significant differences (Table 2; and Witt et.al [16]).

No significant overall group effect was found between homoeopathy and conventional treatment in the repeated measures analysis when analyzing SCORAD differences to baseline for the subset of patients with SCORAD data available for all time points ($p = 0.908$). However, SCORAD values in general decreased significantly over time ($p<0.001$). This change in time seemed different for the two groups with a faster improvement in the conventional treatment group at 6 months, and a catching up of the homoeopathy group after 12 months ($p = 0.055$, Fig. 4).

No significant differences could be observed at any time point for adjusted response rates based on SCORAD values. At 36 months a 33% response (defined as an improvement of at least 33% in the SCORAD) of 63.9% was seen in the homoeopathic and 64.5% in the conventional group ($p = 0.949$). A 50% response was seen at 36 months in 52.0% of patients in the homoeopathic and 52.3% of patients in the conventional group ($p = 0.974$).

At 36 months the quality of life of the children and parents was similar in both groups in the short and long-term (Table 2).

Conventional Treatment

At 36 months the frequency of daily basic skin care was reduced compared to baseline, and comparable in both groups, as was the number of different medications (including corticosteroids and antihistamines) according to the patients' documentation (Table 2).

Table 1. Baseline characteristics of study participants.

	Homoeopathy			Conventional			
	n	mean±SD or n (%)	Median	n	mean±SD or n (%)	Median	P-value
PATIENTS							
Age (years)	48	4.3±2.9	4.0	87	3.9±3.0	3.0	0.300
Gender female	48	26 (54.2%)		87	39 (44.8%)		0.369
Siblings	47	1.1±1.0	1.0	84	1.0±1.2	1.0	0.530
Symptom duration (years)	48	3.5±2.6	3.0	86	2.9±2.7	2.0	0.057
Treatment duration (years)	46	3.0±2.7	2.0	83	2.7±2.9	1.0	0.364
Additional atopic disease							
Allergic rhinitis	47	4 (8.5%)		84	8 (9.5%)		1.000
Allergic asthma	47	2 (4.3%)		84	8 (9.5%)		0.330
Food allergy	47	10 (21.3%)		84	10 (11.9%)		0.205
Other	47	6 (12.8%)		84	8 (9.5%)		0.568
Allergy test	48	21 (43.8%)		87	36 (41.4%)		0.856
Allergen positive	19	11 (57.9%)		30	14 (46.7%)		0.561
Three item severity score (TIS) (0–9)[a]	48	3.8±1.6	3.0	87	4.5±1.5	4.0	0.010
Therapy for AE during previous 12 months							
Basic skin care	47	40 (85.1%)		84	73 (86.9%)		0.795
Avoidance of certain food	47	25 (53.2%)		84	33 (39.3%)		0.144
Alternative therapies	47	19 (40.4%)		84	3 (3.6%)		<0.001
Drug therapy	47	42 (89.4%)		84	71 (84.5%)		0.598
Number of different medications	47	2.2±1.7	2.0	84	2.3±1.9	2.0	0.852
Corticosteroids	47	12 (25.5%)		84	40 (47.6%)		0.016
Topical calcineurin inhibitors	47	18 (38.3%)		84	26 (31.0%)		0.443
Antihistamines	47	9 (19.1%)		84	18 (21.4%)		0.825
SCORAD Total score[b]	48	31.3±14.1	30.9	87	22.8±13.4	19.9	0.001
SCORAD Extent	48	18.7±19.4	13.3	87	12.9±16.0	7.0	0.066
SCORAD Intensity	48	6.1±2.7	6.5	87	4.1±2.6	3.0	<0.001
SCORAD Subjective symptoms	48	6.1±4.6	5.0	87	5.9±5.0	5.0	0.856
Children's QoL CDLQI[c]	28	3.8±2.6	3.5	49	4.8±3.6	4.0	0.189
ACCOMPANYING PARENT							
Age (years)	47	36.7±6.1	36.0	84	32.7±6.3	32.5	<0.001
Gender female	47	41 (87.2%)		84	76 (90.5%)		0.568
Single parent	47	7 (14.9%)		84	21 (25.0%)		0.192
Education	47			84			<0.001
A-level		31 (66.0%)			22 (26.2%)		
University, College		20 (42.6%)			13 (15.5%)		
Net income per month	38			61			<0.001
<2000 Euro		16 (42.1%)			41 (67.2%)		
2000–4000 Euro		18 (47.4%)			20 (32.8%)		
>4000 Euro		4 (10.5%)			0 (0.0%)		
Social class	47			84			<0.001
Low		2 (4.3%)			29 (34.5%)		
Middle		17 (36.2%)			34 (40.5%)		
High		28 (59.6%)			21 (25.0%)		
Parents' QoL[d]							
Psychosomatic wellbeing	47	65.0±20.9	69.4	84	64.4±21.3	69.4	0.890
Effects on social life	47	87.2±16.7	91.7	84	84.6±15.4	87.5	0.384
Confidence in medical treatment	45	62.8±21.6	60.0	84	67.4±18.1	65.0	0.195

Table 1. Cont.

Emotional coping	47	72.9±19.3	75.0	84	71.7±21.5	75.0	0.762
Acceptance of the disease	46	70.4±22.1	75.0	84	68.6±24.4	75.0	0.682
Expected symptom improvement (0–6)[e]	46	4.4±1.2	4.0	83	3.8±1.2	4.0	0.013
Costs during 12 months before study [in EURO]		**mean±SD**	**95% CI**		**mean±SD**	**95% CI**	
Medication	48	119.5±146.5	77.0;162.1	87	109.6±150.7	77.5;141.7	0.493
Hospital	48	22.6±156.2	−22.8;67.9	87	12.4±81.6	−5.0;29.8	0.950
Physician contact	48	86.6±68.0	66.9;106.4	87	102.3±95.0	82.1;122.6	0.190
Medical aids and adjuvant therapies	48	254.6±563.2	91.0;418.1	87	113.5±264.2	57.1;169.8	0.032
Indirect costs	48	134.0±460.9	0.2;267.9	87	32.2±105.1	9.8;54.5	0.527
Total	48	617.3±841.2	373.0;861.6	87	370.0±380.8	288.8;451.1	0.164

[a]high score = high intensity;
[b]<25 mild, 25–50 moderate, >50 severe disease;
[c]high score = low QoL (only children of age 3 to 16 could be questioned, because CDLQI was only validated for that age group);
[d]high score = high QoL;
[e]0 = not sure, 6 = very sure;
AE: atopic eczema, QoL: quality of life, SD: standard deviation, CI: confidence interval.

One patient (2.6%) in the homoeopathic group and one patient (1.6%) in the conventional group took corticosteroids of the weak group (group I according [19]), while one patient (1.6%) in the in the conventional group took moderately potent corticosteroids (group II). Three patients (7.9%) in the homoeopathic and 11 patients (18.0%) in the conventional group took potent corticosteroids (group III). Details of the homeopathic treatment within the first 12 months of the study have previously been described [16].

Subgroups

Considering only patients still treated by the study doctor they have chosen at study start at 36 months (n = 62), SCORAD values showed no differences between the groups (homeopathic 14.28±3.46, 95% CI [7.36–21.21] vs. conventional group 15.89±2.72 [10.46–21.33], p = 0.722). Similar results were found for patients no longer receiving study therapy at 36 months (n = 33) (homeopathic 12.26±4.17 [3.92–20.60] vs. conventional group 14.33±3.09 [8.16–20.50], p = 0.686). A test of interaction (effect modification) from still receiving study therapy was not significant (p = 0.937).

Adverse Events

The number of patients reporting adverse events at 36 months was similar in both groups. Two patients (5.3%) in the homoeopathy group and five (8.2%) in the conventional group reported adverse events (p = 0.704). The following eight adverse events were reported in the homoeopathy group: pruritus (n = 2),

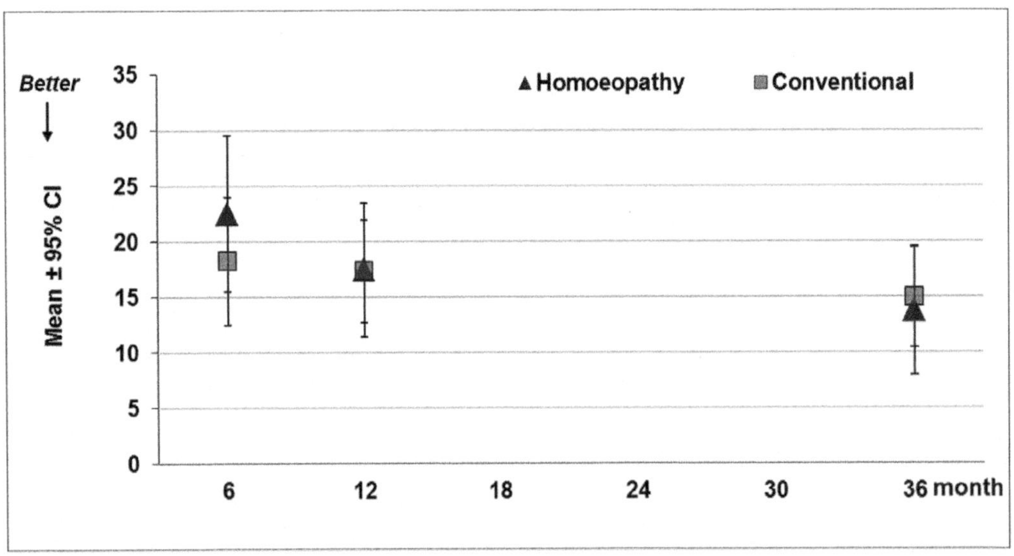

Figure 3. SCORAD at 6, 12 and 36 months, adjusted mean ±95% confidence interval (CI) per group from multilevel models (ANCOVA) with fixed effects age, gender, baseline value, TIS-score, social status, expectation of the parents, and random effect physician (lower values indicate lower disease severity).

Table 2. Intention to treat analyses of SCORAD and secondary outcomes at 36 months (adjusted means or proportions and confidence intervals (CI) from multilevel models (ANCOVA or GEE) with fixed effects age, gender, baseline value, TIS-score, social status, expectation of the parents, and random effect physician).

	Homoeopathy n = 37		**Conventional n = 61**		
	Mean	**95% CI**	**Mean**	**95% CI**	**P-value**
PATIENTS					
SCORAD Total score[a]	13.7	7.9–19.5	14.9	10.4–19.4	0.741
SCORAD Extent	5.0	2.1–7.8	3.4	1.1–5.8	0.406
SCORAD Intensity	3.1	1.9–4.4	3.4	2.4–4.3	0.777
SCORAD Subjective symptoms	2.0	0.8–3.2	2.3	1.4–3.3	0.682
Children's QoL CDLQI (0–30)[b]	2.2	1.4–3.4	1.8	1.2–2.8	0.627
Different medications per patient	0.7	0.4–1.4	0.7	0.5–0.9	0.904
Other physician visits	1.7	0.4–3.0	1.5	0.5–2.4	0.754
MEDICATION (31–36 months)	Proportion of patients (%)	95% CI	Proportion of patients (%)	95% CI	P-value
Corticosteroids	9.5	2.9–27.1	10.2	3.8–24.8	0.889
Topical calcineurin inhibitors	n.c.	n.c.	n.c.	n.c.	n.c.
Antihistamines	1.3	0.2–10.9	4.0	1.7–9.1	0.304
Basic skin care	66.9	53.0–78.4	61.0	50.0–70.9	0.557
Still treated by study doctor	71.7	47.6–87.6	62.9	50.1–74.0	0.5068
ACCOMPANYING PARENT	Mean	95% CI	Mean	95% CI	P-value
Parents' QoL[c]					
Psychosomatic wellbeing	82.4	76.8–88.0	77.1	73.0–81.1	0.136
Effects on social life	94.8	91.8–97.9	94.1	91.8–96.5	0.726
Confidence in medical treatment	77.7	71.1–84.3	77.5	72.7–82.4	0.959
Emotional coping	87.0	81.1–92.8	85.0	80.8–89.2	0.597
Acceptance of the disease	83.3	76.0–90.6	84.0	78.4–89.6	0.869
COSTS (31–36 months)					
Medication	36.0	7.3–64.7	36.7	14.4–59.1	0.969
Hospital	n.c.	n.c.	n.c.	n.c.	n.c.
Physician contact	119.8	95.1–144.5	45.4	27.5–63.4	<0.001
Study doctor	83.8	63.8–103.9	17.1	0.8–33.5	<0.001
Other physicians	35.1	12.8–57.5	26.6	10.3–43.0	0.546
Medical aids and adjuvant therapies	53.0	18.6–87.3	16.1	0.0–41.0	0.093
Indirect costs	9.3	0.0–22.1	1.9	0–11.7	0.369
Total costs	217.0	154.1–279.9	99.9	53.7–146.1	0.005

[a]<25: mild, 25–50: moderate, >50: severe disease.
[b]higher scores refer to lower QoL.
[c]higher scores refer to higher QoL.
SCORAD: Scoring atopic dermatitis; CDLQI: Children Dermatology Life Quality Index; QoL: quality of life; CI: confidence interval, n.c.: not computable.

burning sensation (1), reddening (1), dry skin/flaky skin (2), burns (1), herpes zoster (1); and 12 adverse events in the conventional group: pruritus (3), burning sensation (3), reddening (2), dry skin/flaky skin (3), and allergic reaction (1). The number of adverse events reported was also similar in the two groups at six and 12 months, with one child in the conventional group needing hospitalisation due of a worsening of the atopic eczema with additional streptococcal infection [16].

Economic Analyses

Economic data from the patients' questionnaires were available for 135 patients at baseline and for 98 patients for the study period from 31 to 36 months. During the 12 months before baseline costs were 617.28 Euro 95%CI [373.02–861.55] in the homoeopathic group and 369.96 Euro [288.80–451.13] in the conventional group ($p = 0.164$, Table 1).

Cost-comparison analyses

Significant total cost differences were found at the long-term follow-up from 31 to 36 months after baseline (homoeopathic group: 216.99 Euro [154.12–279.87]; conventional group: 99.93 Euro [53.75–146.12], $p = 0.004$; Table 2). The respective physician's contacts were one of the main cost drivers (homoeopathic group: Euro 119.77 [95.06–144.49]; conventional group: Euro 45.44 [27.48–63.41], $p<0.001$), particularly contacts with the study doctor (homoeopathic group: 83.84 Euro [63.84–103.85];

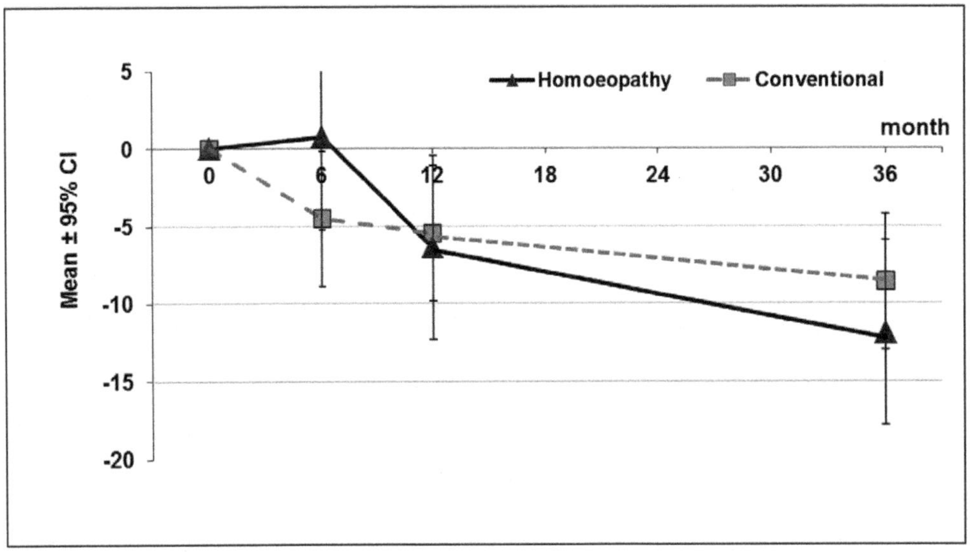

Figure 4. SCORAD differences to baseline at 6, 12, and 36 months, adjusted mean ±95% confidence interval (CI) per group from repeated measures multilevel model with time and time-by-group interaction and fixed effects age, gender, baseline value, TIS-score, social status, expectation of the parents, and random effect physician; post-hoc analysis on complete cases (patients with SCORAD data available for all time points); lower mean values indicate greater improvement.

conventional group: 17.12 Euro [0.75–33.49], $p<0.001$). In the sensitivity analysis the total costs were 183.17 Euro [119.65–246.69] in the homoeopathic, and 100.18 Euro [53.19–147.17] in the conventional group ($p = 0.043$).

Discussion

In this observational comparative effectiveness study, no significant long-term outcome differences were seen after 36 months in children with atopic eczema when treated conventionally compared to homoeopathic treatment; neither were short-term differences seen (at six or 12 months [16]). Both groups substantially improved during the observation period and in both groups every tenth patient used corticoids. Patients in the conventional groups showed a trend towards earlier improvements. Costs, however, were higher in the homoeopathic group.

The design of the study (observational, usual-care and multi-centre setting) allows evaluation of a therapy's comparative effectiveness considering the patients' own preferences and therapy choices. In our study the treatment was individualised and to reflect a more realistic care additional medication was not forbidden. Data collection was performed using a variety of sources including the affected child, their parents, study doctors and external blinded raters, to improve the objectivity and validity of the study outcomes.

The aim of this study was to reflect the real world situation and to compare conventional and homeopathic care provided by physicians in a usual care setting. Thus, we chose to take patients' and/or parents' therapy preferences into account, making randomisation not possible. The observational design resulted in relevant baseline differences between the two groups. In the homoeopathic group severity of disease appeared higher compared to the conventional group. Eczema conditions according to the SCORAD were less favourable (especially the intensity and extent of atopic eczema) and the disease duration was longer. In addition, parents in the homoeopathic group were older, had a higher social class background and a higher treatment expectation. To take baseline differences into account, we adjusted our analyses for these factors. However, it is possible that other unknown and unmeasured factors might have influenced the results. If other confounding factors were present but not accounted for, or if the performed adjustments were not sufficient (e.g. due to broad value categories or measurement error), residual confounding might be present. If adjustments did not sufficiently balance disease severity, then results might be biased in favour of either the conventional or the homoeopathic group. Therefore, the non-randomised design is a clear limitation of our study regarding the internal validity of our results [16].

At six, 12 and 36 months SCORAD severity was comparable in both groups, although patients in the conventional group took more conventional medication in the first year, e.g. corticosteroids, antihistamines or pimecrolimus and tacrolimus [16]. Baseline use of pimecrolimus and tacrolimus was comparable in both groups, in contrast to less use of corticosteroids in the homoeopathic group than in the conventional group. While at six months, the use of these anti-inflammatory drugs was lower in the homoeopathic group, after 36 months around ten percent of patients in both groups used corticoids. Overall medication use decreased during the trial in both groups compared to baseline values. In both groups the frequency of basic skin care was comparable. However when interpreting these results, one should also take into account that atopic eczema can improve spontaneously in young children.

Although disease specific costs in both groups appear lower in the third year compared to the first year, the long-term costs were more than twice as high in the homeopathy group compared to the conventional group. Costs were mainly driven by doctors' fees and paying for medical aids. As described in the methods section, the mean costs during months 7–12 of the study were used to estimate the costs for the outpatient contact at the long-term follow-up for the main analysis. We chose this method as it also seems to be a conservative approach, in assuming that the intensity of medical contact (especially for homeopathic treatment) is much higher during the first year of treatment, and that the use of these costs for estimating follow-up expenditures might lead to an overestimation of costs. Data from another prospective observational study that included 3981 patients with different diagnoses showed that children with atopic eczema [18] visited their homeopathic doctor between month 7–12 40% more often (1.5±1,7 times) than a year later (0.9±1.2 times in months 19–24). These findings were used as the basis for a sensitivity analysis, resulting still in higher costs in the homoeopathic group.

The substantial and statistically significant cost-differences between the groups found during the first year of treatment were stable over time. The follow-up between 31 and 36 months lead to a comparable result compared to the analysis in the first year. While interpreting these differences, potential limitations should be kept in mind, particularly in regard to how the outpatient costs were estimated. Within the 31–36 months follow-up detailed therapeutic documentation was not available. However, the method of calculating the outpatient costs during the first year of the study was based on this kind of documentation.

Conclusion

In this long-term observational study after three years, while unable to rule out residual confounding but taking patient preferences into account, treatment at homoeopathic doctors was similar, yet not superior to treatment at conventional doctors for children with mild to moderate atopic eczema, but still had higher costs.

Acknowledgments

We would like to thank Beatrice Eden for her excellent performance at the study office, data collection, and rating. We also thank Angelina Bockelbrink for drafting the background section of the manuscript.

Author Contributions

Conceived and designed the experiments: CMW BB SNW. Performed the experiments: CMW BB DP DS TJ. Analyzed the data: SR TR KI KW. Wrote the paper: SR TR DP BB KW DS TJ KI SNW CMW.

References

1. Committee on Comparative Effectiveness Research Prioritization (2009) What is Comparative Effectiveness Research? In: Institute of Medicine, ed. Initial National Priorities for Comparative Effectiveness Research. Washington D.C.: The National Academies Press. 29.
2. Fineberg H (2009) Foreword. In: Institute of Medicine, ed. Initial National Priorities for Comparative Effectiveness Research. Washington D.C.: The National Academies Press.
3. Hoare DY, Wan Po AL, Williams H (2000) Systematic Review of treatment of atopic eczema. Health Technol Assess 4: 1–191.
4. Odhiambo JA, Williams HC, Clayton TO, Robertson CF, Asher MI (2009) Global variations in prevalence of eczema symptoms in children from ISAAC Phase Three. J Allergy Clin Immunol 124: 1251–1258.
5. Schlaud M, Atzpodien K, Thierfelder W (2007) Allergische Erkrankungen. Bundesgesundheitsblatt - Gesundheitsforschung - Gesundheitsschutz 50: 701–710.
6. Emerson RM, Williams HC, Allen BR (2001) What is the cost of atopic dermatitis in preschool children? Br J Dermatol 144: 514–522.
7. Herd RM (2002) The financial impact on families of children with atopic dermatitis. Arch Dermatol 138: 819–820.
8. Augustin M, Zschocke I (2001) Lebensqualität und Ökonomie bei allergischen Hauterkrankungen. Allergologie 24: 433–442.
9. Szucs T (1995) Sozioökonomische Aspekte der Neurodermitis in Deutschland. In: Riedl-Seifert R, ed. Expert Report zu Bufexamac. München: 49–66.
10. Anderson P, Dinulos JG (2009) Atopic dermatitis and alternative management strategies. Current Opinion in Pediatrics 21: 131–138.
11. Keil T, Witt CM, Roll S, Vance W, Weber K, et al. (2008) Homoeopathic versus conventional treatment of children with eczema: a comparative cohort study. Complement Ther Med 16: 15–21.
12. Schäfer T, Riehle A, Wichmann HE, Ring J (2002) Alternative medicine in allergies - prevalence, patterns of use, and costs. Allergy 57: 694–700.
13. Becker-Witt C, Lüdtke R, Weisshuhn TE, Willich SN (2004) Diagnoses and treatment in homeopathic medical practice. Forsch Komplementärmed Klass Naturheilkd 11: 98–103.
14. Linde K, Clausius N, Ramirez G, Melchart D, Eitel F, et al. (1997) Are the clinical effects of homeopathy placebo effects? A meta-analysis of placebo-controlled trials. Lancet 350: 834–843.
15. Siebenwirth J, Lüdtke R, Remy W, Rakoski J, Borelli S, et al. (2009) Wirksamkeit einer klassisch-homöopathischen Therapie bei atopischem Ekzem. Forsch Komplementärmed Klass Naturheilkd 16: 315–323.
16. Witt CM, Brinkhaus B, Pach D, Reinhold T, Wruck K, et al. (2009) Homoeopathic versus Conventional Therapy for Atopic Eczema in Children: Medical and Economic Results. Dermatology 219: 329–340.
17. Schwabe U, Paffrath D (2007) Arzneiverordnungsreport 2007 - Aktuelle Daten, Kosten, Trends und Kommentare. Heidelberg: Springer.
18. Witt CM, Lüdtke R, Willich SN (2009) Homeopathic treatment of children with atopic eczema: a prospcective observational study with 2 years follow-up. Acta Derm Venereol 89: 182–183.
19. WHO Collaborating Centre for Drug Statistics Methodology. Available from: www.whocc.no/atc_ddd_index/?code=D07A. Accessed at 16-7-22012.

Nasal Epithelial Cells Can Act as a Physiological Surrogate for Paediatric Asthma Studies

Surendran Thavagnanam[4]◔, Jeremy C Parker[1]◔, Michael E McBrien[2], Grzegorz Skibinski[1], Michael D Shields[1,3]*¶, Liam G Heaney[1]¶

1 Centre for Infection and Immunity, Queen's University Belfast, Belfast, Northern Ireland, United Kingdom, 2 Department of Anaesthetics, Royal Victoria Hospital, Belfast Health and Social Care Trust, Belfast, Northern Ireland, United Kingdom, 3 Department of Paediatrics, Royal Belfast Hospital for Sick Children, Belfast Health and Social Care Trust, Belfast, Northern Ireland, United Kingdom, 4 Paediatric Department, University Malaya Medical Centre, Kuala Lumpar, Malaysia

Abstract

Introduction: Differentiated paediatric epithelial cells can be used to study the role of epithelial cells in asthma. Nasal epithelial cells are easier to obtain and may act as a surrogate for bronchial epithelium in asthma studies. We assessed the suitability of nasal epithelium from asthmatic children to be a surrogate for bronchial epithelium using air-liquid interface cultures.

Methods: Paired nasal and bronchial epithelial cells from asthmatic children (n = 9) were differentiated for 28 days under unstimulated and IL-13-stimulated conditions. Morphological and physiological markers were analysed using immunocytochemistry, transepithelial-electrical-resistance, Quantitative Real-time-PCR, ELISA and multiplex cytokine/chemokine analysis.

Results: Physiologically, nasal epithelial cells from asthmatic children exhibit similar cytokine responses to stimulation with IL-13 compared with paired bronchial epithelial cells. Morphologically however, nasal epithelial cells differed significantly from bronchial epithelial cells from asthmatic patients under unstimulated and IL-13-stimulated conditions. Nasal epithelial cells exhibited lower proliferation/differentiation rates and lower percentages of goblet and ciliated cells when unstimulated, while exhibiting a diminished and varied response to IL-13.

Conclusions: We conclude that morphologically, nasal epithelial cells would not be a suitable surrogate due to a significantly lower rate of proliferation and differentiation of goblet and ciliated cells. Physiologically, nasal epithelial cells respond similarly to exogenous stimulation with IL-13 in cytokine production and could be used as a physiological surrogate in the event that bronchial epithelial cells are not available.

Editor: Brian Knoll, University of Houston, United States of America

Funding: This study was funded by Northern Ireland Chest Heart and Stroke Association and Surendran Thavagnanam was employed on an Irish Thoracic Soceity/Boehringer Ingleheim Fellowship. The funders had no role in study design, data collection and analysis, decision to publish, or preparation of the manuscript.

Competing Interests: Liam G. Heaney received grant funding from Medimmune, Novartis UK, Roche/Genentech Inc, and Glaxo Smith Kline, has taken part in Advisory Boards and given lectures at meetings supported by Glaxo Smith Kline, Merck Sharpe & Dohme, Nycomed, Boehringer Ingelheim, Novartis and Astra Zeneca. Michael David Shields has received support funding to attend International Respiratory meetings (Astra Zeneca, Chiesi, Novartis, Boehringer Ingelheim and Glaxo Smith Kline) and has taken part in asthma clinical trials (GSK, Schering Pough and Roche/Genentech) for which his Institution was remunerated. Michael David Shields has received honoraria for speaking at educational events from GlaxoSmithKline (GSK), MerckSharp&Dohme (MSD), Novartis, AstraZeneca, Alk Abello. Over the last 5 years Michael David Shields has received sponsorship to attend the ERS and EAACI annual meetings from GSK, MSD, AstraZeneca, Novartis, Alk Abello.

* E-mail: m.shields@qub.ac.uk

◔ These authors contributed equally to this work.

¶ These authors also contributed equally to this work.

Introduction

Airway epithelial cells not only provide a physical barrier to potentially harmful insults but they also play a significant role in the first line of immunological defence. There is increasing evidence that allergic diseases such as asthma are associated with epithelial disorders and, furthermore, that a primary abnormality of the airway epithelium may be central to disease causation [1,2]. Chronic inflammation and airway remodelling are the main characteristics of asthma however they have been observed to occur in young children before asthma has become firmly established [3,4]. In asthma, bronchial epithelial airway remodelling is characterised by goblet cell hyperplasia, reduced ciliated cell numbers and mucus hypersecretion [5], defective repair and proliferation [6], increased basal cell number [7] and impaired barrier function [8,9].

Differentiated ALI cultures using the Transwell system have recently been shown to be an authentic model representing the airway epithelium *ex vivo* [10]. Differentiated ALI cultures from healthy subjects displayed a polarised pseudostratified multi-layered epithelium comprising basal, ciliated and goblet cells whereas cultures from asthmatic subjects displayed a dysfunctional epithelium consistent with the asthmatic airway *in vivo* [5]. The cultures closely mimic *in vivo* airway epithelial physiology in terms of cilia coverage and cilial beating, mucus production and formation of intact tight junctions [5,11].

Samples from the lower airways in children can be obtained at the time of clinically indicated bronchoscopy but it is difficult to justify sampling the lower airways in otherwise healthy control children and in those with milder disease. The nasal epithelium therefore represents an attractive alternative although it is unclear how well the nasal epithelium represents the bronchial epithelium in paediatric asthma. According to the 'united airway concept' there is a close connection between the upper and lower airways [12–16]. This suggests that changes found in the nasal epithelium might mirror similar changes occurring in the lower airways. The link between allergic rhinitis and asthma has been underlined by epidemiological and clinical studies [12–16] which suggest that upper airway inflammation may reflect and provide an additional insight into lower airway involvement. Devalia *et al* have demonstrated that adult human nasal and bronchial epithelial cells cultured *in vitro* resemble the cells *in vivo* [17]. These studies involved using samples from adults and extrapolating data from adult studies cannot accurately represent the paediatric epithelium, especially since functional differences exist between adult and paediatric epithelium [18]. Several studies have shown similar morphology and response to cytokine stimulation between nasal and bronchial epithelium using submerged monolayer cultures, which only poorly represents the epithelium [19,20]. Differentiated ALI cultures on the other hand are more authentic and can be analysed for markers of differentiation including MUC5AC (the major mucus-forming mucin) and SAM-pointed domain containing Ets-transcription factor (SPDEF) (a transcription factor in the goblet cell hyperplasia pathway) production as well as for goblet and ciliated cells and tight junction formation. As a result the differentiated ALI culture model is the most appropriate platform with which to conduct a comparison of paired nasal and bronchial differentiated ALI cultures.

In this study we aimed to compare the morphological and physiological profiles of nasal differentiated ALI cultures (PNECs) with bronchial differentiated ALI cultures (PBECs) under basal unstimulated and IL-13 stimulated conditions to determine the ability of PNECs to act as an *in vitro* surrogate for PBECs in asthma studies.

Methods

Subjects

Children less than 12 years of age (mean age 7.2 years [range: 1 to 12 years]) attending elective surgical procedures at the Royal Belfast Hospital for Sick Children were recruited. A doctor administered pro-forma was used to record the clinical history. Of the nine children with atopic asthma, defined as recurrent wheezing within the last year, 5 children had asthma plus allergic rhinitis and 4 children had asthma plus eczema but no allergic rhinitis (Table 1).

Ethics Statement

Written informed parental consent was obtained. This study was approved by the Office of the Research Ethics Committees of Northern Ireland (ORECNI).

Isolation of PBECs and PNECs

Primary bronchial epithelial cells were obtained from asthmatic children as previously described [21]. Nasal brushings were performed by rotating an endocervical brush in each nostril. Asthmatic PBECs and asthmatic PNECs were cultured as previously described [5]. All brush washings were analysed for viruses using a multi-viral PCR analysis and only uncontaminated cultures were used [22].

Differentiated ALI culture

ALI cultures (n = 9) were grown as previously described [5,11]. Briefly, cells from subjects used in this study were grown at ALI at passage 2 for 28 days. At confluence, ALI was created by removing the apical medium and restricting the culture feeding to the basolateral compartment. The culture medium was changed on alternate days during which the cells differentiated over 28 days to ensure full differentiation as assessed by the presence of beating cilia and mucus on the apical surface of the cultures. We sampled 12 patients in total however 3 of the cultures either did not proliferate due to lack of cells from the initial sample or they did not form a 100% confluent monolayer prior to differentiation and so were rejected from the study.

Stimulation of PBECs and PNECs with IL-13

Following the establishment of ALI, cells were fed basolaterally on alternate days with ALI medium [5] supplemented with recombinant human IL-13 (PeProTech EC Ltd, UK) at 20 ng/ml throughout the duration of the cultures (28 days) starting at day 0 ALI [11,23–30].

Transepithelial Electrical Resistance measurements (TEER)

We used TEER as a measure of 'tight junction' formation in epithelial cultures [31]. TEER was measured weekly using an EVOM meter (World Precision Instruments, FL, USA) [5,11].

Immunocytochemistry (ICC) for goblet and ciliated cell markers

Cytospin slides were made for the detection of goblet and ciliated cells from PBEC and PNEC cultures [5,11]. Negative controls were subjected to routine conditions with the omission of the primary antibody. The results are expressed as the percentage differential goblet or ciliated cell count corrected for cell number from 3 slides per stain per insert per patient.

RNA extraction and Quantitative Real-time PCR for MUC5AC and SPDEF mRNA

RNA extraction and cDNA synthesis were carried out using the RNeasy Mini kit (Qiagen, Crawley, UK) and First Strand cDNA Synthesis Kit (AMV) (Roche, UK) according to the manufacturer's protocol. Quantitative Real time PCR was carried out as previously described [11].

Measurement of MUC5AC secreted apically using ELISA

Production of MUC5AC secreted mucin in the apical washes from PBECs and PNECs was measured as previously described [5,11] using an adapted in-house MUC5AC ELISA [32]. We used mouse monoclonal antibody to MUC5AC [45M1] clone (Abcam, UK) as the primary antibody and Goat anti-mouse IgG HRP secondary antibody (Jackson Laboratories, USA) for detection of primary antibody binding. Results are expressed as the optical density corrected for MUC5AC positive control.

Table 1. Patient details including clinical status and clinical atopy.

Clinical Status	Clinical Atopy (assessed by questionnaire)	Serum IgE Concentration (kU/L)	Age (y)	Gender (M/F)	Treatment
Asthmatic	Allergic Rhinitis, Allergic Conjunctivitis	2258	6	M	ICS/LABA, LTA
Asthmatic	Eczema	154	7	M	ICS/LABA
Asthmatic	Eczema	446	4	F	SABA, when required
Asthmatic	Eczema, Allergic Rhinitis	5158	12	M	ICS/LABA
Asthmatic	Allergic Rhinitis	101	9	M	ICS/LABA
Asthmatic	Eczema	10	2	M	ICS, SABA
Asthmatic	Eczema	627	7	M	ICS/LABA
Asthmatic	Eczema, Allergic Rhinitis	100	11	M	ICS
Asthmatic	Allergic Rhinitis	40	1	M	ICS

Current treatment abbreviations are classed as follows: inhaled corticosteroid (ICS), long-acting beta agonist (LABA), short-acting beta agonist (SABA) and leukotriene antagonist (LTA).

Cytokine Analysis

Apical washings and basolateral supernatants from unstimulated and IL-13-stimulated PBECs and PNECs were analyzed using a 27-plex bead array assay (Bio-Plex Pro Human Cytokine 27-plex) (BioRad, UK) as per manufacturers' instructions. Results are only shown for analytes that were within the limits of detection (IL-1rα, IL-6, IL-7, IL-8, IL-12p70, granulocyte colony–stimulating factor (G-CSF), granulocyte macrophage colony-stimulating factor (GM-CSF), interferon gamma-induced protein 10 (IP-10), monocyte chemoattractant protein-1 (MCP-1), regulated upon activation, normal T cell expressed and secreted (RANTES) and vascular endothelial growth factor (VEGF).

Statistical Analysis

Comparisons between PBECs and PNECs were made using paired t-tests and repeated measures ANOVA, with logarithmic transformation where appropriate. Cytokine concentrations were corrected for total cell number (pg/cell) and then the fold change in cytokine secretion following IL-13 stimulation was compared with unstimulated cytokine secretion (IL-13-stimulated/unstimulated). These results were then plotted on a log axis due to the varying ranges of all analytes involved. Individual cytokine profiles are included as supplemental data (Figures S1, S2, S3, S4, S5, S6) along with additional detail on all of the mentioned methods in the online data supplement (Methods S1).

Results

It is unlikely given the number of passages the cells go through along with the length of time from sampling to completion of culture (7–10 weeks) that there would be any carry-over effect of inhaled corticosteriods in the following results.

TEER

We detected no overall differences in TEER values over time under unstimulated conditions between PBECs and PNECs [Figure 1A]. In contrast, following IL-13 stimulation, there was a significant difference in TEER values on days 7 ($p = 0.02$) & 14 ($p = 0.02$) between PBECs and PNECs with the difference in resistance becoming similar by days 21 & 28 [Figure 1B].

Total Cell Count

On day 28 we found a significantly higher total cell number between PBECs [mean 5.7×10^5 cells/ml (SD 1.2)] and PNECs [mean 3.4×10^5 cells/ml (SD 0.8), ($p = 0.002$)] under unstimulated conditions [Table 2]. However there was no significant difference in the total cell number under IL-13 stimulated conditions [PBECs [mean 5.3×10^5 cells/ml (SD 0.9); PNECs: mean 4.2×10^5 cells/ml (SD 1.1)] [Table 2]. All subsequent results have been adjusted for total cell number.

Goblet Cell Quantification

IL-13 stimulation resulted in a similar increase in the percentage of goblet cells in both PBECs [43.3% (SD 18.1), $p = 0.0036$] and PNECs [19.4% (SD 4.0), $p = 0.0001$] compared with unstimulated controls [PBEC: 27.1% (SD 18.4); PNEC: 8.4% (SD 2.4)] [Figure 2]. In addition there was a significant difference in goblet cell percentage between PNEC unstimulated and PBEC unstimulated [8.4% (SD 2.4) versus 27.1% (SD 18.4) respectively, $p = 0.033$] and PNEC IL-13 stimulated and PBEC IL-13 stimulated [19.4% (SD 4.0) versus 43.3% SD (18.1) respectively, $p = 0.009$].

Real Time PCR

SPDEF mRNA was higher in IL-13 stimulated PNECs ($p = 0.013$) and IL-13 stimulated PBECs ($p = 0.02$) compared with unstimulated PNECs and PBECs demonstrating a similar response to exogenous stimulation between PBECs and PNECs [Figure 3A]. However under IL-13 stimulation there was a similar level of MUC5AC mRNA between stimulated and unstimulated PNECs whereas IL-13 stimulated PBECs had higher levels of MUC5AC mRNA than unstimulated PBECs ($p = 0.04$) [Figure 3B].

Measurement of MUC5AC secreted apically using ELISA

Under IL-13 stimulation similar quantities of apically secreted mucin were measured between PNECs and PBECs [Figure 3C].

Ciliated Cell Quantification

IL-13 stimulated PBECs had lower ciliated cell numbers than unstimulated PBECs [5.9% (SD 1.6) versus 14.8% (SD 2.5) respectively, $p = 0.005$] which was not observed between PNEC IL-13 stimulated and PNEC unstimulated [2.8% (SD 3.4) versus 3.5% (SD 1.7) respectively] [Figure 4]. There was a significant difference between PBEC unstimulated and PNEC unstimulated [14.8% (SD 2.5) versus 3.5% (SD 1.7) respectively, $p = 0.0001$] [Figure 4]. In addition there was a significant difference between PBEC IL-13 stimulated and PNEC IL-13 stimulated [5.9% (SD 1.6) versus 2.8% (SD 3.4) respectively, $p = 0.002$] [Figure 4].

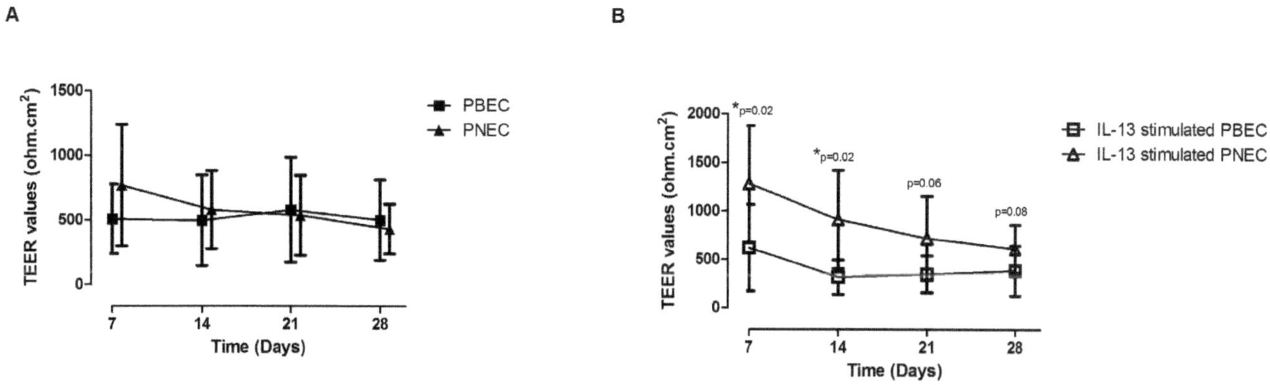

Figure 1. Measurement of Transepithelial Electrical Resistance (TEER). A - TEER of unstimulated PNECs and PBECs cultured for 28 d. Values are expressed as mean ± SD. No significant difference was observed in the TEER values between the groups. B - TEER of PNECs and PBECs cultured with 20 ng/ml IL-13 for 28 d. Values are expressed as mean ± SD. On days 7 and 14 there was a significant difference in TEER values between PNECs and PBECs ($p<0.02$ for each time point) however by the end of the culture period the TEER values were similar between groups.

Cytokine production from PBECs and PNECs

Analytes that were within the limits of detection were IL-1rα, IL-6, IL-7, IL-8, IL-12p70, granulocyte colony–stimulating factor (G-CSF), granulocyte macrophage colony-stimulating factor (GM-CSF), interferon gamma-induced protein 10 (IP-10), monocyte chemoattractant protein-1 (MCP-1), regulated upon activation, normal T cell expressed and secreted (RANTES) and vascular endothelial growth factor (VEGF). The fold change of apically secreted cytokines after IL-13 stimulation [Figure 5A] showed there to be no significant difference between PBECs and PNECs. Similarly, there was no significant difference in basolaterally secreted cytokines between PBECs and PNECs stimulated with IL-13 [Figure 5B] demonstrating an overall similar response to IL-13 stimulation between PNECs and PBECs. Individual cytokine secretion graphs are included in the supplementary data section of this paper.

Discussion

Nasal epithelial cells provide an attractive alternative to bronchial epithelial cells for use in asthma research due to their accessibility without the need for anaesthesia and intubation however it is unclear whether differentiated nasal ALI cultures represent the differentiated bronchial ALI cultures morphologically and physiologically. We have compared paired nasal and bronchial epithelial cells differentiated at ALI from asthmatic children in order to determine whether nasal epithelial cells can act as a surrogate for bronchial epithelial cells. We have found that PNECs exhibit different morphological features such as lower proliferation rates and differentiation of goblet and ciliated cells compared with PBECs however their physiological response of secreted cytokines to exogenous stimulation with IL-13, a key cytokine in the pathogenesis of asthma is strikingly similar when corrected for cell number.

In considering morphology, unstimulated PNECs do not exhibit the constitutive goblet cell hyperplasia seen in unstimulated PBECs [5]. This is to be expected as asthma is a lower airways disease. Mouse models of allergic rhinitis have reported that a goblet cell hyperplasia may only exist following stimulation with ovalbumin [33,34] or TGF-β [35]. IL-13 has been shown to increase goblet cell hyperplasia in non-asthmatic and asthmatic paediatric bronchial epithelium [11] and in this study we have shown that PNECs also respond with a goblet cell increase to IL-13 stimulation along with a significant increase in SAM-pointed domain-containing Ets-like factor (SPDEF) mRNA which is implicated in the goblet cell hyperplasia pathway [36]. Miyahara and colleagues found that although IL-13 is a major contributor to the late nasal response it did not induce a goblet cell hyperplasia [37] however our data is at odds with this finding. The IL-13 mediated reduction of ciliated cells in PBECs is not observed with IL-13 stimulation in PNECs however.

In a previous study by McDougall *et al.* which compared bronchial and nasal epithelial monolayers from adults and children they found the cells to look morphologically similar [19]. However, differentiated nasal ALI cultures display notable morphological differences when compared with the differentiated bronchial ALI cultures which could not have been detected in submerged monolayer cultures. We found that PNECs did not proliferate or differentiate at the same rate as PBECs with a significant lower total cell number at the end of the culture period

Table 2. Total cell count on day 28 of ALI culture.

Sample	Mean number of cells (×10^5 cells/ml)	Standard Deviation	P value	Treatment
PBEC(A)	5.7	1.2	0.002	Unstimulated
PNEC(A)	3.4	0.8		Unstimulated
PBEC(A)	5.3	0.9	>0.05	20 ng/ml IL-13
PNEC(A)	4.2	1.1		20 ng/ml IL-13

Under unstimulated conditions there were significant differences between PBECs and PNECs ($p=0.002$). However under IL-13 stimulated conditions there were no significant differences between the same groups.

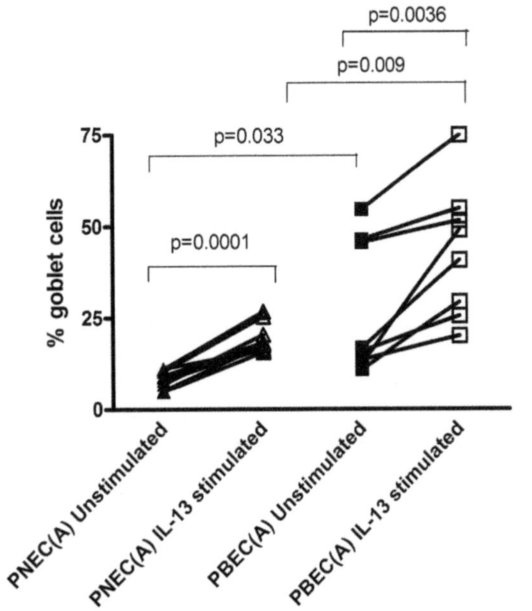

Figure 2. Quantification of Goblet Cell Number. Number of goblet cells from PNECs and PBECs treated with 20 ng/ml IL-13 expressed as the percentage differential goblet cell count corrected for cell number on d 28 of ALI culture. Comparisons of average values between groups were performed using paired t-tests. There was a significant difference seen between unstimulated and IL-13 stimulated PNECs (p = 0.0001) and in IL-13 stimulated PBECs when compared to unstimulated PBECs (p = 0.0036). Additionally, there was a significant difference between PNEC unstimulated and PBEC unstimulated (p = 0.033) and when cells where stimulated with IL-13, the percentage of goblet cells was significantly higher in stimulated PBECs compared to stimulated PNECs (p = 0.009).

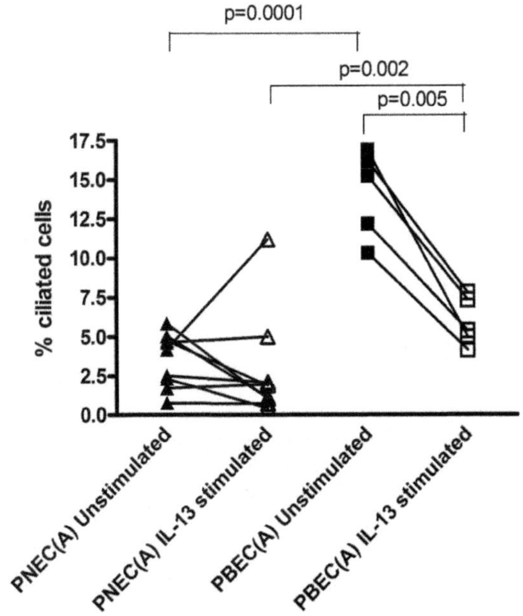

Figure 4. Quantification of Ciliated Cells. Number of ciliated cells from PNECs and PBECs treated with 20 ng/ml IL-13 expressed as the percentage differential ciliated cell count corrected for cell number on d 28 of ALI culture. Comparisons of average values between groups were performed using paired t-tests. In unstimulated conditions, PBEC cultures contained a significantly higher percentage of ciliated cells than PNECs (p = 0.0001). However, when stimulated with IL-13, the percentage of ciliated cells significantly decreased in PBECs (p = 0.005), but IL-13 had no effect on ciliated cell numbers in PNECs. Additionally, IL-13 stimulated PBECs had significantly higher numbers of ciliated cells compared with IL-13 stimulated PNECs (p = 0.002).

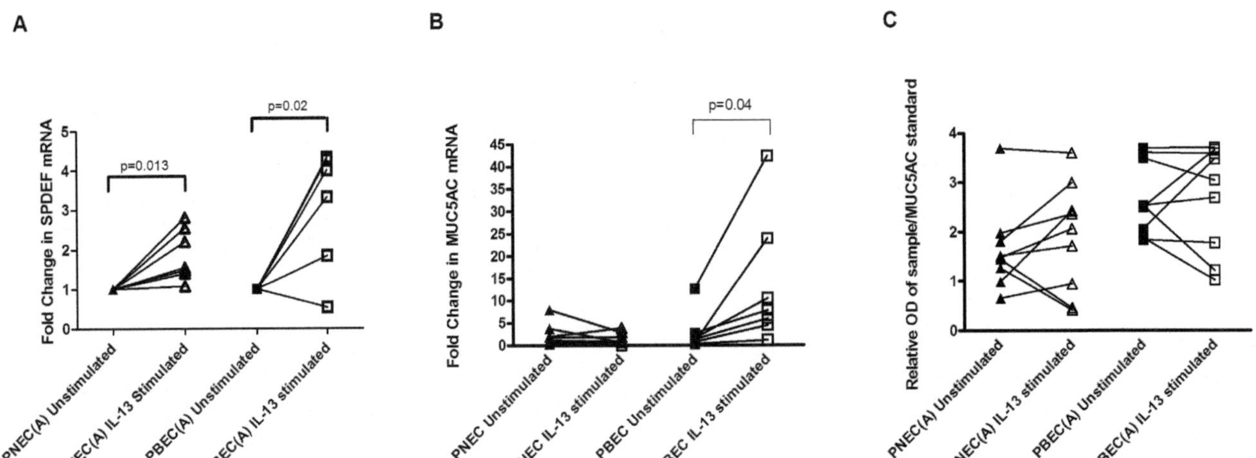

Figure 3. Gene expression of SPDEF & MUC5AC mRNA and ELISA for MUC5AC mucin secretion. A - Gene expression of SPDEF mRNA using comparative quantitation real time PCR in IL-13 stimulated PNECs and PBECs expressed as fold change compared to unstimulated cells. In both cell types, stimulation with IL-13 caused a significant increase in SPDEF mRNA levels (PNECs: p = 0.013; PBECs: p = 0.02). B - Gene expression of MUC5AC mRNA using comparative quantitation real time PCR in IL-13 stimulated PNECs and PBECs expressed as fold change compared to unstimulated cells. There was no significant increase in MUC5AC mRNA levels in PNECs, however, stimulation with IL-13 caused a significant increase in MUC5AC mRNA levels in PBECs (p = 0.04). C - Relative optical density (OD $\lambda = 450$ nm) of MUC5AC secreted apically using ELISA corrected for MUC5AC positive control. There was no significant difference between unstimulated and IL-13 stimulated PNECs or PBECs.

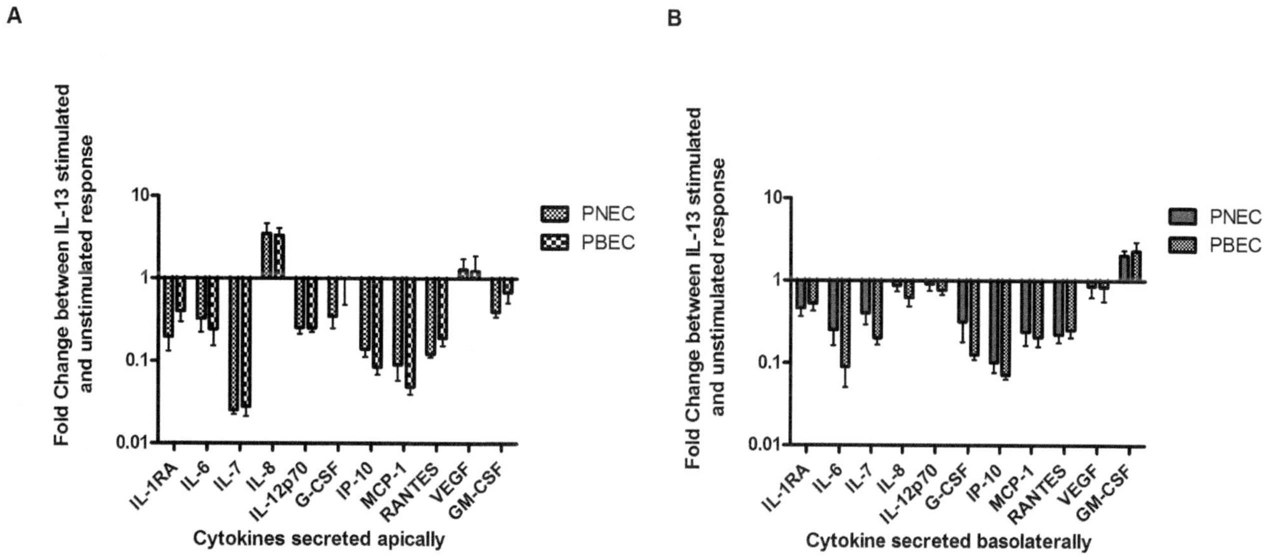

Figure 5. Cytokine Analysis of Apical Washings and Basolateral Supernatants using Bioplex. A – Apical secretion of cytokines in PBEC and PNEC cultures. Results were corrected for cell numbers and a fold change ratio was calculated (IL-13 stimulated/unstimulated). In order to graphically represent all detectable cytokines the results were plotted on a logarithmic axis. There were no significant differences in any of the detected cytokines secreted between PNECs and PBECs. B - Basolateral secretion of cytokines in PBEC and PNEC cultures. Results were corrected for cell number and a fold change ratio was then calculated (IL-13 stimulated/unstimulated). In order to graphically represent all detectable cytokines the results were plotted on a logarithmic axis. There were no significant differences in any of the cytokines secreted between PNECs and PBECs.

in addition to the differences seen in goblet and ciliated cells under basal and stimulated conditions. PBECs appeared to exhibit consistent distinct morphological changes in response to IL-13 stimulation whereas PNECs responded in a variable manner. We did however observe some similarities between PBECs and PNECs: TEER measurements, which is at odds with the TEER data generated by Lopez-Souza and colleagues [38] and MUC5AC secretion under unstimulated conditions. Taken together, morphologically there does not appear to be enough consistency between PBECs and PNECs which would suggest that for studies focussing on the morphology of the asthmatic bronchial epithelium, PNECs would not serve as an appropriate surrogate.

In considering physiological response we examined the effects of an exogenous cytokine, namely IL-13, on cytokine/mediator release from PBECs and PNECs and found a similar response profile when corrected for cell number. McDougall *et al.* found that constitutive and cytokine-stimulated release of particular cytokines (IL-6, IL-8, MMP-9 and RANTES) was significantly higher in nasal monolayer than bronchial monolayer cultures but that on further analysis nasal and bronchial epithelial cells responded in the same way showing significant correlation [19]. In a follow-up study from the same group, looking specifically at mediator release between nasal and bronchial epithelial monolayer cultures from children, Pringle and colleagues found that RANTES, MMP-9, TIMP-1, MCP-1 and VEGF were similar between nasal and bronchial monolayer cultures whereas IL-6, IL-8 and G-CSF were higher [20]. The difference in observations of MMP-9 and RANTES between the studies is proposed to be due to the first study having a mixed population of adult and paediatric epithelial cells. We demonstrated a similar finding to McDougall *et al.* and Pringle *et al.* in those cytokines from our panel that were detectable. Both PNECs and PBECs responded to IL-13 stimulation (corrected for cell numbers) in a similar manner, albeit with PNECs generally expressing higher levels of cytokine. This would suggest that physiologically for the cytokines measured, PNECs could be used as a surrogate for PBECs. Further studies would hope to confirm this observation however it would suggest that the similarities seen in monolayer mediator release are maintained throughout the differentiation process.

In a more recent study using well-differentiated paediatric asthmatic and non-asthmatic paired bronchial and nasal epithelial cells, Lopez-Guisa and colleagues also suggested that there was correlation in mediator release between PBEC and PNEC cultures [39]. This group showed TGF-β2 and VEGF to be significantly increased in asthmatic bronchial and nasal epithelium compared to non-asthmatic under unstimulated conditions. TGF-β2 and periostin were significantly up-regulated in nasal and bronchial asthmatic epithelium under unstimulated and following IL-4/IL-13 stimulation [39]. Unfortunately our study did not have a sample of non-asthmatic children to perform a similar comparison. However, our study broadly agrees with Lopez-Guisa *et al.* in terms of the similarities observed in mediator release between nasal and bronchial asthmatic epithelium.

IL-13 resulted in the reduction of the majority of cytokines, with the exceptions of IL-8 and VEGF, when secreted apically and basolaterally and GM-CSF when secreted basolaterally. Surprisingly, a number of cytokines that we expected to increase actually decreased including IL-1ra, GM-CSF and MCP-1 [40–43]. While there are various studies that have noted increases in these cytokines under stimulation with IL-13 we would add that many used different culture systems, stimulation concentrations and treatment regimens compared to our study, which may go some way to explaining the unexpected decrease in these mediators. We believe this is a true reflection of the epithelium as in both PBECs and PNECs we saw strikingly similar responses to our chronic stimulation.

Our data confirm that characteristics and responses in submerged monolayer cultures differ from differentiated ALI cultures. We believe that our differentiated ALI model authentically represents the true state of the epithelium *in vivo* [10]. A recent study by Ogilvie and colleagues, who compared paired CF nasal and bronchial epithelial brushings using microarray, found that differences in the global gene expression profiles of CF and non-CF nasal and bronchial epithelial cells existed. They recommended not using nasal epithelial cells as a surrogate for pre-screening prior to lung-directed therapies [44]. Whether nasal epithelium should be used in place of bronchial epithelium will inevitably be determined by the focus and design of future studies and with a growing literature on the many comparisons now taking place, we will be much better informed of the benefits or drawbacks of using nasal as a surrogate for bronchial epithelial cells.

Our study was limited in a number of ways. Firstly, we were unable to sample a large enough number of non-asthmatic controls to perform a comparison between health and disease. Secondly, in terms of stimulation only one cytokine (IL-13) was used due to the quantity of cells available. It would be interesting to know if other stimuli in PNECs reflect the response in PBECs. Additional studies are required to further explore the use of nasal epithelial cells as a surrogate.

In conclusion, we have demonstrated that our models of differentiated PNECs and PBECs display notable morphological differences which would question the use of PNECs as a reliable and reproducible morphological surrogate, especially in asthma where characteristic traits such as constitutive goblet cell hyperplasia are absent in PNECs from asthmatics. However, we have also demonstrated that physiologically, both PNECs and PBECs respond in the same way to stimulation with IL-13 suggesting that PNECs could be used as a physiological surrogate for PBECs in asthmatic studies in the event that bronchial epithelial cells are not available.

Supporting Information

Figure S1 Cytokine analysis of IL-1ra, IL-6, IL-7 & IL-8 secreted apically. A - Analysis of IL-1ra secreted apically using the Bioplex system. Results were corrected for cell number and absolute concentrations plotted in pg/cell. IL-13 stimulated PNECs and PBECs secreted significantly less IL-1ra compared with unstimulated PNECs ($p = 0.02$) and PBECs ($p = 0.001$). Additionally unstimulated PNECs secreted higher levels of IL-1ra compared with unstimulated PBECs ($p = 0.04$). B - Analysis of IL-6 secreted apically using the Bioplex system. Results were corrected for cell number and absolute concentrations plotted in pg/cell. IL-13 stimulated PNECs and PBECs secreted significantly less IL-6 compared with unstimulated PNECs ($p = 0.02$) and PBECs ($p = 0.01$). Additionally unstimulated PNECs secreted higher levels of IL-6 compared with unstimulated PBECs ($p = 0.04$). C - Analysis of IL-7 secreted apically using the Bioplex system. Results were corrected for cell number and absolute concentrations plotted in pg/cell. IL-13 stimulated PNECs and PBECs secreted significantly less IL-7 compared with unstimulated PNECs ($p = 0.0003$) and PBECs ($p = 0.0004$). Additionally unstimulated PNECs secreted higher levels of IL-7 compared with unstimulated PBECs ($p = 0.04$). D - Analysis of IL-8 secreted apically using the Bioplex system. Results were corrected for cell number and absolute concentrations plotted in pg/cell. IL-13 stimulated PNECs and PBECs secreted higher levels of IL-8 compared with unstimulated PNECs and PBECs however they did not reach statistical significance. Additionally IL-13 stimulated PNECs secreted higher levels of IL-8 compared with IL-13 stimulated PBECs ($p = 0.03$).

Figure S2 Cytokine analysis of IL-12p70, G-CSF, IP-10 & MCP-1 secreted apically. A - Analysis of IL-12p70 secreted apically using the Bioplex system. Results were corrected for cell number and absolute concentrations plotted in pg/cell. IL-13 stimulated PNECs and PBECs secreted significantly less IL-12p70 compared with unstimulated PNECs ($p = 0.007$) and PBECs ($p = 0.0009$). Additionally unstimulated PNECs secreted higher levels of IL-12p70 compared with unstimulated PBECs although this was not statistically significant ($p = 0.08$). B - Analysis of G-CSF secreted apically using the Bioplex system. Results were corrected for cell number and absolute concentrations plotted in pg/cell. IL-13 stimulated PNECs secreted significantly less G-CSF compared with unstimulated PNECs ($p = 0.03$). There was no significant difference between IL-13 stimulated and unstimulated PBECs. Additionally unstimulated PNECs secreted higher levels of G-CSF compared with unstimulated PBECs although this was not statistically significant. C - Analysis of IP-10 secreted apically using the Bioplex system. Results were corrected for cell number and absolute concentrations plotted in pg/cell. IL-13 stimulated PNECs and PBECs secreted lower levels of IP-10 compared with unstimulated PNECs ($p = 0.006$) and PBECs ($p = 0.01$). Additionally unstimulated PNECs secreted significantly higher levels of IP-10 compared with unstimulated PBECs ($p = 0.047$) and IL-13 stimulated PNECs secreted higher levels of IP-10 compared with IL-13 stimulated PBECs ($p = 0.04$). D - Analysis of MCP-1 secreted apically using the Bioplex system. Results were corrected for cell number and absolute concentrations plotted in pg/cell. IL-13 stimulated PNECs and PBECs secreted lower levels of MCP-1 compared with unstimulated PNECs ($p = 0.005$) and PBECs ($p = 0.01$). Additionally unstimulated PNECs secreted significantly higher levels of IP-10 compared with unstimulated PBECs ($p = 0.001$).

Figure S3 Cytokine analysis of RANTES, VEGF & GM-CSF secreted apically. A - Analysis of RANTES secreted apically using the Bioplex system. Results were corrected for cell number and absolute concentrations plotted in pg/cell. IL-13 stimulated PNECs and PBECs secreted lower levels of RANTES compared with unstimulated PNECs ($p = 0.003$) and PBECs ($p = 0.049$). Additionally unstimulated PNECs secreted significantly higher levels of RANTES compared with unstimulated PBECs ($p = 0.047$). B - Analysis of VEGF secreted apically using the Bioplex system. Results were corrected for cell number and absolute concentrations plotted in pg/cell. There was no significant difference between IL-13 stimulated PNECs and PBECs compared with unstimulated PNECs and PBECs or between PNECs and PBECs. C - Analysis of GM-CSF secreted apically using the Bioplex system. Results were corrected for cell number and absolute concentrations plotted in pg/cell. IL-13 stimulated PNECs secreted lower levels of GM-CSF compared with unstimulated PNECs ($p = 0.009$). There was no significant change in GM-CSF between IL-13 stimulated and unstimulated PBECs. Additionally unstimulated PNECs secreted significantly higher levels of GM-CSF compared with unstimulated PBECs ($p = 0.01$).

Figure S4 Cytokine analysis of IL-1ra, IL-6, IL-7 & IL-8 secreted basolaterally. A - Analysis of IL-1ra secreted basolaterally using the Bioplex system. Results were corrected for cell number and absolute concentrations plotted in pg/cell. IL-13 stimulated PNECs secreted significantly less IL-1ra compared with unstimulated PNECs ($p = 0.04$). There was no significant difference between IL-13 stimulated and unstimulated PBECs. Additionally there was no difference in IL-1ra secretion between PNECs and PBECs. B - Analysis of IL-6 secreted basolaterally using the Bioplex system. Results were corrected for cell number and absolute concentrations plotted in pg/cell. IL-13 stimulated PNECs secreted less IL-6 compared with unstimulated PNECs however, this did not reach statistical significance. There was a significant difference in IL-6 secretion between IL-13 stimulated and unstimulated PBECs ($p = 0.04$). Additionally the IL-13 stimulated PNECs secreted higher levels of IL-1ra compared with IL-13 stimulated PBECs ($p = 0.04$). C - Analysis of IL-7 secreted basolaterally using the Bioplex system. Results were corrected for cell number and absolute concentrations plotted in pg/cell. IL-13 stimulated PNECs and PBECs secreted less IL-7 compared with unstimulated PNECs ($p = 0.06$) and PBECs ($p = 0.05$) but these did not reach statistical significance. Additionally there was no significant difference in IL-7 secretion between PBECs and PNECs. D - Analysis of IL-8 secreted basolaterally using the Bioplex system. Results were corrected for cell number and absolute concentrations plotted in pg/cell. There was no significant difference in IL-8 secretion between IL-13 stimulated PNECs and PBECs compared with unstimulated PNECs and PBECs or between PNECs and PBECs.

Figure S5 Cytokine analysis of IL-12p70, G-CSF, IP-10 & MCP-1 secreted basolaterally. A - Analysis of IL-12p70 secreted basolaterally using the Bioplex system. Results were corrected for cell number and absolute concentrations plotted in pg/cell. There was no significant difference between IL-13 stimulated PNECs and PBECs compared with unstimulated PNECs and PBECs. However unstimulated PNECs secreted higher levels of IL-12p70 compared with unstimulated PBECs ($p = 0.009$). B - Analysis of G-CSF secreted basolaterally using the Bioplex system. Results were corrected for cell number and absolute concentrations plotted in pg/cell. There was no significant difference between IL-13 stimulated PNECs and PBECs compared with unstimulated PNECs and PBECs although there was a large decrease in concentration. However IL-13 stimulated PNECs secreted higher levels of IL-12p70 compared with IL-13 stimulated PBECs ($p = 0.048$). C - Analysis of IP-10 secreted basolaterally using the Bioplex system. Results were corrected for cell number and absolute concentrations plotted in pg/cell. There was no significant difference between IL-13 stimulated PNECs and PBECs compared with unstimulated PNECs and PBECs. However unstimulated PNECs secreted higher levels of IP-10 compared with unstimulated PBECs ($p = 0.009$). D - Analysis of MCP-1 secreted basolaterally using the Bioplex system. Results were corrected for cell number and absolute concentrations plotted in pg/cell. There was lower MCP-1 secretion between IL-13 stimulated PNECs and PBECs compared with unstimulated PNECs and PBECs however this did not reach statistical significance. Unstimulated PNECs secreted significantly higher levels of MCP-1 compared with unstimulated PBECs ($p = 0.003$) as did IL-13 stimulated PNECs compared with IL-13 stimulated PBECs which was close to reaching significance ($p = 0.05$).

Figure S6 Cytokine analysis of RANTES, VEGF & GM-CSF secreted basolaterally. A - Analysis of RANTES secreted basolaterally using the Bioplex system. Results were corrected for cell number and absolute concentrations plotted in pg/cell. There was no significant difference between IL-13 stimulated PNECs and PBECs compared with unstimulated PNECs and PBECs or between PNECs and PBECs. B - Analysis of VEGF secreted basolaterally using the Bioplex system. Results were corrected for cell number and absolute concentrations plotted in pg/cell. There was no significant difference between IL-13 stimulated PNECs and PBECs compared with unstimulated PNECs and PBECs or between PNECs and PBECs. C - Analysis of GM-CSF secreted basolaterally using the Bioplex system. Results were corrected for cell number and absolute concentrations plotted in pg/cell. IL-13 stimulated PNECs secreted significantly more GM-CSF compared with unstimulated PNECs ($p = 0.039$). Additionally there was no significant difference in GM-CSF secretion between IL-13 stimulated and unstimulated PBECs or between PBECs and PNECs.

Methods S1 Full descriptions of each method used in the study are provided in the supplementary methods section.

Acknowledgments

The authors would like to thank the parents and children involved for facilitating this study along with Prof. Madeleine Ennis and Dr. Bettina Schock for their critical comments on this manuscript.

Author Contributions

Conceived and designed the experiments: ST JCP GS MDS LGH. Performed the experiments: ST JCP. Analyzed the data: ST JCP MDS. Contributed reagents/materials/analysis tools: MEMcB. Wrote the paper: ST JCP MDS LGH.

References

1. Cookson W (2004) The immunogenetics of asthma and eczema: a new focus on the epithelium. Nat Rev Immunol 4(12): 978–988.
2. Holgate ST (2011) The sentinel role of the airway epithelium in asthma pathogenesis. Immunol Rev 242(1): 205–219.
3. Saglani S, Payne DN, Zhu J, Wang Z, Nicholson AG, et al. (2007) Early detection of airway wall remodeling and eosinophilic inflammation in preschool wheezers. Am J Respir Crit Care Med 176(9) 858–864.
4. Thavagnanam S, Williamson G, Ennis M, Heaney LG, Shields MD (2010) Does airway allergic inflammation pre-exist before late onset wheeze in children? Pediatr Allergy Immunol 21(7): 1002–1007.
5. Parker J, Sarlang S, Thavagnanam S, Williamson G, O'Donoghue D, et al. (2010) A 3-D well-differentiated model of pediatric bronchial epithelium demonstrates un-stimulated morphological differences between asthmatic and non-asthmatic cells. Ped Res 67:17–22.
6. Puddicombe SM, Torres-Lozano C, Richter A, Bucchieri F, Lordan JL, et al. (2003) Increased expression of p21(waf) cyclin-dependent kinase inhibitor in asthmatic bronchial epithelium. Am J Respir Cell Mol Biol 28(1): 61–68.
7. Hackett TL, Warner SM, Stefanowicz D, Shaheen F, Pechkovsky DV, et al. (2009) Induction of epithelial-mesenchymal transition in primary airway epithelial cells from patients with asthma by transforming growth factor-beta1. Am J Respir Crit Care Med 180(2): 122–133.
8. Hackett TL, Singhera GK, Shaheen F, Hayden P, Jackson GR, et al. (2011) Intrinsic phenotypic differences of asthmatic epithelium and its inflammatory responses to respiratory syncytial virus and air pollution. Am J Respir Cell Mol Biol 45(5): 1090–1100.
9. deBoer WI, Sharma HS, Baelemans SM, Hoogsteden HC, Lambrecht BN, et al. (2008) Altered expression of epithelial junctional proteins in atopic asthma: possible role in inflammation. Can J Physiol Pharmacol 86(3): 105–112.
10. Pezzulo AA, Starner TD, Scheetz TE, Traver GL, Tilley AE, et al. (2011) The air-liquid interface and use of primary cell cultures are important to recapitulate the transcriptional profile of *in vivo* airway epithelia. Am J Physiol Lung Cell Mol Physiol 300: L25–31.
11. Thavagnanam S, Parker JC, McBrien ME, Skibinski G, Heaney LG, et al. (2011) Effects of Interleukin-13 on mucociliary differentiation of pediatric asthmatic bronchial epithelial cells. Ped Res 69: 95–100.
12. Gaga M, Vignola AM, Chanez P (2001) Upper and lower airways: similarities and differences. Eur Respir Monogr 6: 1–15.
13. Hellings PW, Hens G (2009) Rhinosinusitis and the lower airways. Immunol Allergy Clin North Am 29: 733–740.
14. Jeffery PK, Haahtela T (2006) Allergic rhinitis and asthma: inflammation in a one-airway condition. BMC Pulm Med 6: Suppl 1:S5.

15. Brozek JL, Bousquet J, Baena-Cagnani CE, Bonini S, Canonica GW, et al. (2010) Allergic Rhinitis and its Impact on Asthma (ARIA) guidelines: 2010 revision. J Allergy Clin Immunol 126: 466–476.
16. Bousquet J, Vignola AM, Demoly P (2003) Links between rhinitis and asthma. Allergy 58: 691–706.
17. Devalia JL, Davies RJ (1991) Human nasal and bronchial epithelial cells in culture: an overview of their characteristics and function. Allergy Proc 12: 71–79.
18. Legget JJ, Doherty GM, Skibinski G (2004) Susceptibility of bronchial epithelial cells from asthmatics to oxidant injury. Eur Respir J 24: 100.
19. McDougall CM, Blaylock MG, Douglas JG, Brooker RJ, Helms PJ, et al. (2008) Nasal epithelial cells as surrogates for bronchial epithelial cells in airway inflammation studies. Am J Respir Cell Mol Biol 39: 560–568.
20. Pringle EJ, Richardson HB, Miller D, Cornish DS, Devereux GS, et al. (2012) Nasal and bronchial airway epithelial cell mediator release in children. Pediatr Pulmonol 47(12): 1215–1225.
21. Doherty GM, Christie SN, Skibinski G, Puddicombe SM, Warke TJ, et al. (2003) Non-bronchoscopic sampling and culture of bronchial epithelial cells in children. Clin Exp Allergy 33: 1221–1225.
22. Coyle PV, Ong GM, O'Neill HJ, McCaughey C, DeOrnellas D, et al. (2004) A touchdown nucleic acid amplification protocol as an alternative to culture backup for immunofluorescence in the routine diagnosis of acute viral respiratory tract infections. BMC Microbiol 4: 41.
23. Laoukili J, Perret E, Willems T, Minty A, Parthoens E, et al. (2001) IL-13 alters mucociliary differentiation and ciliary beating of human respiratory epithelial cells. J Clin Invest 108: 1817–1824.
24. Skowron M, Perret E, Marano F, Caput D, Tournier F (2003) Interleukin-13 alters mucociliary differentiation of human nasal epithelial cells. Chest (Suppl) 123: 3.
25. Kim CH, Song KS, Koo JS, Kim HU, Cho JY, et al. (2002) IL-13 suppresses MUC5AC gene expression and mucin secretion in nasal epithelial cells. Acta Otolaryngol 122: 638–643.
26. Atherton HC, Jones G, Danahay H (2003) IL-13-induced changes in the goblet cell density of human bronchial epithelial cell cultures: MAP kinase and phosphatidylinositol 3-kinase regulation. Am J Physiol Lung Cell Mol Physiol 285: L730–739.
27. Gomperts BN, Kim LJ, Flaherty SA, Hackett BP (2007) IL-13 regulates cilia loss and foxj1 expression in human airway epithelium. Am J Respir Cell Mol Biol 37: 339–346.
28. Kondo M, Tamaoki J, Takeyama K, Nakata J, Nagai A (2002) Interleukin-13 induces goblet cell differentiation in primary cell culture from Guinea pig tracheal epithelium. Am J Respir Cell Mol Biol 27: 536–541.
29. Malavia NK, Mih JD, Raub CB, Dinh BT, George SC (2008) IL-13 induces a bronchial epithelial phenotype that is profibrotic. Respir Res 9: 27.
30. Zhen G, Park SW, Nguyenvu LT, Rodriguez MW, Barbeau R, et al. (2007) IL-13 and epidermal growth factor receptor have critical but distinct roles in epithelial cell mucin production. Am J Respir Cell Mol Biol 36: 244–253.
31. Denker BM, Nigam SK (1998) Molecular structure and assembly of the tight junction. Am J Physiol 274: F1–9.
32. Takeyama K, Dabbagh K, Lee HM, Agusti C, Lausier JA, et al. (1999) Epidermal growth factor system regulates mucin production in airways. Proc Natl Acad Sci U S A 96: 3081–3086.
33. Nakaya M, Dohi M, Okunishi K, Nakagome K, Tanaka R, et al. (2007) Prolonged allergen challenge in murine nasal allergic rhinitis: nasal airway remodeling and adaptation of nasal airway responsiveness. Laryngoscope 117: 881–885.
34. Wagner JG, Jiang Q, Harkema JR, Ames BN, Illek B, et al. (2008) Gamma-tocopherol prevents airway eosinophilia and mucous cell hyperplasia in experimentally induced allergic rhinitis and asthma. Clin Exp Allergy 38: 501–511.
35. Ouyang Y, Miyata M, Hatsushika K, Ohnuma Y, Katoh R, et al. (2010) TGF-beta signaling may play a role in the development of goblet cell hyperplasia in a mouse model of allergic rhinitis. Allergol Int 59: 313–319.
36. Haitchi HM, Davies DE, Holgate ST, Howarth PH, Whitsett JA, et al. (2011) The SPDEF network regulates mucus cell differentiation in asthma [abstract]. Am J Respir Crit Care Med 183: A2771.
37. Miyahara S, Miyahara N, Matsubara S, Takeda K, Koya T, et al. (2006) IL-13 is essential to the late-phase response in allergic rhinitis. J Allergy Clin Immunol 118: 1110–1116.
38. Lopez-Souza N, Favoreto S, Wong H, Ward T, Yagi S,, et al. (2009) In vitro susceptibility to rhinovirus infection is greater for bronchial than for nasal epithelial cells in human subjects. J Allergy Clin Immunol 123(6): 1384–1390.
39. Lopez-Guisa JM, Powers C, File D, Cochrane E, Jiminez N,, et al. (2012) Airway epithelial cells from asthmatic children differentially express proremodeling factors. J Allergy Clin Immunol 129(4): 990–997.
40. Akdis M, Burgler S, Crameri R, Eiwegger T, Fujita H, et al. (2011) Interleukins, from 1–37, and interferon-γ: Receptors, functions and roles in diseases. J Allergy Clin Immunol 127: 701–721.e70.
41. Levine SJ, Wu T, Shelhamer JH (1997) Extracellular release of the type-1 intracellular receptor antagonist from human airway epithelial cells. J Immunol 158: 5949–5957.
42. Lordan JL, Bucchieri F, Richter A, Konstantinidis A, Holloway JW, et al. (2002) Cooperative effects of Th2 cytokines and allergen on normal and asthmatic bronchial epithelial cells. J Immunol 169(1): 407–414.
43. Ip WK, Wong CK, Lam CWK (2006) Interleukin (IL)-4 and IL-13 up-regulate monocyte chemoattractant protein-1 expression in human bronchial epithelial cells: involvement of p38 mitogen-activated protein kinase, extracellular signal-regulated kinase 1/2 and Janus kinase-2 but not cJun NH2-terminal kinase 1/2 signalling pathways. Clin Exp Allergy 145: 162–172.
44. Ogilvie V, Passmore M, Hyndman L, Jones L, Stevenson B, et al. (2011) Differential global gene expression in cystic fibrosis nasal and bronchial epithelium. Genomics 98(5): 327–336.

11

Variable Food-Specific IgG Antibody Levels in Healthy and Symptomatic Chinese Adults

Qiang Zeng[1*⁹], Sheng-Yong Dong[1⁹], Liu-Xin Wu[2], Hong Li[3], Zhi-Jian Sun[4], Jing-Bo Li[5], Hong-Xia Jiang[6], Zhi-Heng Chen[7], Qi-Bin Wang[8], Wei-Wei Chen[9*]

1 International Medical Center, Chinese PLA General Hospital, Beijing, China, **2** The Second Laboratory, PLA Air Force Institute of Aviation Medicine, Beijing, China, **3** Health Management Center, Fujian Provincial Hospital, Fuzhou, Fujian, China, **4** Health Management Center, Shandong Provincial Hospital, Jinan, Shandong, China, **5** Health Management Center, Southwest Hospital, The Third Military Medical University, Chongqing, China, **6** Health Management Center, Xiangya Hospital, Central South University, Changsha, Hunan, China, **7** Health Management Center, The Third Xiangya Hospital of Central South University, Changsha, Hunan, China, **8** Health Management Center, Shandong Electric Power Center Hospital, Jinan, Shandong, China, **9** Treatment and Research Center for Infectious Diseases, 302 Hospital of PLA, Beijing, China

Abstract

Background: The presence of food-specific IgG antibodies in human serum may be useful for diagnosis of adverse food reactions. However, the clinical utility of tesing for such antibodies remains very controversial. The aim of this study was to evaluate the serum levels and population distribution of food-specific IgGs and their association with chronic symptoms in a large-scale Chinese population.

Methodology/Principal Findings: A total of 21305 adult participants from different regions of China had 14 type of food-specific serum IgG antibodies that were measured by enzyme-linked immunosorbent assay. Amongthese, 5,394 participants were randomly chosen to complete follow-up questionnaire surveys on their dietary characteristics and chronic symptoms. The concentrations of food-specific IgGs against 14 foods ranged from a median (interquartile range) of 7.3 (3.8, 12.6) U/mL of pork-specfic IgG to 42.3 (28.8, 60.2) U/mL of crab-specific IgG. The concentration of food-specific IgGs was closely related to gender; after adjustment for region and age, women had higher concentrations of food-specific IgGs against all of the 14 foods except chicken (regression coefficient (95% CI): 0.01 (−0.003, 0.023); $P=0.129$) and corn (0.002 (−0.013, 0.016); $P=0.825$). Similar results were also found in the relationship of geographic region to the food-specific IgG concentrations for the 14 foods. Chronic symptoms were negatively associated with the concentrations of a few food-specific IgGs, and were positively associated with the concentrations of other food-specific IgGs.

Conclusions: The levels of food-specific IgGs were variable both in healthy and in symptomatic Chinese adults. These findings raise awareness that demographic factors, the type of food and specific chronic symptoms should be considered before food elimination treatment based on IgG testing in patients with chronic symptoms is used in clinical practice.

Editor: Susanne Krauss-Etschmann, Ludwig-Maximilians-University Munich, Germany

Funding: This study was supported by the State Science and Technology Support Program (No. 2012BAI37B04). The funders had no role in study design, data collection and analysis, decision to publish, or preparation of the manuscript.

Competing Interests: The authors have declared that no competing interests exist.

* E-mail: zq301@hotmail.com (QZ); cww302@126.com (WC)

⁹ These authors contributed equally to this work.

Introduction

The prevalence of migraine, asthma, allergic dermatitis and irritable bowel syndrome has been continuously increasing. Etiological studies suggest that these diseases may be related to adverse food reactions (food hypersensitivity) [1,2,3,4,5]. According to a recent report of an expert panel sponsored by the U.S. National Institute of Allergy and Infectious Diseases [6], adverse food reactions include food allergies and food intolerances, and the gold standard for the diagnosis of adverse food reactions remains the double-blind, placebo-controlled food challenge (DBPCFC). However, DBPCFC is difficult to use in large population studies due to the tedious, inconvenient, and costly procedures involved [7]. Other diagnostic tests such as skin prick tests, serum food-specific IgE tests, and atopy patch tests lack specificity and may lead to the unnecessary exclusion of foods from the patient's diet [6].

Previous studies have found that the levels of food-specific IgGs and IgG subclasses in blood serum were significantly higher in individuals with food hypersensitivity [8,9,10], and that IgG-mediated immunologic responses may play an important role in the pathogenesis of adverse food reactions [11,12,13]. However, other studies indicate that the serum level of food-specific IgGs may also be elevated in healthy individuals, suggesting that the elevation of food-specific IgGs and IgG subclasses may merely reflect the presence of immunological tolerance to food-specific antigens, i.e., that it may only reflect a history of exposure to a certain food [14,15]. Therefore, it was determined that food-specific IgGs and IgG subclasses lack diagnostic value for food allergy/intolerance [15,16,17].

Although the diagnostic utility of the presence of food-specific IgGs in patients with adverse food reactions remain controversial, serum food-specific IgG tests have been used in patients with chronic symptoms because of their convenience [18,19]. In addition, selective food elimination based on the results of food-specific IgG testing has been suggested to be effective in the treatment of irritable bowel syndrome and migraine [4,5]. However, the distribution of food-specific IgG concentrations, and the relationship of food-specific IgGs to chronic symptoms has not been reported in any large-scale population studies [18]. The aim of this study was to investigate the factors related to the presence of food-specific IgGs and their association with diet characteristics and chronic symptoms in a large adult population from various regions of China.

Materials and Methods

Study Population

The study population was recruited as patients presented to the clinic and underwent routine physical examination in general hospitals in 23 provinces in China (Figure S1), beginning in August 2008. Participation in the study was voluntary. Individuals aged 18–75 years were randomly selected using a single-blind method;, patients who were pregnancy or had a history of anaphylactic shock, secondary chronic symptoms caused by other known cardiovascular diseases, chronic kidney diseases or organic intestinal diseases were excluded. The concentrations of serum IgGs that reacted with 14 foods that are commonly consumed in China were measured in these individuals. By October 2010, a total of 21305 participants were included after excluding those with incomplete data. From this population, 6000 subjects were randomly selected and contacted for a questionnaire survey. Informed written consent was obtained from all participants, and the study protocol was approved by the Institution Review Board of the Chinese PLA General Hospital, Beijing, China.

Questionnaire Design

A questionnaire was designed with questions adapted to Chinese adults. The questions included consumption frequencies of 14 common foods: beef, chicken, codfish, corn, crab, eggs, mushrooms, cow's milk, pork, rice, shrimp, soybeans, tomatoes and wheat. Regular consumption referred to a consumption frequency of ≥3 times/week, and rare consumption referred to a consumption frequency ≤ one time/3 months; moderate consumption was defined as a consumption frequency that fell between these two extremes. The questionnaire also included information about perceived connections between ingestion of specific foods and chronic symptoms, such as gastrointestinal symptoms (abdominal pain, diarrhea or nausea), eczema, urticaria, rhinitis, asthma, arthritis, migraine headaches or other chronic symptoms (chest pain, or heart discomfort).

Food-specific Serum IgG Assays

Participants' sera were collected and sent, with only numerical identifiers, to authorized hospital laboratories, where enzyme-linked immunosorbent assays (ELISA) were performed to measure the concentrations of 14 different food-specific IgGs using a commercially available kit (Biomerica, Inc. USA). This assay has been described in a previous study [20]. Briefly, the serum samples were diluted 100-fold, and added to reaction wells coated with one of 14 food-specific allergens. After the plate was sealed, incubated at room temperature for 1 hour, washed and patted dry, anti-human IgG antibody conjugated to horseradish peroxidase was added to the wells. After another incubation at room temperature for 30 minutes, washing and patting dry, 100 μl of a substrate mixture consisting of equal proportions of 3,3′,5,5′-tetramethyl-benzidine and hydrogenperoxide was added. The reaction was stopped after 10 minutes, and absorbance was measured at 450 nm. The concentrations of food-specific IgGs (U/mL; 1 U = 1.47 ng) were calculated using the standard curves of 14 types of food-specific IgGs provided by the manufacture. The detection limit was 0.01 U/mL. All authorized laboratories were asked to satisfy several standards of quality assurance for the determinations of these 14 types of food-specific IgGs. The quality assurance standards were as follows: the optical density of the negative controls should be <0.2, the concentrations of IgG in the positive quality controls should be >100 U/mL and the optical density in 50 U/mL, 100 U/mL, 200 U/mL and 400 U/mL standard wells should be 1.2 times more than in negative 50 U/mL, 100 U/mL and 200 U/mL standard wells, respectively. For the great majority of clinically relevant allergens, no standardized reference allergens are available for comparisons between methods. To ensure the reproducibility and accuracy of the ELISA kit assays, each serum sample was tested in duplicate parallel tests, all ELISA kits were required to be used within 10 days of their delivery from the factory, and all testing was performed using an automated spotting system that was supervised by well-trained medical laboratory technologists who were blinded to the clinical data. On average, the intra- and inter-assay coefficients of variant were 2.7% and 5.3%, respectively, in the Chinese PLA General Hospital laboratory, and 8.5% and 12.1% in other authorized laboratories. Before the study, all participating laboratories calibrated food-specific IgG measurements according to the quality control results distributed from the Chinese PLA General Hospital laboratory.

Statistical Analysis

All data were entered into an Epidata 3.0 database through double-blinded entry, followed by automatic check and verification. Continuous variables are reported as median values with the corresponding 25th and 75th percentiles. Discrete variables are summarized in terms of frequencies and percentages. Because the data demonstrated a skewed distribution, serum concentrations of food-specific IgGs were logarithmically transformed; undetectable specific IgG concentrations (<0.01 U/mL) were considered 0.005 U/mL. Maximum likelihood estimation was performed to evaluate the means and standard deviations of food-specific IgG concentrations using R 2.15.2. To visualize the distribution of food-specific IgG concentrations in all subjects and demographic subgroups (sex, geographic region and age group), histograms or line graphs were generated, and one-way analysis of variance (ANOVA) and post-hoc Tukey tests were used for comparison of the resultings curves. *P*-values for trends were calculated when age group-related differences in food-specific IgG concentrations were examined. Pearson correlation was performed to analyze the relationship of food-specific IgG concentrations among the 14 foods. Differences in food consumption frequencies in demographic subgroups were tested using the Pearson chi-square test and *P* values for trends were calculated when differences in the food consumption frequencies of different age group were examined. Differences in food-specific IgG concentrations between subjects with chronic symptoms and subjects without chronic symptoms were also examined with ANOVA. Multivariate linear regression models were applied to evaluate the association of food-specific IgG concentrations of each of the 14 foods with demographic factors and food consumption frequencies. Logistic regression models were performed to analyze the association of chronic symptoms with food-specific IgG concentrations of the 14 foods, and odd ratios (OR) and 95% CI were calculated. All statistical analyses were performed with SPSS 10.0 (SPSS Inc., Chicago, IL, USA). Two-tailed P values <0.05 were considered significant.

Results

Study Population Characteristics

Of the 21305 subjects (mean age: 46.63±10.52 years; 13,426 men and 7,879 women), most (74.0%) were northern Chinese. Questionnaire replies were received from 5394 individuals (89.9% of the randomly selected subjects); of the 5394 individuals who responded to the questionnaire, 32.2% were women and 77.2% were northern Chinese. In the 2353 subjects who reported having chronic symptoms, the most common chronic symptoms were gastrointestinal symptoms (23.6%), rhinitis (11.8%) and migraine (9.5%) (Table 1).

Distribution of Food-specific IgG Concentrations

The distributions of the serum concentrations of food-specific IgG against the 14 foods tested varied significantly (Figure 1). The log-distributed curves for food-specific IgG concentrations of crab, codfish, egg and shrimp are shifed slightly to the right; the medians (interquartile range) of the IgG concentrations against these foods were 42.3 (28.8, 60.2) U/mL, 27.5 (16.9, 44.2) U/mL, 26.6 (11.4, 72.5) U/mL and 22.8 (14.9, 35.2) U/mL, respectively. For pork-specific IgG, the log-distributed curve is shifted slightly to the left; the median and interquartile range of the concentration of pork-specific IgG is 7.3 and 3.8 to 12.6 U/mL. The means and standard deviations of log-transformed food-specific IgG concentrations that were calculated using maximum likelihood estimation are shown in Table S1.

The distribution of food-specific IgG concentration against egg varied more than for other foods. For example, a total of 61 subjects had levels of egg-specific IgG above 1000 U/mL, and the proportion of subjects who had egg-specific IgG levels above 200 U/mL was 8.4%, the highest od the 14 foods. The proportion of subjects who had the egg-specific IgG levels less than 10 U/mL was 21.7%; this level was higher than for other foods against which subjects had similar IgG levels, such as codfish (only 8.8% of the subjects had codfish-specific IgG levels that were less than 10 U/mL). Interestingly, the food-specific IgG levels against the 14 foods tested were all correlated with each other. The strongest relationship between food-specific IgG levels were found for beef and chicken (correlation coefficient, 0.691; $P<0.01$); the next strongest was for codfish and crab (correlation coefficient, 0.561; $P<0.01$) (Table S2).

Relationship of Demographic Factors and Food-specific IgG Concentrations

Compared to the log-distributed curves of the frequencies of food-specific IgG concentrations in men, the log-distributed curves of the frequencies of food-specific IgG concentrations in women were shifted to the right for 10 of the 14 foods; the exceptions were chicken (median (interquartile) men vs. women: 11.5 (7.1, 17.3) U/mL vs. 11.8 (7.4, 17.9) U/mL; $P=0.052$), corn (men vs. women: 11.3 (6.5, 18.5) U/mL vs. 12.0 (6.9, 19.0) U/mL; $P=0.378$), mushrooms (men vs. women: 14.5 (8.1, 22.4) U/mL vs. 14.9 (8.1, 23.9) U/mL; $P=0.065$) and pork (men vs. women: 7.3 (3.8, 12.4) U/mL vs. 7.4 (3.8, 12.8) U/mL; $P=0.432$). When the subjects were grouped according to sex, the greatest difference in food-specific IgG concentrations between men and women was found for egg (men vs. women: 22.4 (10.3, 61.2) U/mL vs. 36.8 (14.2, 93.6) U/mL; $P<0.001$); the next greatest differences were for cow's milk (men vs. women: 14.9 (8.5, 26.2) U/mL vs. 18.2 (10.1,

Table 1. Baseline characteristics of the study population.

	Overall subjects, n = 21305 Number (%)	Subjects with questionnaire survey, n = 5394 Number (%)
Women	7879 (37.0)	1735 (32.2)
Age (year)		
18–34	1585 (7.4)	462 (8.6)
35–44	7526 (35.3)	1751 (32.5)
45–54	8268 (38.8)	2025 (37.5)
55–64	2849 (13.4)	733 (13.6)
≥65	1077 (5.1)	423 (7.8)
Region		
South China	5547 (26.0)	1231 (22.8)
North China	15758 (74.0)	4163 (77.2)
Chronic symptoms		
Gastrointestinal	--	1274 (23.6)
Rhinitis	--	636 (11.8)
Migraine	--	511 (9.5)
Arthritis	--	392 (7.3)
Eczema	--	310 (5.7)
Urticaria	--	259 (4.8)
Asthma	--	153 (2.8)
Other	--	721 (13.4)

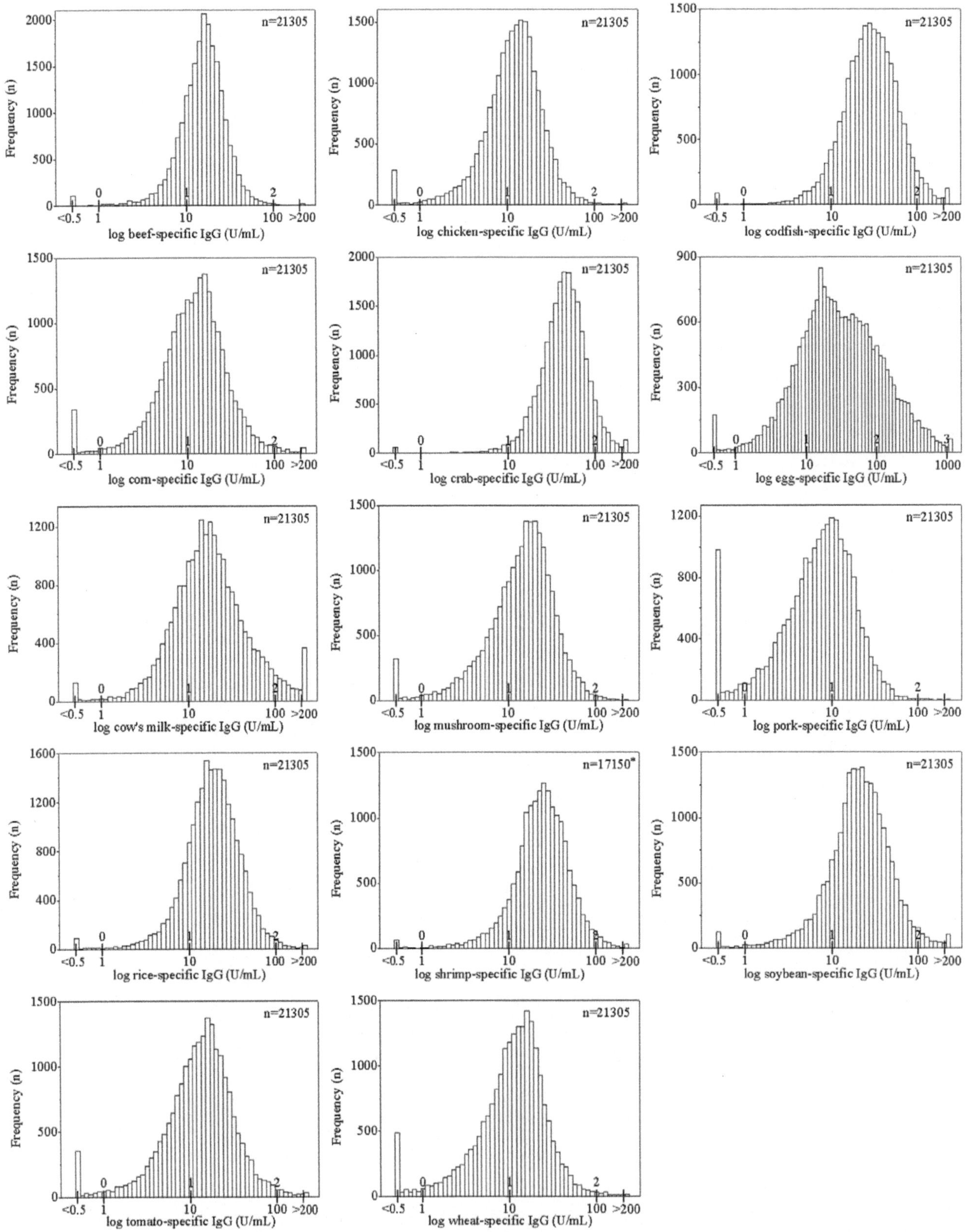

Figure 1. Distribution of serum food-specific IgG concentrations for 14 foods. *The serum concentration of shrimp-specific IgG was recorded as the original value in 17150 subjects and has been classified as negative or positive in remaining 4155 subjects according to the directions provided by the manufacturer of the test kit.

34.3) U/mL; $P<0.001$) and soybean (men vs. women: 18.7 (11.7, 30.1) U/mL vs. 22.4 (13.9, 36.8) U/mL; $P<0.001$) (Figure S2).

Region subgroup histograms also showed that the log-distributed curves for almost all of the 14 foods shifted slightly for South Chinese compared to North Chinese subjects; the exceptions were chicken (south vs. north: 10.7 (7.1, 16.4) U/mL vs. 11.9 (7.3, 17.9) U/mL; $P=0.333$) and soybean (south vs. north: 18.7 (11.5, 30.8) U/mL vs. 20.5 (12.8, 33.0) U/mL; $P=0.062$) (Figure S3). Compared to subjects in North China, subjects in South China had higher mean concentrations of beef-specific IgG (south vs. north: 16.3 (11.6, 22.8) U/mL vs. 14.6 (9.9, 20.1) U/mL; $P<0.001$), corn-specific IgG (south vs. north: 11.7 (6.9, 19.7) U/mL vs. 11.5 (6.5, 18.3) U/mL; $P<0.001$) and shrimp-specific IgG (south vs. north: 24.9 (16.5, 37.6) U/mL vs. 22.6 (14.8, 35.0) U/mL; $P<0.001$). The mean concentrations of food-specific IgG against the other 9 foods were higher in North China than in South China, especially mushroom (south vs. north: 9.9 (5.1, 18.5) U/mL vs. 15.9 (9.6, 24.1) U/mL; $P<0.001$), pork (south vs. north: 4.8 (2.4, 9.1) U/mL vs. 8.3 (4.5, 13.6) U/mL; $P<0.001$) and wheat (south vs. north: 7.8 (4.1, 13.9) U/mL vs. 12.3 (7.3, 18.3) U/mL; $P<0.001$).

With increasing age of the subjects, the mean concentrations of food-specific IgG for almost all of the 14 foods increased. The exceptions were corn (11.9 (6.6, 19.4) U/mL, 11.4 (6.5, 18.7) U/mL, 11.3 (6.6, 18.3) U/mL, 11.8 (6.7, 18.5) U/mL and 13.2 (7.9, 21.7) U/mL for 20–34, 35–44, 45–54, 55–64 and ≥65 years age group, respectively; P for trend = 0.092) and wheat (12.1 (6.5, 20.0) U/mL, 10.5 (5.6, 17.2) U/mL, 10.9 (6.2, 17.3) U/mL, 11.6 (6.8, 17.5) U/mL and 13.4 (8.0, 18.8) U/mL for 20–34, 35–44, 45–54, 55–64 and ≥65 years age groups, respectively; P for trend = 0.115). Although food-specific IgG concentrations for the other 12 foods showed an increasing trend with age, the concentrations of egg-specific IgG and cow's milk-specific IgG were significantly higher in the 18–34 years age group than in the 35–44, 45–54 and 55–64 years age groups (Figure S4).

Multivariate analysis showed that women had higher food-specific IgG concentrations than men against all of the 14 foods except chicken (regression coefficient (95% CI): 0.01 (−0.003, 0.023); $P=0.129$) and corn (0.002 (−0.013, 0.016); $P=0.825$) after adjustment for region and age. Of the other 12 foods, egg-specific IgG concentration showed the strongest relationship to sex (0.184 (0.166, 0.202); $P<0.001$). After adjustment for sex and age, subjects in South China had higher concentrations of beef-specific IgG (−0.079 (−0.089, −0.068); $P<0.001$), corn-specific IgG (−0.047 (−0.063, −0.031); $P<0.001$) and shrimp-specific IgG (−0.052 (−0.071, −0.033); $P<0.001$) than subjects in North China, whereas they had similar chicken-specific IgG concentration (−0.009 (−0.023, 0.005); $P=0.210$) as subjects in North China; food-specific IgG concentrations against the other 11 foods were higher in subjects in North China. After adjustment for sex and region, age also showed strong relationship with to the food-specific IgG concentrations against all foods except corn (0.001 (0, 0.001); $P=0.083$), cow's milk (0.001 (0, 0.001); $P=0.065$) and wheat (0 (−0.001, 0.001); $P=0.910$). Age was inversely associated with egg-specific IgG concentration (−0.002 (−0.003, −0.001); $P<0.001$) and positively associated with food-specific IgG concentrations for the other 10 foods (Figure 2).

Relationship between Consumption Frequency and Food-specific IgG

Of the 5394 subjects who responded to the questionnaire, the majority regularly consumed (≥3 times/week) rice and pork (83.8% and 70.1%, respectively); a minority of subjects regularly consumed shrimp and crab (15.4% and 6.9%, respectively). Men showed higher diet frequencies of codfish and meat, while more women regularly consumed cow's milk and non-meat foods. The proportions of subjects who regularly consumed rice, crab, shrimp and codfish were higher in South than in North China, while the proportion of subjects who regularly consumed wheat was higher in North China population (69.7% vs. 35.4%, respectively; $P<0.001$).Shrimp, chicken, beef and pork were consumed most frequently by the 18–34 yearold age group, and the consumption of egg, cow's milk, soybeans, corn, tomatoes and wheat increased with age (P for trend <0.001) (Table S3).

After adjustment for sex, region and age, the diet frequencies of 9 of the tested foods were not significantly associated with the corresponding food-specific serum IgG concentrations. Dietary consumption frequencies of egg, cow's milk and rice were inversely associated with egg-specific IgG (regression coefficient (95%CI): −0.052 (−0.088, −0.016); $P=0.005$), cow's milk-specific IgG (−0.039 (−0.062, −0.015); $P=0.001$) and rice-specific IgG concentrations (−0.03 (−0.059, −0.002); $P=0.038$), respectively; whereas, the dietary consumption frequencies of chicken and tomato were positively associated with chicken-specific IgG (0.028 (0.001, 0.054); $P=0.042$) and tomato-specific IgG concentrations (0.034 (0.004, 0.064); $P=0.028$), respectively (Figure 3).

Relationship between Food-specific IgGs and Chronic Symptoms

Compared to subjects who reported having no gastrointestinal symptoms, subjects who reported having chronic symptoms had higher concentrations of codfish-specific IgG (median (interquartile) gastrointestinal symptom, yes vs. no: 23.8 (14.3, 45.1) U/mL vs. 20.9 (14.4, 37.9) U/mL; $P=0.013$) and rice-specific IgG (16.7 (9.4, 28.0) U/mL vs. 15.4 (10.9, 22.0) U/mL; $P=0.032$); and lower concentrations of mushroom-specific IgG (8.9 (4.3, 16.0) U/mL vs. 12.0 (6.5, 16.9) U/mL; $P=0.026$), tomato-specific IgG (10.1(5.1, 17.7) U/mL vs. 13.1 (7.2, 18.4) U/mL; $P=0.018$) and wheat-specific IgG (6.8 (3.0, 13.3) U/mL vs. 9.9 (4.6, 15.7) U/mL; $P=0.010$). Subjects who reported having migraine also had lower concentrations of mushroom-specific IgG (8.4 (4.1, 15.7) U/mL vs. 11.8 (6.2, 16.9) U/mL; $P=0.007$) and tomato-specific IgG (9.8 (4.6, 16.2) U/mL vs. 13.0 (7.0, 18.5) U/mL; $P=0.003$) than subjects who reported having no migraine. Subjects who reported having eczema had higher concentrations of crab-specific IgG (44.8 (24.8, 66.5) U/mL vs. 37.3 (21.4, 58.5) U/mL; $P=0.038$) and rice-specific IgG (17.0 (11.7, 27.2) U/mL vs. 15.5 (10.5, 22.9) U/mL; $P=0.009$) than subjects who reported having no eczema. Rice-specific IgG concentration was higher in subjects who reported having urticaria than in subjects who reported having no urticaria (20.9 (13.0, 31.2) U/mL vs. 15.4 (10.5, 22.7) U/mL; $P=0.006$); whereas, cow's milk-specific IgG concentration was lower in subjects who reported having asthma than in subjects who reported having no asthma (14.2 (6.6, 23.7) U/mL vs. 15.3 (9.0, 27.7) U/mL; $P=0.042$). The concentrations of food-specific IgG for cow's milk, pork and wheat were also lower in subjects who reported having other symptoms than in those who reported having no other symptoms (Figure S5).

The association of chronic symptoms with serum levels of specific IgGs against the 14 foods tested is shown in Figure 4. After adjustment for sex, region and age, gastrointestinal symptom were inversely associated with mushroom-specifi (OR (95% CI): 0.85 (0.72, 0.99); $P=0.048$), tomato-specific (0.82 (0.70, 0.97); $P=0.020$) and wheat-specific (0.84 (0.73, 0.95); $P=0.007$) IgG levels; and positively associated with codfish-specific (1.47 (1.11, 1.94); $P=0.007$), rice-specific (1.45 (1.08, 1.95); $P=0.015$) and shrimp-specific (1.40 (1.06, 1.85); $P=0.017$) IgG levels. Rhinitis was inversely associated with the serum concentration of tomato-

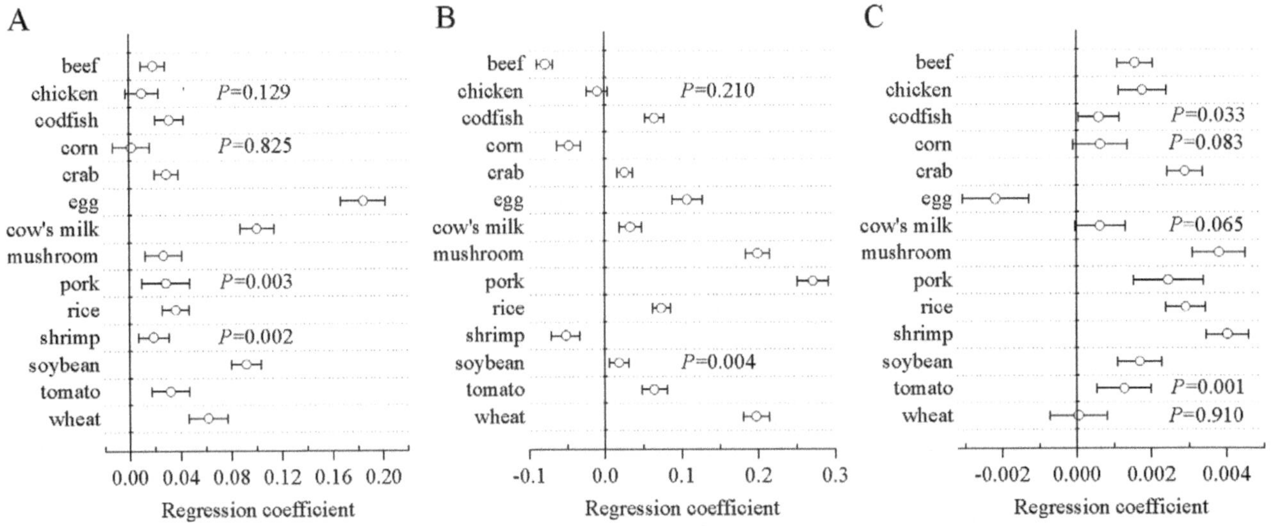

Figure 2. Association of demographic subgroups with serum food-specific IgG concentrations for 14 foods. (A) sex, (B) geographic region, (C) age. Regression coefficients and *P* values were derived from multivariate linear regression models that set sex (men, 0; women, 1), geographic region (South China, 0; North China, 1) and age as independent variables and the logarithmically transformed serum food-specific IgG concentrations for 14 foods as dependent variables. The food items for which *P* values are not shown yielded mean *P* values less than 0.001.

specific IgG (0.82 (0.66, 0.99); $P = 0.049$) and positively associated with the concentration of rice-specific IgG (1.49 (1.01, 2.19); $P = 0.044$). Migraine was inversely associated with mushroom-specific (0.78 (0.64, 0.95); $P = 0.016$) and tomato-specific IgG levels (0.74 (0.61, 0.91); $P = 0.004$) and positively associated with rice-specific IgG levels (1.57 (1.01, 2.43); $P = 0.043$). Arthritis was inversely associated with wheat-specific IgG levels (079 (0.63, 0.98); $P = 0.035$). Eczema was positively associated with food-specific concentrations of beef-specific (2.01 (1.07, 3.75); $P = 0.030$), crab-specific (1.90 (1.12, 3.20); $P = 0.017$) and rice-specific (2.23 (1.27, 3.93); $P = 0.005$) IgG levels. Urticaria was positively associated with rice-specific (3.71 (1.76, 7.86); $P = 0.001$) and shrimp-specific (2.15 (1.11, 4.18); $P = 0.024$) IgG levels. Asthma was inversely associated with milk-specific IgG levels (0.63 (0.41, 0.98); $P = 0.042$). Other symptoms were inversely associated with pork-specific (075 (0.64, 0.89); $P = 0.001$) and wheat-specific (0.80 (0.69, 0.93); $P = 0.004$) IgG levels and positively associated with crab-specific IgG levels (1.53 (1.07, 2.17); $P = 0.019$).

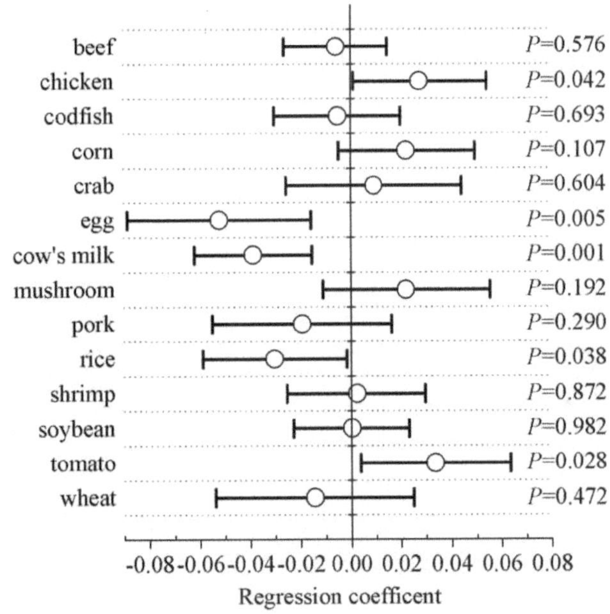

Figure 3. Association of various dietary frequencies of 14 foods with corresponding serum food-specific IgG concentrations. Regression coefficients and *P* values were derived from multivariate linear regression models in which the dietary frequencies of 14 foods (rare, 0; moderate, 1; regular, 2) were used as independent variables and the corresponding and logarithmically transformed serum food-specific IgG concentrations for 14 foods were the dependent variables. Demographic factorsincluding sex, region and age were adjusted for in these models.

Discussion

Although commercial laboratories worldwide are currently offering broad-scale = testings for serum levels of food-specific IgGs to the public, to our knowledge, the study described here is the first representative cross-sectional study to address the distribution of food-specific IgGs and its relationship to chronic symptoms in a large population. Previous studies have either involved \ research on the potential involvement of various IgG subclasses in food allergy/intolerance [9,21] or have addressed food elimination based on IgG testing [4,5].

Although testing for the presence of food-specific IgGs has been regarded as a potential tool for the diagnosis of food allergy/intolerance, it's the accuracy and clinical utility of such testing remain unclear. In our study, serum concentrations of food-specific IgGs against the 14 foods tested varied widely. Different foods have different proteins and components, and this may induce different immune reactions and lead to the presence of variable amounts of food-specific IgG. The completeness of extraction of different food proteins and other components of the 14 foods tested and the relative coupling efficiency of different extracted food components/antigens to the ELISA plate would also be expected to influence the accuracy of measurement of serum concentrations of food-specific IgGs. Although the levels of

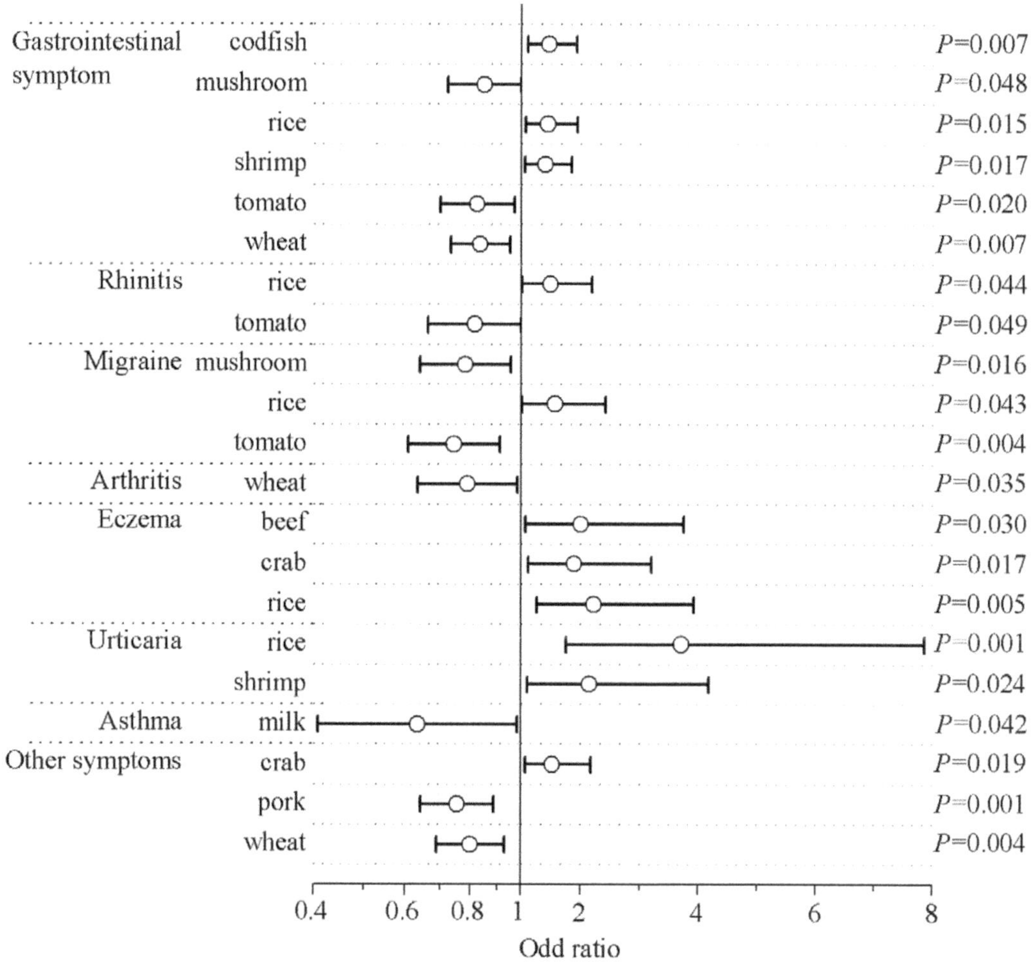

Figure 4. Association of chronic symptoms with food-specific IgG concentrations for 14 foods. Only the foods for which food-specific IgG levels were significantly associated with certain chronic symptoms ($P<0.05$) are listed. Odds ratios and *P* values were derived from logistic regression models that set logarithmically transformed serum food-specific IgG concentrations for the 14 foods as the independent variables and the presence of various chronic symptoms (No, 0; Yes, 1) as the dependent variables. Demographic factors including sex, region and age were adjusted for in these models.

food-specific IgG against the 14 tested foods were significantly different, the concentrations of all 14 food-specific IgGs, especially IgGs directed against beef and chicken, were correlated with one another. Similar results were reported by Kanagawa et al [22] in an analysis of food antigens in 6549 subjects; the results of that study suggested that the appearance of food antigens clusters may be a result of immune cross-reaction between similar food antigens [6].

In our study, the distribution of food-specific IgG levels varied as a function of demographic subgroups (sex, region and age). Women had higher concentrations offood-specific IgGs against almost all of the tested foods than men. It has been consistently reported that the prevalence of food allergy/intolerance is significantly higher in women than in men [23,24,25]. In childhood, boys suffer from asthma, urticaria, anaphylaxis and food allergies to eggplant and peanuts more frequently than girls, while the sex difference is reversed after puberty [26,27,28,29]. Studies suggest that some female sex steroids are pro-inflammatory and increase the susceptibility of atopy, while testosterone is a powerful inhibitor of histamine and known to inhibit mast cell degranulation [26,30]. Moreover, for the first time, our study demonstrated that the distribution of food-specific IgGs against almost all of the 14 foods tested were significantly different between Southern and Northern Chinese. In the present study, this difference is not related to the subject's gender, age or dietary habits; however, it may be due to the different genetic backgrounds of subjects of different ethnicities [31,32]. Our study also showed that the serum concentrations of all food-specific IgGs except egg-specific IgG were positively associated with age. Previous studies have suggested that older people may be more likely than younger people to experience allergic reactions to foods [33]. It is not clear whether the higher levels of foods-specific IgGs in older persons indicates a higher probability of food allergies with increasing age. It is also unclear why egg-specific IgG concentrations were highest in the 20–34-year-old subjects and lowest in the 35–44-yearold subjects.

Previous studies have shown that abdominal discomforts self-attributed to food hypersensitivity is not related to eating habits or meal patterns [34]. Our study also showed that although the dietary frequencies of the 14 foods differed significantly in the demographic subgroups, only the dietary frequencies of chicken, egg, cow's milk, rice and tomato were associated with the corresponding food-specific IgG serum levels after adjustment for demographic factors. The immunological mechanism responsible for the association of chicken, egg, cow's milk, rice and tomato eating patterns with food-specific serum IgG concentrations is unclear, and further studies of this phenomenon are needed.

Previous studies have shown that chronic symptoms are closely related to food hypersensitivity [2,6]. In our study, we found the food-specific concentrations of a few IgGs to be associated with a variety of chronic symptoms; the levels of some food-specific IgG were inversely associated with chronic symptoms, while the levels of other food-specific IgG were positively associated with chronic symptoms. Chronic symptoms were positively related to the serum levels of certain food-specific IgG. This may be a result of chronic inflammatory responses induced by elevated IgG or IgG subclasses in highly sensitive individuals [5]. For instance, gliadins and glutenins in wheat may increase specific IgG levels and may lead to chronic symptoms [35]. Our study also revealed negative associations between the level of rice-specific IgG and gastrointestinal symptoms, rhinitis, migraine, urticaria and eczema; such associations may result from different (protective or negative) roles of different IgG antibodies. Similarly, Tay et al [36] found that strong IgG responses to ovalbumin may be a normal physiological response to protein ingestion frequently shown in infancy, whereas up-regulated IgG responses that occur in peanut allergy may be indicative of a dysregulated immune response to peanut allergens. The normal physiological response reflected by the presence of food-specific IgG subclasses may be immunological tolerance due to the secretion of IL-10 by the activation of regulatory T cells upon prolonged exposure to food antigen [37].

The present study has several limitations. First, because food-specific IgG antibody testing is popular in China, we only tested for the presence of IgGs against commonly consumed foods, and did not measure levels of specific IgGs against pollen, fruits, nuts or food additives [1,24,25]. However, it should be kept in mind that self-reported chronic symptoms may result from the presence of IgGs specific for the latter foods and substances rather than from the presence of IgGs against the 14 tested food allergens. Second, in our study, the prevalence of chronic symptoms was determined by self-reporting of such symptoms on a questionnaire. The chronic symptoms reported by the patients in this study have not been confirmed by the adjudication of professional doctors. Thus, misclassification of chronic symptoms is possible, and the conclusions of the study regarding the associations of specific chronic symptoms with certain food-specific IgG levels should be regarded cautiously. Third, children and adolescents 0–17 years of age were not included in our study. It has been reported that the presence of food-specific IgGs in serum is more common in children and adolescents than in adults [15]. In children and adolescents, high levels of specific IgG are not significantly associated with clinical symptoms, and are likely to represent a protective mechanism that can result in immune tolerance to the corresponding foods later in life [38]. However, a similar protective role of food-specific IgG and IgG subclasses in adults has not been confirmed [15,21]. Finally, the study does not provide an answer to the question of whether food-specific IgGs play a protective role or an allergic role in adults. The immunological mechanisms by which food-specific IgGs are induced are also unclear. A complete understanding of the importance of the presence of food-specific IgGs requires further accumulation of epidemiologic and experimental data.

In summary, the present study demonstrates for the first time that food-specific IgG serum concentrations are variable in both healthy and symptomatic Chinese adults. These findings raise awareness that demographic factors, types of food and the presence or absence of specific chronic symptoms should be considered before food elimination treatment based on IgG testing in patients with chronic symptoms is used in clinical practice. Further elucidation of the role played by food-specific IgGs in food allergies and tolerance should be an objective of future studies.

Supporting Information

Figure S1 Map of China with participating sites and numbers of subjects. The middle line represents the boundary between southern China and northern China. The dots and triangles represent the participating sites in northern China and southern China, respectively.

Figure S2 Distribution of serum food-specific IgG concentrations for 14 foods in subgroups according to sex. The white and gray columns represent men and women, respectively. * See Figure 1.

Figure S3 Distribution of serum food-specific IgG concentrations for 14 foods in subgroups according to geographic region. The white and gray columns represent participants in South China and North China, respectively. * See Figure 1.

Figure S4 Distribution of serum food-specific IgG concentrations for 14 foods according to age group. CI, confidence interval.

Figure S5 Differences in serum food-specific IgG concentrations in subjects with and without chronic symptoms. * *P* value <0.05. CI, confidence interval.

Table S1 Means and standard deviations of log-transformed food-specific IgG concentrations. *The means and standard deviations of log-transformed food-specific IgG concentrations were calculated after the undetectable food-specific IgG concentrations were set as the half-value of the limit of detection. †The means and standard deviations of log-transformed food-specific IgG concentrations were calculated using maximum likelihood estimation.

Table S2 Correlation of food-specific IgG concentrations among 14 foods*. *The Pearson correlation was used to analyze possible correlations among the food-specific IgG concentrations for 14 foods. **Indicates that the correlation is significant at the 0.01 level (2-tailed).

Table S3 Regular intake (≥3 times/week) of 14 foods in 5394 subjects (number (%)).

Acknowledgments

We thank the staffs of China Health Management Association, Medical Center of the First Affiliated Hospital of China Medical University, Medical Center of Sichuan Provincial People's Hospital, Medical Center of the Health Ministry Beijing Hospital, Beijing Xiaotangshan Hospital, The First Affiliated Hospital of Chongqing Medical University, Bethune International Peace Hospital, Xinjiang Uygur Autonomous Region People's Hospital, Zhongshan Hospital Xiamen University, General Hospital of Guangzhou Military Command of PLA, and Shuguang

Hospital Affiliated to Shanghai University of Traditional Chinese Medicine for their commitment, and all subjects who participated in the study.

Author Contributions

Conceived and designed the experiments: QZ WC. Performed the experiments: LW HL ZS JL HJ. Analyzed the data: SD WC. Contributed reagents/materials/analysis tools: QZ LW ZC QW. Wrote the paper: QZ SD.

References

1. Sicherer SH (2011) Epidemiology of food allergy. J Allergy Clin Immunol 127: 594–602.
2. Sampson HA (2004) Update on food allergy. J Allergy Clin Immunol 113: 805–819; quiz 820.
3. Penard-Morand C, Raherison C, Kopferschmitt C, Caillaud D, Lavaud F, et al. (2005) Prevalence of food allergy and its relationship to asthma and allergic rhinitis in schoolchildren. Allergy 60: 1165–1171.
4. Atkinson W, Sheldon TA, Shaath N, Whorwell PJ (2004) Food elimination based on IgG antibodies in irritable bowel syndrome: a randomised controlled trial. Gut 53: 1459–1464.
5. Alpay K, Ertas M, Orhan EK, Ustay DK, Lieners C, et al. (2010) Diet restriction in migraine, based on IgG against foods: a clinical double-blind, randomised, cross-over trial. Cephalalgia 30: 829–837.
6. Boyce JA, Assa'ad A, Burks AW, Jones SM, Sampson HA, et al. (2010) Guidelines for the diagnosis and management of food allergy in the United States: report of the NIAID-sponsored expert panel. J Allergy Clin Immunol 126: S1–58.
7. Chafen JJ, Newberry SJ, Riedl MA, Bravata DM, Maglione M, et al. (2010) Diagnosing and managing common food allergies: a systematic review. JAMA 303: 1848–1856.
8. Host A, Husby S, Gjesing B, Larsen JN, Lowenstein H (1992) Prospective estimation of IgG, IgG subclass and IgE antibodies to dietary proteins in infants with cow milk allergy. Levels of antibodies to whole milk protein, BLG and ovalbumin in relation to repeated milk challenge and clinical course of cow milk allergy. Allergy 47: 218–229.
9. Zar S, Benson MJ, Kumar D (2005) Food-specific serum IgG4 and IgE titers to common food antigens in irritable bowel syndrome. Am J Gastroenterol 100: 1550–1557.
10. Dreskin SC, Tripputi MT, Aubrey MT, Mustafa SS, Atkins D, et al. (2010) Peanut-allergic subjects and their peanut-tolerant siblings have large differences in peanut-specific IgG that are independent of HLA class II. Clin Immunol 137: 366–373.
11. Crowe SE, Perdue MH (1992) Gastrointestinal food hypersensitivity: basic mechanisms of pathophysiology. Gastroenterology 103: 1075–1095.
12. Shreffler WG, Lencer DA, Bardina L, Sampson HA (2005) IgE and IgG4 epitope mapping by microarray immunoassay reveals the diversity of immune response to the peanut allergen, Ara h 2. J Allergy Clin Immunol 116: 893–899.
13. Scott-Taylor TH, J OBH, Strobel S (2010) Correlation of allergen-specific IgG subclass antibodies and T lymphocyte cytokine responses in children with multiple food allergies. Pediatr Allergy Immunol 21: 935–944.
14. Johansson SG, Bieber T, Dahl R, Friedmann PS, Lanier BQ, et al. (2004) Revised nomenclature for allergy for global use: report of the Nomenclature Review Committee of the World Allergy Organization, October 2003. J Allergy Clin Immunol 113: 832–836.
15. Stapel SO, Asero R, Ballmer-Weber BK, Knol EF, Strobel S, et al. (2008) Testing for IgG4 against foods is not recommended as a diagnostic tool: EAACI Task Force Report. Allergy 63: 793–796.
16. Ahrens B, Lopes de Oliveira LC, Schulz G, Borres MP, Niggemann B, et al. (2010) The role of hen's egg-specific IgE, IgG and IgG4 in the diagnostic procedure of hen's egg allergy. Allergy 65: 1554–1557.
17. Hochwallner H, Schulmeister U, Swoboda I, Twaroch TE, Vogelsang H, et al. (2011) Patients suffering from non-IgE-mediated cow's milk protein intolerance cannot be diagnosed based on IgG subclass or IgA responses to milk allergens. Allergy 66: 1201–1207.
18. Hunter JO (2005) Food elimination in IBS: the case for IgG testing remains doubtful. Gut 54: 1203; author reply 1203.
19. Pelsser LM, Frankena K, Toorman J, Savelkoul HF, Dubois AE, et al. (2011) Effects of a restricted elimination diet on the behaviour of children with attention-deficit hyperactivity disorder (INCA study): a randomised controlled trial. Lancet 377: 494–503.
20. Zuo XL, Li YQ, Li WJ, Guo YT, Lu XF, et al. (2007) Alterations of food antigen-specific serum immunoglobulins G and E antibodies in patients with irritable bowel syndrome and functional dyspepsia. Clinical and experimental allergy : journal of the British Society for Allergy and Clinical Immunology 37: 823–830.
21. Antico A, Pagani M, Vescovi PP, Bonadonna P, Senna G (2011) Food-Specific IgG4 Lack Diagnostic Value in Adult Patients with Chronic Urticaria and Other Suspected Allergy Skin Symptoms. Int Arch Allergy Immunol 155: 52–56.
22. Kanagawa Y, Matsumoto S, Koike S, Imamura T (2009) Association analysis of food allergens. Pediatr Allergy Immunol 20: 347–352.
23. Young E, Stoneham MD, Petruckevitch A, Barton J, Rona R (1994) A population study of food intolerance. Lancet 343: 1127–1130.
24. Schafer T, Bohler E, Ruhdorfer S, Weigl L, Wessner D, et al. (2001) Epidemiology of food allergy/food intolerance in adults: associations with other manifestations of atopy. Allergy 56: 1172–1179.
25. Zuberbier T, Edenharter G, Worm M, Ehlers I, Reimann S, et al. (2004) Prevalence of adverse reactions to food in Germany - a population study. Allergy 59: 338–345.
26. Harish Babu BN, Mahesh PA, Venkatesh YP (2008) A cross-sectional study on the prevalence of food allergy to eggplant (Solanum melongena L.) reveals female predominance. Clinical and experimental allergy : journal of the British Society for Allergy and Clinical Immunology 38: 1795–1802.
27. Poulos LM, Waters AM, Correll PK, Loblay RH, Marks GB (2007) Trends in hospitalizations for anaphylaxis, angioedema, and urticaria in Australia, 1993–1994 to 2004–2005. J Allergy Clin Immunol 120: 878–884.
28. Sicherer SH, Munoz-Furlong A, Sampson HA (2003) Prevalence of peanut and tree nut allergy in the United States determined by means of a random digit dial telephone survey: a 5-year follow-up study. J Allergy Clin Immunol 112: 1203–1207.
29. Chen Y, Stewart P, Johansen H, McRae L, Taylor G (2003) Sex difference in hospitalization due to asthma in relation to age. J Clin Epidemiol 56: 180–187.
30. Zaitsu M, Narita S, Lambert KC, Grady JJ, Estes DM, et al. (2007) Estradiol activates mast cells via a non-genomic estrogen receptor-alpha and calcium influx. Molecular immunology 44: 1977–1985.
31. Hong X, Wang G, Liu X, Kumar R, Tsai HJ, et al. (2011) Gene polymorphisms, breast-feeding, and development of food sensitization in early childhood. J Allergy Clin Immunol 128: 374–381 e372.
32. Campos Alberto EJ, Shimojo N, Suzuki Y, Mashimo Y, Arima T, et al. (2008) IL-10 gene polymorphism, but not TGF-beta1 gene polymorphisms, is associated with food allergy in a Japanese population. Pediatr Allergy Immunol 19: 716–721.
33. Harduar-Morano L, Simon MR, Watkins S, Blackmore C (2011) A population-based epidemiologic study of emergency department visits for anaphylaxis in Florida. The Journal of allergy and clinical immunology 128: 594–600 e591.
34. Carvalho RV, Lorena SL, Almeida JR, Mesquita MA (2010) Food intolerance, diet composition, and eating patterns in functional dyspepsia patients. Dig Dis Sci 55: 60–65.
35. Battais F, Pineau F, Popineau Y, Aparicio C, Kanny G, et al. (2003) Food allergy to wheat: identification of immunogloglin E and immunoglobulin G-binding proteins with sequential extracts and purified proteins from wheat flour. Clin Exp Allergy 33: 962–970.
36. Tay SS, Clark AT, Deighton J, King Y, Ewan PW (2007) Patterns of immunoglobulin G responses to egg and peanut allergens are distinct: ovalbumin-specific immunoglobulin responses are ubiquitous, but peanut-specific immunoglobulin responses are up-regulated in peanut allergy. Clin Exp Allergy 37: 1512–1518.
37. Satoguina JS, Weyand E, Larbi J, Hoerauf A (2005) T regulatory-1 cells induce IgG4 production by B cells: role of IL-10. J Immunol 174: 4718–4726.
38. Skripak JM, Nash SD, Rowley H, Brereton NH, Oh S, et al. (2008) A randomized, double-blind, placebo-controlled study of milk oral immunotherapy for cow's milk allergy. J Allergy Clin Immunol 122: 1154–1160.

Allergies and Risk of Head and Neck Cancer: An Original Study plus Meta-Analysis

Jenn-Ren Hsiao[1]⁹, Chun-Yen Ou[1]⁹, Hung-I Lo[1], Cheng-Chih Huang[1], Wei-Ting Lee[1], Jehn-Shyun Huang[2], Ken-Chung Chen[2], Tung-Yiu Wong[2], Sen-Tien Tsai[1], Chia-Jui Yen[3], Yuan-Hua Wu[4], Wei-Ting Hsueh[4], Ming-Wei Yang[4], Shang-Yin Wu[3], Jang-Yang Chang[3,5], Kwang-Yu Chang[3,5], Chen-Lin Lin[6], Fang-Ting Wang[1], Yi-Hui Wang[5], Ya-Ling Weng[5], Han-Chien Yang[5], Jeffrey S. Chang[5]*

1 Department of Otolaryngology, National Cheng Kung University Hospital, College of Medicine, National Cheng Kung University, Tainan, Taiwan, **2** Department of Stomatology, National Cheng Kung University Hospital, College of Medicine, National Cheng Kung University, Tainan, Taiwan, **3** Division of Hematology/Oncology, Department of Internal Medicine, National Cheng Kung University Hospital, College of Medicine, National Cheng Kung University, Tainan, Taiwan, **4** Department of Radiation Oncology, National Cheng Kung University Hospital, College of Medicine, National Cheng Kung University, Tainan, Taiwan, **5** National Institute of Cancer Research, National Health Research Institutes, Tainan, Taiwan, **6** Department of Nursing, National Cheng Kung University Hospital, College of Medicine, National Cheng Kung University, Tainan, Taiwan

Abstract

Background: Although the relationship between allergy and cancer has been investigated extensively, the role of allergy in head and neck cancer (HNC) appears less consistent. It is not clear whether allergies can independently influence the risk of HNC in the presence of known strong environmental risk factors, including consumption of alcohol, betel quid, and cigarette.

Methods: The current paper reports results from: 1) an original hospital-based case-control study, which included 252 incident cases of HNC and 236 controls frequency-matched to cases on sex and age; and 2) a meta-analysis combining the results of the current case-control study and 13 previously published studies (9 cohort studies with 727,569 subjects and 550 HNC outcomes and 5 case-control studies with 4,017 HNC cases and 10,928 controls).

Results: In the original case-control study, we observed a strong inverse association between allergies and HNC [odds ratio = 0.41, 95% confidence interval (CI): 0.27–0.62]. The meta-analysis also indicated a statistically significant inverse association between HNC and allergies [meta-relative risk (RR) = 0.76, 95% CI: 0.63–0.91], particularly strong for allergic rhinitis (meta-RR = 0.55, 95% CI: 0.40–0.76). In addition, the inverse association between allergies and HNC was observed only among men (meta-RR = 0.67, 95% CI: 0.54–0.84) but not among women (meta-RR = 0.98, 95% CI: 0.81–1.18).

Conclusions: These findings suggest that immunity plays an influential role in the risk of HNC. Future studies investigating immune biomarkers, including cytokine profiles and genetic polymorphisms, are warranted to further delineate the relationship between allergies and HNC. Understanding the relationship between allergies and HNC may help devise effective strategies to reduce and treat HNC.

Editor: Michael Scheurer, Baylor College of Medicine, United States of America

Funding: This work was funded by the National Health Research Institutes (CA-101-PP-07), the National Research Program for Biopharmaceuticals (100CAP1015-6, NSC100-2325-B-400-013), the National Science Council (NSC99-2314-B-006-018-MY3, NSC101-2325-B-006-009) and the Establishment of Cancer Research System Excellence Program funded by the Department of Health, Executive Yuan (DOH101-TD-C-111-003, DOH101-TD-C-111-004), Taiwan. The funders had no role in study design, data collection and analysis, decision to publish, or preparation of the manuscript.

Competing Interests: The authors have declared that no competing interests exist.

* E-mail: jeffreychang@nhri.org.tw

⁹ These authors contributed equally to this work.

Introduction

Head and neck cancer (HNC), including cancers of the oral cavity, oropharynx and larynx, is one of the leading cancers worldwide. Each year, approximately 400,000 cases of oral and oropharyngeal cancer and 160,000 cases of laryngeal cancer are diagnosed worldwide [1]. HNC is also a leading cancer among Taiwanese men, who have the second highest incidence of HNC in the world [2]. According to the Department of Health of Taiwan, HNC was the fourth most common cancer among Taiwanese men in 2009, with an annual incidence of 41 per 100,000 persons [3].

The occurrence of most HNC can be attributed to the consumption of alcohol, cigarette, and betel quid [4,5], although human papillomavirus infection also plays a role, particularly for oropharyngeal cancer [6]. Although alcohol, cigarette, and betel quid are the causes for the majority of the HNC cancer cases, most people who consume these three agents will not develop HNC in their lifetimes, which suggests the roles of other environmental and genetic factors [7,8]. Other potential risk factors for HNC include occupational exposures, poor oral hygiene, mouthwashes containing alcohol, and low fruit and vegetable intake [1,9]; however, there is insufficient knowledge regarding the pathogenesis of HNC.

Immune reactions manifested in the form of allergies have been extensively studied for their relationship with cancer risk [10–12]. Allergies usually result from an overactive immune response to substances in the environment among people with atopic tendency, who are genetically predisposed to produce immunoglobulin E (IgE) against common allergens [13–15]. The cross-linking of IgE on the surface of mast cells and basophils leads to a series of events resulting in allergic diseases, including allergic rhinitis, asthma, eczema, and food allergy [14].

Two hypotheses have been proposed to explain the inverse association between allergies and cancer, the "immunosurveillance hypothesis" and the "prophylaxis hypothesis" [11]. In the "immunosurveillance hypothesis", allergy does not play a direct role to reduce the risk of cancer but is merely a side effect of a more active immune function that effectively detects and eradicates malignant cells [11]. In contrast, allergy plays a direct role to reduce the risk of cancer in the "prophylaxis hypothesis" by expelling toxins or pathogens from the body [11]. A reduced risk associated with allergies has been consistently observed for glioma and pancreatic cancer [16,17], two cancers with largely unknown environmental risk factors. Compared to glioma and pancreatic cancer, the role of allergy in HNC appears less consistent. It is not clear whether allergies can independently influence the risk of HNC in the presence of known strong environmental risk factors, including alcohol, betel quid, and cigarette. In addition, only one previous study has examined the interaction between lifestyle factors (cigarette smoking and alcohol drinking) and allergies on the risk of HNC [18]. To this end, we conducted a hospital-based study to examine the association between allergies and HNC, including the interaction between allergies and alcohol, betel quid, or cigarette on the development of HNC. In addition, a comprehensive literature search was performed to conduct a meta-analysis, combining results from the published literature with the current study in order to explore the different aspects of the relationship between allergies and HNC and to generate new hypotheses for further investigations.

Materials and Methods

Original Study

This hospital-based case-control study was approved by the institutional review boards of the National Cheng Kung University Hospital and the National Health Research Institutes. All participants of the study signed a written informed consent.

Study subjects. All of the study subjects were recruited from the Department of Otolaryngology and the Department of Stomatology at the National Cheng Kung University Hospital from September 1, 2010 to June 30, 2012. The case subjects were patients newly diagnosed with HNC, including cancers of the oral cavity, oropharynx, and larynx, had no cancer history, aged 20 to 80 years, and had the ability to give informed consent. All HNC cases were pathologically confirmed squamous cell carcinoma. The controls subjects were patients who required surgery for non-cancerous diseases unrelated to cigarette smoking, alcohol drinking, or area nut/betel quid chewing, had no cancer history, had the ability to give informed consent, and frequency-matched to the cases on age (±5 years) and sex.

Data collection. In-person interview was conducted with each study subject by a trained interviewer using a standardized questionnaire. Demographic information, including sex, age, and educational level were collected. Detailed information (dose and duration) of the three major risk factors of HNC, including alcohol, betel quid, and cigarette, was ascertained. Study subjects were asked whether they had any of the five types of allergies, including allergic rhinitis, skin allergy, food allergy, drug allergy, and asthma. Those that responded positive were further asked about the age of onset for these allergies.

Statistical analysis. To assess for the differences in demographic variables and lifestyle habits (alcohol drinking, betel quid chewing, and cigarette smoking) between cases and controls, t-tests and chi-squared tests were performed for continuous variables and categorical variables, respectively. Multivariable unconditional logistic regression was performed to estimate the odds ratio (OR) and 95% confidence interval (CI) of HNC associated with allergies adjusted for age, sex, education, alcohol drinking (frequency), betel quid use (pack-years), and cigarette smoking (pack-years). Although, no pack-year definition has been established for betel-quid use, in order to adjust for the amount and the duration of betel quid use, a pack-year definition similar to the pack-year of cigarette of smoking was used, with 1 pack-year of betel quid use = 1 pack of betel quid (20 betel quids) use per day ×1 year. The analysis was first performed with all allergies combined (yes/no to any of the five allergies, number of allergies, duration of allergies, and age of allergic symptom onset). Subsequent analyses were performed to assess the association between HNC risk and individual types of allergies. To evaluate for the influence of allergy on the association between alcohol, betel quid, or cigarette and HNC, unconditional logistic regression was performed stratified by allergy status (yes/no). The heterogeneity of the association between alcohol, betel quid or cigarette and HNC risk by allergy status was assessed by the log-likelihood ratio test comparing the unconditional logistic regression model with the interaction term (allergy × alcohol, allergy × betel quid, or allergy × cigarette) to the model without the interaction term.

Meta-analysis

Literature search. A literature search was conducted until July 18, 2012 using the PubMed database and Thomson Reuters Web of Science with the search terms: "cancer AND ("allergies" OR "allergy" OR "atopy" OR "atopic" OR "asthma" OR "allergic rhinitis" OR "atopic dermatitis" OR "hive" OR "eczema") AND risk". A total of 1,463 articles were identified using the search terms (Figure 1). Articles were excluded if they had the following characteristics: 1) did not study allergy and cancer risk (n = 1,248); 2) commentary or response to commentary (n = 4); 3) review articles (n = 9); or 4) did not include HNC or did not report separate results for HNC (n = 191). Eleven articles were identified from this initial literature search.[18–28] No additional articles were identified by reviewing the reference lists of the 11 articles identified from the literature search. Two articles by Ericsson had overlapping information and only the most recent article was included in the current meta-analysis [21,22]. Three more articles [29–31] were identified by searching through the reference lists of four review articles [10–12,32]. Along with our original case-control study, a total of 14 studies (9 cohort studies with 727,569 subjects and 550 HNC outcomes and 5 case-control studies with 4,017 HNC cases and 10,928 controls) (Table S1) was included in the meta-analysis.

Data abstraction and calculation of summary statistics. The data extracted from each article included authors, year of publication, types of study (cohort or case-control

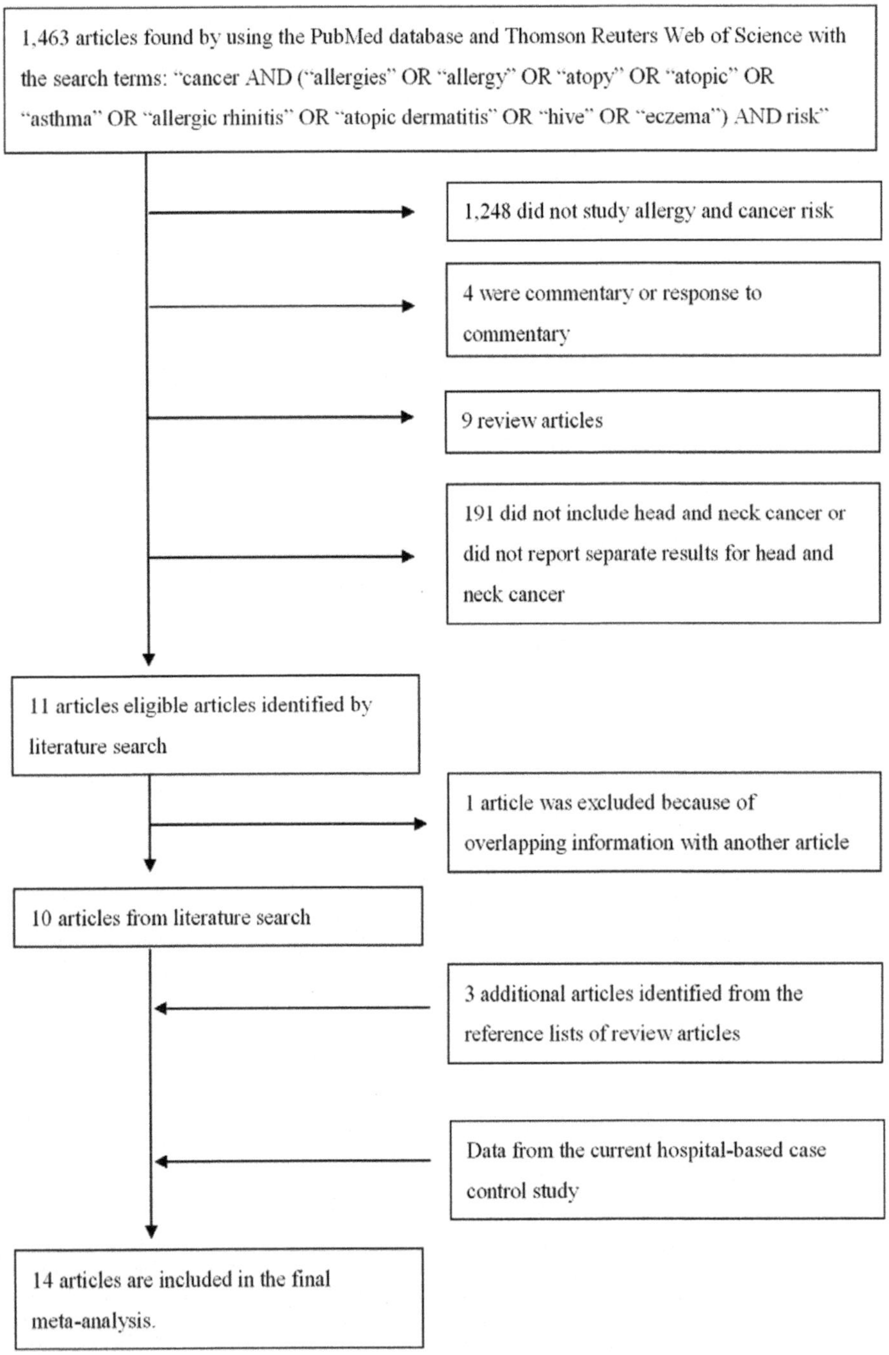

Figure 1. Process of article exclusion.

studies), number of study subjects, variables used for matching and for statistical adjustments, and relative risk (RR, which includes incidence ratio or standardize mortality ratio for cohort studies and odds ratio for case-control studies) with corresponding 95% CIs. For studies that presented only frequency data, RRs and 95% CIs were calculated using the exact method. If a study only reported RRs separately by gender, specific types of allergy or HNC sites, a meta-analysis with a fixed effects model was performed to combine stratum-specific RRs into an overall RR of HNC.

Statistical analysis. STATA software (version 11.0; Stata-Corp, College Station, TX, USA) was used to perform analyses of the current meta-analysis. Summary RRs (meta-RRs) was generated by the "metan" command [33]. The RRs of individual studies are displayed in a forest plot. I^2 statistic was used to evaluate inconsistencies between studies [34]. $I^2 = 0$–24.9%, 25–49.9%, and 50% or more represent low, moderate and high heterogeneity between studies, respectively. The summary RR was generated by a random effects model using the DerSimonian and Laird method if the heterogeneity was moderate to high ($I^2 \geq 25\%$) [35] and by a fixed effects model if the heterogeneity was low

Table 1. Demographic and lifestyle characteristics of the head and neck cancer patients and control subjects.

Characteristics	Cases N = 252 n (%)	Controls N = 236 n (%)	*P*
Age (years)			
Mean (SE)	55.3 (0.7)	53.5 (0.7)	0.05
Sex			
Male	238 (94.4)	220 (93.2)	0.57
Female	14 (5.6)	16 (6.8)	
Education			
≦ Elementary school	81 (32.1)	40 (16.9)	<0.0001
Junior high	77 (30.6)	42 (17.8)	
High school/Technical school	74 (29.4)	96 (40.7)	
Some college or more	20 (7.9)	58 (24.6)	
Alcohol			
Never+occasional	69 (27.4)	100 (42.4)	0.002
Former regular	49 (19.4)	33 (14.0)	
Current regular	134 (53.2)	103 (43.6)	
Never	62 (24.9)	85 (36.2)	<0.0001
1 drink per month	14 (5.6)	29 (12.3)	
1–2 drinks per week	10 (4.1)	14 (6.0)	
3–5 drinks per week	21 (8.4)	31 (13.2)	
Daily drinkers	142 (57.0)	76 (32.3)	
Betel quid			
Never	90 (35.7)	181 (76.7)	<0.0001
Former	103 (40.9)	36 (15.2)	
Current	59 (23.4)	19 (8.1)	
Pack-years (SE)	27.3 (2.9)	7.1 (1.3)	<0.0001
Cigarette			
Never	35 (13.9)	66 (28.0)	0.0001
Former	56 (22.2)	58 (24.6)	
Current	161 (63.9)	112 (47.4)	
Pack-years (SE)	35.1 (1.8)	23.5 (1.6)	<0.0001

Abbreviation: N, number; SE, standard error.

(I^2<25%). The analysis was first performed to generate an overall meta-RR measuring the association between all allergies combined and HNC risk. Additional analyses were performed by study design (cohort vs. case-control), by sex, by HNC sites, and by specific types of allergies (allergic rhinitis, skin allergy, or asthma). Sensitivity analysis was performed using the "metainf" command by excluding one study at a time to examine whether any individual study had a dominant effect on the summary RR. Publication bias was examined by viewing the funnel plot and by Egger's regression asymmetry test [36,37].

Results

Original Study

From September 1, 2010 to June 30, 2012, 252 HNC cases (166 oral cancers, 61 oropharyngeal cancers, and 25 laryngeal cancers) and 236 controls were successfully recruited with a participation of 74.3% and 86.5% for the cases and controls, respectively. The HNC cases were slightly older than controls (55.3 years vs. 53.5 years, P = 0.05) (Table 1). HNC cases and controls were similar in the distribution of sex (Table 1). Compared to controls, cases had lower educational levels (37% with ≥ high school education among cases vs. 65% with ≥ high school education among controls, P<0.0001) (Table 1). Cases had higher consumptions of alcohol, betel quid, and cigarette compared to controls in frequency, duration, and amount (Table 1).

Having any allergy was associated with a reduced risk of HNC (OR = 0.41, 95% CI: 0.27–0.62) (Table 2). This reduced risk was observed across all three HNC sites (oral cancer: OR = 0.36, 95% CI: 0.22–0.57; oropharyngeal cancer: OR = 0.49, 95% CI: 0.25–0.96; laryngeal cancer: OR = 0.48, 95% CI: 0.19–1.18). An inverse association between allergies and HNC was observed among both genders and was particularly strong for men (OR = 0.42, 95% CI: 0.27–0.64) but not statistically significant for women (OR = 0.67, 95 CI: 0.08–5.46), although the result for women was based on small numbers (14 cases and 16 controls). No clear trend in HNC risk was observed with the number of allergies or the duration of allergies (Table 2). In addition, the association between HNC risk and allergies did not differ by the age of allergy onset (<21 years vs. 21 years or older) (Table 2).

The most common type of allergy reported by the study subjects was allergic rhinitis (20% of cases and 41% of controls), which was

Table 2. The association between allergies and head and neck cancer.

Allergy	Head and neck cancer N = 252 n (%)	Control N = 236 n (%)	OR (95% CI)*	*P*
No	164 (65.1)	95 (40.3)	Referent	
Yes	88 (34.9)	135 (57.2)	0.41 (0.27–0.62)	<0.0001
Unknown	0 (1.2)	6 (2.5)	–	–
Number of allergies				
0	164 (65.1)	95 (40.2)	Referent	
1	54 (21.4)	80 (33.9)	0.39 (0.24–0.64)	0.0002
2	23 (9.1)	32 (13.6)	0.54 (0.28–1.02)	0.06
3 or more	10 (4.0)	17 (7.2)	0.40 (0.16–1.03)	0.06
unknown	1 (0.4)	12 (5.1)	–	–
Allergy duration				
No allergy	164 (65.1)	95 (40.3)	Referent	
<10 years	18 (7.1)	25 (10.6)	0.48 (0.23–0.99)	0.05
10–20 years	10 (4.0)	23 (9.7)	0.32 (0.14–0.75)	0.008
>20 years	48 (19.0)	67 (28.4)	0.45 (0.27–0.74)	0.002
Unknown	12 (4.8)	26 (11.0)	–	–
Age of allergy onset				
No allergy	164 (65.1)	95 (40.3)	Referent	
<21 years old	27 (10.7)	52 (22.0)	0.38 (0.21–0.68)	0.001
21 years or older	53 (21.0)	75 (31.8)	0.42 (0.26–0.69)	0.0005
Unknown	8 (3.2)	14 (5.9)	–	–

*OR was adjusted for age, sex, education, alcohol drinking (frequency), betel quid chewing (pack-years), and cigarette smoking (pack-years).
Abbreviations: CI, confidence interval; N, number; OR, odds ratio.

associated with a reduced risk of HNC (OR = 0.32, 95 CI: 0.20–0.52) (Table 3). A consistent reduction in the risk of HNC was seen with the other four types of allergies, including skin allergy, food allergy, drug allergy, and asthma.

The increased risk of HNC associated with alcohol drinking, betel quid chewing or cigarette smoking appeared stronger among those without history of allergies, although the tests for heterogeneity were not statistically significant (Table 4).

Meta-analysis (Table 5)

Combining the data from 14 studies (9 cohort and 5 case-control studies), the meta-analysis showed a reduced risk of HNC associated with having allergies (meta-RR = 0.76, 95% CI: 0.63–0.91, $I^2 = 76.5\%$) (Figure 2). Sensitivity analysis by dropping one study at a time did not indicate a dominant influence of any one individual study on the summary RR. The Egger's regression asymmetry test indicated no evidence of publication bias (p = 0.07). Funnel plot (Figure 3) showed that there may be minor evidence of publication bias with a slight over-representation of smaller studies (n = 2) [22,31] with a RR value greater than the meta-RR. However, the meta-analysis excluding those two smaller studies generated a result (meta-RR = 0.74, 95% CI: 0.62–0.90, $I^2 = 79.0\%$) that was nearly identical to the result that combined all 14 studies, which indicated that the possibility of publication bias was minimal.

The combined analysis of 9 cohort studies with 727,569 subjects with allergies and 550 HNC outcomes showed a 9% reduction in HNC risk associated with allergies, although not statistically significant (meta-RR = 0.91, 95% CI: 0.71–1.17, $I^2 = 74.0\%$). The combined analysis of 5 case-control studies with 4,017 HNC cases and 10,928 controls showed a statistically significant inverse association between allergies and HNC (meta-RR = 0.58, 95% CI: 0.44–0.78, $I^2 = 76.1\%$).

When stratified by sex, the inverse association between allergies and HNC was only observed among men (meta-RR = 0.67, 95% CI: 0.54–0.84, $I^2 = 68.2\%$) but not among women (meta-RR = 0.98, 95% CI: 0.81–1.18, $I^2 = 20.2\%$). In the analysis with specific types of allergies, the strongest reduced risk of HNC was observed for allergic rhinitis (meta-RR = 0.55, 95% CI: 0.40–0.76, $I^2 = 46.1\%$) and a weaker reduction in HNC risk was observed for skin allergy (meta-RR = 0.84, 95% CI: 0.62–1.14, $I^2 = 43.0\%$) and asthma (meta-RR = 0.86, 95% CI: 0.71–1.05, $I^2 = 63.1\%$). A reduced risk associated with allergies was observed across all three sites of HNC (meta-RR for oral cancer = 0.78, 95% CI: 0.61–1.00, $I^2 = 72.2\%$; meta-RR for oropharyngeal cancer = 0.69, 95% CI: 0.58–0.82, $I^2 = 33.6\%$; meta-RR for laryngeal cancer = 0.66, 95% CI: 0.47–0.92, $I^2 = 53.0\%$) (Table 5); however, similar to the results of all sites combined, the inverse association between allergies and subsites of HNC occurred predominantly among men.

Discussion

A statistically significant inverse association between allergies and HNC was observed in our hospital-based case-control study. Combining the results of our study and those from the 13 published studies, the meta-analysis also indicated a statistically significant inverse association between HNC and allergies, particularly for allergic rhinitis and predominantly among men.

The inverse association between allergies and cancer may be explained by two hypotheses, the "immunosurveillance hypothe-

Table 3. The association between head and neck cancer and specific types of allergies.

Allergies	Cases N = 252	Controls N = 236	OR (95% CI)*	P
Nasal allergy				
No allergy	164 (65.1)	95 (40.2)	Referent	
Yes	51 (20.2)	97 (41.1)	0.32 (0.20–0.52)	<0.0001
Other allergies	36 (14.3)	36 (15.3)	0.67 (0.37–1.20)	0.18
Unknown	1 (0.4)	8 (3.4)	–	–
Skin allergy				
No allergy	164 (65.1)	95 (40.2)	Referent	
Yes	39 (15.5)	40 (17.0)	0.67 (0.38–1.17)	0.16
Other allergies	49 (19.4)	92 (39.0)	0.32 (0.20–0.52)	<0.0001
Unknown	0 (0.0)	9 (3.8)	–	–
Food allergy				
No allergy	164 (65.1)	95 (40.2)	Referent	
Yes	20 (7.9)	23 (9.8)	0.63 (0.30–1.31)	0.21
Other allergies	68 (27.0)	112 (47.5)	0.38 (0.24–0.58)	<0.0001
Unknown	0 (0.0)	6 (2.5)	–	–
Drug Allergy				
No allergy	164 (65.1)	95 (40.2)	Referent	
Yes	16 (6.3)	29 (12.3)	0.44 (0.21–0.92)	0.03
Other allergies	72 (28.6)	105 (44.5)	0.41 (0.27–0.64)	<0.0001
Unknown	0 (0.0)	7 (3.0)	–	–
Asthma				
No allergy	164 (65.1)	95 (40.2)	Referent	
Yes	7 (2.8)	17 (7.2)	0.26 (0.09–0.73)	0.01
Other allergies	81 (32.1)	118 (50.0)	0.44 (0.29–0.67)	0.0001
Unknown	0 (0.0)	6 (2.6)	–	–

*OR was adjusted for age, sex, education, alcohol drinking (frequency), betel quid chewing (pack-years), and cigarette smoking (pack-years).
Abbreviations: CI, confidence interval; N, number; OR, odds ratio.

sis" and the "prophylaxis hypothesis" [11]. In the "immunosurveillance hypothesis", allergy is a side effect of an overactive immune function that effectively detects and eradicates malignant cells and does not play a direct role to reduce the risk of cancer [11]. In contrast, in the "prophylaxis hypothesis", allergy is directly involved in cancer prevention by expelling toxins or pathogens from the body [11]. A review by Sherman *et al.* observed that the inverse association between allergies and cancer was more commonly found among tissues or organ systems that interface with the external environment (*i.e.* glia, mouth and throat, colon and rectum, pancreas, skin, uterus and cervix, lung, bladder, and gastrointestinal tract) than among those that do not (*i.e.* ovaries, meninges, prostate, breast, and blood cells); this led them to conclude that the "prophylaxis hypothesis" may be the more appropriate explanation for the site-specific inverse association between allergies and certain cancers [11]. Although the results from our case-control study and meta-analysis appear to be consistent with the "prophylaxis hypothesis" because the three sites of HNC, oral cavity, oropharynx, and larynx, directly interface with the external environment, the role of "immunosurveillance hypothesis" cannot be ruled out by the evidence from this analysis. Further investigation is needed to delineate the underlying biological mechanism for the inverse association between allergies and HNC risk.

IgE plays a key role in most allergic reactions and evidence shows that IgE itself may possess anti-tumor activities [38]. An immunohistochemical study by Neuchrist *et al.* examined the distribution of immunoglobulins in squamous cell carcinoma of head and neck by comparing tumor and normal tissues [39]. They found that the distribution of IgE showed the largest difference, with significantly higher number of IgE-positive cells found in the tumor tissue compared to the normal tissue [39], which suggested that IgE may participate in tumor surveillance. In addition, IgE may also bind to cell surface IgE receptors, FcεRI and CD23, and engage several types of effector cells in antibody-dependent cellular cytotoxicity and antibody-dependent cellular phagocytosis against cancer cells [38]. Overall, the possible anti-tumor activities of IgE may partially explain the inverse association between allergies and cancer, including HNC.

In our original case-control study, there was a suggestion that allergies may attenuate the carcinogenic effect of alcohol, betel quid, or cigarette on the development of HNC risk, although the results were not statistically significant likely due to a sample size without sufficient statistical power. A possible explanation for the attenuating effect of allergies on HNC risk due to alcohol, betel quid, or cigarette may be a hyperactive immune function that can detect and destroy malignant cells before they have a chance to grow and expand. Alternatively, allergy-associated immune activities may rid body of the carcinogens before they have a chance to induce the oncogenic transformation of normal cells. However, in a previous study by Michaud *et al.* the association between allergies and HNC risk did not differ by smoking status (never smoker: OR = 0.75, 95% CI:0.54–1.04; former smoker: OR = 0.80, 95% CI: 0.62–1.02) or drinking status (less than 7 drinks per week: OR = 0.78, 95% CI: 0.60–1.01; greater than 25 drinks per week: OR = 0.59, 95% CI: 0.37–0.95) [18]. Unfortunately, among the studies to date, only Michaud *et al.* [18] and our study had examined the interaction between allergies and lifestyle factors (cigarette smoking, alcohol drinking, or betel quid chewing) on HNC risk, and thus, we were unable to explore this topic further in the meta-analysis.

The results from the meta-analysis showed that the inverse association between allergies and HNC was stronger among the case-control studies (meta-RR = 0.58, 95% CI: 0.44–0.78) compared to that among the cohort studies (meta-RR = 0.91, 95% CI: 0.71–1.17). All except one of the cohort studies on the association between allergies and HNC used data from medical records or clinical tests, whereas all of the case-control studies used self-reported data of allergies. Self-reported data might be more inaccurate due to recall errors associated with false memory or misinterpretation of non-allergic symptoms (*e.g.* common cold) as allergies. These recall errors were likely non-differential and would have biased the results toward the null; thus, the actual inverse association between allergies and HNC should be stronger in the absence of non-differential recall errors. Self-reported data in a case-control study can also be subject to differential recall bias. Usually, case subjects are more likely to ruminate about the possible causes of their diseases and may thus report more allergic symptoms, leading to a false positive association between allergies and HNC. However, the current meta-analysis indicated an inverse association between allergies and HNC for the case-control studies. In addition, the potential association between allergies and cancer is not well-known to the public; therefore, the inverse

Table 4. The association between lifestyle factors and head and neck cancer by allergy status.

Characteristics	Allergy = Yes OR (95% CI)*	Allergy = No OR (95% CI)*	Interaction *P*
Alcohol			
Never+non-daily drinkers	Referent	Referent	
Ever daily drinker	1.47 (0.76–2.85)	2.65 (1.37–5.13)	0.17
Never+non-daily drinkers	Referent	Referent	
Former daily drinker	1.18 (0.40–3.51)	2.23 (0.62–8.10)	
Current daily drinkers	1.56 (0.77–3.18)	2.73 (1.37–5.45)	0.39
Betel quid			
Never	Referent	Referent	
Ever	4.25 (2.14–8.42)	5.62 (2.84–11.12)	0.49
Never	Referent	Referent	
Former	3.82 (1.82–7.99)	6.31 (2.88–13.82)	0.49
Current	5.48 (2.08–14.45)	4.57 (1.80–11.59)	
Pack-years			
Never	Referent	Referent	
<20 pack-years	3.29 (1.44–7.49)	3.97 (1.66–9.50)	
≥20 pack-years	4.76 (2.04–11.09)	6.51 (2.84–14.95)	0.80
Cigarette			
Never	Referent	Referent	
Ever	0.98 (0.41–2.38)	2.63 (1.17–5.93)	0.09
Never	Referent	Referent	
Former	0.87 (0.31–2.41)	2.60 (1.05–6.42)	0.28
Current	1.05 (0.42–2.62)	2.66 (1.11–6.39)	
Pack-years			
Never	Referent	Referent	
<20 pack-years	0.62 (0.21–1.77)	3.17 (1.15–8.73)	0.11
≥20 pack-years	1.28 (0.51–3.22)	(1.04–5.62)	

*OR was adjusted for age, sex, education, alcohol drinking (frequency), betel quid chewing (pack-years), and cigarette smoking (pack-years).
Abbreviations: CI, confidence interval; OR, odds ratio.

association between allergies and HNC among the case-control studies is unlikely due to differential recall bias. Compared to the cohort studies, the case-control studies were more likely to suffer from reverse causality, since the information on allergies was ascertained after the diagnosis of HNC and the immune function might be affected by the oncogenic process. In our original hospital-based case-control study, even when we considered allergies occurring more than 10 years before the diagnosis of cancer (or before the interview date for the controls), a strong inverse association between allergies and HNC still existed. In a hospital-based case-control by Vena et al. which considered only allergies diagnosed five years before the hospital admission, a reduced risk of HNC associated with allergies was observed among men [26]. These indicate that reverse causality might not play a major role in the inverse relationship between allergies and HNC. Although cohort studies do not suffer from recall bias or reverse causality, they are not without limitations. A major limitation of cohort studies, especially when studying a rare disease or a disease with a long latency period (*e.g.* cancer), is that there may not be enough outcomes during the follow-up period to produce a precise effect estimate [40].

An alternative method to study the association between allergies and HNC is "Mendelian Randomization", which utilizes a functional genetic polymorphism as an instrumental variable to study the relationship between modifiable exposures and disease in observational studies [41]. Genetic polymorphisms are not subject to recall or selection biases and therefore may serve as a more objective marker. For example, interleukin-4 is a key cytokine that induces naïve T-helper cells to differentiate into T-helper 2 cells, which play a major role in the development of allergies [42]. The T allele of a promoter single nucleotide polymorphism of the interleukin-4 gene, C-589T (also known as C-590T or rs2243250), has been associated with a higher level of serum IgE and a higher risk of allergy [43]. To date, three studies have examined the relationship between rs2243250 and HNC, specifically oral cancer [44–46]. Two of the three studies showed an increased risk of oral cancer with either the C allele [45] or the CC genotype [46], consistent with an inverse association between allergies and HNC. However, one study reported an opposite finding with an increased risk of oral cancer associated with the TT genotype [44]. With more investigations of rs2243250 and other genetic polymorphisms associated with allergies, the true association and the underlying biological mechanism between allergies and HNC may be clarified.

The current meta-analysis suggests that the inverse association between allergies and HNC may be particularly strong for allergic rhinitis. It has been long observed that not all people with atopic tendency will develop allergic symptoms and those who develop

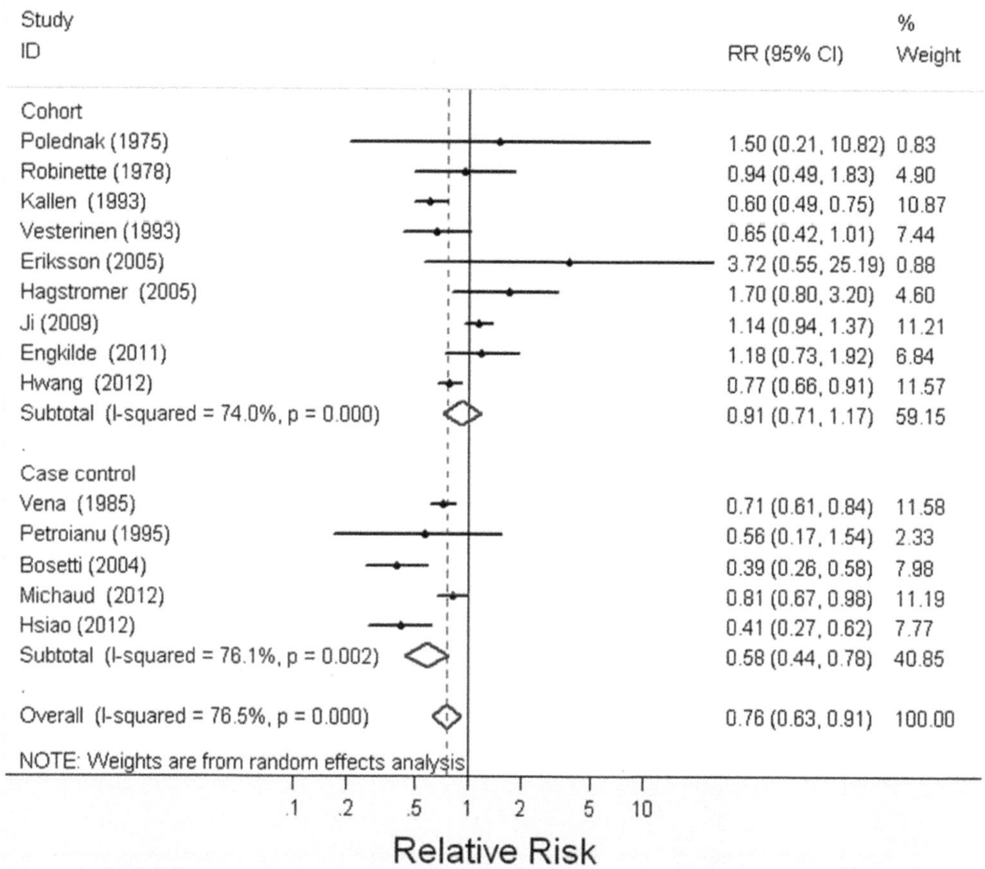

Figure 2. Meta-analysis assessing the association between allergies and head and neck cancer Risk.

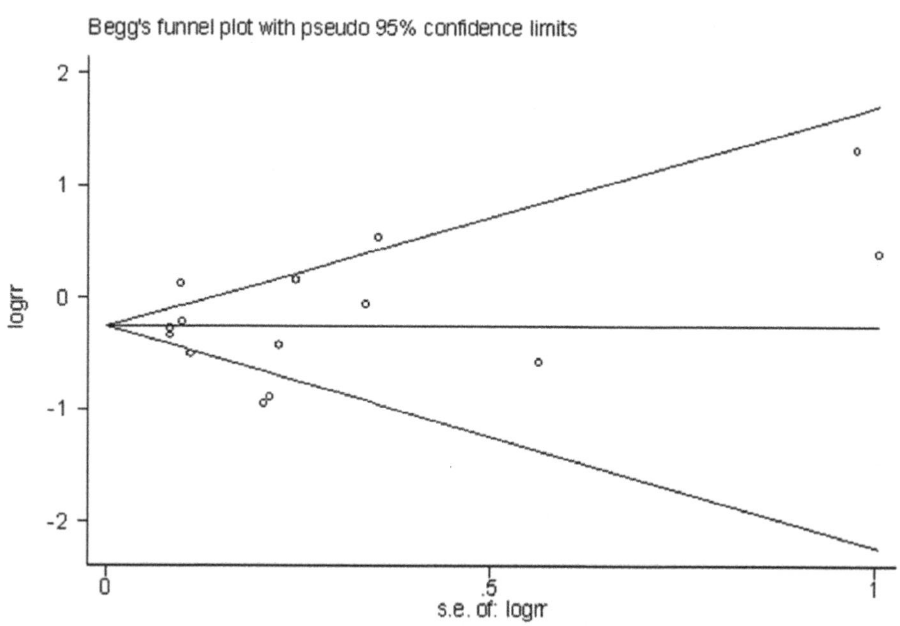

Figure 3. Funnel plot of the 14 studies assessing the association between allergies and head and neck cancer risk.

Table 5. Meta-analysis on the association between allergy and head and neck cancer.

	Both genders combined			Male			Female		
	n	Meta-RR (95% CI)*	I^2	n	Meta-RR (95% CI)*	I^2	n	Meta-RR (95% CI)*	I^2
Head and neck cancer									
All allergy combined	14	0.76 (0.63–0.91)	76.5	9	0.67 (0.54–0.84)	68.2	7	0.98 (0.81–1.18)	20.2
Study designs									
Cohort	9	0.91 (0.71–1.17)	74.0	5	0.80 (0.60–1.07)	34.7	3	0.89 (0.48–1.65)	47.2
Case–control	5	0.58 (0.44–0.78)	76.1	4	0.56 (0.39–0.81)	83.4	4	0.98 (0.79–1.21)	19.6
Allergic rhinitis	3	0.55 (0.40–0.76)	46.1	3	0.53 (0.42–0.66)	20.0	3	1.25 (0.77–2.04)	0.0
Skin allergy	5	0.84 (0.62–1.14)	43.0	4	0.82 (0.62–1.08)	0.0	3	0.78 (0.50–1.21)	0.0
Asthma	9	0.86 (0.71–1.05)	63.1	6	0.79 (0.61–1.02)	35.8	3	1.55 (1.02–2.38)	0.0
Oral cancer									
All allergy combined	9	0.78 (0.61–1.00)	72.2	7	0.64 (0.45–0.91)	69.1	4	1.06 (0.76–1.50)	33.7
Allergic rhinitis	3	0.56 (0.36–0.88)	66.6	3	0.48 (0.31–0.75)	48.8	2	1.31 (0.79–2.16)	0.0
Skin allergy	5	0.84 (0.52–1.34)	64.8	4	0.77 (0.48–1.25)	42.7	2	0.68 (0.42–1.12)	0.0
Asthma	6	0.88 (0.74–1.04)	0.0	5	0.76 (0.57–1.02)	0.0	2	1.59 (0.97–2.61)	0.0
Pharynx									
All allergy combined	10	0.69 (0.58–0.82)	33.6	7	0.67 (0.45–1.00)	61.4	4	1.12 (0.60–2.12)	49.5
Allergic rhinitis	3	0.43 (0.23–0.80)	37.1	3	0.49 (0.22–0.83)	41.7	0	–	–
Skin allergy	4	0.92 (0.65–1.30)	0.0	4	0.97 (0.62–1.50)	17.9	2	0.75 (0.33–1.74)	42.4
Asthma	7	0.67 (0.56–0.79)	0.0	5	0.79 (0.54–1.15)	0.0	2	2.06 (0.70–6.10)	0.0
Larynx									
All allergy combined	7	0.66 (0.47–0.92)	53.0	5	0.64 (0.42–0.96)	56.7	2	0.67 (0.22–2.04)	0.0
Allergic rhinitis	2	0.39 (0.13–1.13)	42.2	2	0.40 (0.15–1.08)	33.1	0	–	–
Skin allergy	2	1.07 (0.61–1.85)	0.0	2	1.10 (0.63–1.92)	0.0	0	–	–
Asthma	4	0.86 (0.58–1.28)	38.8	3	0.92 (0.48–1.74)	67.3	1	–	–

*The Meta-RR was generated by a random effects model using the DersSimonian and Laird method if the heterogeneity was high to moderate ($I^2 \geq 25\%$) and by a fixed effects model if the heterogeneity was low ($I^2 < 25\%$).
Abbreviations: CI, confidence interval; meta-RR, meta-relative risk; n, number of studies.

allergies can have different symptoms with some develop asthma while others develop allergic rhinitis or different combinations of symptoms [13,15]. Studies have detected IgE to specific allergens in the nasal washing among patients with allergic rhinitis regardless of their systemic allergy test status, suggesting the importance of local IgE production in the development of allergic rhinitis [15]. It is possible that allergic rhinitis may be an indicator for a more active local immunity in the upper aerodigestive tract against foreign substances, leading to a reduced HNC risk; however, this needs to be confirmed with further investigations.

The inverse association between allergies and HNC was present predominantly among men as indicated by the results of the current meta-analysis. While there is no obvious explanation for this observation, several HNC differences between men and women may provide clues. The incidence of HNC is higher among men than women, ranging from 1.6 times to 9.8 times higher depending on the anatomical sites and the regions of the world. Studies have shown that a higher proportion of HNC among men (74–82%) can be attributed to alcohol and cigarette compared to women (50–61%) [7,47,48], suggesting that HNC in women may have other causes that are less common among men. Although cigarette smoking may explain more of the HNC cases among men than among women, women appear to be more susceptible to the carcinogenic effect of cigarette. For those who smoked up to one cigarette pack per day, the HNC risk was higher in women (hazard ratio: 3.08, 95% CI: 1.77–5.36) than in men (hazard ratio: 1.26, 95% CI: 0.99–1.61) [49]. The possible differences in the causes of and the susceptibility to HNC between men and women may have contributed to their disparity in the association between allergies and HNC. More investigations on these gender differences may help establish the biological mechanism underlying the relationship between allergies and HNC.

Several limitations must be considered when interpreting the results of the current analysis. Because our case-control study is hospital-based, it is difficult to determine whether the cases and controls arise from the same source population. Our recruiting hospital is a major medical center in Southern Taiwan, and over 95% of our study subjects came from the county where the hospital is located. Even though we tried to exclude controls with diseases related to the use of alcohol, betel quid, and cigarette smoking, the possibility remains that our controls may not be representative of the background population for the cases. For the meta-analysis, studies were heterogeneous in design, patient population, disease sites, and types of allergies assessed. We explored the sources of heterogeneity by performing subgroup analyses by study design, disease sites, types of allergies, and gender. In addition, random-effect models were used to account for the heterogeneity across studies. Finally, the association between allergies and HNC was only assessed qualitatively with a binary status (yes vs. no) in the current analysis. More studies with quantitative measures of allergies (*e.g.* severity as indicated by the level of serum IgE, numbers of allergy-associated genetic variants, cytokine profiles) may provide a clearer picture to describe the relationship between allergies and HNC.

In summary, we observed an inverse association between allergies and HNC, particularly among men, in our original case-control study and meta-analysis. This suggests that immunity may play an important role to influence the risk of HNC. Future studies may investigate immune biomarkers, including cytokine profiles and genetic polymorphisms to further delineate the relationship between allergies and HNC. In addition, more studies are needed to determine whether allergies can reduce the risk HNC associated with alcohol, betel quid, or cigarette. Understanding the relationship between allergies and HNC may help devise effective strategies to reduce and treat HNC.

Supporting Information

Table S1 Fourteen studies (9 cohort studies and 5 case-control studies) included in the meta-analysis for the association between allergies and head and neck cancer.

Checklist S1 PRISMA Checklist.

Acknowledgments

We thank Dr. Neela Guha of the International Agency for Research on Cancer for her careful editing of the manuscript.

Author Contributions

Conceived and designed the experiments: JRH JSC. Performed the experiments: JRH JSC CLL FTW Y. Wang YLW HCY JSC. Analyzed the data: JRH CYO JSC. Contributed reagents/materials/analysis tools: JSC. Wrote the paper: JRH CYO JSC. Acquisition of data: JRH CYO HIL CCH WTL JSH KCC TYW STT CJY Y. Wu WTH MWY SYW JYC KYC CLL FTW Y. Wang YLW HCY JSC. Interpretation of data: JRH CYO HIL CCH WTL JSH KCC TYW STT CJY Y. Wu WTH MWY SYW JYC KYC CLL FTW Y. Wang YLW HCY JSC. Critically evaluated or revised the content of the manuscript: JRH CYO HIL CCH WTL JSH KCC TYW STT CJY Y. Wu WTH MWY SYW JYC KYC CLL FTW Y. Wang YLW HCY JSC. Approved the final manuscript: JRH CYO HIL CCH WTL JSH KCC TYW STT CJY Y. Wu WTH MWY SYW JYC KYC CLL FTW Y. Wang YLW HCY JSC.

References

1. Boyle P, Levin B, editors (2008) World Cancer Report. Lyon: International Agency for Research on Cancer.
2. International Agency for Research on Cancer. Globocan 2008. Available: http://globocan.iarc.fr/. Accessed 2012 Aug 1.
3. Department of Health, Taiwan, R.O.C. Annual Cancer Report, Year 2009. Available: http://www.bhp.doh.gov.tw. Accessed 2012 Aug 1.
4. Bouvard V, Baan R, Straif K, Grosse Y, Secretan B, et al. (2009) A review of human carcinogens–Part B: biological agents. Lancet Oncol 10: 321–322.
5. Secretan B, Straif K, Baan R, Grosse Y, El Ghissassi F, et al. (2009) A review of human carcinogens–Part E: tobacco, areca nut, alcohol, coal smoke, and salted fish. Lancet Oncol 10: 1033–1034.
6. Mehanna H, Beech T, Nicholson T, El-Hariry I, McConkey C, et al. (2012 Jan 20. doi: 10.1002/hed.22015. [Epub ahead of print]) Prevalence of human papillomavirus in oropharyngeal and nonoropharyngeal head and neck cancer-systematic review and meta-analysis of trends by time and region. Head Neck.
7. Hashibe M, Brennan P, Chuang SC, Boccia S, Castellsague X, et al. (2009) Interaction between tobacco and alcohol use and the risk of head and neck cancer: pooled analysis in the International Head and Neck Cancer Epidemiology Consortium. Cancer Epidemiol Biomarkers Prev 18: 541–550.
8. de Andrade M, Amos CI, Foulkes WD (1998) Segregation analysis of squamous cell carcinoma of the head and neck: evidence for a major gene determining risk. Ann Hum Genet 62: 505–510.
9. Guha N, Boffetta P, Wunsch Filho V, Eluf Neto J, Shangina O, et al. (2007) Oral health and risk of squamous cell carcinoma of the head and neck and esophagus: results of two multicentric case-control studies. Am J Epidemiol 166: 1159–1173.
10. Merrill RM, Isakson RT, Beck RE (2007) The association between allergies and cancer: what is currently known? Ann Allergy Asthma Immunol 99: 102–116; quiz 117–109, 150.
11. Sherman PW, Holland E, Sherman JS (2008) Allergies: their role in cancer prevention. Q Rev Biol 83: 339–362.
12. Turner MC, Chen Y, Krewski D, Ghadirian P (2006) An overview of the association between allergy and cancer. Int J Cancer 118: 3124–3132.
13. Kay AB (2000) Overview of 'allergy and allergic diseases: with a view to the future'. Br Med Bull 56: 843–864.
14. Durham SR, Smurthwaite L, Gould HJ (2000) Local IgE production. Am J Rhinol 14: 305–307.
15. Hoddeson EK, Pratt E, Harvey RJ, Wise SK (2010) Local and systemic IgE in the evaluation and treatment of allergy. Otolaryngol Clin North Am 43: 503–520, viii.
16. Linos E, Raine T, Alonso A, Michaud D (2007) Atopy and risk of brain tumors: a meta-analysis. J Natl Cancer Inst 99: 1544–1550.
17. Gandini S, Lowenfels AB, Jaffee EM, Armstrong TD, Maisonneuve P (2005) Allergies and the risk of pancreatic cancer: a meta-analysis with review of epidemiology and biological mechanisms. Cancer Epidemiol Biomarkers Prev 14: 1908–1916.
18. Michaud DS, Langevin SM, Eliot M, Nelson HH, McClean MD, et al. (2012) Allergies and risk of head and neck cancer. Cancer Causes Control 23: 1317–1322.
19. Bosetti C, Talamini R, Franceschi S, Negri E, Giacosa A, et al. (2004) Allergy and the risk of selected digestive and laryngeal neoplasms. Eur J Cancer Prev 13: 173–176.
20. Engkilde K, Thyssen JP, Menne T, Johansen JD (2011) Association between cancer and contact allergy: a linkage study. BMJ Open 1: e000084.
21. Eriksson NE, Holmen A, Hogstedt B, Mikoczy Z, Hagmar L (1995) A prospective study of cancer incidence in a cohort examined for allergy. Allergy 50: 718–722.
22. Eriksson NE, Mikoczy Z, Hagmar L (2005) Cancer incidence in 13811 patients skin tested for allergy. J Investig Allergol Clin Immunol 15: 161–166.
23. Hagstromer L, Ye W, Nyren O, Emtestam L (2005) Incidence of cancer among patients with atopic dermatitis. Arch Dermatol 141: 1123–1127.
24. Hwang CY, Chen YJ, Lin MW, Chen TJ, Chu SY, et al. (2012) Cancer risk in patients with allergic rhinitis, asthma and atopic dermatitis: a nationwide cohort study in Taiwan. Int J Cancer 130: 1160–1167.
25. Kallen B, Gunnarskog J, Conradson TB (1993) Cancer risk in asthmatic subjects selected from hospital discharge registry. Eur Respir J 6: 694–697.
26. Vena JE, Bona JR, Byers TE, Middleton E Jr, Swanson MK, et al. (1985) Allergy-related diseases and cancer: an inverse association. Am J Epidemiol 122: 66–74.
27. Vesterinen E, Pukkala E, Timonen T, Aromaa A (1993) Cancer incidence among 78,000 asthmatic patients. Int J Epidemiol 22: 976–982.
28. Ji J, Shu X, Li X, Sundquist K, Sundquist J, et al. (2009) Cancer risk in hospitalised asthma patients. Br J Cancer 100: 829–833.
29. Petroianu A, Chaves DN, De Oliveira O Jr (1995) Comparative incidence of allergy in the presence or absence of cancer. J Int Med Res 23: 358–363.
30. Robinette CD, Fraumeni JF Jr (1978) Asthma and subsequent mortality in World War II veterans. J Chronic Dis 31: 619–624.
31. Polednak AP (1975) Letter: Asthma and cancer mortality. Lancet 2: 1147–1148.
32. Wang H, Diepgen TL (2005) Is atopy a protective or a risk factor for cancer? A review of epidemiological studies. Allergy 60: 1098–1111.
33. Harris RJ, Bradburn MJ, Deeks JJ, Harbord RM, Altman DG, et al. (2008) Metan: fixed- and random-effects meta-analysis. The Stata Journal 8: 3–28.
34. Higgins JP, Thompson SG, Deeks JJ, Altman DG (2003) Measuring inconsistency in meta-analyses. Bmj 327: 557–560.
35. DerSimonian R, Laird N (1986) Meta-analysis in clinical trials. Control Clin Trials 7: 177–188.
36. Sterne JAC, Egger M, Smith GD (2005) Investigating and dealing with publication and other biases. In: Egger M, Smith GD, Altman DG, editors. Systematic Reviews in Health: Care Meta-Analysis Context. London: BMJ Books, 285–312.
37. Egger M, Davey Smith G, Schneider M, Minder C (1997) Bias in meta-analysis detected by a simple, graphical test. BMJ 315: 629–634.
38. Jensen-Jarolim E, Achatz G, Turner MC, Karagiannis S, Legrand F, et al. (2008) AllergoOncology: the role of IgE-mediated allergy in cancer. Allergy 63: 1255–1266.
39. Neuchrist C, Kornfehl J, Grasl M, Lassmann H, Kraft D, et al. (1994) Distribution of immunoglobulins in squamous cell carcinoma of the head and neck. Int Arch Allergy Immunol 104: 97–100.
40. Grimes DA, Schulz KF (2002) Cohort studies: marching towards outcomes. Lancet 359: 341–345.
41. Davey Smith G, Ebrahim S (2003) 'Mendelian randomization': can genetic epidemiology contribute to understanding environmental determinants of disease? Int J Epidemiol 32: 1–22.

42. Sokol CL, Barton GM, Farr AG, Medzhitov R (2008) A mechanism for the initiation of allergen-induced T helper type 2 responses. Nat Immunol 9: 310–318.
43. de Guia RM, Ramos JD (2010) The -590C/TIL4 single-nucleotide polymorphism as a genetic factor of atopic allergy. Int J Mol Epidemiol Genet 1: 67–73.
44. Vairaktaris E, Yannopoulos A, Vassiliou S, Serefoglou Z, Vylliotis A, et al. (2007) Strong association of interleukin-4 (−590 C/T) polymorphism with increased risk for oral squamous cell carcinoma in Europeans. Oral Surg Oral Med Oral Pathol Oral Radiol Endod 104: 796–802.
45. Gaur P, Mittal M, Mohanti B, Das S (2011) Functional variants of IL4 and IL6 genes and risk of tobacco-related oral carcinoma in high-risk Asian Indians. Oral Dis 17: 720–726.
46. Tsai MH, Chen WC, Tsai CH, Hang LW, Tsai FJ (2005) Interleukin-4 gene, but not the interleukin-1 beta gene polymorphism, is associated with oral cancer. J Clin Lab Anal 19: 93–98.
47. Anantharaman D, Marron M, Lagiou P, Samoli E, Ahrens W, et al. (2011) Population attributable risk of tobacco and alcohol for upper aerodigestive tract cancer. Oral Oncol 47: 725–731.
48. Blot WJ, McLaughlin JK, Winn DM, Austin DF, Greenberg RS, et al. (1988) Smoking and drinking in relation to oral and pharyngeal cancer. Cancer Res 48: 3282–3287.
49. Freedman ND, Abnet CC, Leitzmann MF, Hollenbeck AR, Schatzkin A (2007) Prospective investigation of the cigarette smoking-head and neck cancer association by sex. Cancer 110: 1593–1601.

13

Anti-Allergic Role of Cholinergic Neuronal Pathway via α7 Nicotinic ACh Receptors on Mucosal Mast Cells in a Murine Food Allergy Model

Takeshi Yamamoto[1], Toshihisa Kodama[1], Jaemin Lee[1], Naho Utsunomiya[1], Shusaku Hayashi[1], Hiroshi Sakamoto[2], Hirofumi Kuramoto[3], Makoto Kadowaki[1]*

1 Division of Gastrointestinal Pathophysiology, Institute of Natural Medicine, University of Toyama, Toyama, Toyama, Japan, **2** Department of Physical Therapy, Health Science University, Fujikawaguchiko, Yamanashi, Japan, **3** Department of Applied Biology, Kyoto Institute of Technology, Kyoto, Kyoto, Japan

Abstract

The prevalence of food allergy (FA) has increased in developed countries over the past few decades. However, no effective drug therapies are currently available. Therefore, we investigated cholinergic anti-inflammatory pathway as a regulatory system to ameliorate disrupted mucosal immune homeostasis in the gut based on the pathophysiological elucidation of mucosal mast cells (MMCs) in a murine FA model. BALB/c mice sensitized with ovalbumin received repeated oral ovalbumin for the development of FA. FA mice developed severe allergic diarrhea and exhibited enhanced type 2 helper T (Th2) cell immune responses in both systemic immunity and mucosal immunity, along with MMCs hyperplasia in the colon. MMCs were localized primarily in the strategic position of the mucosal epithelium. Furthermore, the allergic symptoms did not develop in p85α disrupted phosphoinositide-3 kinase-deficient mice that lacked mast cells in the gut. Vagal stimulation by 2-deoxy-D-glucose and drug treatment with nicotinic ACh receptor (nAChR) agonists (nicotine and α7 nAChR agonist GTS-21) alleviated the allergic symptoms in the FA mice. Nicotine treatment suppressed MMCs hyperplasia, enhanced MPO and upregulated mRNA expression of Th1 and Th2 cytokines in the FA mice colon. MMCs, which are negatively regulated by α7 nAChRs, were often located in close proximity to cholinergic CGRP-immunoreactive nerve fibers in the FA mice colon. The present results reveal that the cholinergic neuroimmune interaction via α7 nAChRs on MMCs is largely involved in maintaining intestinal immune homeostasis and can be a target for a new therapy against mucosal immune diseases with homeostatic disturbances such as FA.

Editor: Kenji Hashimoto, Chiba University Center for Forensic Mental Health, Japan

Funding: This research was supported by a Grant-in-Aid for Scientific Research from the Ministry of Education, Culture, Sports, Science and Technology of Japan (http://www.jsps.go.jp/j-grantsinaid/index.html) to T. Yamamoto (No. 25460891) and M. Kadowaki (No. 24590879). The funders had no role in study design, data collection and analysis, decision to publish, or preparation of the manuscript.

Competing Interests: The authors have declared that no competing interests exist.

* E-mail: makotok@inm.u-toyama.ac.jp

Introduction

Food allergy (FA) is an abnormal immunologic reaction to food proteins, and its prevalence has increased in developed countries over the past few decades. However, the pathogenic mechanisms underlying FA are not fully understood, and no effective drug therapies are yet available. The only way to avoid allergic reactions to food is to avoid the foods that trigger these responses [1].

It is well known that type 2 helper T (Th2) cell-biased immune responses are responsible for allergic diseases. There is a growing body of work that has examined the interaction between T cells and mast cells and how these relationships might alter immunity to foreign antigens [2]. Th2 cell-associated cytokines, such as IL-4, IL-5, IL-9 and IL-13, are involved in B cell class switching to IgE and in the differentiation and maturation of mast cells and Th2 cells [3,4,5].

In the pathological Th2 cell-biased immunological environment, mast cells are usually positioned close to the external environment to respond to the pathogens, and mast cells play a central role as an effector cell and a conductor cell in the pathogenesis of various allergic diseases [5,6]. The activation of mast cells results in the release of various inflammatory mediators, such as proteases, eicosanoids, biogenic amines, cytokines and chemokines [2]. Despite their strategic location in the mucosa of the intestinal microenvironment, the role of mast cells in FA has not been well investigated.

We previously demonstrated that the number of mucosal mast cells (MMCs) is greatly increased in the colonic mucosa of ovalbumin (OVA)-induced FA mice [7]. Mast cells are classified as MMCs or connective tissue mast cells (CTMCs). Considerable evidence has demonstrated that MMCs are morphologically, biochemically and functionally distinct from CTMCs [2]. CTMCs reside in connective tissues, such as the skin, whereas MMC progenitors migrate to intestinal or bronchial mucosal tissues, where MMCs are able to mature following antigen exposure. CTMCs contain high concentrations of histamine in their granules and mainly contribute to allergic symptoms, such as congestion, itch, urticaria and anaphylaxis, whereas MMCs contain low concentrations of histamine [8]. Consequently, anti-histamine agents have no effect on FA. Furthermore, CTMC stabilizers (e.g., tranilast, ketotifen, and cromolyn) are frequently used for the treatment of various allergic disorders, while these stabilizers fail to exert therapeutic effects on FA, which is supported by our finding that these stabilizers are not able to suppress MMC activation [9].

Recent advances in neuroscience and immunology have revealed a bidirectional interaction between the nervous and immune systems. Therefore, the function of the intestine may be modulated by neuro-immune interactions, but this interaction is not fully understood. Mast cells are ubiquitous in the body, and these cells are often found in close proximity to nerve fibers in various tissues, including the lamina propria of the intestine [3,4,10,11]. Mast cells and nerves are assumed to communicate bilaterally to modulate neuro-physiological effects and mast cell functions [12], which suggests that the neuro-immune interaction may be involved in the pathology of allergic diseases.

Until now, findings on the cholinergic regulation of immune responses have been accumulated in various inflammatory experimental models [13,14,15,16], while there has been little information obtained on the cholinergic control in allergic models, especially in FA models. We have already shown that nicotine exerts an inhibitory effect on antigen-induced degranulation in mucosal-type murine bone marrow-derived mast cells (mBMMCs) through α7 nicotinic ACh receptors (nAChRs), which is reversed by the α7 nAChR antagonist methyllycaconitine [17].

Therefore, an elucidation of the cholinergic regulatory pathway has provided new concepts in understanding and treating FA.

Materials and Methods

Ethics statement

This study was carried out in strict accordance with the recommendations in the Guide for the Care and Use of Laboratory Animals of the National Institutes of Health. The Animal Experiment Committee at the University of Toyama approved all of the animal care procedures and experiments (authorization no. S-2009 INM-9).

Animals

Male BALB/c mice, C57BL/6 mice and BALB/c nude (nu/nu) mice (5 weeks old) were purchased from Japan SLC (Shizuoka, Japan). BALB/c background p85α subunit-disrupted class Ia phosphoinositide-3 kinase (PI3K)-deficient ($PI3K^{-/-}$) mice were gifted from Drs. Shigeo Koyasu (Keio University, Tokyo, Japan) and Takashi Kadowaki (the University of Tokyo, Tokyo, Japan). All mice were housed in the experimental animal facility at the University of Toyama and were provided free access to food and water.

Induction of food allergy

The murine model of FA was initiated as described previously.8 Briefly, male BALB/c mice (5 weeks old) were sensitized twice at 2-week intervals using an intraperitoneal injection of 50 μg OVA (fraction V; Sigma-Aldrich, St. Louis, MO) in the presence of 1.3 mg/100 μl aluminium hydroxide gel adjuvant (Sigma-Aldrich). Two weeks after systemic priming, the mice received repeated oral administrations of 50 mg/0.3 ml OVA every other day. Diarrhea resulting from FA was assessed by visual monitoring for up to 1 hour following oral challenge. Profuse liquid stool was detected as allergic diarrhea, and the diarrhea-presenting mice were considered to be FA mice.

For the pharmacological evaluation of an activation of nicotinic AChRs (nAChRs) in the FA model, a non-selective nAChR agonist nicotine (Sigma-Aldrich) or a selective α7 nAChR agonist GTS-21 (10 mg/kg, Taiho, Tokushima, Japan) was subcutaneously administered to mice 1 hour before the oral OVA challenges. A central vagal stimulant 2-deoxy-D-glucose (2-DG, 200 mg/kg, Sigma-Aldrich) was intraperitoneally administered 30 minutes before OVA challenges. Furthermore, hexamethonium (C6, 100 mg/kg, Sigma-Aldrich) as a non-selective nAChR antagonist was intraperitoneally administered 30 minutes before 2-DG administration. A CTMC stabilizer disodium cromoglycate (cromolyn, 100 mg/g, Sigma-Aldrich), a CTMC and MMC stabilizer doxantrazole (10 mg/kg, Sigma-Aldrich) or an anti-inflammatory drug prednisolone (10 mg/kg, Sigma-Aldrich) was administered 1 hour before OVA challenges.

One hour after the 6th oral OVA challenge, the proximal colon and spleen were used for morphological and biological analyses, and plasma was for measurement of OVA-specific IgE and mouse mast cell protease (mMCP)-1 (a marker of mouse MMCs) levels. Plasma OVA-specific IgE level was measured using an ELISA kit (DS Pharma Biomedical, Osaka, Japan). Plasma mMCP-1 level was measured using an ELISA kit (Moredun Scientific). These measurements were performed according to the manufacturers' instructions.

Measurement of myeloperoxidase activity

One hour after the 6th oral OVA challenge, the entire colon of each mouse was excised. Each colon was weighed and cut into small pieces. The colon was homogenized on ice in 1 ml of 0.5% hexadecyltrimethylammonium bromide in 50 mM potassium phosphate buffer (pH 6.0) using a Polytron homogenizer (Kinematica, Littau, Switzerland) and fortified with an additional quantity of the same buffer to 100 mg of the colon in 1 ml. The homogenate was frozen and thawed three times and then was vortex-mixed. The suspension was centrifuged at 15,000×*g* for 20 minutes at 4°C. Myeloperoxidase (MPO) activity of the resulting supernatant was measured. The supernatant (100 μl) was vortex-mixed with 2.87 ml of 0.5 mM *o*-dianisidine in 50 mM potassium phosphate buffer (pH 6.0) and 30 μl of 0.05% hydrogen peroxide. The mixture was measured spectrophotometrically at 460 nm for 4 minutes of incubation. MPO activity is expressed as units per wet weight of the colon in grams (gwwt).

Expression of cytokine mRNA

One hour after the 6th oral OVA challenge, 2 cm of the proximal colon and spleen were excised. Total RNA was extracted from the tissues using Sepasol Super (Nacalai Tesque, Kyoto, Japan) according to the manufacturer's instructions. Reverse transcription was performed using the Exscript RT reagent kit (Takara Bio, Ohtsu, Japan) and random primers, followed by real-time PCR. Real-time PCR amplification of IL-4, IL-5, IFN-γ and GAPDH was performed using SYBR Premix Ex Taq (Takara Bio). The following primer pairs were used:

IL-4, forward 5′-GGTCTCAACCCCCAGCTAGT-3′ and reverse 5′-GCCGATGATCTCTCTCAAGTGAT-3′;

IL-5, forward 5′-GAAGTGTGGCGAGGAGAGAC-3′ and reverse 5′-GCACAGTTTTGTGGGGTTTT-3′;

IFN-γ, forward 5′-CGGCACAGTCATTGAAAGCCTA-3′ and reverse 5′-GTTGCTGATGGCCTGATTGTC-3′;

GAPDH, forward 5′-TGACCACAGTCCATGCCATC-3′ and reverse 5′-GACGGACACATTGGGGGTAG-3′.

The PCR reaction conditions consisted of 10 seconds at 95°C followed by 40 cycles of 5 seconds at 95°C and 20 seconds at 63°C. Target mRNA levels were normalized to those of GAPDH as an internal control in each sample. The results are expressed as the ratio relative to the naïve group average.

Morphological analysis

One hour after the 6th oral OVA challenge, the proximal colon was excised. The proximal colon was fixed with 4% paraformaldehyde (w/v) in 0.1 M sodium phosphate buffer (PB; pH 7.3) and immersed for 12–18 hours at 4°C. The tissue was washed with 0.01 M phosphate-buffered saline (PBS; pH 7.3), cryoprotected with 30% sucrose in 0.01 M PBS and embedded in OCT compound. Frozen sections (25 μm) were cut at −20°C using a cryostat microtome (Leica Microsystems, Nussloch, Germany). The sections were soaked for 12–18 hours in 0.01 M PBS containing 0.3% Triton X-100 to increase permeability, and they were then exposed to normal donkey serum (1:10; Jackson Immunoresearch Laboratories, West Grove, PA) for 30 minutes to reduce the nonspecific binding of antisera and washed in 0.01 M PBS. The sections were exposed to each primary antibody for 12–18 hours, washed with 0.01 M PBS and incubated with the appropriate secondary antibody for 2 hours. All incubations were performed at room temperature. The following primary antibodies were used: goat anti-choline acetyltransferase (ChAT) (1:200; Chemicon, Temecula, CA), sheep anti-mouse mast cell protease (mMCP)-1 (1:5,000; Moredun Scientific, Midlothian, UK) and rabbit anti- CGRP (1:10,000; Chemicon). Cy3-conjugated donkey anti-sheep IgG (1:200; Jackson Immunoresearch Laboratories, West Grove, PA) and Alexa 488-conjugated donkey anti-rabbit IgG (1:200; Jackson Immunoresearch Laboratories) were used as secondary antibodies. The preparations were examined using a fluorescence microscope (IX71 system; Olympus, Tokyo, Japan) with a U-MWIG3 filter set (Olympus) and photographed using an Olympus digital camera (DP70; Olympus). The preparations were also observed using confocal laser-scanning microscopy (LSM700; Carl Zeiss, Oberkochen, Germany) to examine the proximity between mMCP-1-positive cells and CGRP-immunoreactive (IR) nerve fibers in the colonic mucosa of the FA mice. Stacks of confocal sections were three-dimensionally reconstructed and observed using Imaris software (Bitplane, Zurich, Switzerland). Surface rendering of each channel was performed in an optimal intensity threshold setting. The intensity threshold setting was optimized by visual comparison between the original and the three-dimensional rendered result.

Furthermore, a segment of the proximal colon was opened along the mesenteric border and fixed with 4% paraformaldehyde. The whole-mount preparation of longitudinal muscle with adherent enteric plexus was dissected from the proximal colon, and the aforementioned immunohistochemical procedures were performed to examine the ChAT and CGRP immunoreactivities in nerve cell bodies of the enteric neurons.

Sections (1 μm thick) of the fixed colon embedded in LR white resin (Sigma-Aldrich) were stained with 1% toluidine blue and observed with light microscopy for the analysis of mast cells.

The brightness and contrast of the images were modified using Adobe Photoshop Elements 2.0 (Adobe Systems, San Jose, CA).

Electron microscopy

For electron microscopy, the FA mice were perfusion-fixed with 2% paraformaldehyde and 2.5% glutaraldehyde in 0.1 M PB and the proximal colon was removed. The colon was transversely sectioned into 0.5–1.0 mm thick sections with a razor blade. The sections were post-fixed for 1 hour by 1% OsO_4 in 0.1 M PB, dehydrated in graded ethanol and embedded in EPON 812 (Shell Chemical, Houston, Tex). Ultrathin sections were cut using an LKB 2088-V ultramicrotome (LKB, Bromma, Sweden). The ultrathin sections were collected on copper grids, stained with lead citrate and uranyl acetate and examined with an electron microscope (H-7500, Hitachi, Tokyo, Japan).

Statistical analysis

The data are expressed as the means ±SE. The statistical comparisons were performed using Student's unpaired *t*-test, the chi-squared test and one-way repeated measures ANOVA followed by Tukey's HSD. A significant difference was defined as $P<0.05$.

Results

Induction of food allergy in mice

Repeated oral OVA challenges to systemically OVA primed mice produced FA associated with allergic diarrhea in Th2-prone BALB/c mice (FA mice, $n=5$–7), but not in Th1-prone C57BL/6 mice ($n=8$) (Figure 1A). The occurrence of allergic diarrhea reached about 80.0% after the 6th OVA challenge. However, repeated OVA challenges without systemic OVA priming did not induce allergic diarrhea in BALB/c mice ($n=5$) (Figure 1A).

The plasma level of OVA-specific IgE was elevated after the systemic OVA priming, and subsequent repeated oral OVA challenges caused a remarkable elevation of the OVA-specific IgE level (naïve mice 0.0±0.0 μg/ml, OVA primed mice

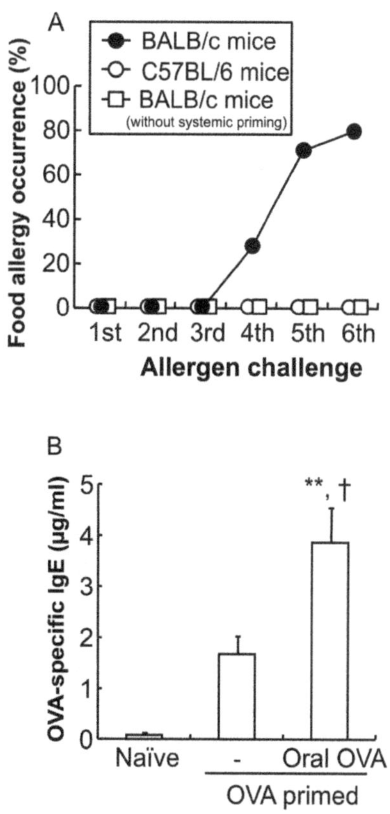

Figure 1. Induction of Th2-mediated food allergy. The allergic responses were induced by two instances of systemic OVA priming and repeated oral OVA (50 mg) challenges. *A*: Systemically primed BALB/c mice (closed circle) and C57BL/6 mice (open circle) and non-systemically primed BALB/c mice (open square) were subjected to food allergy (FA)-inducing oral OVA challenges ($n=5$–8 mice per group). *B*: The level of OVA-specific IgE in the plasma of naïve mice, systemically primed mice, and systemically primed and repeated oral OVA challenged mice is shown. The level of OVA-specific IgE in the plasma was determined using an ELISA kit. Data are expressed as means ±SE. **$P<0.01$ vs. naïve mice. †$P<0.05$ vs. systemically primed mice ($n=5$ mice per group).

1.7±0.2 μg/ml, oral OVA challenged OVA primed mice 3.8±0.7 μg/ml; **$P<0.01$ vs. naïve mice, †$P<0.05$ vs. OVA primed mice; $n=5$ mice per group) (Figure 1B).

Systemic and mucosal immune responses in food allergy mice

The expression of Th1 and Th2 cytokine mRNA was measured using real-time PCR. In systemic immunity (spleen, Figure 2A), mRNA levels of Th2 cytokines (IL-4 and IL-5) were significantly increased in the FA mice (IL-4: naïve mice 1.0±0.2, FA mice 3.7±0.8, *$P<0.05$ vs. naïve mice; IL-5: naïve mice 1.0±0.4, FA mice 3.2±0.9, *$P<0.05$ vs. naïve mice; $n=5$–6 mice per group), whereas the Th1 cytokine (IFN-γ) mRNA level was significantly decreased in the FA mice (naïve mice 1.0±0.1, FA mice 0.5±0.1; **$P<0.01$ vs. naïve mice; $n=6$ mice per group). On the other hand, in mucosal immunity (proximal colon, Figure 2B), Th2 cytokine (IL-4 and IL-5) mRNA levels were significantly increased in the FA mice (IL-4: naïve mice 1.0±0.7, FA mice 2.9±0.6, *$P<0.05$ vs. naïve mice; IL-5: naïve mice 1.0±0.2, FA mice 11.3±1.4, **$P<0.01$ vs. naïve mice; $n=4$ mice per group), and the Th1 cytokine (IFN-γ) mRNA level exhibited a tendency to be increased in the FA mice (naïve mice 1.0±0.3, FA mice 2.4±0.8; $n=5$–8 mice per group).

Mucosal mast cell hyperplasia in the colon of food allergy mice

We investigated mucosal mast cells in the proximal colon by immunohistochemistry. As shown in Figure 3A, very few MMCs (mMCP-1-positive cells) were scattered in the lamina propria and submucosal layer of the mice colon two weeks after twice systemic OVA priming. The distribution of MMCs was similar to that in the proximal colon of the vehicle-treated control mice. MMCs began to occur in the mucosal epithelium of the primed mice proximal colon two days after the second oral OVA administration, and the number of MMCs was dramatically elevated in the mucosal epithelium of the primed mice colon in proportion to the OVA challenge time. MMCs were localized primarily in the mucosal epithelium of the upper half of the crypts throughout the primed mice colon two days after the fifth oral OVA administration.

To investigate the degranulation of mucosal mast cells, we measured the concentration of plasma mMCP-1 by ELISA (Figure 3B). There was no detectable plasma mMCP-1 in naïve mice. In contrast, the repeated OVA challenges resulted in a dramatic increase in the plasma mMCP-1 level (naïve mice 0.0±0.0 μg/ml, FA mice 29.0±8.0 μg/ml; **$P<0.01$ vs. naïve mice; $n=5$ mice per group).

Involvement of T cell in the development of food allergy in mice

In the FA mouse model, we used BALB/c nude mice that lack functional T cells due to their thymus deficiency. The nude mice did not exhibit any sign of allergic responses following exposure to

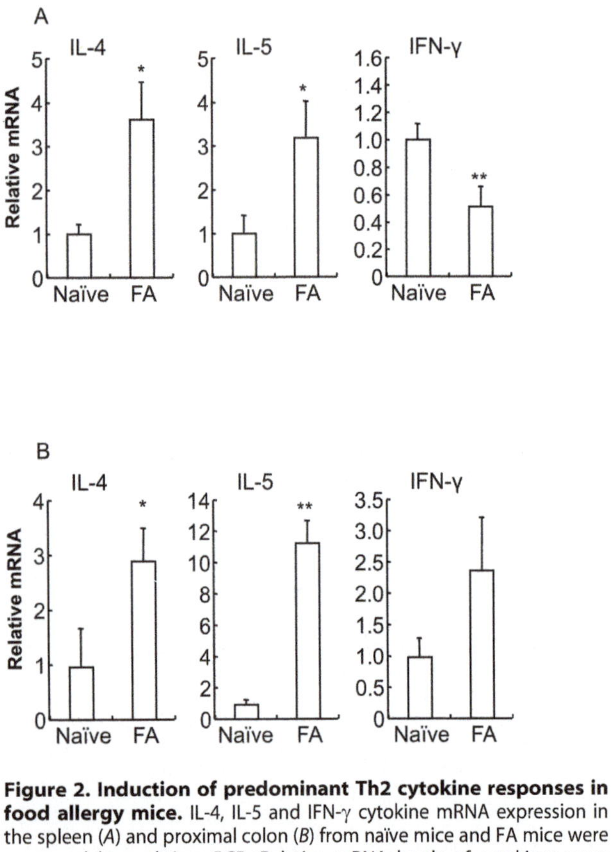

Figure 2. Induction of predominant Th2 cytokine responses in food allergy mice. IL-4, IL-5 and IFN-γ cytokine mRNA expression in the spleen (*A*) and proximal colon (*B*) from naïve mice and FA mice were measured by real-time PCR. Relative mRNA levels of cytokines were normalized to GAPDH expression. Data are expressed as means ±SE. *$P<0.05$, **$P<0.01$ vs. naïve mice ($n=4$–8 mice per group).

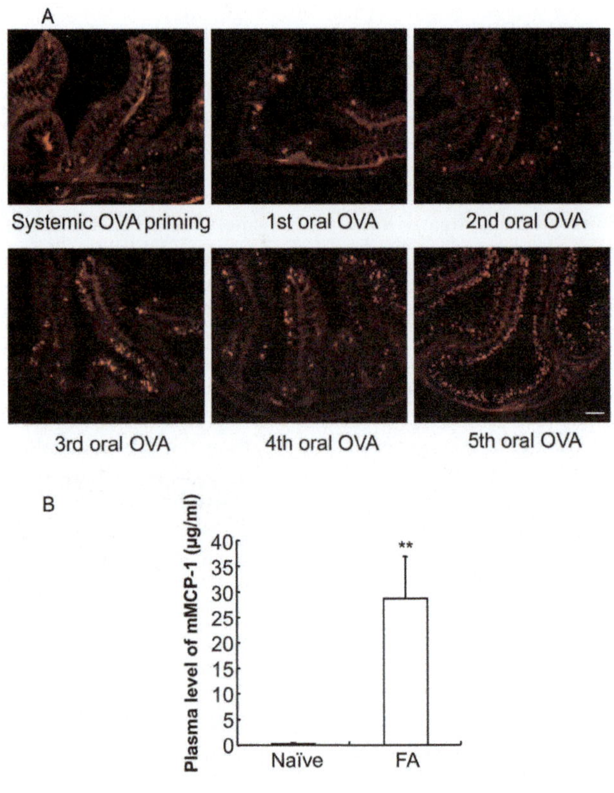

Figure 3. Mucosal mast cell hyperplasia and degranulation in the colon of food allergy mice. *A*: The proximal colons of systemically OVA primed mice and oral OVA-challenged mice after each oral OVA challenge were stained with anti-mouse mast cell protease-1 (mMCP-1) antibodies. Scale bar represents 200 μm. *B*: The concentration of mMCP-1 in the plasma of naïve mice and FA mice is shown. The concentration of mMCP-1 in the plasma was determined using an ELISA kit. Data are expressed as means ±SE. **$P<0.01$ vs. naïve mice ($n=5$ mice per group).

repeated oral allergen challenges (Figure 4A, $n = 5$ mice per group) and that OVA-specific IgE and mMCP-1 were not detected in the plasma of nude naïve mice and nude FA mice (Figure 4B: $^{**}P < 0.01$ vs. wild-type (WT) naïve mice, ††$P < 0.01$ vs. WT FA mice: $n = 3$–5 mice per group; Figure 4C: $^{*}P < 0.05$ vs. WT naïve mice, ††$P < 0.01$ vs. WT FA mice: $n = 3$–5 mice per group). Furthermore, no increase of mucosal mast cells was observed in the mucosal layer of the proximal colons of nude FA mice as compared to those of WT mice in the FA model (Figure 4D).

Characteristics of mast cells in the colon of food allergy mice

Mast cells were observed in the proximal colon of the FA mice and contained many granules intensely stained with toluidine blue (Figure 5A). Only a few mast cells were observed in the lamina propria. These mast cells contained numerous granules in the cytoplasm, most of which exhibited reddish violet metachromasia with toluidine blue (Figure 5B), indicating that these mast cells exhibit properties of CTMCs because in rodents, CTMC granules stain purple, and MMC granules stain blue with toluidine blue [18]. However, a few granules in these mast cells in the lamina propria were nonmetachromatic and were larger than metachromatic granules (Figure 5B; arrows).

Many MMCs were observed in the mucosal epithelium, and the majority of MMC granules were larger (Figure 5C) and were spherical or polymorphic in shape (Figure 5C; arrows). In addition, these MMC granules, which exhibited nonmetachromasia, were strongly stained with toluidine blue, but some were weakly stained.

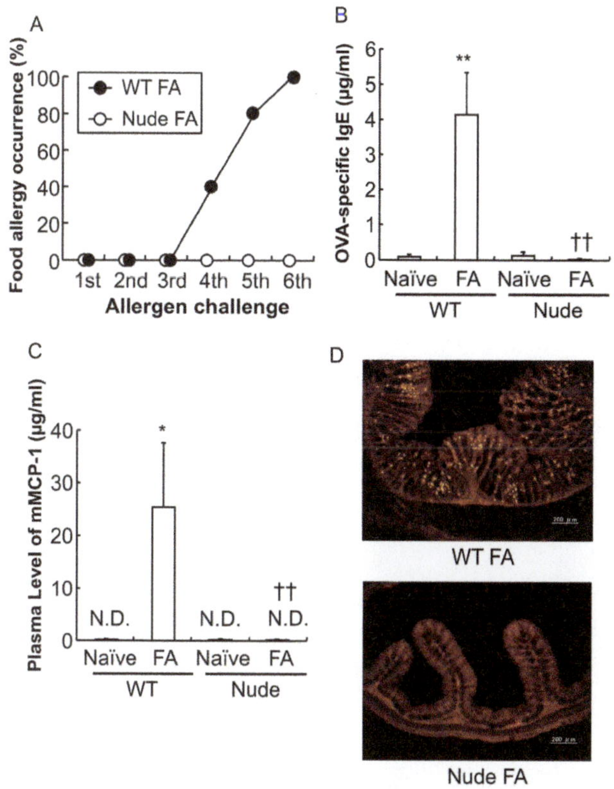

Figure 4. Induction of food allergy in athymic nude mice. *A*: The occurrence of allergic diarrhea in wild-type (WT) FA mice and nude FA mice after each oral OVA challenge is shown ($n = 5$ mice per group). *B*: The level of OVA-specific IgE in the plasma of WT naïve mice, WT FA mice, nude naïve mice and nude FA mice is shown. The level of OVA-specific IgE in the plasma was determined using an ELISA kit. $^{**}P < 0.01$ vs. WT naïve mice, ††$P < 0.01$ vs. WT FA mice ($n = 3$–5 mice per group). *C*: The level of mMCP-1 in the plasma of WT naïve mice, WT FA mice, nude naïve mice and nude FA mice is shown. The level of mMCP-1 in the plasma was determined using an ELISA kit. $^{*}P < 0.05$ vs. WT naïve mice, ††$P < 0.01$ vs. WT FA mice ($n = 3$–5 mice per group). *D*: The proximal colon of WT FA mice and nude FA mice after the 6th oral OVA challenge was stained with anti-mMCP-1 antibodies. Scale bars represent 200 μm.

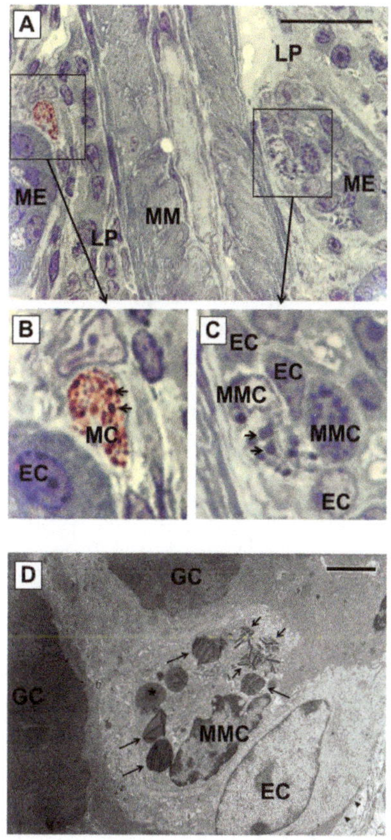

Figure 5. Morphology of mast cells in the colon of food allergy mice. Sections (1 μm thick) of the fixed colon embedded in resin were stained with 1% toluidine blue and were observed with light microscopy for the analysis of mast cells. *A*: On the left hand side of the picture, a mast cell (surrounded by a square) with metachromatic granules was observed in the lamina propria. On the other side, two mast cells (surrounded with another square) with nonmetachromatic granules were localized in the mucosal epithelium. ME: mucosal epithelium, LP: lamina propria, MM: muscularis mucosa. Scale bar represents 50 μm. *B*: An image of higher magnification of the mast cell in the lamina propria. Most of granules of the mast cell exhibited metachromasia, but a few granules (arrows) were nonmetachromatic. MC: mast cell, EC: epithelial cell. *C*: An image of higher magnification of mucosal mast cells (MMCs) in the mucosal epithelium. The granules in MMCs did not exhibit metachromasia and some of the granules were polymorphic in shape (arrows). MMC: mucosal mast cell. *D*: Electron microscopic analysis of mucosal mast cells in the proximal colon of food allergy mice. A variety of morphologies of granules was seen in a MMC: one (asterisk) showed amorphous inner structure, some (long arrows) showed crystals with amorphous matrix and others (short arrows) seemed to be occupied by the crystalline structure. Arrowheads indicate basement membrane. GC: goblet cell. Scale bar represents 4 μm.

Ultrastructural characteristics of mucosal mast cells in food allergy mice

MMCs in the mucosal epithelium of the FA mice proximal colon have been examined with the electron microscope (Figure 5D). Many MMCs were observed within the mucosal epithelium, and they were characterized by the presence of peculiar large granules (0.5–2.5 μm) in the cytoplasm. MMCs had specific granules of varying size, shape and electron-density. Many of the granules (Figure 5D, long arrows) contained crystalline inclusions with cylindrical shape and had irregular contours and showed polymorphic shapes. Other granules seemed to be occupied by crystalline structures (Figure 5D, short arrows). Some of the granules had relatively homogeneous matrix with round or oval contours without the crystalline inclusion (Figure 5D, asterisk).

Critical involvement of mast cells in the pathogenesis of food allergy in mice

Mice that specifically lack only mast cells have not been reported/generated; two mouse strains, WBB6F1/J-$Kit^{W}/Kit^{W\text{-}v}$ and C57BL/6-$Kit^{W\text{-}sh}/Kit^{W\text{-}sh}$ are profoundly deficient in mast cells. These mice are most frequently used to analyze the *in vivo* functions of mast cells, but we could not employ these strains to examine the role of mast cells in the induction of FA because the genetic background of these mice is not BALB/c and these mice have other phenotypic abnormalities, such as gastric ulcer and intestinal motility disorder.

Therefore, in this study, we employed $PI3K^{-/-}$ mice with a BALB/c genetic background that exhibit a selective loss of gastrointestinal mast cells [19]. As a result, $PI3K^{-/-}$ mice failed to develop allergic diarrhea ($PI3K^{-/-}$ FA mice) (Figure 6A, $n=5$ mice per group). As shown in Figure 6B, immunohistochemical staining with the mMCP-1 antibody revealed that MMCs were dramatically increased in the proximal colon of WT FA mice, whereas only a few mast cells were observed in the mucosal layer of $PI3K^{-/-}$ FA mice. Plasma mMCP-1 was almost undetectable in $PI3K^{-/-}$ naïve mice and $PI3K^{-/-}$ FA mice (Figure 6C: $^{**}P<0.01$ vs. WT naïve mice, $^{††}P<0.01$ vs. WT FA mice; $n=3$–5 mice per group).

Furthermore, in systemic immunity (spleen, Figure 6D), mRNA levels of Th2 cytokines (IL-4 and IL-5) were increased in $PI3K^{-/-}$ FA mice as compared to $PI3K^{-/-}$ naïve mice (IL-4: $^{*}P<0.05$ vs. WT naïve mice, $^{**}P<0.01$ vs. $PI3K^{-/-}$ naïve mice; IL-5: $^{**}P<0.01$ vs. WT naïve mice; $n=4$–7 mice per group), which is similar to those in WT FA mice. On the other hand, in mucosal immunity (proximal colon, Figure 6E, lower expression of mRNA for Th2 cytokines was found in $PI3K^{-/-}$ FA mice as compared to WT FA mice (IL-4: $^{*}P<0.05$ vs. WT naïve mice, $^{††}P<0.01$ vs. WT FA mice; IL-5: $^{*}P<0.05$ vs. WT naïve mice; $n=4$–7 mice per group).

Effect of mast cell stabilizers on the induction of food allergy in mice

The critical involvement of MMCs in the pathogenesis of FA was pharmacologically investigated in the FA model. The subcutaneous administration of a CTMC and MMC dual stabilizer doxantrazole (10 mg/kg) completely prevented the allergic responses following exposure to repeated oral allergen challenges, whereas the oral treatment with cromolyn (100 mg/kg), a CTMC stabilizer failed to suppress these responses (Figure 7: $^{**}P<0.01$ vs. FA mice; $n=10$–15 mice per group). In addition, mice treated with an anti-inflammatory drug prednisolone (10 mg/kg) did not exhibit any sign of allergic diarrhea in the FA model.

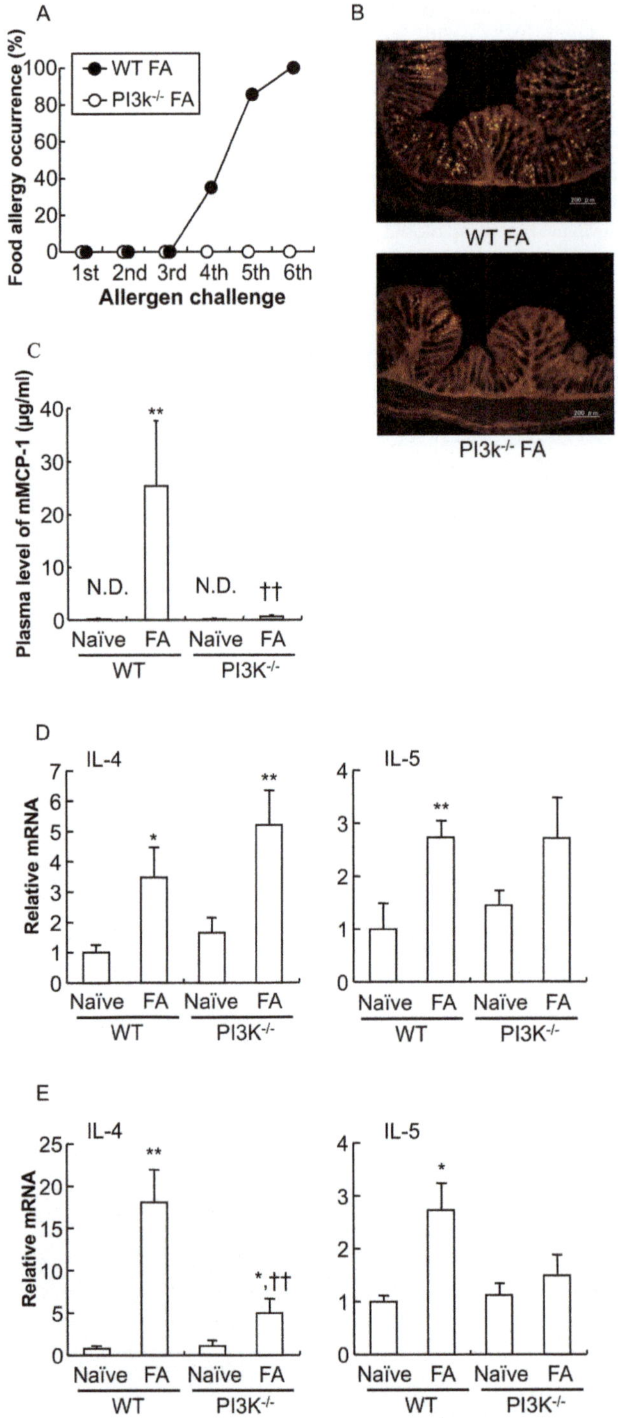

Figure 6. Induction of food allergy in PI3K-deficient mice. $PI3K^{-/-}$ mice as a gastrointestinal mast cell-deficient murine model were subjected to FA-inducing oral OVA challenges. *A*: The occurrence of allergic diarrhea in WT mice (WT FA mice) and $PI3K^{-/-}$ mice ($PI3K^{-/-}$ FA mice) after each oral OVA challenge is shown ($n=5$ mice per group). *B*: The proximal colon of FA-induced $PI3K^{-/-}$ mice after oral OVA challenge was stained with anti- mMCP-1 antibodies. Scale bars represent 200 μm. *C*: The level of mMCP-1 in the plasma of $PI3K^{-/-}$ naïve mice and $PI3K^{-/-}$ FA mice is shown. The level of mMCP-1 in the plasma was determined using an ELISA kit. Data are expressed as means ±SE. $^{**}P<0.01$ vs. WT naïve mice, $^{††}P<0.01$ vs. WT FA mice ($n=3$–5 mice per group). IL-4 and IL-5 cytokine mRNA expression in the spleen (*D*) and proximal colon (*E*) from WT naïve mice, WT FA mice, $PI3K^{-/-}$

naïve mice and PI3K$^{-/-}$ FA mice were measured by real-time PCR. Relative mRNA levels of cytokines were normalized to GAPDH expression. *$P<0.05$, **$P<0.01$ vs. each naïve mice, ††$P<0.01$ vs. WT FA mice (n = 4–7 mice per group).

Cholinergic anti-inflammatory pathway in food allergy mice

To investigate whether vagal activity influences the development of FA, we examined the effect of 2-deoxy-D-glucose (2-DG), a central vagal stimulant on the FA model. Intraperitoneal injection of 2-DG (200 mg/kg) significantly ameliorated allergic diarrhea. After the 6th OVA challenge, the occurrence of allergic diarrhea was significantly decreased from 100.0% to 54.5% (Figure 8A: *$P<0.05$ vs. vehicle, n = 11–18 mice per group). The therapeutic effect of 2-DG was significantly blocked by the subcutaneous injection of the non-selective nAChR antagonist hexamethonium (C6) at 32 mg/kg (Figure 8A: †$P<0.05$ vs. 2-DG, n = 11 mice per group).

We next examined the therapeutic effect of nAChR activation on the development of FA. The subcutaneous injection of nicotine attenuated the induction of allergic diarrhea at 1 and 3.2 mg/kg (Figure 8B: *$P<0.05$, **$P<0.01$ vs. FA mice, n = 10–74 mice per group). The selective α7 nAChR agonist GTS-21 was used to determine whether α7 nAChR mediated the therapeutic effect of nicotine. The subcutaneous injection of GTS-21 (10 mg/kg) resulted in a significant suppression of allergic diarrhea (Figure 8C: *$P<0.05$, **$P<0.01$ vs. FA mice, n = 23–40 mice per group).

Effect of nicotine treatment on the systemic and mucosal immune responses in food allergy mice

The number of MMCs that was dramatically increased in the proximal colon of the FA mice was significantly decreased in that of nicotine-treated FA mice (Figure 9A).

MPO activity in the colon of the FA mice was significantly increased approximately 2.5-fold compared to that in the naïve mice colon, and the subcutaneous injection of nicotine significantly suppressed the increment of MPO activity in the FA mice (Figure 9B: naïve mice 534.8±56.5 units/gwwt, FA mice 1285.7±123.5 units/gwwt, nicotine-treated FA mice 740.5±138.4 units/gwwt; *$P<0.05$ vs. naïve mice, †$P<0.05$ vs. FA mice; n = 3–10 mice per group).

In contrast, the plasma level of OVA-specific IgE remained unchanged in nicotine-treated FA mice compared to the FA mice (Figure 9C: naïve mice 0.1±0.0 μg/ml, FA mice 3.8±0.7 μg/ml, nicotine-treated FA mice 4.3±0.4 μg/ml; **$P<0.01$ vs. naïve mice; n = 5 mice per group).

To investigate the effects of nicotine treatment on the cytokine profile in the FA mice, cytokine mRNA expression was detected by real-time PCR. In systemic immunity (spleen), the upregulated Th2 cytokine (IL-4 and IL-5) mRNA expression observed in the FA mice was not significantly changed by nicotine treatment (Figure 9D: n = 6 mice per group), which is almost consistent with no effect of nicotine on the enhanced plasma OVA-specific IgE level in the FA mice (Figure 9C). In contrast, the downregulated Th1 cytokine (IFN-γ) mRNA expression observed in the FA mice was significantly increased in nicotine-treated FA mice (Figure 9D: *$P<0.01$ vs. FA mice, n = 6 mice per group). On the other hand, in mucosal immunity (proximal colon), the upregulated mRNA expression of both Th1 (IFN-γ) and Th2 (IL-4 and IL-5) cytokines was significantly suppressed in nicotine-treated FA mice (Figure 9E: *$P<0.05$, **$P<0.01$ vs. FA mice, n = 3–6 mice per group).

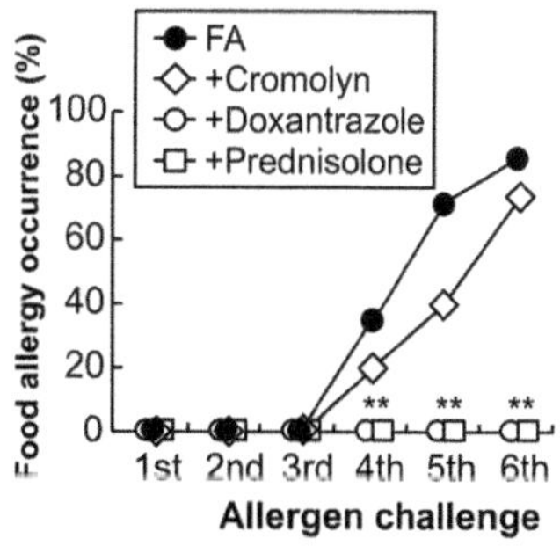

Figure 7. Effect of mast cell stabilizers on the induction of food allergy in mice. The occurrence of allergic diarrhea in FA mice (closed circle) and cromolyn-treated mice (open diamond) after each oral OVA challenge is shown (n = 14–15 mice per group). In addition, mice treated with the subcutaneous administration of doxantrazole (open circle, 10 mg/kg) or the oral administration of prednisolone (open square, 10 mg/kg) did not exhibit any sign of allergic responses in the FA model. **$P<0.01$ vs. FA mice (n = 10 mice per each group).

Morphological analysis of mucosal mast cell–cholinergic nerve interactions in the colon of food allergy mice

We have demonstrated that α7 nAChRs are expressed in mBMMCs and that the stimulation of α7 nAChRs can negatively regulate the activation of mBMMCs [17]. Therefore, we investigated the morphological interaction of MMCs and cholinergic nerve fibers in the lamina propria of the FA mouse proximal colon. It was difficult to investigate the morphological interaction of MMCs and cholinergic nerve fibers using two-dimensional images with fine-resolution in the colon. Therefore, digital images acquired by confocal laser-scanning microscopy were three-dimensionally reconstructed and observed using Imaris software (Figure 10A). The majority of mMCP-1-positive MMCs (green) were located in close vicinity of the CGRP-IR cholinergic nerve fibers (red) in the FA mouse proximal colon (Figure 10B, C, D: arrows). Furthermore, we verified that CGRP-IR neurons (Figure 10E: arrows) exhibited ChAT immunoreactivities in the myenteric and submucosal neurons of the mouse enteric nervous system.

Discussion

In this study, we provide evidence that MMCs are primarily responsible for the pathology of the FA model and that the cholinergic neuro-immune interaction via α7 nAChRs on MMCs play a crucial role in controlling pathological immune activation to restore the homeostasis in the intestine.

The neuro-immune interaction can be targeted for the design of novel therapeutic agents for the treatment of intestinal immune diseases.

Our murine FA model exhibited various features of type 1 hypersensitive allergic reactions, such as allergic diarrhea within 1 hour after oral antigen exposure, antigen-specific IgE hyperproduction and MMC hyperplasia and degranulation. In addition, Th1-prone C57BL/6 mice did not develop the allergic diarrhea.

Taken together, these data suggest that enhanced Th2-mediated immune responses are responsible for the pathology of our murine FA model.

In the mRNA analysis of cytokines, the FA mice exhibited Th2-biased immune responses in systemic immunity. On the other hand, in mucosal immunity, Th2 immune responses were significantly enhanced, whereas Th1 immune responses were not decreased, but rather increased, indicating that there is a

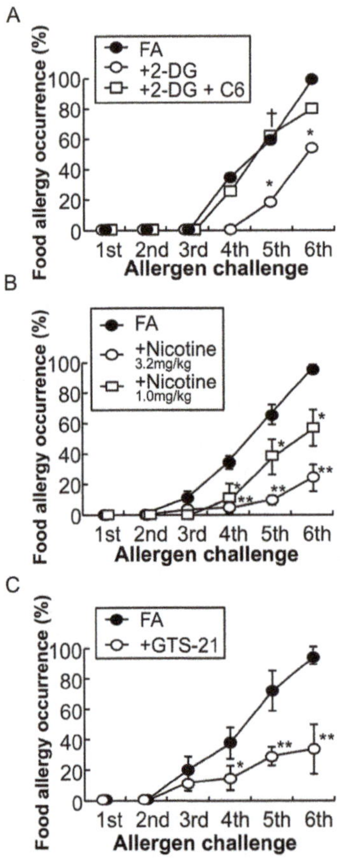

Figure 8. Cholinergic control of food allergy in mice. *A*: The occurrence of allergic diarrhea in FA mice (closed circle), 2-deoxy-d-glucose (2-DG)-treated mice (open circle) and hexamethonium (C6)-treated mice prior to 2-DG administration (open square) after each oral OVA challenge is shown. *$P<0.05$ vs. FA mice. †$P<0.05$ vs. 2-DG mice ($n = 11–18$ mice per group). *B*: The occurrence of allergic diarrhea in FA mice (closed circle) and nicotine-treated mice (3.2 mg/kg; open circle, 1.0 mg/kg; open square, and 0.32 mg/kg; open diamond) after each oral OVA challenge is shown. *$P<0.05$, **$P<0.01$ vs. FA mice ($n = 10–74$ mice per group). *C*: The occurrence of allergic diarrhea in FA mice (closed circle) and GTS-21-treated mice (open circle) after each oral OVA challenge is shown. *$P<0.05$, **$P<0.01$ vs. FA mice ($n = 23–40$ mice per group).

difference between the systemic immune responses and the mucosal immune responses in the FA mice. Furthermore, these enhanced Th2 responses were almost consistent with those observed in other murine OVA-induced FA models, but Th1 responses in the mucosal immunity were different from those in the other models [20,21]. Kweon et al. observed increased IFN-γ production in the spleen and no IFN-γ production in the colon using ELISA in another murine FA model with allergic diarrhea [21], and Brandt et al. reported no change of IFN-γ mRNA expression in the jejunum of their FA mice with allergic diarrhea [20]. These discrepancies may be due to differences in immunization protocols, cytokine measurement methods and tissue segments. Thus, our murine FA model is characterized by the activation of not only Th2 but also Th1 immune responses in the mucosal immunity of the FA mice colon [7].

Furthermore, to determine whether T cells have a pathological role in the development of FA, we examined whether food allergic diarrhea was induced in nude mice that lack functional T cells due

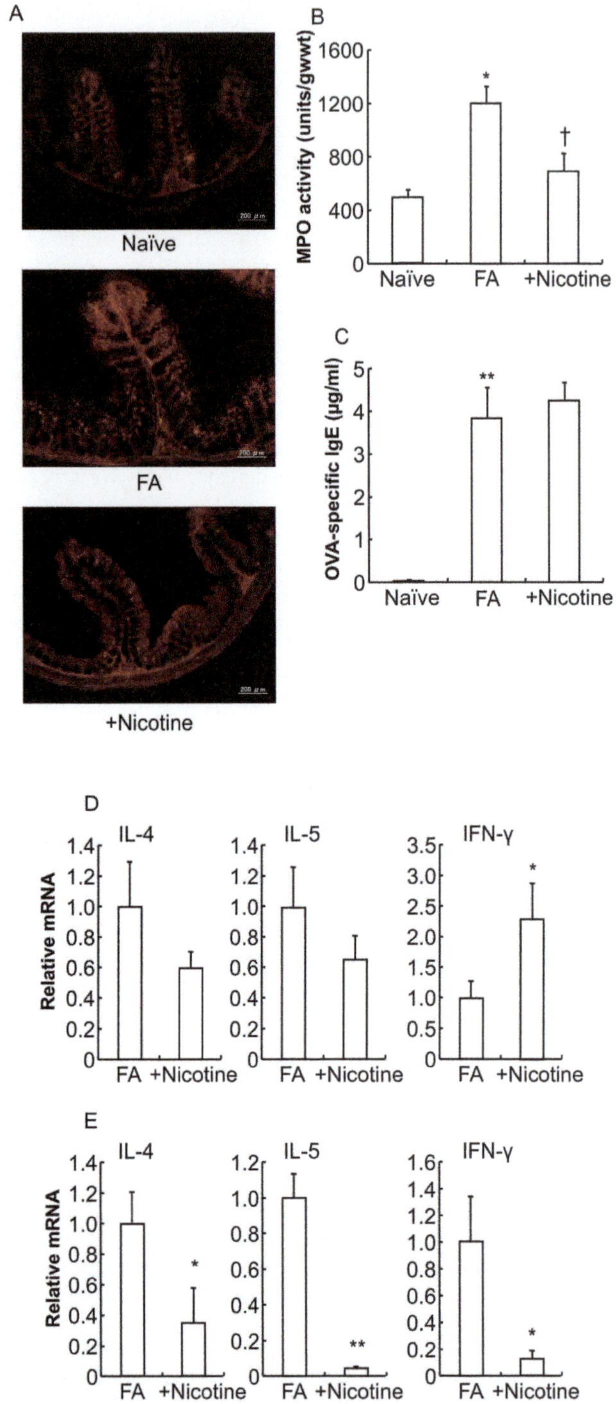

Figure 9. Effect of nicotine on the pathology of food allergy in mice. *A*: The proximal colons of naïve mice, FA mice, and mice treated with the subcutaneous administration of nicotine were stained with mMCP-1 antibodies. Scale bars represent 200 μm. *B*: MPO activity was measured in the colon of naïve mice, FA mice and nicotine-treated FA mice. *$P<0.01$ vs. naïve mice. †$P<0.05$ vs. FA mice ($n = 3–10$ mice per group). *C*: The level of OVA-specific IgE in the plasma of naïve mice, FA mice and nicotine-treated FA mice is shown. The level of OVA-specific IgE in the plasma was determined using an ELISA kit. **$P<0.01$ vs. naïve mice ($n = 5$ mice per group). IL-4, IL-5 and IFN-γ cytokine mRNA expression in the spleen (*D*) and proximal colon (*E*) from FA mice and nicotine-treated FA mice were measured by real-time PCR. Relative mRNA levels of cytokines were normalized to GAPDH expression. *$P<0.05$, **$P<0.01$ vs. FA mice ($n = 3–6$ mice per group).

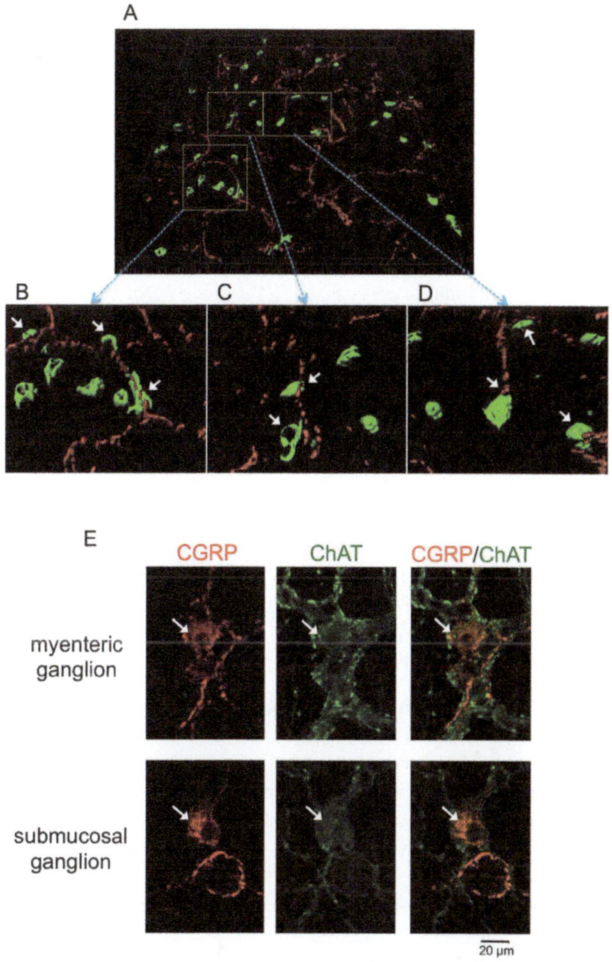

Figure 10. Spatial relationship of mucosal mast cells and cholinergic nerve fibers in the FA mouse colon. *A*: Three-dimensional reconstruction of the confocal images reveals the morphological interaction of mMCP-1-positive MMCs (green) and cholinergic CGRP- immunoreactive nerve fibers (red). Major grid space represents 20 µm. *B–D*: High-magnification images of three boxed regions in (*A*). *E*: CGRP- immunoreactive neurons (arrows) exhibited ChAT immunoreactivities in the myenteric and submucosal ganglion of the mouse enteric nervous system. Scale bar represents 20 µm.

to their thymus deficiency. We found that nude mice failed to exhibit allergic responses in the FA mouse model and that increased OVA-specific IgE and mMCP-1 levels in the plasma and mastocytosis in the mucosa of the proximal colon were not detected in nude naïve mice and nude FA mice. In addition, in this study, OVA-challenged mice without systemic priming failed to exhibit allergic diarrhea. Thus, these results indicate that the T-cell-mediated immune responses in the systemic immunity are essentially required for the development of the allergic responses in our FA model.

This study revealed that mMCP-1 immunoreactive MMCs increased in the mucosal epithelium of the FA mice colon, which is similar to previous reports on the appearance of mast cells in the jejunal mucosa of oral allergen–induced diarrhea mice [20] and parasite-infected mice [22,23]. Thus, these findings suggest that MMCs are localized in the strategic position to enhance a rapid expulsion of food antigens or parasites from the gut by bioactive products released from MMCs.

The toluidine blue staining revealed a difference between mast cells in the lamina propria and MMCs in the mucosal epithelium of the FA mice colon. Most of the granules of mast cells in the lamina propria, but not MMCs exhibited metachromasia presumably caused by sulfate radicals of proteoglycan such as heparin, suggesting that the difference results from chemical properties of substances contained in the granules of mast cells and that the granules of MMCs in the mucosal epithelium have depleted the reactive substances.

In the previous studies with mMCP-1-deficient mice in the parasite infection model, the light microscopic analysis reveals that MMCs in the jejunal mucosa of the deficient mice have smaller, less intensely toluidine blue-positive granules than those in WT mice and that the granules of MMCs in the deficient mice are uniformly round, whereas those in WT mice are irregularly shaped [23]. Furthermore, previous ultrastructural analysis demonstrates that crystalline inclusions with a cylindrical shape abundantly exist in the irregularly shaped granules of MMCs in the jejunal mucosa of the murine parasite infection model [23], which is consistent with the present findings using the electron microscopy in the granules of MMCs in the mucosal epithelium of the FA mice colon. However, in the mMCP-1 deficient mice, the shapes of MMC granules are regular and oval, and no crystalline structures are observed within the granules in the parasite infection model [23]. Taken all together, it is suggested that the disappearance of matrix constituents such as chondroitin sulfate in the granules of mast cells may be related to the formation of crystalline structures of chymases such as mMCP-1.

The PI3K family is involved in signal transduction that regulates cell proliferation, survival and differentiation. In particular, PI3K is involved in many functions of immune cells [24], and in mast cells, the activation of class Ia PI3K is required in the downstream signaling cascades initiated by the stimulation of high-affinity IgE receptor FcεRI. $PI3K^{-/-}$ mice are observed to be deficient in gastrointestinal mast cells but still have abundant dermal mast cells [19], indicating that the p85α subunit of PI3K is required for the development of gastrointestinal mast cells, but not dermal mast cells.

$PI3K^{-/-}$ mice failed to develop FA in our FA model, which were attributed to a deficiency of mast cells in the intestine, because: 1) mast cells can promote T-cell migration by producing chemokines [25,26], 2) mast cell products can promote dendritic cells to acquire a Th2 cell-inducing phenotype [2,27], and 3) mast cells themselves can produce Th2 cytokines, such as IL-4, 5 and 13 [2,25].

Furthermore, despite our finding that nicotine treatment atteuated allergic diarrhea in the FA mouse model, nicotine had no effect on the enhanced plasma IgE level.

Thus, these data suggest that the pathogenesis of FA is mainly attributed to mast cell hyperplasia in the intestine, but not antigen-specific IgE hyperproduction. Taken all together, our results indicate that MMCs critically contribute to the development of FA through orchestrating Th2 immune responses in the mucosal immunity of the FA mice.

The cross-talk between the autonomic nervous system and immune system is becoming increasingly elucidated to be of great importance for the maintenance of immune homeostasis. Several lines of evidence indicate that parasympathetic vagus nerve, through release of acetylcholine, plays a counter-regulatory role to restore immune homeostasis in diverse inflammatory disease models, such as ischemia-reperfusion injury [28], pancreatitis [29], peritonitis [30], DSS-induced colitis [31] and postoperative ileus [32,33]. The anti-inflammatory properties of the vagus nerve in these mouse models are primarily attributed to the suppression of macrophage activation that leads to the induction of inflammation through the release of the central inflammatory mediator TNF-α. Recently, it has become clear that nAChRs are expressed in various immune cells [14,32] as well as macrophages [34]. However, it still remains unclear whether the stimulation of nAChRs on these immune cells ameliorates diverse inflammatory diseases. In particular, it is worth noting that it is unknown whether cholinergic activation via nAChRs serves as an anti-inflammatory pathway in Th2-related diseases, especially allergic diseases.

In this FA study, vagal stimulation with 2-DG ameliorated the development of FA, which was reversed by the nAChR antagonist C6, indicating that vagus nerves exhibit anti-allergic properties via nAChRs. The therapeutic potential of the cholinergic agonist nicotine in inflammatory diseases has recently been demonstrated. In fact, nicotine has been shown to suppress inflammatory responses in various clinical studies, animal models and in vitro studies [12,35,36,37]. Notably, in a randomized double-blind study, nicotine patches in combination with conventional therapy have ameliorated ulcerative colitis, in which Th2-mediated phenomena tend to predominate, as compared to placebo patches and conventional therapy; however, nicotine patch treatment has caused adverse side effects, such as nausea, dizziness, headache and addiction due to non-selectivity of nicotine for subtypes of nAChRs [38].

In this study, nicotine treatment significantly ameliorated FA, mainly due to the suppression of upregulated mucosal immune responses via α7 nAChRs on immune cells. Therefore, the therapeutic effects of nicotine and GTS-21 on the FA model raise the possibility that a strategy for drug discovery against FA by targeting α7 nAChRs could potentially have therapeutic benefits.

Moreover, we have demonstrated that mBMMCs express α7 nAChRs and that their activation exerts inhibitory effects on antigen-IgE-mediated degranulation in mBMMCs [17]. In addition, our results in this study reveal that MMCs can orchestrate the allergic and inflammatory responses in the mucosal immune environment of the FA mice colon. Therefore, it is suggested that nicotine treatment suppresses the activation of MMCs through α7 nAChRs on MMCs, thereby reducing the number of MMCs and the plasma mMPC-1 level, which results in the significant amelioration of FA.

Furthermore, to examine whether the cholinergic anti-allergic pathway is a hard-wired connection between the immune and nervous systems closely interacting to regulate FA, we undertook morphological analysis in the mucosa of the FA mouse colon. Previous reports and this study demonstrate that in the mouse enteric nervous system, CGRP is exclusively contained in intrinsic primary afferent neurons that are immunoreactive for choline acetyltransferase [39,40], indicating that CGRP-IR neurons contain ACh as a neurotransmitter in the mouse colon. Our morphological findings of the close proximity between MMCs and CGRP-IR cholinergic nerve fibers in the colonic mucosa of the FA mice imply that the neural cholinergic regulation of immune responses occurs via nAChRs on immune cells, which is consistent with previous reports [14,32]. Collectively, it is suggested that cholinergic nerve fibers closely communicate with MMCs to regulate mast cell functions in the FA mice colon.

Further investigation of this cholinergic counter-regulatory nerve-immune interactions in the intestine will provide new insights to elucidate FA. In addition, new strategies for drug discovery that target the hard-wired connection via α7 nAChRs can lead to novel drug therapies against diverse intestinal immune diseases.

Supporting Information

Figure S1 α7 nAChR-mediated control of food allergy in mice. The occurrence of allergic diarrhea in FA mice (closed circle), GTS-21-treated mice (open circle; 10 mg/kg, p.o.) and MLA-treated mice prior to GTS-21 administration (open square; 1 mg/kg, s.c.) after each oral OVA challenge is shown. *$P<0.05$, **$P<0.01$ vs. FA mice. †$P<0.05$ vs. GST-21-treated mice ($n=6$–18 mice per group).

Author Contributions

Conceived and designed the experiments: MK. Performed the experiments: TY TK JL NU SH HS HK MK. Analyzed the data: JL TY. Contributed reagents/materials/analysis tools: TY JL HS HK. Wrote the paper: MK JL TY.

References

1. Sicherer SH, Sampson HA (2010) Food allergy. J Allergy Clin Immunol 125: S116–125.
2. Abraham SN, St John AL (2010) Mast cell-orchestrated immunity to pathogens. Nat Rev Immunol 10: 440–452.
3. Eigenmann PA, Frossard CP (2003) The T lymphocyte in food-allergy disorders. Curr Opin Allergy Clin Immunol 3: 199–203.
4. MacDonald TT, Di Sabatino A (2009) The immunologic basis for gastrointestinal food allergy. Curr Opin Gastroenterol 25: 521–526.
5. Paul WE, Zhu J (2010) How are T(H)2-type immune responses initiated and amplified? Nat Rev Immunol 10: 225–235.
6. Dawicki W, Marshall JS (2007) New and emerging roles for mast cells in host defence. Curr Opin Immunol 19: 31–38.
7. Yamamoto T, Fujiwara K, Yoshida M, Kageyama-Yahara N, Kuramoto H, et al. (2009) Therapeutic effect of kakkonto in a mouse model of food allergy with gastrointestinal symptoms. Int Arch Allergy Immunol 148: 175–185.
8. Metcalfe DD, Baram D, Mekori YA (1997) Mast cells. Physiol Rev 77: 1033–1079.
9. Kageyama-Yahara N, Suehiro Y, Maeda F, Kageyama S, Fukuoka J, et al. (2010) Pentagalloylglucose down-regulates mast cell surface FcepsilonRI expression in vitro and in vivo. FEBS Lett 584: 111–118.
10. Bienenstock J, Goetzl EJ, Blennerhassett MG (2003) Autonomic neuroimmunology. London: CRC Press. 392 p.
11. van Diest SA, Stanisor OI, Boeckxstaens GE, de Jonge WJ, van den Wijngaard RM (2012) Relevance of mast cell-nerve interactions in intestinal nociception. Biochim Biophys Acta 1822: 74–84.
12. Bauer O, Razin E (2000) Mast Cell-Nerve Interactions. News Physiol Sci 15: 213–218.
13. de Jonge WJ, Ulloa L (2007) The alpha7 nicotinic acetylcholine receptor as a pharmacological target for inflammation. Br J Pharmacol 151: 915–929.
14. Rosas-Ballina M, Tracey KJ (2009) Cholinergic control of inflammation. J Intern Med 265: 663–679.
15. Tracey KJ (2009) Reflex control of immunity. Nat Rev Immunol 9: 418–428.
16. van Der Zanden EP, Boeckxstaens GE, de Jonge WJ (2009) The vagus nerve as a modulator of intestinal inflammation. Neurogastroenterol Motil 21: 6–17.
17. Kageyama-Yahara N, Suehiro Y, Yamamoto T, Kadowaki M (2008) IgE-induced degranulation of mucosal mast cells is negatively regulated via nicotinic acetylcholine receptors. Biochem Biophys Res Commun 377: 321–325.
18. Miller HR, Walshaw R (1972) Immune reactions in mucous membranes. IV. Histochemistry of intestinal mast cells during helminth expulsion in the rat. Am J Pathol 69: 195–208.
19. Fukao T, Yamada T, Tanabe M, Terauchi Y, Ota T, et al. (2002) Selective loss of gastrointestinal mast cells and impaired immunity in PI3K-deficient mice. Nat Immunol 3: 295–304.
20. Brandt EB, Strait RT, Hershko D, Wang Q, Muntel EE, et al. (2003) Mast cells are required for experimental oral allergen-induced diarrhea. J Clin Invest 112: 1666–1677.
21. Kweon MN, Yamamoto M, Kajiki M, Takahashi I, Kiyono H (2000) Systemically derived large intestinal CD4(+) Th2 cells play a central role in STAT6-mediated allergic diarrhea. J Clin Invest 106: 199–206.
22. Friend DS, Ghildyal N, Austen KF, Gurish MF, Matsumoto R, et al. (1996) Mast cells that reside at different locations in the jejunum of mice infected with Trichinella spiralis exhibit sequential changes in their granule ultrastructure and chymase phenotype. J Cell Biol 135: 279–290.

23. Wastling JM, Knight P, Ure J, Wright S, Thornton EM, et al. (1998) Histochemical and ultrastructural modification of mucosal mast cell granules in parasitized mice lacking the beta-chymase, mouse mast cell protease-1. Am J Pathol 153: 491–504.
24. Koyasu S (2003) The role of PI3K in immune cells. Nat Immunol 4: 313–319.
25. Galli SJ, Nakae S, Tsai M (2005) Mast cells in the development of adaptive immune responses. Nat Immunol 6: 135–142.
26. Nakajima T, Inagaki N, Tanaka H, Tanaka A, Yoshikawa M, et al. (2002) Marked increase in CC chemokine gene expression in both human and mouse mast cell transcriptomes following Fcepsilon receptor I cross-linking: an interspecies comparison. Blood 100: 3861–3868.
27. Mazzoni A, Siraganian RP, Leifer CA, Segal DM (2006) Dendritic cell modulation by mast cells controls the Th1/Th2 balance in responding T cells. J Immunol 177: 3577–3581.
28. Bernik TR, Friedman SG, Ochani M, DiRaimo R, Ulloa L, et al. (2002) Pharmacological stimulation of the cholinergic antiinflammatory pathway. J Exp Med 195: 781–788.
29. van Westerloo DJ, Giebelen IA, Florquin S, Bruno MJ, Larosa GJ, et al. (2006) The vagus nerve and nicotinic receptors modulate experimental pancreatitis severity in mice. Gastroenterology 130: 1822–1830.
30. van Westerloo DJ, Giebelen IA, Florquin S, Daalhuisen J, Bruno MJ, et al. (2005) The cholinergic anti-inflammatory pathway regulates the host response during septic peritonitis. J Infect Dis 191: 2138–2148.
31. Ghia JE, Blennerhassett P, Kumar-Ondiveeran H, Verdu EF, Collins SM (2006) The vagus nerve: a tonic inhibitory influence associated with inflammatory bowel disease in a murine model. Gastroenterology 131: 1122–1130.
32. Dhawan S, Cailotto C, Harthoorn LF, de Jonge WJ (2012) Cholinergic signalling in gut immunity. Life Sci 91: 1038–1042.
33. The FO, Boeckxstaens GE, Snoek SA, Cash JL, Bennink R, et al. (2007) Activation of the cholinergic anti-inflammatory pathway ameliorates postoperative ileus in mice. Gastroenterology 133: 1219–1228.
34. Wang H, Yu M, Ochani M, Amella CA, Tanovic M, et al. (2003) Nicotinic acetylcholine receptor alpha7 subunit is an essential regulator of inflammation. Nature 421: 384–388.
35. Andersson U, Tracey KJ (2012) Reflex principles of immunological homeostasis. Annu Rev Immunol 30: 313–335.
36. Lakhan SE, Kirchgessner A (2011) Anti-inflammatory effects of nicotine in obesity and ulcerative colitis. J Transl Med 9: 129.
37. Yoshikawa H, Kurokawa M, Ozaki N, Nara K, Atou K, et al. (2006) Nicotine inhibits the production of proinflammatory mediators in human monocytes by suppression of I-kappaB phosphorylation and nuclear factor-kappaB transcriptional activity through nicotinic acetylcholine receptor alpha7. Clin Exp Immunol 146: 116–123.
38. Pullan RD, Rhodes J, Ganesh S, Mani V, Morris JS, et al. (1994) Transdermal nicotine for active ulcerative colitis. N Engl J Med 330: 811–815.
39. Furness JB, Robbins HL, Xiao J, Stebbing MJ, Nurgali K (2004) Projections and chemistry of Dogiel type II neurons in the mouse colon. Cell Tissue Res 317: 1–12.
40. Qu ZD, Thacker M, Castelucci P, Bagyanszki M, Epstein ML, et al. (2008) Immunohistochemical analysis of neuron types in the mouse small intestine. Cell Tissue Res 334: 147–161.

14

Antigenic Proteins Involved in Occupational Rhinitis and Asthma Caused by Obeche Wood (*Triplochiton Scleroxylon*)

Ana Aranda[1], Paloma Campo[2*], Arantxa Palacin[3], Inmaculada Doña[2], Cristina Gomez-Casado[3], Luisa Galindo[2], Araceli Díaz-Perales[3], Miguel Blanca[2]

1 Allergy Research Laboratory, Carlos Haya Hospital, Málaga, Spain, 2 Unidad de Gestión Clínica Allergy, Carlos Haya Hospital, Málaga, Spain, 3 Biotechnology Department, Center for Plant Biotechnology and Genomics, Pozuelo de Alarcon, Madrid, Spain

Abstract

Background: Obeche wood dust is a known cause of occupational asthma where an IgE-mediated mechanism has been demonstrated.

Objective: To characterize the allergenic profile of obeche wood dust and evaluate the reactivity of the proteins by *in vitro*, *ex vivo* and *in vivo* assays in carpenters with confirmed rhinitis and/or asthma

Materials and methods: An in-house obeche extract was obtained, and two IgE binding bands were purified (24 and 12 kDa) and sequenced by N-terminal identity. Specific IgE and IgG, basophil activation tests and skin prick tests (SPTs) were performed with whole extract and purified proteins. CCD binding was analyzed by ELISA inhibition studies.

Results: Sixty-two subjects participated: 12 with confirmed occupational asthma/rhinitis (ORA+), 40 asymptomatic exposed (ORA−), and 10 controls. Of the confirmed subjects, 83% had a positive SPT to obeche. There was a 100% recognition by ELISA in symptomatic subjects vs. 30% and 10% in asymptomatic exposed subjects and controls respectively ($p<0.05$). Two new proteins were purified, a 24 kDa protein identified as a putative thaumatin-like protein and a 12 kDa gamma-expansin. Both showed allergenic activity *in vitro*, with the putative thaumatin being the most active, with 92% recognition by ELISA and 100% by basophil activation test in ORA+ subjects. Cross-reactivity due to CCD was ruled out in 82% of cases.

Conclusions: Two proteins of obeche wood were identified and were recognized by a high percentage of symptomatic subjects and by a small proportion of asymptomatic exposed subjects. Further studies are required to evaluate cross reactivity with other plant allergens.

Editor: Vladimir N. Uversky, University of South Florida College of Medicine, United States of America

Funding: Financial Support: Ministry of Health grant FIS/PI071175; Andalusian Health Division grants PI-0182/2008; grant from the Spanish Society of Allergy, Ministry of Science and Innovation-DGI, Spain (grant BIO2009-07050); and Thematic Network FIS-RIRAAF (RD07/0064). The funders had no role in study design, data collection and analysis, decision to publish, or preparation of the manuscript.

Competing Interests: None of the authors has any conflict of interest, nor have they received any money from a biotechnology and/or pharmaceutical manufacturer for the present study.

* E-mail: campomozo@yahoo.com

Introduction

Wood is a known sensitizer widely extended in the construction and furniture industries worldwide [1,2]. Exposure to wood dust has been associated with the risk of developing asthma, an increase in airway hyperresponsiveness and decreased FEV_1 [3,4], even in apprentices [5]. The obeche (*Triplochiton scleroxylon*) is a tree from West Africa belonging to the *Sterculiaceace* family [6]. Several cases of occupational asthma due to inhalation of obeche dust have been reported, with positive skin prick tests (SPTs), specific IgE to wood extracts and positive bronchial challenges suggesting an IgE-mediated mechanism [6–10]. However, there is no standardized extract for accurate diagnosis and the nature of the IgE-binding components in obeche is not fully known. Two reports [6–9] first described IgE binding bands by means of SDS-PAGE and immunodetection assays. In the study by Quirce *et al*, allergic subjects mostly recognized a 28 kDa band [6], while other bands of 64, 57.8, and 17 kDa were recognized with less intensity. In addition, IgE reactivity was reduced only by 8.6% when a deglycosylated extract was used, which indicates a non-carbohydrate nature of these IgE binding proteins. The same 28 and 17 kDa reactive components were also found in two other studies [9,11]. One of these, that of Vidal *et al*, described the presence of the 28 kDa protein in both obeche and in fruit extracts (*Cyphomandra betacea Sendth* or tamarillo), and this protein was recognized *in vitro* by a carpenter with occupational asthma due to obeche who suffered anaphylaxis after ingestion of tamarillo [11]. However, no further experiments were conducted to identify these components. Later on, a high molecular weight class I chitinase was described (Trip s1), and still remains the only allergen identified so far [10]. This 38 kDa protein shares a high molecular similarity with Prs a 1 (avocado allergen) and with Hev b 6, and cross reactivity has been demonstrated in a small group of sensitized subjects [10,12]. However, this allergen was not recognized by most subjects in the aforementioned studies [6,9,11], so its relevance in other populations remains unknown. Thus, the allergenic content of obeche wood needs to be analyzed in detail.

The aim of this study was to further characterize the allergenic profile of obeche wood dust. We also evaluated the reactivity of the potentially allergenic proteins by *in vitro*, *ex vivo* and *in vivo* assays in a well-characterized population of carpenters with confirmed rhinitis and/or asthma due to obeche wood exposure and two control populations.

Materials and Methods

Production of in-house obeche extract

Obeche wood dust was extracted with phosphate-buffered saline (PBS) buffer for 1 h at 4°C, centrifuged at 10000× g for 30 min at 4°C. The supernatant was dialysed (cut-off point, 3.5 kDa) against H_2O and freeze-dried. The protein concentration was quantified according to the method of Bradford (Pierce Biotechnology, In. Rockford, USA).

Study population

This study involved carpenters and carpentry apprentices with respiratory symptoms (nasal and/or bronchial) due to occupational exposure to obeche wood, and with a diagnosis of occupational rhinitis/asthma confirmed by specific inhalation challenge with the in-house obeche extract at 1 mg/ml. Nasal challenges were performed according to published methods [13], and responses were monitored by acoustic rhinometry, visual analogue scale and symptoms score. Bronchial challenges were performed using a DeVilbiss nebulizer and responses were monitored by serial spirometry [14]. Nasal and bronchial challenges were performed with the same extract in 5 controls showing negative responses. A group of asymptomatic exposed subjects, with negative SPT to obeche extract who worked in the same factories or school as the symptomatic subjects were invited to participate, and a number of them were randomly selected for the study. A group of non-exposed asymptomatic subjects was also recruited as a control group. All participants completed an occupational questionnaire, as described [15]. Spirometry was performed using a Spirobank spirometer (RDSM, Hasselt, Belgium) following the guidelines [16]. Skin prick tests (SPTs) (ALK-Abelló, Spain) were performed [17] with a battery of common aeroallergens that included grass pollen, trees, dust mites, molds, dog/cat dander and latex. Also, SPT with thaumatin-containing food extracts (banana, peach, hazelnut, chestnut, kiwi, apple and melon, ALK-Abelló, Spain) were performed. Written informed consent was obtained from all subjects and the ethical committee of our institution approved the study.

Isolation of allergens

Obeche extract was fractionated by anion-exchange chromatography on a Bio-Scale™ Mini Macro-Prep® High Q column (BioRad, Hercules, CA, USA) equilibrated 20 mM ethalonamine, pH 9, and eluted with 1 M NaCl in the same buffer. Retained fractions were identified by SDS-PAGE and immunodetection with a serum pool from confirmed obeche-sensitised patients. The non-retained material was separated by RP-HPLC on Europa protein C4 column (25×0.7 mm; particle size 5 µm; Teknokroma, Barcelona, Spain). Elution was performed with a linear gradient of acetonitrile in 0.1% (v/v) trifluoroacetic acid (0–10% for 15 min and 10–100% for 150 min, at a flow rate of 0.5 ml/min). Peaks were processed along with the retained ion exchange fractions. The purified proteins were quantified by a commercial bicinchoninic acid test (Pierce, Cheshire, UK) and their purity was tested by SDS-PAGE, N-terminal amino acid sequencing with an Applied Biosystems 477A gas-phase sequencer (Applied Biosystems, CA, USA), and mass spectrophotometric analysis with a Biflex III Spectrometer (Bruker-Franzen Analytik, Bremen, Germany), using standard methods.

SDS-PAGE and immunodetection

Obeche extract (30 µg) and purified proteins (5 µg) were separated on SDS-PAGE [18]. Proteins were electrotransferred to polyvinylidene difluoride membranes. Blocked membranes (Blocking solution, Sigma, St.Louis, USA) were incubated with a pool of sera from symptomatic exposed subjects with positive specific IgE to obeche (1:5 dilution). The IgE binding was revealed with anti-human IgE-peroxidase conjugate (Biosource, Camarillo, CA, USA; 1:3000 dilution) and chemiluminiscence (Amersham Supersignal West Pico Chemiluminutoescent Substrate, Rockford, USA). Further, blocked membranes were incubated with different polyclonal antibodies and then treated with goat anti-rabbit IgG-peroxidase conjugate (Dako, Carpinteria, CA, USA; 1:10000 dilution) and revealed by means of chemiluminiscence.

Skin prick tests with obeche extract and purified allergens

SPTs with the in-house obeche dust extract (1 mg/ml protein in a 1:1 [v/v] PBS buffer/glycerol solution) or with purified proteins (20 µg/ml) were carried out [17]. Histamine dihydrochloride (10 mg/ml) and PBS buffer/glycerol solution served as positive and negative controls, respectively. Ten non-exposed asymptomatic subjects were tested with this obeche extract and purified proteins, and the responses were all negative.

Specific immunoglobulin E and G determination

Specific IgE and IgG antibodies to obeche wood dust extract were determined in each individual serum in triplicate by direct ELISA method [19]. Obeche extract was tested at 20 µg/ml and purified proteins at 5 µg/ml as solid phase, and serum at 1:10 dilution for measurement of IgE and at 1:50 dilution for measurement of IgG. Blocking solution was used as a negative control. Specific IgE levels greater than 0.19 OD units and specific IgG levels greater than 0,25 OD units (mean [OD]+3× S.D. to blocking) were considered positive. Sera from subjects with confirmed occupational rhinitis and/or asthma were selected to analyze the IgE binding activity of the purified proteins as solid phase following the same protocol described above.

ELISA inhibition studies with CCD determinants

Sera from subjects with confirmed occupational asthma/rhinitis were pre-incubated with different inhibitors (in-house obeche extract and bromelain, Sigma, St. Louis, USA) at final concentrations of 100, 10 and 1 µg/ml at room temperature for 3 h [19]. Later on, the inhibitor mixtures (including sera with no inhibitor as a positive control) were added to plates coated with obeche extract a 20 µg/ml and incubated at 37°C overnight. The assay was completed by incubating with rabbit anti-human IgE antibody (1:3000; DAKO A/S, Denmark). IgE binding was detected using o-phenylenediamine tablets (OPD, DAKO) and the reaction was stopped by adding 2 M chloric acid. The absorbance (OD) in each well was measured at 490 nm. The percentage inhibition of IgE binding was calculated using the following formula: % inhibition = (serum not inhibited-serum inhibited/serum not inhibited) ×100.

Basophil activation test

The basophil activation test (BAT) was performed as described [20], using different concentrations of obeche extract (50, 25, 12.5 and 6.25 μg/ml) and of purified proteins (10, 5 and 2,5 μg/ml). The optimal concentrations of extract and purified proteins were chosen based on dose-response curves and cytotoxicity studies. Results were considered as positive when the stimulation index (SI), calculated as the ratio between the percentage of degranulated basophils with the allergens and the negative control, was >2 in at least one of the dilutions.

Statistical analysis

Differences between groups were compared by the Student t test for continuous variables and by Chi square test for categorical variables using the SPSS software package (SPSS Corporation, Chicago, IL); p values<0.05 were considered statistically significant.

Results

Clinical characteristics of study population

Sixty-two subjects participated in the study:

1. Subjects with confirmed occupational rhinitis and/or asthma (n = 12). These subjects had a diagnosis of either occupational rhinitis (n = 7) or asthma (n = 5) as confirmed by specific nasal or bronchial challenges, all having immediate isolated nasal or bronchial responses. These subjects comprised the occupational rhinitis/asthma group (ORA+).
2. Subjects who were occupationally exposed to obeche wood without any respiratory symptoms and with a negative SPT to obeche extract (n = 40). These subjects comprised the non occupational rhinitis/asthma (ORA−) group.
3. Control group of non-exposed, asymptomatic subjects (CG, n = 10).

The characteristics of the ORA+ subjects were compared to the ORA- group and the control group (see **Table 1**). ORA+ subjects were older and had a significantly longer exposure time when compared with the asymptomatic group (p<0.05). ORA+ subjects had higher total IgE levels compared to ORA− and CG although this difference was not significant. The percentage of smokers and the FEV_1 were similar in all groups. Both ORA+ and ORA− subjects had a high percentage of positive SPT to pollen (ORA+:75%, 67% grass pollen; ORA−: 49%, 60% grass pollen).

Measurement of specific IgE antibodies against obeche wood

Specific IgE antibodies to obeche wood were measured by ELISA in all ORA+, ORA− and CG subjects. As shown in **Figure 1a**, 100% of the ORA+ subjects had specific IgE antibodies against obeche extract, with the highest mean OD of the three groups (solid line shows the positivity cut-off point, dotted lines show mean OD for each group). On the other hand, only 30% of the ORA− subjects had specific IgE antibodies (p<0.05 ORA+ *vs.* ORA−). The control group of unexposed subjects showed the lowest mean value, below the cut-off point of positivity, with only one serum showing a positive value. Thus, detection of specific IgE antibodies was significantly higher (p<0.05) in symptomatic subjects as compared to asymptomatic subjects and controls. **Figure 1b** shows the measurement of specific IgG. We observed 100% positive results in ORA+ subjects and 80% in ORA− subjects. However, 40% of unexposed subjects also showed positive results, with the mean value of this group below the threshold of positivity (p<0.05).

In-house obeche extract showed two principal IgE binding bands

To better characterize the molecular basis of obeche sensitization, the in-house extract was separated by SDS-PAGE and stained with Coomassie (**Figure 2A**). Replicas were electrotransferred and incubated with a pool of sera of sensitized subjects. Two principal bands seemed to be recognized with the highest intensity by serum pool: a 24 kDa and a band with an apparent molecular weight of 12 kDa. In order to identify the nature of these IgE-binding bands, their purification was investigated through different ionic exchange chromatographic techniques. The high molecular weight protein was the most difficult to purify since it was extremely unstable. For this reason, the amount of this purified protein was very small and therefore it was not possible to obtain enough protein to analyze its allergic activity *in vivo* by skin prick test in all subjects. However, the two proteins were purified in sufficient quantity to demonstrate their allergenic activity by *in vitro* (ELISA and BAT) assays. Their purity was checked sequencing their N-terminal amino acids and analyzing their real molecular weight by mass spectrometry.

A gamma-expansin was identified as new allergen of obeche

The protein with the lowest molecular weight (12 kDa) presented 11642.5 Da by mass spectrometry, and its N-terminal amino acid was sequenced and rendered IQGTATFYTPPYVPS. This sequence matched in homology with gamma-expansins of alder (*Alnus glutinasa*; GU06293.1) and of lemon tree (*Citrus jambluri*; AF015782). Members of the same protein family have been associated with grass pollen allergy (group 1 of grass allergens) although their sequence identity with the new allergen is poor [21].

The 24 kDa IgE binding protein could belong to the thaumatin-like family

The highest protein showed 23590.3 Da and its N-terminal corresponded to AQITVTYNGQNG. However, the number of residues was not enough to find identity with known sequences deposited in data banks. For this reason, SDS-PAGE bands were excised and in-gel trypsin digestion followed by offline LC-MALDI-TOF/TOF analysis was performed, but results did not add any relevant information about the identity of the proteins. Since attempts to characterize the purified proteins were not successful, an indirect strategy was attempted. Several protein-specific antibodies were used against the 24 kDa protein. These included rabbit polyclonal antibodies to chestnut TLP (1:30,000 dilution; 1 h; anti-TLP; kindly provided by Dr. L. Gómez, ETSIM, UPM, Madrid) or chestnut chitinases antibodies (dilution 1: 500; 1 h; anti-Chi), or with anti-complex asparagine-linked glycan serum (1:30,000 dilution; 1 h; anti-CCD). The 24 kDa band was recognized by a pool of sera (anti-IgE) (**Figure 2B**), by anti-thaumatin-like proteins (anti-TLP) (**Figure 2C**), antibodies and by anti-carbohydrate complex determinant (anti-CCD) (**Figure 2E**). In contrast, we detected no positive recognition with other antibodies, such as antibodies produced against chestnut-chitinases (anti-Chi) (**Figure 2D**). This result suggested that a TLP could be implicated in the obeche dust sensitization,

Table 1. Demographic and clinical characteristics of subjects with confirmed occupational rhinitis/asthma (ORA+) *vs.* asymptomatic exposed (ORA−) and controls (CG). SPT: skin prick test; SD: standard deviation; *: $p<0.05$.

	ORA+	ORA−	CG
	n = 12	n = 40	n = 10
Age, mean (SD)*	42,3 (13)	20,05 (2,8)	36,33 (7,2)
Sex, M/F*	10/2	40/0	2/8
Smokers, (%)	41,7%	29,3%	30%
Total IgE, mean (range)	250 (54–688)	192 (3–1270)	64 (3–270)
Mean exposure to wood, months*	238	42	0
Mean FEV$_1$, %	93%	94%	95%
Positive SPTs to pollen, %	75% (67% grass)	49% (60% grass)	30% (33% grass)

and its recognition by anti-CCD could confirm this possibility. In order to clarify this aspect, two control proteins were used: Prs a1, class I chitinase and avocado allergen; and Act d2, TLP and kiwi allergen. Both were incubated with the corresponding antibodies and with the pool of obeche sensitized sera (**Figure 2B**). The avocado-protein was not recognized by IgE, nor could we detect any positive band when the extract was incubated with anti-chitinase antibodies. However, Act d 2 was recognized by the obeche-sensitized serum pool, and a reactive band was observed when the extract was incubated with anti-TLP antibodies. Thus, the 24 kDa band may be a TLP.

Relevance of CCD determinants in the measurement of specific IgE to obeche wood

In order to determine the influence of cross-reactive carbohydrate determinants (CCDs) in the measurement of specific IgE to obeche wood in symptomatic subjects, ELISA inhibition studies were performed using obeche extract as solid phase and CCDs as inhibitors in all ORA+ patients (n = 12). Results were obtained in 11 cases, but in one case the correct interpretation of results was not possible, probably due to the low levels of IgE. A significant number of sera (9/11, 82% of cases) showed no inhibition of specific IgE binding when incubated with bromelain, but showed a specific IgE binding to obeche proteins in more than 80% of the

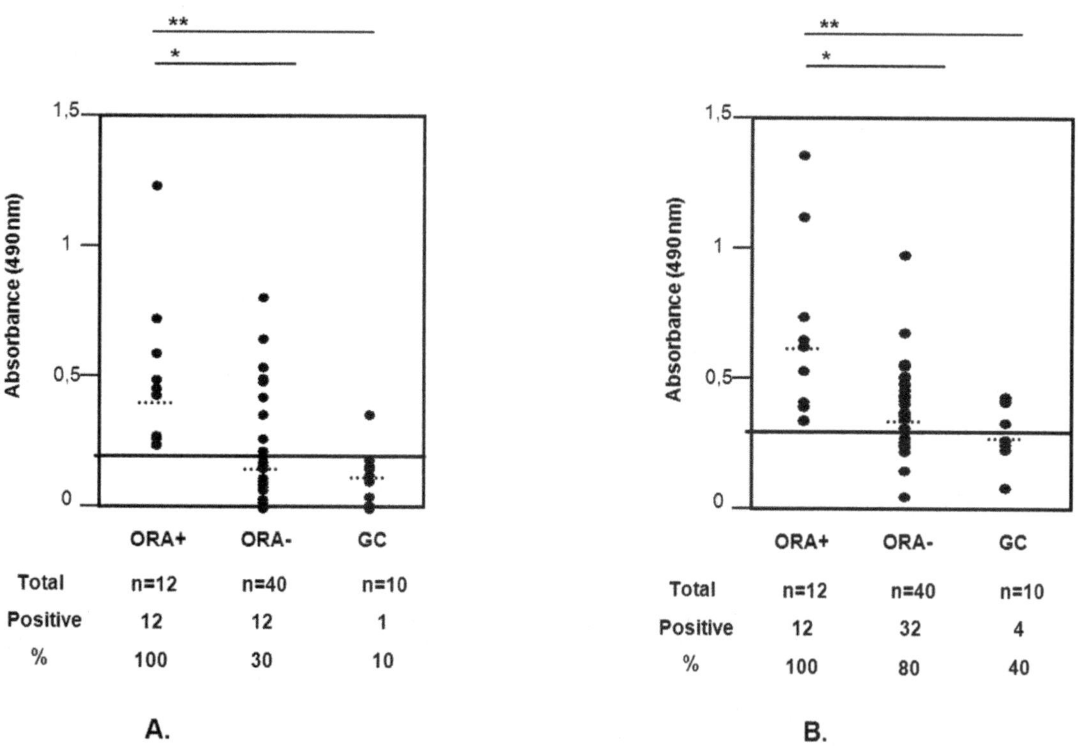

Figure 1. Measurement of specific antibodies to obeche wood dust. Means are represented by dotted lines and a horizontal line indicates cut-off value. *$p<0.05$ symptomatic vs asymptomatics; **$p<0.05$ symptomatic vs controls. **1A**. Levels of specific IgE in ORA+, ORA− and CG subjects; **1B**. Levels of specific IgG in ORA+, ORA− and CG subjects.

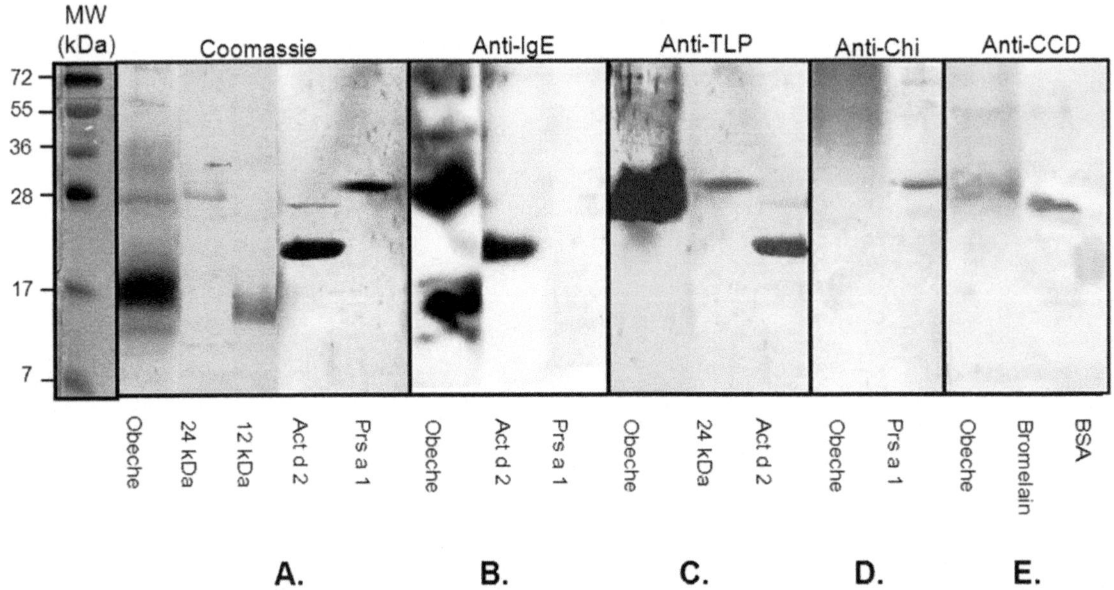

Figure 2. Immunodetection of proteins in obeche wood dust. 2A. *In-house* obeche wood dust extract (40 µg; Obeche), purified protein (5 µg; 24 kDa; 12 kDa) or purified allergens Act d 2 and Prs a 1 (5 µg) were separated by SDS-PAGE and stained with Coomassie blue (Coomassie). Replicas from the extract were electrotransferred and incubated with serum pool of selected exposure subjects (anti-IgE) (**2B**) or with antibodies produced against chestnut thaumatin-like protein (anti-TLP) (**2C**), against chestnut chitinases (anti-Ch) (**2D**) or anti N-glycan antibodies (anti-CCD) with bromelain and bovine serum albumin (BSA) as positive and negative controls (**2E**).

cases. Only two sera showed significant percentage of inhibition of specific IgE binding ≥50% when incubated with bromelain (subjects #4 and 10, see **Table 2**), showing that in these two cases the positive results may be attributed to cross-reactivity with CCDs (see **Figure 3**).

Purified IgE binding proteins of obeche were recognized by exposed subjects

Allergenic activity of purified proteins was studied by ELISA using individual sera from the 12 symptomatic subjects (**Figure 4A**). The putative TLP was recognized by 92% of the subjects, and the gamma-expansin showed a positive response in 67%. This result was confirmed when the proteins were used in BAT (**Figure 4B**) in symptomatic subjects with total extract and with purified proteins (24 and 12 kDa). A positive activation of basophils was observed in 90% of ORA+ subjects in the presence of the obeche extract. The putative TLP protein was again the most active when it was incubated with basophils from exposed subjects, being recognized by 100% of the symptomatic subjects. The 12 kDa protein showed less activation capacity (70%). The optimal concentrations were chosen based on dose-response curves and cytotoxicity studies. Results of ELISA and BAT measurements for each subject are summarized in **Table 2**. Also, results were analyzed considering whether ORA+ subjects had rhinitis or rhinitis and asthma. As shown in Table 2, subjects with rhinitis recognized more the 12 kD band by ELISA compared to subjects with asthma (75% vs.50% respectively). However, rhinitis subjects recognized less the 12 kD band by BAT than asthmatic subjects (43% vs 100%). Also, the 24 kD band was recognized similarly by both groups regarding the technique used. Therefore, there are no significant differences between both groups.

Skin prick testing with in-house extract and purified proteins

Skin prick testing with whole obeche extract at 1 mg/ml was positive in 83% of the ORA+ subjects, with no positive responses in the non-exposed asymptomatic controls. The allergenic capacity of the obeche-purified proteins was confirmed by SPT in 9 out of 12 ORA+ workers, obtaining 44% of positive responses to the purified putative TLP protein, while 11% recognized the gamma-expansin protein. Results of SPTs for each subject are summarized in **Table 2**.

Reactivity of SE subjects to thaumatin-containing food extracts

Since the identified 24 kDa protein was a potential TLP, as demonstrated by specific antibodies, the presence of cross-reactivity with thaumatin-containing foods and food allergy was investigated. ORA+ workers were questioned about food allergy history, and SPTs were performed with commercial banana, peach, hazelnut, chestnut, kiwi, apple and melon extracts. Almost half of ORA+ patients reported a history of food allergy (see **Table 2**). SPTs to food extracts were positive in 40% of these subjects, mostly to peach, chestnut, hazelnut and kiwi extracts.

Discussion

Occupational asthma is the most common occupational respiratory disease in developed countries [22]. Wood dust has been identified as a risk factor for the development of asthma [23], and in some cases it is caused by IgE-mediated sensitization to protein compounds of wood dust [6–10,24–26]. In the present study, an in-house obeche extract was produced that was recognized by SPT in 83% and by ELISA in 100% of subjects with confirmed occupational rhinitis and/or asthma, and by a small subset of asymptomatic exposed subjects (30% by ELISA).

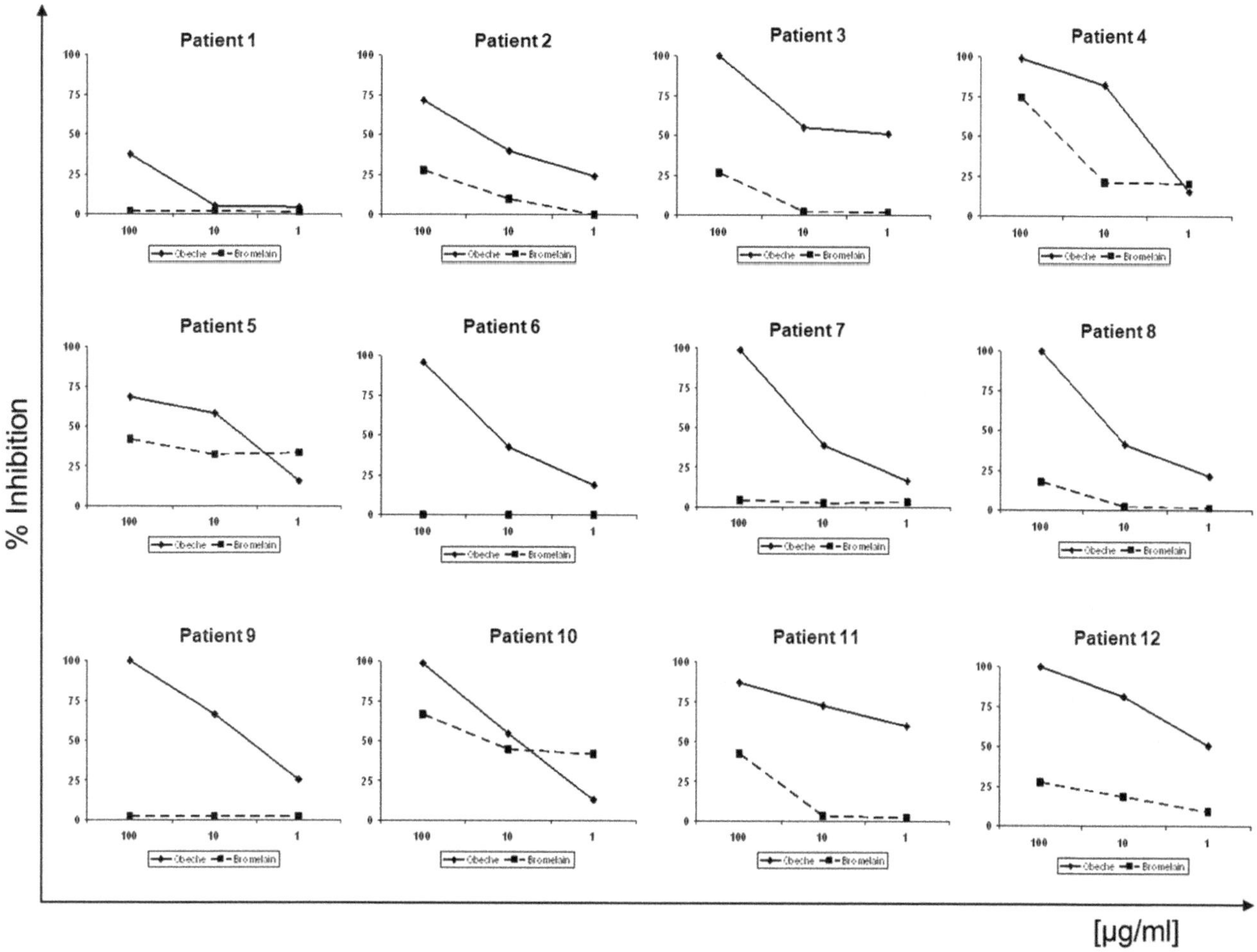

Figure 3. ELISA inhibition studies in ORA+ subjects. Bromelain (CCD, solid line) and obeche (dotted line) are inhibitors and obeche extract is the solid phase.

The detailed characterization of the allergenic activity of obeche wood dust revealed two principal bands of 24 and 12 kDa, which were recognized by ELISA in 92% and 67% of the ORA+ subjects, respectively. Unfortunately, there was not a sufficient amount of protein to test the asymptomatic subjects to obtain the reactivity to these proteins in that group. As reported, bands with apparent molecular weight of 28 and 17 kDa have been identified as principal IgE-binding proteins related to obeche sensitization [6,9], and these could correspond to our bands of 24 and 12 kDa. Surprisingly, no major IgE-binding band was observed that could be identified as Trip s1 in the present study. In addition, no recognition was shown when the in-house extract of obeche was incubated with antibodies produced against chestnut chitinase. This difference in protein recognition may be explained by several hypotheses; the first possibility is that the allergen recognition profile may differ depending on geographic characteristics, as has been described in some food allergens such as LTPs [27]. Another possible explanation is that methodological differences in dust extraction and the fact that chitinases are highly thermolabile proteins may result in the absence of 38 kDa IgE-bands in the present study and others [6,9–11]. And finally, the geographical origin of the wood may influence the protein content of the extract, SDS-Page demonstrated that Trip s1 was mostly detected in wood samples coming from Ghana (*wawa*) but not in the samples coming from Cameroon (*ayous*) [28]. However, protein bands of 28 and 12 kDa were detected in dust samples from both wawa and ayous woods.

Identification of the 12 kDa protein revealed that it belonged to the gamma-expansin family [29], showing homology with tree-members of this family. Expansins refer to a family of non-enzymatic proteins found in the plant cell wall [30], and which includes small proteins grouped in two large (alpha and beta-expansins) and two small (gamma-, and epsilon- expansins) subfamilies [31]. A subset of beta-expansins has evolved a special role in grass pollen, where they are known as group 1 grass pollen allergens [21]. In contrast, the amino acid N-terminal and the trypsin-peptides obtained from the putative TLP had no correspondence with any known sequence deposited in the data bank. However, its recognition by anti-chestnut TLP antibodies suggests that it could belong to the thaumatin-like family, although more experimental analysis will be necessary to clarify its nature. Thaumatins are proteins described as plant defence proteins (PR5) against pathogen attacks and as panallergens responsible for cross-reactivity among foods and pollens [31], which may explain why some asymptomatic exposed subjects recognized the proteins mostly *in vitro* in our study [32–34]. For this reason, food allergy was also investigated in the ORA+ group, where 42% of the subjects reported a history of food allergy, and 40% had positive

Table 2. Results of *in vivo* and *in vitro* tests with obeche extract and purified proteins in subjects with confirmed occupational rhinitis and asthma (ORA+; R = rhinitis; R+A = rhinitis and asthma).

Subjects #	Symptoms	SPT extract	SPT 12 kDa	SPT 24 kDa	ELISA extract	ELISA 12 kDa	ELISA 24 kDa	BAT extract	BAT 12 kDa	BAT 24 kDa	+SPT grass	Food allergy history	SPT TLP-related food	SPT+ food	CCD recognition
1	R+A	+	−	+	+	−	+	+	+	+	+	no	−	−	n/a
2	R	+	nd	nd	+	+	+	nd	nd	nd	+	no	nd	nd	no
3	R+A	+	nd	nd	+	+	−	nd	nd	nd	+	no	nd	nd	no
4	R+A	+	−	−	+	−	+	+	+	+	+	no	+	Peach,chestnut,hazelnut,kiwi, melon	yes
5	R+A	+	−	−	+	+	+	+	+	+	−	yes	+	Peach,chestnut,apple	no
6	R	+	+	+	+	+	+	+	+	+	+	no	−	−	no
7	R	+	−	+	+	+	+	+	−	+	−	yes	+	banana,kiwi	no
8	R	−	−	−	+	−	+	−	−	+	+	yes	+	hazelnut	no
9	R	+	−	+	+	+	+	+	+	+	−	yes	−	chestnut	no
10	R	−	−	−	+	+	+	+	−	+	−	yes	−	−	yes
11	R	+	−	−	+	−	+	+	+	+	−	no	−	−	no
12	R	+	nd	nd	+	+	+	+	+	+	−	no	−	−	no

Results regarding food allergy assessment and CCD recognition are also included.

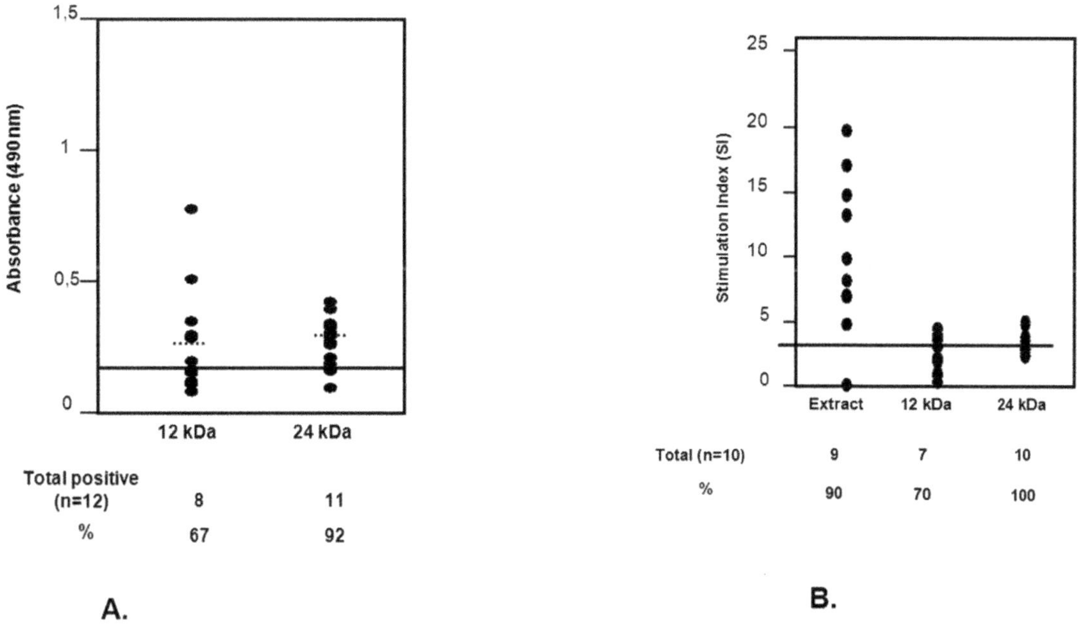

Figure 4. Allergenic activity of purified proteins of obeche wood dust. 4A. IgE-binding (ELISA) to purified obeche proteins (24 and 12 kDa). Solid line shows the positivity cut-off point, dotted lines show mean OD for each group. **4B.** Basophil activation tests using the *in-house* obeche wood dust extract and purified proteins (24 and 12 kDa). The solid line shows the threshold of positivity.

SPTs to several TLP-containing foods including peach, chestnut, hazelnut and kiwi, although the structural similarity among these TLPs and the 24 kDa protein in obeche is still unknown.

Regardless of their biochemical nature, the putative TLP and the obeche gamma-expansin were recognized by ELISA in 92% and 67% of workers with confirmed occupational rhinitis or asthma (ORA+), obtaining similar results in the BAT (100% for 24 kDa and 70% for 12 kDa protein, respectively). The results show that the protein with the highest molecular weight is the most active. However, the *in vivo* recognition was lower for both proteins, obtaining percentages of positive responses in the ORA+ group of 44% for the 24 kDa protein and only 11% for the 12 kDa protein.

The role of the cross-reactive carbohydrate determinants (CCDs) in sensitization allergy to wood proteins has been evaluated in other woods [35], showing a high rate of sensitization to CCDs in workers with *in vitro* sensitization to several woods but not among workers with a single sensitization or clinically relevant symptoms [36]. The putative thaumatin described in the present study may be glycosilated, based on the results of the incubation with anti-CCD antibodies. However, in our study, more than 80% of cases showed a specific IgE binding to obeche proteins that were not inhibited by bromelain, as demonstrated by ELISA-inhibition studies. A previous study that also described the 28 kDa as the most relevant protein in a very similar population showed that the use of a deglycosylated extract only reduced the IgE binding activity by 8.6%. Therefore, in the case of these obeche wood proteins, CCD sensitization does not seem relevant in most patients.

In conclusion, a 24 kDa putative TLP and a 12 kDa gamma-expansin were identified in obeche wood, showing a high percentage of recognition by *in vitro* studies and a modest *in vivo* recognition by subjects with confirmed rhinitis/asthma caused by obeche wood. This study will contribute to better characterize this wood, since there is a need of standardized, well-characterized extracts to correctly diagnose this disease, which is currently underestimated. Consequently, further studies are needed to establish the sensitivity and specificity parameters of these diagnostic techniques and further characterization of these and other wood allergens.

Acknowledgments

The authors would like to thank Ian Johnson Johnstone for his help with the final English version of this manuscript. They also thank Mrs. Arias and Mr. García-Montes, and the staff and students from CEMER School (Cordoba, Spain) for their support and collaboration in this study.

Author Contributions

Designed and coordinated the study and the protocol to collect sera: PC AD-P MB. Corrected the manuscript and suggested important contributions to define the final version: PC AD-P MB. Carried out the allergen purification: AA AP CG-C. Collected patients' sera and performed challenge tests: PC ID LG. Performed the experiments: AA AP CG-C. Analyzed the data: AA AP CG-C. Wrote the paper: AA PC AD-P.

References

1. Chan-Yeung M, Malo JL (2006) Western Red cedar (*Thuja plicata*) and other wood dusts. IN: "Asthma in the workplace" 3rd edition Pages 505–524 Bernstein IL, Chan-Yeung M, Bernstein D, editors Taylor & Francis Group Publishers NY
2. Kauppinen T, Vincent R, Liukkonen T, Grzebyk M, Kauppinen A, et al. (2006) Occupational exposure to inhaled wood dust in the member status of the European Union. Ann Occup Hyg; 50: 549–61
3. Malmberg PO, Rask-Andersen A, Larsson KA, Stjernberg N, Sundblad BM, et al. (1996) Increased bronchial responsiveness in workers sawing Scots pine. Am J Respir Crit Care Med; 153(3): 948–52
4. Schlünssen V, Jacobsen G, Erlandsen M, Mikkelsen AB, Schaumburg I, et al. (2008) Determinants of wood dust exposure in the Danish furniture industry-Cross sectional studies 6 years apart. Ann Occup Hyg; 52(4): 227–238

5. Campo P, Aranda A, Rondon C, Doña I, Diaz-Perales A, et al. (2010) Work-related sensitization and respiratory symptoms in carpentry apprentices exposed to wood dust and diisocyanates. Ann Allergy Asthma Immunol, 105: 24–30
6. Quirce S, Hinojosa M, Marañón F, Ferrer A, Fernández-Caldas E, et al. (2000) Identification of obeche wood (Triplochiton scleroxylon) allergens associated with occupational asthma. J Allergy Clin Immunol; 106: 400–1
7. Hinojosa M, Losada E, Moneo I, Dominguez J, Carrillo T, et al. (1986) Occupational asthma caused by African maple (Obeche) and Ramin: evidence of cross reactivity between these two woods. Clin Allergy; 16:145–53
8. Reijula K, Kujala V, Latvala J (1994) Sauna builder's asthma caused by obeche (Triplochiton scleroxylon) dust. Thorax; 49:622–3
9. Ferrer A, Marañón F, Casanovas M, Fernández-Caldas E (2001) Asthma from inhalation of Triplochiton scleroxylon (Samba) wood dust. J Investig Allergol Clin Immunol.; 11: 199–203.
10. Kespohl S, Sander I, Merget R, Petersen A, Meyer HE, et al. (2005) Identification of an obeche (Triplochiton scleroxylon) wood allergen as a class I chitinase. Allergy; 60: 808–14
11. Vidal C, González-Quintela A, Rodriguez V, Armisén M, Liñares T, et al. (2006) Anaphylaxis to Cyphomandra betacea Sendth (tamarillo) in an obeche wood (*Triplochiton scleroxylon*) allergic patient. Ann Allergy Asthma Immunol.;96: 870–3.
12. Venturini M, Gastaminza G, Kespohl S, Bernedo N, Garmendia M, et al. (2004) Cross-reactivity between obeche wood *(Triplochiton scleroxylon)* and natural rubber latex. Allergy; 59: 225–8
13. Rondon C, Romero JJ, Lopez S, Antunez C, Martin-Casañez E, et al. (2007) Local IgE production and positive nasal provocation test in patients with persistent nonallergic rhinitis. J Allergy Clin Immunol.; 119(4): 899–905
14. Fernandez-Nieto M, Quirce S, Carnes J, Sastre J (2006) Occupational asthma due to chromium and nickel salts. Int Arch Occup Environ Health.; 79(6):483–6
15. Burney PG, Laitinen LA, Perdrizet S, Huckauf H, Tattersfield AE, et al. (1989) Validity and repeatability of the IUATLD (1984) bronchial symptoms questionnaire: an international comparison. Eur Resp J; 940–945
16. Miller MR, Hankinson J, Brusasco V, Burgos F, Casaburi R, et al. (2005) Series "ATS/ERS Task Force: standarization of lung function testing" Standardization of Spirometry. Eur Resp J; 26: 319–338.
17. Dreborg S, Frew A (1993) EAACI Position Paper: Allergen Standardization and skin tests; 48: 49–54.
18. Laemmli UK (1970) Cleavage of structural proteins during the assembly of the head of bacteriophage T4. Nature; 227:680–5
19. Díaz-Perales A, Lombardero M, Sánchez-Monge R, García-Selles FJ, Pernas M, et al. (2000) Lipid-transfer proteins as potential plant panallergens: cross-reactivity among proteins of Artemisia pollen, Castanea nut and Rosaceae fruits, with different IgE-binding capacities. Clin Exp Allergy; 30:1403–10
20. Torres MJ, Padial A, Mayorga C, Fernández T, Sanchez-Sabate E, et al. (2004) The diagnostic interpretation of basophil activation test in immediate allergic reactions to betalactams. Clin Exp Allergy; 34:1768–75.
21. Cosgrove DJ, Bedinger P, Durachko DM (1997) Group I allergens of grass pollen as cell wall-loosening agents. Proc. Natl. Acad. Sci. USA; 94: 6559–6564.
22. Kauppinen T, Vincent R, Liukkonen T, Grzebyk M, Kauppinen A, et al. (2006) Occupational exposure to inhalable wood dust in the member states of the European Union. Ann Occup Hyg.; 50: 549–61
23. Pérez-Ríos M, Ruano-Ravina A, Etminan M, Takkouche B (2010) A meta-analysis on wood dust exposure and risk of asthma. Allergy; 65: 467–73
24. Tse KS, Chan H, Chan Yeung M (1982) Specific IgE antibodies in workers with occupational asthma due to Western red cedar. Clin Allergy; 12: 249–258.
25. Quirce S, Parra A, Antón E, Fernández-Nieto M, Jerez J, et al. (2004) Occupational asthma caused by tali and jatoba wood dusts. J Allergy Clin Immunol; 113: 361–3.
26. Skovsted TA, Schlünssen V, Schaumburg I, Wang P, Staun-Olsen P, et al. (2003) Only few workers exposed to wood dust are detected with specific IgE against pine wood. Allergy;58: 772–9
27. Fernández-Rivas M, Bolhaar S, González-Mancebo E, Asero R, van Leeuwen A, et al. (2006) Apple allergy across Europe: how allergen sensitization profiles determine the clinical expression of allergies to plant foods. J Allergy Clin Immunol Aug; 118(2): 481–8
28. Kespohl S, Sander I, Schulze J, Poppe M, Brüning T, et al. (2008) Development of an obeche wood allergen quantification assay for the assessment of allergen exposure in workplaces. Scand J Work Environ Health; 34:387–95.
29. Ceccardi TL, Barthe GA, Derrick KS (1998) A novel protein associated with citrus blight has sequence similarities to expansin. Plant Mol Biol, 38:775–783
30. Sampedro J, Cosgrove D (2005) The expansin superfamily. Genome Biology; 6:242–253
31. Li Y, Darley C, Ongaro V, Fleming A, Schipper O, et al. (2002) Plant Expansins Are a Complex Multigene Family with an Ancient Evolutionary Origin. Plant Physiol; 128: 854–864.
32. Breiteneder H (2004) Thaumatin-like proteins: a new family of pollen and fruit allergens. Allergy; 59: 479–481
33. Gavrovic-Jankulovic M, Cirkovic T, Vuckovic O, Atanaskovic-Markovic M, Petersen A, et al. (2002) Isolation and biochemical characterization of a thaumatin-like kiwi allergen. J Allergy Clin Immunol; 110: 805–810
34. Palacín A, Tordesillas L, Gamboa P, Sanchez-Monge R, Cuesta-Herranz J, et al. (2010) Characterization of peach thaumatin-like proteins and their identification as major peach allergens. Clin Exp Allergy; 40:1422–30
35. Kespohl S, Kotschy-Lang N, Tomm JM, von Bergen M, Maryska S, et al. (2012) Occupational IgE-mediated softwood allergy: characterization of the causative allergen. Int Arch Allergy Immunol.;157: 202–8.
36. Kespohl S, Schlünssen V, Jacobsen G, Schaumburg I, Maryska S, et al. (2010) Impact of cross-reactive carbohydrate determinants on wood dust sensitization. Clin Exp Allergy; 40(7): 1099–106

15

The Course of Asthma in Young Adults: A Population-Based Nine-Year Follow-Up on Asthma Remission and Control

Lucia Cazzoletti[1]*, Angelo Guido Corsico[2], Federica Albicini[3], Eti Maria Giulia Di Vincenzo[3], Erica Gini[3], Amelia Grosso[3], Vanessa Ronzoni[3], Massimiliano Bugiani[4], Pietro Pirina[5], Isa Cerveri[3]

1 Unit of Epidemiology and Medical Statistics, University of Verona, Verona, Italy, **2** Department of Molecular Medicine, University of Pavia, Pavia, Italy, **3** Division of Respiratory Diseases, Istituto di Ricovero e Cura a Carattere Scientifico "San Matteo" Hospital Foundation, University of Pavia, Pavia, Italy, **4** Unit of Respiratory Medicine, National Health Service, Turin, Italy, **5** Institute of Respiratory Diseases, University of Sassari, Sassari, Italy

Abstract

Background: Only few longitudinal studies on the course of asthma among adults have been carried out.

Objective: The aim of the present prospective study, carried out between 2000 and 2009 in Italy, is to assess asthma remission and control in adults with asthma, as well as their determinants.

Methods: All the subjects with current asthma (21–47 years) identified in 2000 in the Italian Study on Asthma in Young Adults in 6 Italian centres were followed up. Asthma remission was assessed at follow-up in 2008–2009 (n = 214), asthma control at baseline and follow-up. Asthma remission and control were related to potential determinants by a binomial logistic and a multinomial logistic model. Separate models for remission were used for men and women.

Results: The estimate of the proportion of subjects who were in remission was 29.7% (95%CI: 14.4%;44.9%). Men who were not under control at baseline had a very low probability of being in remission at follow-up (OR = 0.06; 95%CI:0.01;0.33) when compared to women (OR = 0.40; 95%CI:0.17;0.94). The estimates of the proportion of subjects who were under control, partial control or who were not under control in our sample were 26.3% (95%CI: 21.2;31.3%), 51.6% (95%CI: 44.6;58.7%) and 22.1% (95%CI: 16.6;27.6%), respectively. Female gender, increasing age, the presence of chronic cough and phlegm and partial or absent asthma control at baseline increased the risk of uncontrolled asthma at follow-up.

Conclusion: Asthma remission was achieved in nearly 1/3 of the subjects with active asthma in the Italian adult population, whereas the proportion of the subjects with controlled asthma among the remaining subjects was still low.

Editor: Thomas Behrens, Universität Bochum, Germany

Funding: The Agenzia Italiana del Farmaco (AIFA) (FARM5JYS5A). The funders had no role in study design, data collection and analysis, decision to publish, or preparation of the manuscript.

Competing Interests: The authors have declared that no competing interests exist.

* E-mail: lucia.cazzoletti@univr.it

Introduction

Asthma is a major chronic respiratory disease [1] whose prevalence is still on the increase in Italy [2]. Unlike most chronic diseases, which start in adulthood and tend to progress over time, asthma may develop at any age and remittance is relatively common [3], especially during adolescence [4]. However, only few studies on the course of asthma among adults [5–7] have been carried out.

Progress in asthma treatment has reduced the symptoms of asthma and the frequency of severe life–threatening exacerbations of the disease. Asthma is now a treatable disease, but it is not curable. At present, most discussions on asthma treatment goals revolve around disease control [8,9], and little attention is paid to remission as an achievable therapeutic goal [10].

Detecting the factors related to asthma remission or control could have clinical and public health implications. Few longitudinal studies have focused on these implications and many of them have been limited to short follow-up studies [11,12,6].

The aim of the present prospective study, carried out between 2000 and 2009 in Italy, was to assess asthma remission and control in adult subjects with asthma and their determinants.

Methods

Study design

A screening questionnaire investigating the presence of respiratory symptoms and asthma management was sent to random samples of people aged 20–44 years at the time of recruitment, in the frame of the Italian Study on Asthma in Young Adults (ISAYA) carried out between 1998 and 2000 [5,13].

All the subjects in the 6 Italian centres (Verona, Torino, Pavia, Sassuolo, Pisa, Sassari), who reported current asthma at the screening questionnaire (self-reported physician's diagnosis of asthma and at least one asthma attack in the last 12 months and/or current use of anti-asthma drugs), between April and June 2000, were invited to participate in a phone interview aimed at collecting information on symptoms and treatment [14]. Out of the 458 eligible subjects with current asthma at the postal survey, 354 (77.3%) subjects participated in the telephone survey. These subjects were re-surveyed by telephone or in a face to face interview between 2008 and 2009, and 214 subjects (response rate: 60.4%) participated in the follow-up.

Ethics approval

Local ethics committees at each center approved the local study protocols and the follow-up study was approved by the ethic committee of the University of Pavia.

Definition of asthma remission

Remission was defined as no current use of asthma medication, no asthma-like symptoms (wheezing, tightness in the chest, shortness of breath) and no asthma attacks in the last 12 months, as reported by the subjects at follow-up.

Definition of asthma control

Asthma control was defined by using a customized version of the asthma control definition provided in the Global Initiative for Asthma (GINA) guidelines [15,16]. The definition of asthma control was mainly based on the frequency of diurnal and nocturnal symptoms, the limitations in daily activities and the need for reliever/rescue treatment. According to this definition, asthma was considered to be controlled if all the following features were present: diurnal symptoms less than once a week and no asthma attacks in the last 3 months, no activity limitations in the last 12 months, no nocturnal symptoms in the last 3 months, short-acting β_2-agonists twice or less per week in the last 3 months and no use of oral steroids in the last 12 months. Asthma was considered to be partly controlled if 1 or 2 of the above features were absent. Asthma was considered to be uncontrolled if more than 2 features were absent or if asthma, shortness of breath, or wheezing had caused hospital/emergency department admissions in the last 12 months; oral steroids were used in short courses or continuously in the last 3 months; or the subject had more than 12 asthma attacks in the last 3 months.

Information on lung function was not available.

Classification of treatment

Treatment was classified in one of five steps according to the average daily dose of inhaled corticosteroids (ICS) based on the last 3 months [17]:

STEP 1: As needed short-acting β_2-agonist;

STEP 2: Sustained release theophylline OR Leukotriene modifier OR budesonide <400 µg (low-dose) OR an equipotent dose of other ICS;

STEP 3: Budesonide < = 400 µg or an equipotent dose of other ICS plus long-acting β_2-agonist OR

Budesonide < = 400 µg or an equipotent dose of other ICS plus leukotriene modifier OR

Budesonide < = 400 µg or an equipotent dose of other ICS plus sustained release theophylline OR

Budesonide >400 µg (medium or high dose) or an equipotent dose of other ICS;

STEP 4: Budesonide >400 µg or an equipotent dose of other ICS plus long-acting β_2-agonist OR

Budesonide >400 µg or an equipotent dose of other ICS plus leukotriene modifier OR

Budesonide >400 µg or an equipotent dose of other ICS plus sustained release theophylline;

STEP 5: Oral corticosteroids or Anti-IgE treatment

The equipotent doses of other ICS – beclomethasone dipropionate, flunisolide, fluticasone, mometasone, ciclesonide and triamcinolone – were the ones reported in the GINA guidelines [17].

Statistical analysis

Data were summarized as means with standard deviations (s.d.), or as medians with interquartile ranges (IQRs), when appropriate, for continuous variables and as percentages for categorical variables. Comparison of variables across strata was performed by using the χ^2 test for categorical variables and the t-test or the Wilcoxon test for continuous variables. The conventional 5% level of statistical significance was used.

We addressed the problem of unit non-response by the assignment of statistical weights to the participants [18,19]. First, we fitted a logistic stepwise regression model (backward approach) to all the participants at baseline, the resulting fitted model was then used to predict a response propensity for each respondent, and the inverse of the predicted response propensity was the nonresponse adjustment associated with each respondent. The significance level for removal from the stepwise model was 0.20 and the variables included in the final model were smoking habits, asthma attacks in the last 12 months, allergic rhinitis and hospital or emergency department admissions because of asthma, shortness of breath, or wheezing in the last 12 months. Age, gender, age at asthma onset, current asthma drug use, asthma-like symptoms in the last 12 months, chronic cough and phlegm, activity limitations in the last 12 months were excluded from the final model. We trimmed the upper 5% of our weights to control for a possible large variation of the weights (to 2.233) [20,21].

To identify the factors associated with asthma remission, a logistic regression model was fitted to the data, using a dummy indicator as the dependent variable (presence/absence of remission at follow-up). The logistic regression model was weighted by using the mentioned non-response adjustment. We assessed the association between several determinants (gender, smoking habits, allergic rhinitis, age, age at asthma onset, ICS use in the last 3 months) measured at baseline and asthma remission at follow-up, adjusting for the effect of the type of survey (telephone/face to face). Moreover, we assessed the interactions between gender and the other covariates, and the presence of interactions was assessed using the Wald test. The interactions between gender and smoking habits (p for the interaction = 0.023), gender and control at baseline ($p = 0.003$) and gender and age at asthma onset ($p = 0.023$) were statistically significant. The complete model included the significant interaction terms, and 2 separate models were used for men and women. Multivariate associations of potential determinants with asthma remission were expressed by odds ratios (OR) and their 95% Confidence Intervals (95%CIs).

To identify the factors associated with asthma control, a multinomial regression model was fitted to the data, using a 3-level dependent variable (controlled, partially controlled and uncontrolled asthma at follow-up). The multinomial regression model was weighted by using the inverse of the predicted response propensity. Multivariate associations of potential determinants with asthma control were expressed by relative risk ratios (RRRs; using controlled asthma as the reference category) and their 95%CIs.

The multivariate models identified centers as clustering factors, and the Huber/White sandwich estimate of variance was used to adjust for within-center correlation [22].

The statistical analyses were performed using STATA software, release 12.0 (StataCorp, College Station, TX, USA).

Results

Participants and non participants

Gender, age and smoking habits were not significantly different between subjects who did participate in the follow-up and subjects who did not (Table 1). Participants and non participants did not differ with regard to asthma-like symptoms in the previous 12 months, current asthma drug use, chronic cough and phlegm, activity limitations in the last 12 months and hospital/emergency department admissions because of asthma, shortness of breath, or wheezing in the last 12 months, as reported at baseline. Subjects participating in the follow-up were significantly more likely to report allergic rhinitis (76.2%), with respect to subjects who did not participate (65.5%) (p = 0.029). Furthermore, they were significantly less likely to report asthma attacks in the last 12 months (79.0%), with respect to subjects who did not participate (90.0%) (p = 0.006).

Asthma remission and its determinants

Asthma remission could not be defined for 4 subjects at follow-up due to missing information on current asthma drug use, asthma symptoms or attacks in the last 12 months. After adjusting for non-response and for the effect of covariates, the estimate of the proportion of subjects who were in remission was 29.7% (95%CI: 14.4%;44.9%). A regression model for remission at follow-up was estimated separately for men and women (Table 2 and 3). The direction of the association between asthma control at baseline and remission was consistent in men and women, but men who were not under control at baseline had a very low probability of being in remission at follow-up (OR = 0.06; 95%CI:0.01;0.33, Table 2) when compared to women (OR = 0.40; 95%CI:0.17;0.94, Table 3). Age at asthma onset was not significantly associated with remission in men (OR = 1.02; 95%CI:0.96;1.08, Table 2); whereas, in the case of women, as age at onset of the disease increased, the likelihood of being in remission at follow-up increased (OR = 1.07; 95%CI:1.00;1.14, Table 3).

Smoking was associated with asthma remission in women (p for the overall association<0.0001, Table 3), but not in men (p = 0.5896, Table 2).

GINA-based asthma control in subjects with active asthma

Sufficient data to define asthma control at baseline were available for 147 subjects with active asthma at follow-up: 41 (27.9%) of them had controlled, 60 (40.8%) partially controlled and 46 (31.3%) uncontrolled asthma.

Asthma control was defined for 138 subjects with active asthma at follow-up: 38 (27.5%) of them had controlled, 69 (50.0%) partially controlled and 31 (22.5%) uncontrolled asthma.

The distribution of asthma control at follow-up was significantly associated with asthma control at baseline (p = 0.016) (Figure 1): the percentage of subjects with uncontrolled asthma at follow-up was higher for subjects with uncontrolled (31%) or partially

Table 1. Main baseline characteristics of the subjects participating and not participating in the follow-up survey.

	Non participants	Participants	All subjects at baseline	p-value
	n = 140	n = 214	n = 354	
Mean age (years), (sd)	33.2 (7.0)	34.2 (7.5)	33.8 (7.3)	0.242
Gender (%)				0.577
Male	49.3	46.3	47.5	
Female	50.7	53.7	52.5	
Smoking habits (%)				0.125
Non smoker	42.9	48.6	46.3	
Ex-smoker	16.4	21.0	19.2	
Current smoker	40.7	30.4	34.5	
Age at onset of asthma (years), median	14.0	13.0	14.0	0.738
Age at onset of asthma (IQR)*	(5.0–25.0)	(6.0–22.0)	(6.0–24.0)	
Asthma attacks in the last 12 months (%)	90.0	79.0	83.3	0.006
Current asthma drug use (%)	66.4	69.2	68.1	0.590
Asthma-like symptoms (wheezing, tightness, shortness of breath) in the last 12 months (%)	84.9	87.8	86.7	0.434
Chronic cough and phlegm (%)	33.1	33.3	33.2	0.963
Allergic rhinitis (%)	65.5	76.2	71.9	0.029
Lost work days in the last 12 months (%)	18.3	14.8	16.2	0.408
Impaired days in the last 12 months (%)	22.2	19.4	20.5	0.531
Hospital or emergency department admissions because of asthma, shortness of breath, or wheezing in the last 12 months (%)	10.4	5.6	7.4	0.099

*IQR, Interquartile Range: (1st quartile–3rd quartile).
P-values refer to the comparison between non participants and participants.

Table 2. Main baseline characteristics of the men with non remittent asthma and with remittent asthma at follow-up and adjusted Odds Ratios* (CI95%) for the effects of these variables reported at baseline on asthma remission at follow-up.

	Non remittent asthma n = 68	Remittent asthma n = 28	Unadjusted p-value	Adjusted OR* (CI95%)
Age at baseline (years), mean(sd)	33.4 (7.8)	33.2 (6.9)	0.893	0.95 (0.88,1.02)
Smoking habits (%)£			0.772	
Non smoker	42.6	46.4		1.00
Ex-smoker	20.6	14.3		1.18 (0.15;9.25)
Current smoker	36.8	39.3		0.85 (0.22;3.25)
Age at onset of asthma (years), median	10	10	0.842	1.02 (0.96;1.08)
Age at onset of asthma (years), (IQR)§	(6–16)	(5–20)		
ICS use in the last 3 mo. at baseline (%)	43.9	11.1	**0.002**	0.36 (0.08;1.58)
Asthma control at baseline (%)‡			**<0.001**	
Total control	23.5	75.0		1.00
Partial control	53.0	21.4		**0.16 (0.07;0.62)**
No control	23.5	3.6		**0.06 (0.01;0.33)**
Allergic rhinitis (%)	82.4	71.4	0.231	0.56 (0.11;2.91)

*Also adjusted for the type of interview (telephone vs face to face).
£ Overall adjusted p-value for smoking = 0.5896.
§IQR, Interquartile Range: (1st quartile–3rd quartile).
‡Overall adjusted p-value for asthma control at baseline <0.0001.
Significant unadjusted p-value and adjusted OR ($p<0.05$) are reported in bold.

controlled (20%) compared to subjects with controlled (16%) asthma at baseline. The percentage of subjects with controlled asthma at follow-up was higher for subjects with controlled (45%) as compared to subjects with partially controlled (30%) or uncontrolled (11%) asthma at baseline. It is noteworthy to mention that for more than 50% of the subjects who had controlled asthma at baseline, asthma was no longer under control at follow-up.

Table 3. Main baseline characteristics of the women with non remittent asthma and with remittent asthma at follow-up and adjusted Odds Ratios* (CI95%) for the effects of these variables reported at baseline on asthma remission at follow-up.

	Non remittent asthma n = 81	Remittent asthma n = 33	Unadjusted p-value	Adjusted OR* (CI95%)
Age at baseline (years), mean(sd)	34.6 (6.9)	35.9 (8.5)	0.431	1.00 (0.94;1.06)
Smoking habits (%)£			0.452	
Non smoker	54.3	48.5		1.0
Ex-smoker	23.5	18.2		0.39 (0.03;5.66)
Current smoker	22.2	33.3		3.82 (0.56;26.27)
Age at onset of asthma (years), median	14	19.5	**0.027**	**1.07 (1.00;1.14)**
Age at onset of asthma (years), (IQR)§	(5–25)	(12–31.5)		
ICS use in the last 3 mo. at baseline (%)	39.2	21.98	0.081	0.53 (0.27;1.06)
Asthma control at baseline (%)‡			0.425	
Total control	31.6	37.5		1.00
Partial control	30.4	37.5		0.71 (0.20;2.47)
No control	38.0	25.0		**0.40 (0.17;0.94)**
Allergic rhinitis (%)	72.8	72.7	0.990	1.49 (0.78;2.85)

*Also adjusted for the type of interview (telephone vs face to face).
£ Overall adjusted p-value for smoking <0.0001.
§IQR, Interquartile Range: (1st quartile–3rd quartile).
‡Overall adjusted p-value for asthma control at baseline = 0.0791.
Significant unadjusted p-value and adjusted OR ($p<0.05$) are reported in bold.

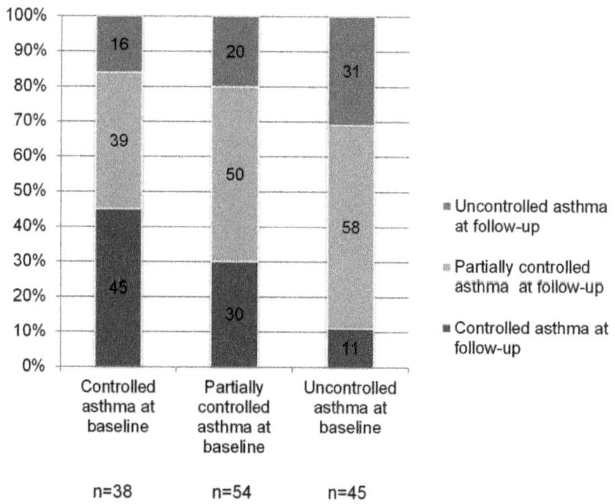

Figure 1. Distribution of GINA-based asthma control at follow-up according to GINA-based asthma control measured at baseline. The percentage of subjects in each category of GINA-based asthma control at follow up is reported inside histograms. The numbers of subjects with controlled, partially controlled and uncontrolled asthma at baseline are different from those reported in the result section due to missing data on control at follow-up.

After adjusting for non-response and for the effect of covariates, the estimates of the proportion of subjects who were under control, partial control or who were not under control were 26.3% (95%CI: 21.2%;31.3%), 51.6% (95%CI: 44.6%;58.7%) and 22.1% (95%CI: 16.6%;27.6%), respectively.

Determinants of asthma control at follow up

At follow-up, women were more likely to have partially controlled (OR = 4.87; 95%CI:2.66,8.93) or uncontrolled asthma (OR = 4.28; 95%CI:1.94,9.42) than controlled asthma with respect to men. Increasing age, the presence of chronic cough and phlegm and partial or absent asthma control at baseline increased the risk of uncontrolled asthma at follow-up (Table 4).

Asthma control and asthma management at follow-up

At follow-up, the percentage of subjects who were not on controller therapy, i.e. who were using at most short-acting β_2-agonists when needed, was 68%, 58% and 42% in subjects with controlled, partially controlled and uncontrolled asthma, respectively (Figure 2).

Discussion

Asthma remission and its determinants

It has been reported that remission prevalence in follow-up studies in adults with asthma range from 5 to 40%, depending on the period of follow-up and the definition of remission [10]. There are only few population-based longitudinal studies on asthma remission in adults [5–7,11,12]. In the present prospective longitudinal study, we estimated that nearly 1/3 (29.7%) of the subjects with current asthma sampled from the Italian adult population aged 20–44 years recover from their asthma after about 10 years. In a postal survey with a similar follow-up period and remission definition, Ekerljung and colleagues found that the 10-year remission was 14.6% in subjects with asthma aged 20–69 years [7]. The difference with respect to our study, could be due to the different age range of the studied population, as there is evidence that the remission rate decreases with increasing age [23].

In contrast to other chronic inflammatory diseases, such as rheumatoid arthritis, there is no clear consensus on what constitutes remission of asthma [10]. In most publications, asthma remission is defined as the absence of asthma symptoms without current pharmacological therapy for a prolonged period of time [6,24–26], although normal lung function and no airway hyperresponsiveness are sometimes included in the definition of asthma remission [27]. If the absence of symptoms is central to the definition of remission, it is very important to establish how long the symptoms should be absent. In the present study, we have defined asthma remission as the absence of asthma symptoms and of the use of asthma medicines in the last 12 months. It could be argued that this period is too short to unambiguously identify the occurrence of asthma remission. However, other investigators used the same time frame [7,11,12,25], and a longer period could raise the problem of recall bias. One year without symptoms has been accepted as the minimum, given the frequent seasonal variability of asthma, but the different observation period chosen in other studies can be responsible, at least in part, for the different results [6]. On the other hand, we cannot exclude that the short time interval we took into consideration to assess asthma remission could have led to an overestimation of the proportion of subjects with asthma in remission at follow-up.

To our knowledge, no studies have assessed the relationship between asthma control, as defined by the GINA guidelines and measured at baseline, and asthma remission at follow-up. Previous studies have noted that markers of asthma control like the presence and the frequency of most respiratory symptoms were correlated with the persistence of asthma, suggesting that subjects with a mild form of the disease are more likely to experience asthma remission [6,11,12,23]. In this study, the lack of asthma control as defined by the GINA guidelines at baseline was associated with the persistence of asthma but we found that gender modified this relationship: men who were not under control at baseline had a very low probability of being in remission at follow-up when compared to women.

Previous studies found early onset asthma to be more likely to remit than later onset asthma [28,29]. In our study, we found a differential effect of gender on the association between age at onset and asthma. As the age at onset of the disease increased, the likelihood of women being in remission at follow-up increased.

It is well known that the relationship between smoking habits and asthma remission is not clear. Some evidence has been found that quitting smoking favours the remission of asthma [6,12]. On the contrary, also a direct association between smoking and remission has been documented and has been associated to the 'healthy smoker' effect, meaning that those subjects with more susceptible airways do not take up smoking or quit early [26,28]. In our study, we found a differential effect of gender on the association between smoking habits and asthma. In particular, smoking was not associated with asthma remission in men, whereas in the case of women the 'healthy smoker' effect was manifest.

Asthma remission and asthma control

Recently, it has been argued that asthma remission rather than control should be regarded as the true goal of treatment [10]. A few studies have considered the natural history and the remission of asthma over very long periods, even as long as 2 or 3 decades or more [23,24,26,28], but the majority of the studies on asthma control were cross-sectional studies [16,30–32] or clinical studies

Table 4. Adjusted RRRs* (CI95%) for the effects of several variables reported at baseline or at follow-up on asthma control (partial control or no control) at follow-up, in subjects with non remittent asthma (n = 127).

		Partial control		No control	
		RRR	CI95%	RRR	CI95%
Age (years)		1.00	0.93;1.08	**1.04**	**1.02;1.05**
Gender	Male	1.00		1.00	
	Female	**4.87**	**2.66;8.93**	**4.28**	**1.94;9.42**
Smoking habits at baseline	No smoker	1.00		1.00	
	Ex-smoker	0.85	0.14;5.02	1.31	0.32;5.31
	Current smoker	2.40	0.72;7.95	1.64	0.75;3.58
Age at onset of asthma (years) at baseline		1.05	0.99;1.11	1.01	0.94;1.09
Asthma control at baseline	Total control	1.00		1.00	
	Partial control	1.79	0.81;3.96	**2.66**	**1.00;7.05**
	No control	3.83	1.01;14.51	**7.67**	**3.47;16.95**
Allergic rhinitis	No	1.00		1.00	
	Yes	0.57	0.11;3.07	2.85	0.17;46.61
Chronic cough and phlegm	No	1.00		1.00	
	Yes	1.35	0.73;2.47	**2.96**	**1.63;5.37**
ICS use in the last 3 months at baseline	No	1.00		1.00	
	Yes	4.30	0.79;23.52	2.31	0.35;15.54
ICS use in the last 3 months at follow-up	No	1.00		1.00	
	Yes	0.57	0.30;1.06	0.46	0.10;2.08

The reference category is control.
*RRRs were obtained through a multinomial logistic regression model with the controlled group as the reference category. RRRs were also adjusted for the type of interview (telephone vs face to face).
RRRs significantly different from 1 are reported in bold ($p<0.05$).

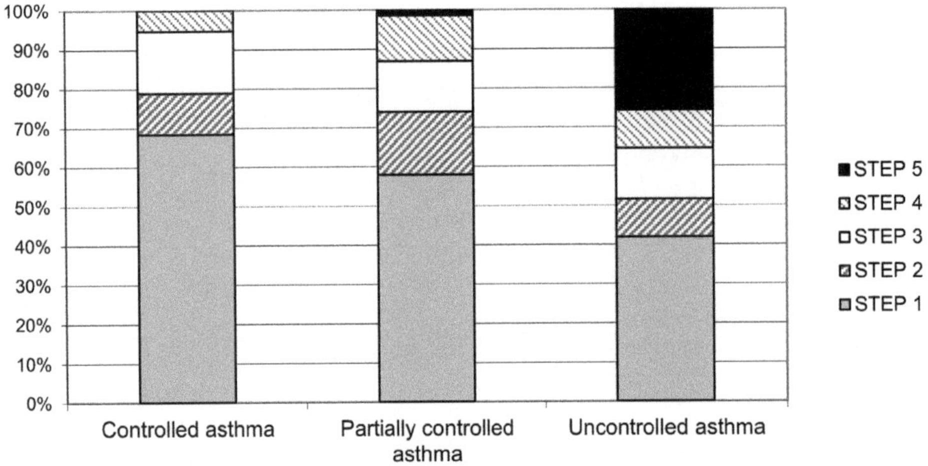

Figure 2. Distribution of treatment step* according to GINA classification in subjects with controlled asthma, partially controlled asthma and uncontrolled asthma, at follow-up. * STEP 1: As needed short-acting β_2-agonist; STEP 2: Sustained release theophylline OR Leukotriene modifier OR Low-dose Inhaled Corticosteroids (ICS); STEP 3: Low-dose ICS plus long-acting β_2-agonist OR Low-dose ICS plus leukotriene modifier OR Low-dose ICS plus sustained release theophylline OR Medium or high dose ICS; STEP 4: Medium or high dose ICS plus long-acting β_2-agonist OR Medium or high dose ICS plus leukotriene modifier OR Medium or high dose ICS plus sustained release theophylline; STEP 5: Oral corticosteroids or Anti-IgE treatment.

[8] conducted over short time intervals, so the information available on the long-term control of asthma is scarce.

In agreement with previous studies, we found that the subjects with controlled asthma at baseline were more likely to have controlled asthma at follow-up. Combescure et al. have found that patients with severe asthma had difficulty in leaving unacceptable control [33]. Our data, according to the study of Koster et al [34], consider a much longer time interval with respect to this study, and indicate a certain instability in asthma control.

Determinants of asthma control

It has already been reported in cross-sectional and/or clinical studies that women have less controlled [13,35] and more severe [36] asthma, greater bronchial responsiveness [37], use more healthcare services [38] and have a poorer health-related quality of life [39] than men with asthma. Our study supplements this evidence by showing that, after adjusting for asthma control at baseline, female gender is an independent predictor of worse asthma control 9 years later.

Current smoking has been found to be associated with uncontrolled asthma [40], but we did not find a significant association between smoking habits at baseline and asthma control nine years later. We found that smoking habits were associated with asthma control at baseline, suggesting a higher level of asthma control in non-smokers compared to ex- and current smokers (data not shown). This is likely to be the reason why, after controlling for asthma control at baseline, smoking is no longer associated with asthma control at follow-up.

In our study, subjects with chronic cough and phlegm at baseline were more likely to have uncontrolled asthma nine years later than subjects without chronic cough and phlegm at baseline, regardless of smoking. A positive association between chronic cough and phlegm and uncontrolled asthma has been previously reported in cross-sectional studies [16,35].

Rhinitis has been shown to be associated with the lack of asthma control [41]. We did not find a significant association between rhinitis at baseline and asthma control 9 years later, probably due to our incomplete diagnosis of allergic rhinitis.

Asthma treatment and control

We found that a considerable part of the subjects with partially controlled or uncontrolled asthma at follow-up (58% and 42%, respectively) was not following a therapy aimed at keeping asthma under control: such large proportions of subjects with partially controlled or uncontrolled asthma who were not using anti-inflammatory drugs raise some concern. This evidence is supported from the results of an Italian study, where the authors found that Italian general practitioners did not use ICS to treat a large number of patients with persistent asthma [42]. Nevertheless, even a poor adherence to the GINA guidelines in asthma patients must be taken into account [43].

Limitations of the study

Some caveats should be considered in the interpretation of our results because of the impossibility to assess the level of the control of asthma through objective measures, as the baseline and follow-up surveys were based on telephone interviews [14]. Control refers to the control of the manifestations of asthma at a multidimensional level [44]. However, it is noteworthy to consider that the assessment of lung function could only have led to a worsening of asthma control. In fact, if a subject had had a normal lung function, his/her level of asthma control would have been dependent on the other markers of control used in the definition and so it would have remained unchanged. Otherwise, if a subject had had reduced lung function, his/her level of control could have remained unchanged or could have been worse. Lung function assessment is also important in the definition of remission. A more stringent definition of asthma remission could require not only a prolonged absence of symptoms, but also an objective demonstration of normal airway function and responsiveness [27]. Another limitation of the study is related to the definition of allergic rhinitis, as allergological tests were not available.

Strengths of the study

To our knowledge, this is one of the few cohort studies evaluating asthma control according to the GINA classification over a nine-year period in a relatively large, random sample of subjects with current asthma in Italy. Furthermore, we had the opportunity to simultaneously evaluate changes in asthma control and asthma remission. Unlike the studies carried out on hospital patients or outpatients, this study was based on subjects with asthma sampled from the general population. Therefore, even subjects with mild forms of the disease could have been included in the survey.

Conclusion

In conclusion, in the present study we found that nearly 1/3 (29.7%) of the subjects with current asthma sampled from the Italian adult population aged 20–44 years had recovered from their asthma after about 10 years, whereas only 26.3% of the subjects with active asthma showed controlled asthma. Asthma control at baseline seems to be an important predictor of asthma remission and asthma control at follow up.

Clinical asthma control is highly relevant at individual and societal levels, and measures of control (which to some extent reflect severity) are related to remission probability.

Author Contributions

Conceived and designed the experiments: LC AGC IC. Analyzed the data: LC. Wrote the paper: LC AGC IC. Each of the following author contributed to the interpretation of data and revised the paper critically for important intellectual content: LC AGC FA EMGDV EG AG VR MB PP IC.

References

1. Bahadori K, Doyle-Waters MM, Marra C, Lynd L, Alasaly K, et al. (2009) Economic burden of asthma: a systematic review. BMC Pulm Med 19: 9–24.
2. de Marco R, Cappa V, Accordini S, Rava M, Antonicelli L, et al. (2012) Trends in the prevalence of asthma and allergic rhinitis in Italy between 1991 and 2010. Eur Respir J 39: 883–92.
3. Gershon A, Guan J, Victor JC, Wang C, To T (2012) The course of asthma activity: a population study. J Allergy Clin Immunol 129: 679–86.
4. Braman SS (2010) Growing old with asthma: what are the changes and challenges? Expert Rev Respir Med 4: 239–48.
5. de Marco R, Poli A, Ferrari M, Accordini S, Giammanco G, et al. (2002) The impact of climate and traffic-related NO2 on the prevalence of asthma and allergic rhinitis in Italy. Clin Exp Allergy 32: 1405–12.
6. Holm M, Omenaas E, Gíslason T, Svanes C, Jõgi R, et al. (2007) Remission of asthma: a prospective longitudinal study from northern Europe (RHINE study). Eur Respir J 30: 62–5.
7. Ekerljung L, Rönmark E, Larsson K, Sundblad BM, Bjerg A, et al. (2008) No further increase of incidence of asthma: incidence, remission and relapse of adult asthma in Sweden. Respir Med 102: 1730–6.
8. Bateman ED, Bousquet J, Busse WW, Clark TJ, Gul N, et al. (2008) Stability of asthma control with regular treatment: an analysis of the Gaining Optimal Asthma controL (GOAL) study. Allergy 63: 932–8.
9. Taylor DR, Bateman ED, Boulet LP, Boushey HA, Busse WW, et al. (2008) A new perspective on concepts of asthma severity and control. Eur Respir J 32: 545–54.

10. Upham JW, James AL. Remission of asthma: The next therapeutic frontier? (2011) Pharmacol Ther 130: 38–45.
11. Bronnimann S, Burrows B (1986) A prospective study of the natural history of asthma. Remission and relapse rates. Chest 90: 480–4.
12. Rönmark E, Jönsson E, Lundbäck B (1999) Remission of asthma in the middle aged and elderly: report from the Obstructive Lung Disease in Northern Sweden study. Thorax 54: 611–13.
13. de Marco R, Bugiani M, Cazzoletti L, Carosso A, Accordini S, et al. (2003) The control of asthma in Italy. A multicentre descriptive study on young adults with doctor diagnosed current asthma. Allergy 58: 221–8.
14. de Marco R, Cazzoletti L, Cerveri I, Corsico A, Bugiani M, et al. (2005) Are the asthma guideline goals achieved in daily practice? A population-based study on treatment adequacy and the control of asthma. Int Arch Allergy Immunol 138: 225–34.
15. Global Initiative for Asthma (2006) Global strategy for asthma management and prevention. NHLBI/WHO workshop report. Bethesda (MD): National Institutes of Health. National Heart Lung and Blood Institute publication no. 02-3659.
16. Cazzoletti L, Marcon A, Janson C, Corsico A, Jarvis D, et al. (2007) Asthma control in Europe: a real-world evaluation based on an international population-based study. J Allergy Clin Immunol 120: 1360–7.
17. Global Initiative for Asthma. Global strategy for asthma management and prevention 2011 update. Available at: http://www.ginasthma.org/uploads/users/files/GINA_Report_2011.pdf. Accessed January 15, 2012.
18. Little RJA, Rubin DB (2002) Statistical Analysis with missing data. (2nd edn). New York: John Wiley & Sons, Inc.
19. Höfler M, Pfister H, Lieb R, Wittchen HU (2005) The use of weights to account for non-response and drop-out. Soc Psychiatry Psychiatr Epidemiol 40: 291–9.
20. Potter FJ (1990) A study of procedures to identify and trim extreme sampling weights. Proceedings of the Survey Research Methods Section of the American Statistical Association, 225–230.
21. Elliott MR, Little RJA (2000) Model-based alternatives to trimming survey weights. J Off Stat 16: 191–209.
22. Williams RL (2000) A note on robust variance estimation for cluster-correlated data. Biometrics 56: 645–646.
23. Panhuysen CI, Vonk JM, Koëter GH, Schouten JP, van Altena R, et al. (1997) Adult patients may outgrow their asthma: a 25-year follow-up study. Am J Respir Crit Care Med 155: 1267–72.
24. Horak E, Lanigan A, Roberts M, Welsh L, Wilson J, et al. (2003) Longitudinal study of childhood wheezy bronchitis and asthma: outcome at age 42. BMJ 326: 422–3.
25. Sears MR, Greene JM, Willan AR, Wiecek EM, Taylor DR, et al. (2003) A longitudinal, population-based, cohort study of childhood asthma followed to adulthood. N Engl J Med 349: 1414–22.
26. Vonk JM, Postma DS, Boezen HM, Grol MH, Schouten JP, et al. (2004) Childhood factors associated with asthma remission after 30 year follow up. Thorax 59: 925–9.
27. Broekema M, Volbeda F, Timens W, Dijkstra A, Lee NA, et al. (2010) Airway eosinophilia in remission and progression of asthma: accumulation with a fast decline of FEV(1). Respir Med 104: 1254–62.
28. Burgess JA, Matheson MC, Gurrin LC, Byrnes GB, Adams KS, et al. (2011) Factors influencing asthma remission: a longitudinal study from childhood to middle age. Thorax 66: 508–13.
29. de Marco R, Locatelli F, Cerveri I, Bugiani M, Marinoni A, et al. (2002) Incidence and remission of asthma: a retrospective study on the natural history of asthma in Italy. J Allergy Clin Immunol 110: 228–35.
30. Rabe KF, Adachi M, Lai CK, Soriano JB, Vermeire PA, et al. (2004) Worldwide severity and control of asthma in children and adults: the global asthma insights and reality surveys. J Allergy Clin Immunol 114: 40–7.
31. Peters SP, Jones CA, Haselkorn T, Mink DR, Valacer DJ, et al. (2007) Real-world Evaluation of Asthma Control and Treatment (REACT): findings from a national Web-based survey. J Allergy Clin Immunol 119: 1454–61.
32. Demoly P, Annunziata K, Gubba E, Adamek L (2012) Repeated cross-sectional survey of patient-reported asthma control in Europe in the past 5 years. Eur Respir Rev 21: 66–74.
33. Combescure C, Chanez P, Saint-Pierre P, Daurès JP, Proudhon H, et al. (2003) Assessment of variations in control of asthma over time. Eur Respir J 22: 298–304.
34. Koster ES, Raaijmakers JA, Vijverberg SJ, Koenderman L, Postma DS, et al. (2011) Limited agreement between current and long-term asthma control in children: the PACMAN cohort study. Pediatr Allergy Immunol 22: 776–83.
35. Siroux V, Boudier A, Bousquet J, Bresson JL, Cracowski JL, et al. (2009) Phenotypic determinants of uncontrolled asthma. Allergy Clin Immunol 124: 681–7.
36. Bottema RW, Reijmerink NE, Koppelman GH, Kerkhof M, Postma DS (2005) Phenotype definition, age, andgender in the genetics of asthma and atopy. Immunol Allergy Clin North Am 25: 621–639.
37. Leynaert B, Bousquet J, Henry C, Liard R, Neukirch F (1997) Is bronchial hyperresponsiveness more frequent in women than in men? A population-based study. Am J Respir Crit Care Med 156: 1413–1420.
38. Lee JH, Haselkorn T, Chipps BE, Miller DP, Wenzel SE (2006) Gender differences in IgE-mediated allergic asthma in the epidemiology and natural history of asthma: Outcomes and Treatment Regimens (TENOR) study. J Asthma 43: 179–184.
39. Braido F, Baiardini I, Balestracci S, Ghiglione V, Stagi E, et al. (2009) Does asthma control correlate with quality of life related to upper and lower airway real life study. Allergy 64: 937–943.
40. Chauhuri R, McSharry C, McCoard A, Livingston E, Hothersall E, et al. (2008) Role of symptoms and lung function in determining asthma control in smokers with asthma. Allergy 63: 132–135.
41. Ponte EV, Franco R, Nascimento HF, Souza-Machado A, Cunha S, et al. (2008) Lack of control of severe asthma is associated with co-existence of moderate-to-severe rhinitis. Allergy 63: 564–9.
42. Baldacci S, Maio S, Simoni M, Cerrai S, Sarno G, et al. (2012) The ARGA study with general practitioners: impact of medical education on asthma/rhinitis management. Respir Med 106: 777–85.
43. Corsico AG, Cazzoletti L, de Marco R, Janson C, Jarvis D, et al. (2007) Factors affecting adherence to asthma treatment in an international cohort of young and middle-aged adults. Respir Med 101: 1363–7.
44. Lundbäck B, Dahl R. (2007) Assessment of asthma control and its impact on optimal treatment strategy. Allergy 62: 611–9.

Natural History of Perceived Food Hypersensitivity and IgE Sensitisation to Food Allergens in a Cohort of Adults

Antonios Patelis[1]*, Maria Gunnbjörnsdottir[1], Magnus P. Borres[2,6], Peter Burney[7], Thorarinn Gislason[3], Kjell Torén[4], Bertil Forsberg[5], Kjell Alving[6], Andrei Malinovschi[8,9], Christer Janson[1,9]

1 Department of Medical Sciences: Respiratory Medicine and Allergology, Uppsala University, Uppsala, Sweden, 2 Immunodiagnostics, Thermo Fischer Scientific, Uppsala, Sweden, 3 University of Iceland, Medical Faculty and Department of Respiratory Medicine and Sleep, Landspitali University Hospital, Reykjavik, Iceland, 4 Section of Occupational and Environmental Medicine, Institute of Medicine, University of Gothenburg, Gothenburg, Sweden, 5 Division of Occupational and Environmental Medicine, Umeå University, Umeå, Sweden, 6 Department of Women's and Children's Health, Uppsala University, Uppsala, Sweden, 7 Respiratory Epidemiology and Public Health, Imperial College, London, United Kingdom, 8 Department of Medical Sciences: Clinical Physiology, Uppsala University, Uppsala, Sweden

Abstract

Background: No longitudinal studies exist on the natural history of food hypersensitivity and IgE sensitisation to food allergens in adults.

Objective: To examine the natural history of food hypersensitivity, the natural history of IgE sensitisation to food allergens and to investigate the risk factors for new onset food hypersensitivity.

Methods: Food hypersensitivity was questionnaire-assessed in 2307 individuals (aged 20–45 years) from Iceland and Sweden during the European Community Respiratory Health Survey both at baseline and follow-up 9 years later. IgE food and aeroallergen sensitisation were assessed in a subgroup of these individuals (n = 807). Values of 0.35 kU/L and above were regarded as positive sensitisation.

Results: Food hypersensitivity was reported by 21% of the subjects and this proportion remained unchanged at follow-up (p = 0.58). Fruits, nuts and vegetables were the three most common causes of food hypersensitivity, with a similar prevalence at baseline and follow-up. The prevalence IgE sensitisation to food allergens decreased in general by 56% (p<0.001) and IgE sensitisation to peanut decreased in particular by 67% (p = 0.003). The prevalence of timothy grass IgE sensitisation decreased by 15% (p = 0.003) while cat, mite and birch IgE sensitisation did not decrease significantly. Female sex, rhinitis, eczema and presence of IgE sensitisation to aeroallergens were independently associated with new onset food hypersensitivity.

Conclusion: The prevalence of food hypersensitivity remained unchanged while the prevalence of IgE sensitisation to food allergens decreased in adults over a 9-year follow-up period. The decrease in prevalence of IgE sensitisation to food allergens was considerably larger than the change in prevalence of IgE sensitisation to aeroallergens.

Editor: Giuseppe Remuzzi, Mario Negri Institute for Pharmacological Research and Azienda Ospedaliera Ospedali Riuniti di Bergamo, Italy

Funding: This study was supported financially by the Swedish Heart and Lung Foundation, the Vårdal Foundation for Health Care Science and Allergy Research, the Swedish Association against Asthma and Allergy, Agnes and Mac Rudberg's Foundation and the Bror Hjerpstedt Foundation. The funders had no role in study design, data collection and analysis, decision to publish, or preparation of the manuscript.

Competing Interests: Kjell Alving is an employee and minority shareholder of Aerocrine AB and has received funds for research from the same company. Magnus Borres is an employee of ThermoFisher Scientific (which manufactures kits to measure IgE antibodies against allergens).

* E-mail: antonios.patelis@medsci.uu.se

9 These authors contributed equally to this work.

Introduction

Several population surveys in the 1990s have estimated the prevalence of perceived food hypersensitivity, e.g. self-reported adverse reactions after food ingestion, regardless of the underlying mechanism [1], at 12% to 20% in adults [2–4]. The majority of adverse reactions to food are not IgE-mediated [5] and there is limited information on the prevalence and distribution of IgE food sensitisation. About 15% to 20% of the population has IgE to at least one food allergen over the detection limit [6,7] e.g. food IgE sensitisation. However, only a small fraction of subjects with IgE antibodies against food allergens have clinical IgE-mediated food allergy. As an example, Liu et al [7] reported that the prevalence of food IgE sensitisation was 15% whereas the prevalence of IgE-mediated food allergy was only 2%.

Aeroallergen IgE sensitisation, especially against perennial allergens, is linked to asthma and airway inflammation [8–11]. The natural history of prevalence of aeroallergen IgE sensitisation has been examined in longitudinal studies in adults [12–18], but the results are contradictory and show the prevalence decreasing

[15,18], remaining stable [12,19] or increasing [13,14,16,17] over time.

To the best of our knowledge, no study exists about the natural history of food hypersensitivity and IgE sensitisation to food allergens in adults. Another reason for studying IgE sensitisation to food allergens and IgE-mediated food allergy is that not only aeroallergen sensitisation, but also food IgE sensitisation, is linked to increased exhaled nitric oxide levels and increased risk for asthma [6,7,20].

The aim of this study was to examine the natural history food hypersensitivity symptoms and IgE sensitisation to food allergens and to investigate the risk factors for new onset food hypersensitivity and sensitisation.

Methods

Population

The study was based on the European Community Respiratory Health Survey (ECRHS) I (1991–92) and II (2000–01) [21] from four participating centres (Reykjavík, Uppsala, Gothenburg and Umeå). Each participant in ECRHS I was sent a brief questionnaire (Stage 1) and among those who responded, both a random and a "symptomatic" sample (consisting of subjects with symptoms of asthma or asthma medication), were invited to undergo a more detailed clinical examination (Stage 2). Subjects from Stage 2 of ECRHS I were invited to participate in the follow-up study, ECRHS II, and answered a standardized questionnaire and underwent a clinical visit [21]. A total of 2,307 individuals answered questions about food hypersensitivity symptoms both at ECRHS I and II. No difference in age, sex, BMI, prevalence of asthma, rhinitis, total IgE, food IgE sensitisation, aeroallergen IgE sensitisation and smoking history were found between subjects with and without follow-up data about food hypersensitivity symptoms (all $p>0.05$). A subgroup of ECRHS participants in Iceland (Reykjavík) and Sweden (Uppsala, Gothenburg and Umeå) from the random sample ($n = 807$) was examined against IgE to food allergens at ECRHS I [22] [23] and ECRHS II (Figure 1).

Questionnaires

The main questionnaire used in ECRHS I and II http://www.ecrhs.org [24] gathered information about respiratory symptoms, exposure to investigated allergens, and smoking history.

Diagnosis of asthma

A person was defined as asthmatic if he/she had ever been diagnosed with asthma and had an asthma attack or one of the following symptoms: nocturnal chest tightness, attack of shortness of breath, chest wheezing or whistling during the last 12 months [25].

Definition of food hypersensitivity

An individual was considered having food hypersensitivity [1] if he/she answered yes to the following questions "Have you ever had an illness or trouble caused by eating a particular food or foods?" and if so, "Have you nearly always had the same illness or trouble after eating this type of food?" Respondents were then asked to list the food(s) and symptoms [2].

Measurements of IgE to aeroallergens and food allergens and total IgE

Venous blood samples were drawn from all participants in the clinical visits and frozen at $-20°C$ for measurement of total serum IgE (total IgE) and serum IgE antibodies to cat, *D. pteronyssinus*, timothy grass, birch, and *Cladosporium*, as part of the ECRHS I and II protocol [21]. Measurement of IgE antibodies against birch was performed in all centres in the ECRHS I and in the Uppsala centre in ECRHS II. In addition, IgE antibodies to a mix of food allergens (containing egg white, milk, cod fish, wheat, peanut, and soybean) were measured in the subgroup of ECRHS participants in Iceland (Reykjavík) and Sweden (Uppsala, Gothenburg and Umeå) from the random sample by same technique and reagents at ECRHS I and II (Pharmacia CAP System, MultiCap fx5, Thermo Fisher Scientific, Uppsala, Sweden). Serum with a positive reaction to the food panel (fx5) was further analysed for the single allergens in the panel. The results are presented in kU/L, and values of 0.35 kU/L and above were regarded as positive sensitisation [26]. A titre below the detection level (<0.35 kU/L) was arbitrarily given the value 0.17 kU/L). All samples from ECRHS I from Reykjavík, Uppsala, Gothenburg and Umeå were analysed in Uppsala, as previously described [22] while samples from the random sample of ECRHS II (depending on availability of residual samples) were analysed within the frame of Euro-PREVALL in Manchester, as described elsewhere [27].

Statistics

Statistical analyses were performed using STATA 12.1 software (Stata Corp., 2011, Texas, USA). IgE titres (both total and specific) were log transformed before analysis. Mc Nemar's test was used to compare prevalence of food hypersensitivity, various food related symptoms and IgE sensitisation in ECRHS I and II. Chi-squared test (for categorical variables) and unpaired t-test (for numerical variables) were used to compare individuals with new onset and no food hypersensitivity and prevalence of IgE sensitisation to food, cat/mite and timothy grass allergens. Chi-squared test was also used to compare prevalence of IgE sensitisation to food in subjects according to age (< or > median age). Paired t-test was used to compare levels of IgE to specific allergens between ECRHS I and II in subjects sensitised to each respective allergen at either ECRHS I or II and unpaired t-test was used to compare levels of IgE against food allergens at ECRHS I in subjects with persistence and remission of IgE sensitisation to food allergens. Multiple logistic regression models were used when examining predictors for new onset food hypersensitivity, and persistent food sensitisation. These models always included age, gender, body mass index, rhinitis, current asthma, total IgE, IgE against food allergens, sample and IgE against aeroallergens. A p–value of <0.05 was considered statistically significant.

Ethics

All subjects consented to the utilization of personal data for the purpose of this study. The study was approved by the Ethics Committee at the Medical Faculty at Uppsala University and University of Iceland.

Results

The study population comprised of 2,307 individuals who answered questions about food hypersensitivity symptoms in both ECRHS I and II. Of these, 53% were women. The group characteristics of the participants are presented in Table 1.

Natural history of food hypersensitivity symptoms

Around 21% of the interviewed subjects reported food hypersensitivity symptoms in both ECRHS I and II (Table 2). The most common foods related to these symptoms were fruits followed by nuts and then vegetables. The prevalence of food

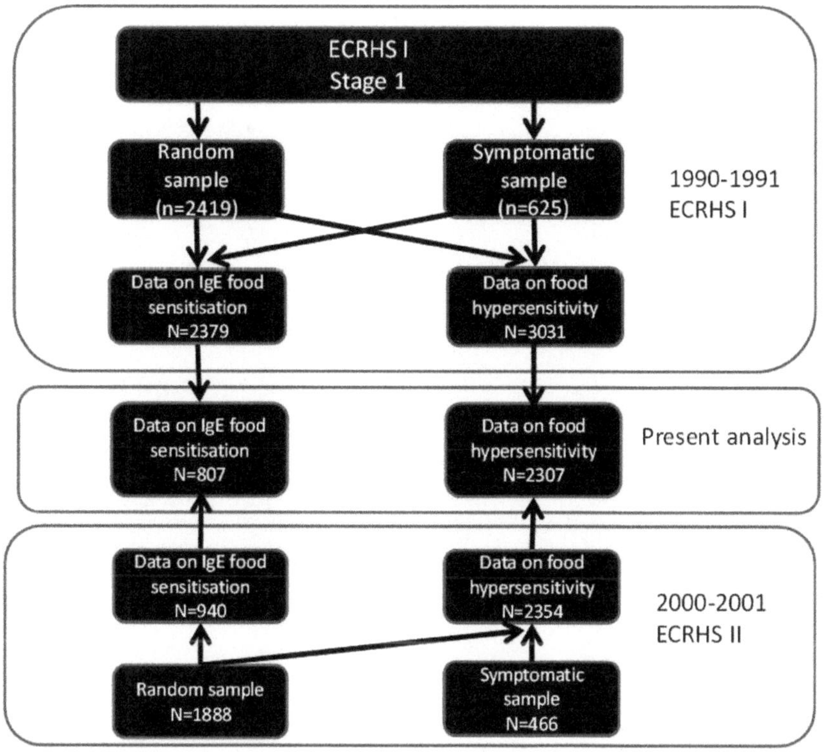

Figure 1. Flow chart explaining the selection of the studied population.

hypersensitivity in relation to ingestion of fish (including seafood and shellfish) increased significantly from ECRHS I to II and become, together with vegetables, the fourth most common cause of food hypersensitivity. Food hypersensitivity symptoms due to dairy products, wheat products (gluten, cereal and wheat) and spices (herbs, chili, and garlic) also increased significantly from ECRHS I to II (Table 2).

Skin reactions were the most common reported symptoms both at baseline and follow-up (Table 3). No significant change in the prevalence of the different symptoms was found during the 9-year period between ECRHS I and II.

Table 1. Characteristics of the participants (n = 2,307; mean ± SD and n (%)).

	ECRHS I 1991–92	ECRHS II 2000–01	p value
Age	33.6 ±7.3	42.4 ±7.2	<0.001
BMI	23.8 ±3.6	25.7 ±4.2	<0.001
Current asthma	314 (13.4)	428 (18.3)	<0.001
Rhinitis	783 (33.3)	904 (38.5)	<0.001
Smoking history			<0.001
Never	1093 (46.6)	1044 (45.9)	
Ex	54 (23.1)	730 (32.2)	
Current	711 (30.3)	497 (21.9)	

Natural history of prevalence of IgE sensitisation to food and aeroallergens

Prevalence of IgE sensitisation to at least one food allergen decreased by 56% during the study (Figure 2A). Prevalence of peanut IgE-sensitisation was the highest among food allergens and decreased by 67%. The prevalence of soy IgE sensitisation decreased significantly between ECRHS I and II, whereas similar prevalence of IgE sensitisation to wheat, milk, egg and fish was found at both time points (Figure 2B). No significant change of prevalence of cat, birch and mite IgE sensitisation was found, whereas prevalence of timothy grass IgE sensitisation decreased by 15% (from 17% to 15%) (Figure 2A).

The prevalence of IgE sensitisation to food allergens decreased from ECRHS I to ECRHS II by 63% (from 6% to 2%) ($p<0.001$) in subjects younger than 31 years and by 44% (from 4% to 2%) ($p<0.001$) in subjects older than 31 years (median age of cohort in ECRHS I).

Changes over time of levels of IgE against food- and aeroallergens and total IgE

Significant decreases of IgE antibodies against peanut ($p<0.001$, Figure 3a) and soy ($p<0.001$ Figure 3b), but not against wheat ($p=0.12$, Figure 3c), milk ($p=0.9$), egg ($p=0.4$) were found between ECRHS I and II among individuals who were IgE-sensitised to the respective allergen either at baseline or follow-up.

Similarly, among the aeroallergens, the levels of IgE antibodies against timothy grass decreased ($p<0.001$) whereas levels of IgE against cat ($p=0.18$), birch ($p=0.43$) and mite ($p=0.12$) remained stable between ECRHS I and II among individuals who were IgE-sensitised to the respective allergen either at baseline or follow-up.

Table 2. Prevalence (n (%)) of type of food reported as cause of food hypersensitivity (n = 2,307).

	ECRHS I 1991–92	ECRHS II 2000–01	p value
Any food	496 (21.5)	508 (22.0)	0.58
Fruits	195 (8.5)	215 (9.3)	0.19
Nuts	126 (5.5)	135 (5.9)	0.47
Vegetables	78 (3.4)	97 (4.2)	0.11
Fish, seafood, shellfish	56 (2.4)	97 (4.2)	<0.001
Chocolate	27 (1.2)	23 (1.0)	0.65
Egg	24 (1.0)	19 (0.8)	0.34
Milk and dairy products	22 (1.0)	57 (2.5)	<0.001
Meat	11 (0.4)	19 (0.8)	0.14
Herbs, chilli, garlic	9 (0.3)	20 (0.9)	0.004
Gluten, cereal, wheat products	5 (0.3)	14 (0.6)	0.049

Total IgE increased between ECHRS I and II (17.7 (16.0, 19.7) vs. 25.7 (23.4, 28.2) kU/L (geometric mean) ($p<0.001$)).

Incidence of food hypersensitivity

The incidence of food hypersensitivity was 11.7% during this 9-year study. The incidence in the symptomatic sample was higher than the random sample (20.6% vs. 9.9%, $p<0.001$). Female sex, rhinitis, eczema, asthma and presence of IgE sensitisation to aeroallergens were associated with new onset food hypersensitivity (Table 4) and these associations were consistent in a multiple logistic regression model (Figure 4).

Incidence and persistence of IgE sensitisation to food allergens

New onset IgE food sensitisation (n = 8) was not associated with age, gender, BMI, current rhinitis, current asthma, current smoking and IgE sensitisation to aeroallergens (data not shown). Persistent IgE food sensitisation was associated with higher total IgE levels at baseline (Table 5) and this association remained significant also after adjusting for age, gender, BMI, current rhinitis, current asthma, current smoking and IgE sensitisation to aeroallergens (OR (95% CI) = 9.8 (1.6, 60.5) per unit of natural logarithm-transformed total IgE). No relation between persistence of IgE sensitisation to food allergens and specific IgE levels to food allergens or aeroallergens or prevalence of IgE sensitisation to aeroallergens at baseline was found (Table 5).

Discussion

The main findings in the present investigation are that one in five adults reported food hypersensitivity symptoms after food intake and this proportion remained unchanged during this 9-year longitudinal study. The prevalence of IgE-sensitisation to food allergens decreased during that 9-year period whereas the prevalence of sensitisation to aeroallergens remained relatively unchanged.

To our knowledge this is the first study that analysed longitudinal changes of perceived self-reported food hypersensitivity in adults. The prevalence of food hypersensitivity reported here is in line with reports from previous cross-sectional studies [2–4,28]. Our results showing an unchanged prevalence of food hypersensitivity over time are opposite to what is known about the natural history of food hypersensitivity in children, where major remission of symptoms has been reported [29–31].

Table 3. Prevalence (n (%)) of symptoms reported after food intake (n = 2,307).

	ECRHS I 1991–92	ECRHS II 2000–01	p value
Rash or itchy skin	101 (4.4)	112 (4.9)	0.39
Diarrhoea or vomiting	40 (1.7)	47 (2.0)	0.26
Runny or stuffy nose	42 (1.8)	48 (2.1)	0.42
Severe headache	18 (0.8)	25 (1.1)	0.21
Breathlessness	54 (2.3)	56 (2.4)	0.87
Other	131 (5.7)	149 (6.5)	0.047

The two most common reported symptoms of food hypersensitivity were skin reactions and gastrointestinal reactions. Reactions occurring at the skin or mucosa were also the most prevalent in a previous study [4]. Fruits, nuts and vegetables were the three

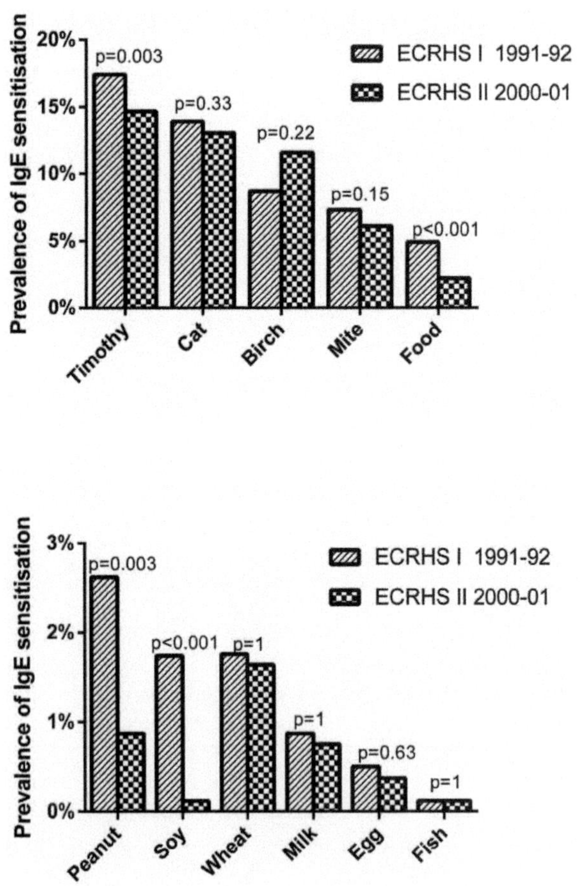

Figure 2. Prevalence (number of individuals of the study population who have IgE for respective allergen ≥0.35 KU/L) of sensitisation to food (n = 807) and aeroallergens (n = 804) (upper panel) and prevalence (number of individuals of the study population who have IgE for respective allergen ≥0.35 KU/L) of IgE sensitisation to individual food allergens (lower panel) in ECRHS I and II. Birch pollen was measured only in Uppsala (n = 138).

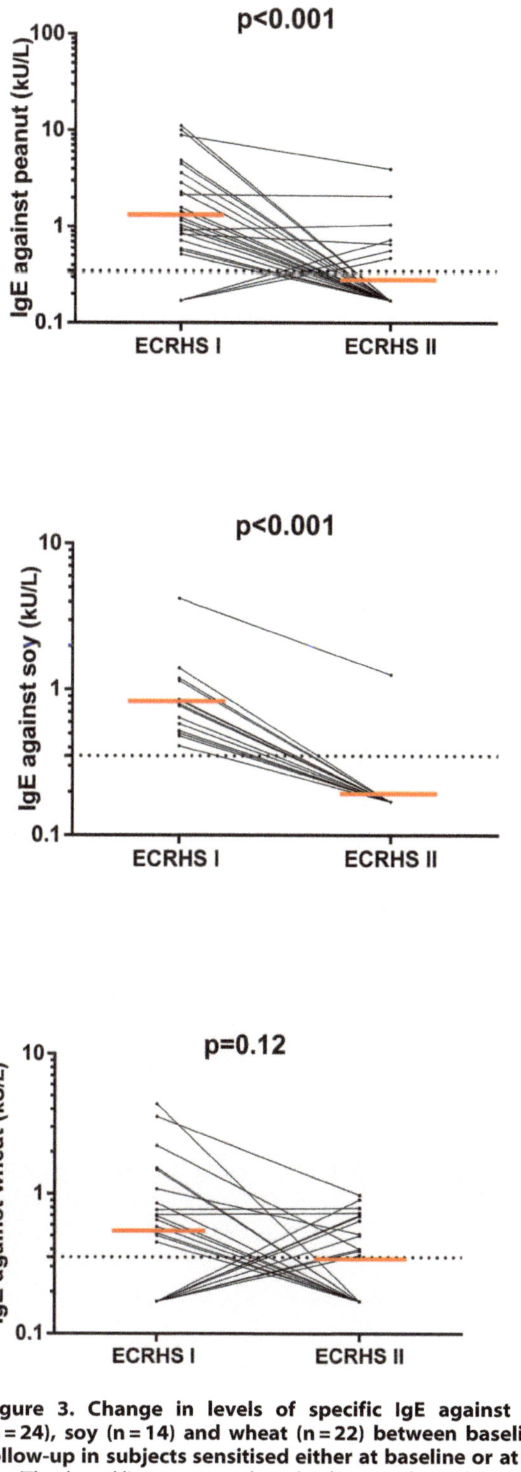

Figure 3. Change in levels of specific IgE against peanut (n = 24), soy (n = 14) and wheat (n = 22) between baseline and follow-up in subjects sensitised either at baseline or at follow-up. (The dotted line corresponds to the detection limit of 0.35 kU/L and the red lines correspond to the geometrical mean of levels of specific IgE against each respective allergen).

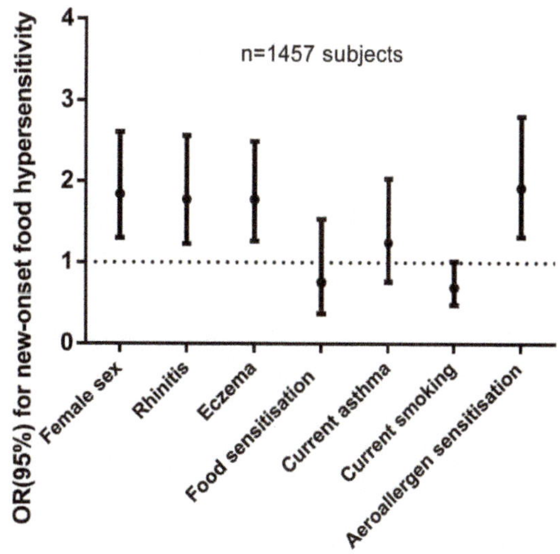

Figure 4. Risk factors (Odds Ratios (95%CI)) for new onset food hypersensitivity. Odds ratios are adjusted for the variables in the figure and age, body mass index, current smoking, sample and total IgE.

most common causes of food hypersensitivity in our population, with a similar prevalence at baseline and follow-up. A previous study [4] showed the same major causes of adverse reactions to foods.

The risk factors for new onset food hypersensitivity in the present study were female sex, rhinitis, eczema, asthma and presence of IgE sensitisation to aeroallergens. Thus, incidence of food hypersensitivity seems to be related to the atopic trait of an individual. We are not aware of any published longitudinal study to compare our results with. However, there are cross-sectional studies showing that food hypersensitivity in adults is often associated with concomitant sensitisation to aeroallergens [4], IgE sensitisation to food allergens [32] and other manifestations of atopy, especially rhinitis [4].

A novel finding of the study was the marked reduction of prevalence of IgE sensitisation to food allergens over time in adults. The natural history of prevalence of IgE sensitisation to food allergens has previously been studied only in children [33] where sensitisation rates to food allergens remained stable during the first 6 years of life (10%). The majority of children outgrow their allergies to milk, soy, egg, and wheat, and some to peanut also [34]. The decrease in the prevalence of IgE sensitisation to food allergens does not appear to be related to the initial age of the subjects, which tends to preclude the possibility that the effect is related to a specific birth cohort. Reductions of similar size could be observed in both younger and older subjects. This probably signals that the decreasing prevalence is somehow related to aging. Previous longitudinal studies [12,14,16,17] on the prevalence of IgE sensitisation to aeroallergens in relation to age report inconsistent results.

In the present study the prevalence of sensitisation to aeroallergens decreased to a much lesser extent than sensitisation to food allergens. However, the levels of IgE antibodies decreased during the 9-year follow-up period for both food and aeroallergens, whereas the levels of total IgE increased. Most of the longitudinal studies have analysed changes in the prevalence of IgE sensitisation without reporting changes in the degree of IgE sensitisation. A decrease of IgE titres to mite in a long-term follow-up of subjects with house-dust allergic asthma has been reported [35]. Karakaya and Kalyoncu [18] reported that the wheal diameter in response to skin prick test decreased under a two-year period for two of the studied allergens, timothy grass and mite. The reason why specific IgE decreased and total IgE increased in the present study is unclear. However our finding of increase total IgE is consistent with an increase of total IgE in all ECRHS centres [36] even if other longitudinal studies reported stable levels

Table 4. Population characteristics in different population strata, subdivided according to presence/absence of food hypersensitivity at ECRHS I and II.

	No food hypersensitivity (n = 1601)	New-onset food hypersensitivity (n = 211)	p value*
Age (years)	33.8±7.3	33.4±7.3	0.35
Female sex	48.8	61.6	<0.001
BMI (kg/m²)	23.7±3.3	23.5±3.4	0.43
Current smoker	31.6	26.5	0.133
Rhinitis	23.0	43.1	<0.001
Eczema	46.6	62.6	<0.001
Asthma	8.8	16.1	0.001
Total IgE (kU/L)	19.0 (18–20)	23.0 (18–29)	0.09
IgE sensitisation to food allergen	5.0	6.8	0.32
IgE sensitisation to aeroallergens	26.5	46	<0.001

Results presented as either prevalence (%), mean±SD or geometric mean (95% CI).
*p-value for comparison new-onset food hypersensitivity vs. no food hypersensitivity

over time [17], [37]. The total IgE levels reflect more than the sum of specific IgE towards a broad panel of allergens [38]. Moreover the fraction of total IgE not-related to specific sensitisations was not related to the specific IgE fraction of total IgE [38]. The factors that control the fraction of total IgE that are not related to specific IgE sensitisation are not fully understood.

Subjects with higher total IgE levels at baseline were more likely to have persistent sensitisation to food allergens in our study. Increased levels of total IgE have been reported to predict the development of IgE sensitisation to aeroallergens and asthma symptoms in children [39]. As far as we know, no study has analysed the relation between baseline total IgE levels and persistence of IgE sensitisation to food allergens, whereas increased total IgE at baseline related [37] to persistence of aeroallergen IgE sensitisation in previous longitudinal studies.

The strength of this study is the population setting and the long follow-up period. This is the first study to our knowledge assessing food hypersensitivity and IgE levels against food allergens in a longitudinal setting. A weakness of the present study is that we were not able to assess the persistence/remission of food hypersensitivity as the questions refer to ever having food hypersensitivity. A limitation is the fairly limited number of participants for whom we had data from repeated measurements of IgE against food allergens. Another limitation is that several of the most common food allergens in adulthood, such as hazelnut, shrimp, peach and apple [27], were not analysed at both time points. The different freezing times before analysis of IgE for samples from ECRHS I and II and that measurements were performed in different laboratories (Uppsala for ECRHS I and Manchester for ECRHS II) does not appear to influence the measured IgE levels [40,41]. Cross reactivity with IgE antibodies against birch or timothy grass can influence the measured IgE sensitisation to food allergens, and the lower prevalence of IgE sensitisation to food allergens at follow-up could have been due to a reduced prevalence of IgE sensitisation to birch at the follow-up. However, the prevalence of IgE sensitisation to birch did not decrease in the present study while the prevalence of IgE sensitisation to timothy grass decreased to a much lesser degree than IgE sensitisation to food allergens.

In conclusion, the prevalence of food hypersensitivity remained unchanged while IgE sensitisation to food allergens decreased in this 9 year follow up study performed in adults. The prevalence of IgE sensitisation towards food allergens decreased to a larger extent than the prevalence and persistence of IgE sensitisation to

Table 5. Baseline characteristic of subjects with persistent IgE food sensitisation compared to those with remission.

	Persistent IgE food sensitisation (n = 10)	Remission of IgE food sensitisation (n = 30)	p value*
Female sex	60.0	43.0	0.36
Age (years)	29.7 ±1.9	30.3 ±0.8	0.74
BMI (kg/m²)	23.2 ±1	24 ±0.6	0.55
Smoking	20.0	17.0	0.81
Rhinitis	50.0	80.0	0.07
Asthma	10.0	23.0	0.36
Food hypersensitivity	44.4	40.0	0.81
Total IgE (kU/L)	370 (110–1242)	106 (72–155)	0.008
IgE sensitisation to aeroallergens	9.0 (90)	24.0 (80)	0.47

Results presented as either prevalence (%), mean ± SD or geometric mean (95% CI).
*p-value for comparison persistent IgE food sensitisation and remission of IgE food sensitisation

aeroallergens. The biological explanation for the high prevalence of food hypersensitivity should be further investigated.

Acknowledgments

We would like to acknowledge Colin Summers for his contribution to EuroPrevall.

Author Contributions

Conceived and designed the experiments: AP CJ AM. Performed the experiments: CJ PB TG KT BF MG. Analyzed the data: AP CJ AM. Contributed reagents/materials/analysis tools: CJ MB KA. Wrote the paper: AP AM CJ. Revised critically: AP MG MB PB TG KT BF KA AM CJ. Final approval: AP MG MB PB TG KT BF KA AM CJ.

References

1. Johansson SG, Bieber T, Dahl R, Friedmann PS, Lanier BQ, et al. (2004) Revised nomenclature for allergy for global use: Report of the Nomenclature Review Committee of the World Allergy Organization, October 2003. J Allergy Clin Immunol 113: 832–836.
2. Woods RK, Abramson M, Bailey M, Walters EH (2001) International prevalences of reported food allergies and intolerances. Comparisons arising from the European Community Respiratory Health Survey (ECRHS) 1991–1994. Eur J Clin Nutr 55: 298–304.
3. Altman DR, Chiaramonte LT (1996) Public perception of food allergy. Journal of Allergy and Clinical Immunology 97: 1247–1251.
4. Schafer T, Bohler E, Ruhdorfer S, Weigl L, Wessner D, et al. (2001) Epidemiology of food allergy/food intolerance in adults: associations with other manifestations of atopy. Allergy 56: 1172–1179.
5. Taylor SL (1986) Food allergies and sensitivities. J Am Diet Assoc 86: 599–600.
6. Patelis A, Gunnbjornsdottir M, Malinovschi A, Matsson P, Onell A, et al. (2012) Population-based study of multiplexed IgE sensitization in relation to asthma, exhaled nitric oxide, and bronchial responsiveness. J Allergy Clin Immunol 130: 397–402 e392.
7. Liu AH, Jaramillo R, Sicherer SH, Wood RA, Bock SA, et al. (2010) National prevalence and risk factors for food allergy and relationship to asthma: results from the National Health and Nutrition Examination Survey 2005–2006. J Allergy Clin Immunol 126: 798–806 e713.
8. Sears MR, Herbison GP, Holdaway MD, Hewitt CJ, Flannery EM, et al. (1989) The relative risks of sensitivity to grass pollen, house dust mite and cat dander in the development of childhood asthma. Clin Exp Allergy 19: 419–424.
9. Malinovschi A, Janson C, Holmkvist T, Norback D, Merilainen P, et al. (2006) IgE sensitisation in relation to flow-independent nitric oxide exchange parameters. Respir Res 7: 92.
10. Sporik R, Ingram J, Price W, Sussman J, Honsinger R, et al. (1995) Association of asthma with serum IgE and skin test reactivity to allergens among children living at high altitude. Tickling the dragon's breath. Am J Respir Crit Care Med 151: 1388–1392.
11. Peat JK, Tovey E, Toelle BG, Haby MM, Gray EJ, et al. (1996) House dust mite allergens. A major risk factor for childhood asthma in Australia. Am J Respir Crit Care Med 153: 141–146.
12. Jarvis D, Luczynska C, Chinn S, Potts J, Sunyer J, et al. (2005) Change in prevalence of IgE sensitization and mean total IgE with age and cohort. J Allergy Clin Immunol 116: 675–682.
13. Barbee RA, Kaltenborn W, Lebowitz MD, Burrows B (1987) Longitudinal changes in allergen skin test reactivity in a community population sample. J Allergy Clin Immunol 79: 16–24.
14. Linneberg A, Nielsen NH, Madsen F, Frolund L, Dirksen A, et al. (2002) Is the increase in allergic respiratory disease caused by a cohort effect? Clin Exp Allergy 32: 1702–1705.
15. Warm K, Backman H, Lindberg A, Lundback B, Ronmark E (2012) Low incidence and high remission of allergic sensitization among adults. J Allergy Clin Immunol 129: 136–142.
16. Broadfield E, McKeever TM, Scrivener S, Venn A, Lewis SA, et al. (2002) Increase in the prevalence of allergen skin sensitization in successive birth cohorts. J Allergy Clin Immunol 109: 969–974.
17. Oryszczyn MP, Annesi I, Neukirch F, Dore MF, Kauffmann F (1995) Longitudinal observations of serum IgE and skin prick test response. Am J Respir Crit Care Med 151: 663–668.
18. Karakaya G, Kalyoncu AF (2006) The natural course of atopy determined by skin prick tests in patients with bronchial asthma and/or rhinitis. Allergol Immunopathol (Madr) 34: 257–262.
19. Linneberg A, Friedrich N, Husemoen LL, Thuesen B, Gonzalez-Quintela A, et al. (2010) Incidence and remission of specific IgE aeroallergen sensitization from age of 40 to 60 years, and association with alcohol consumption. Int Arch Allergy Immunol 151: 142–148.
20. Hughes JL, Brown T, Edgar JD, Shields MD (2010) Peanut allergy and allergic airways inflammation. Pediatr Allergy Immunol 21: 1107–1113.
21. Burney PG, Luczynska C, Chinn S, Jarvis D (1994) The European Community Respiratory Health Survey. Eur Respir J 7: 954–960.
22. Bjornsson E, Janson C, Plaschke P, Norrman E, Sjoberg O (1996) Prevalence of sensitization to food allergens in adult Swedes. Ann Allergy Asthma Immunol 77: 327–332.
23. Gislason D, Bjornsson E, Gislason T, Janson C, Sjoberg O, et al. (1999) Sensitization to airborne and food allergens in Reykjavik (Iceland) and Uppsala (Sweden) - a comparative study. Allergy 54: 1160–1167.
24. (2002) The European Community Respiratory Health Survey II. Eur Respir J 20: 1071–1079.
25. Olafsdottir IS, Gislason T, Thjodleifsson B, Olafsson I, Gislason D, et al. (2005) C reactive protein levels are increased in non-allergic but not allergic asthma: a multicentre epidemiological study. Thorax 60: 451–454.
26. Bousquet J, Chanez P, Chanal I, Michel FB (1990) Comparison between RAST and Pharmacia CAP system: a new automated specific IgE assay. J Allergy Clin Immunol 85: 1039–1043.
27. Burney P, Summers C, Chinn S, Hooper R, van Ree R, et al. (2010) Prevalence and distribution of sensitization to foods in the European Community Respiratory Health Survey: a EuroPrevall analysis. Allergy 65: 1182–1188.
28. Young E, Stoneham MD, Petruckevitch A, Barton J, Rona R (1994) A population study of food intolerance. The Lancet 343: 1127–1130.
29. Sampson HA (1996) Epidemiology of food allergy. Pediatr Allergy Immunol 7: 42–50.
30. Eggesbo M, Halvorsen R, Tambs K, Botten G (1999) Prevalence of parentally perceived adverse reactions to food in young children. Pediatr Allergy Immunol 10: 122–132.
31. Sicherer SH, Leung DY (2013) Advances in allergic skin disease, anaphylaxis, and hypersensitivity reactions to foods, drugs, and insects in 2012. J Allergy Clin Immunol 131: 55–66.
32. Skypala I (2011) Adverse food reactions–an emerging issue for adults. J Am Diet Assoc 111: 1877–1891.
33. Kulig M, Bergmann R, Klettke U, Wahn V, Tacke U, et al. (1999) Natural course of sensitization to food and inhalant allergens during the first 6 years of life. J Allergy Clin Immunol 103: 1173–1179.
34. Ramesh S (2008) Food allergy overview in children. Clin Rev Allergy Immunol 34: 217–230.
35. Rawle FC, Burr ML, Platts-Mills TA (1983) Long-term falls in antibodies to dust mite and pollen allergens in patients with asthma or hay fever. Clin Allergy 13: 409–417.
36. Carsin AE, Zock JP, Jarvis D, Basagana X, Heinrich J, et al. (2013) Serum total immunoglobulin E is a surrogate of atopy in adult-onset asthma: a longitudinal study. Int Arch Allergy Immunol 160: 387–392.
37. Barbee RA, Halonen M, Kaltenborn W, Lebowitz M, Burrows B (1987) A longitudinal study of serum IgE in a community cohort: correlations with age, sex, smoking, and atopic status. J Allergy Clin Immunol 79: 919–927.
38. Jackola DR, Blumenthal MN, Rosenberg A (2004) Evidence for two independent distributions of serum immunoglobulin E in atopic families: cognate and non-cognate IgE. Hum Immunol 65: 20–30.
39. Sherrill DL, Stein R, Halonen M, Holberg CJ, Wright A, et al. (1999) Total serum IgE and its association with asthma symptoms and allergic sensitization among children. J Allergy Clin Immunol 104: 28–36.
40. Linneberg A, Nielsen NH, Madsen F, Frolund L, Dirksen A, et al. (2000) Increasing prevalence of specific IgE to aeroallergens in an adult population: two cross-sectional surveys 8 years apart: the Copenhagen Allergy Study. J Allergy Clin Immunol 106: 247–252.
41. Paganelli R, Ansotegui IJ, Sastre J, Lange CE, Roovers MH, et al. (1998) Specific IgE antibodies in the diagnosis of atopic disease. Clinical evaluation of a new in vitro test system, UniCAP, in six European allergy clinics. Allergy 53: 763–768.

Beyond Labelling: What Strategies Do Nut Allergic Individuals Employ to Make Food Choices?

Julie Barnett[1]*, Konstantina Vasileiou[1], M. Hazel Gowland[2], Monique M. Raats[3], Jane S. Lucas[4]

Department of Information Systems and Computing, Brunel University, Middlesex, United Kingdom, **2** Allergy Action, Farnborough, United Kingdom, **3** School of Psychology, Faculty of Arts and Human Sciences, University of Surrey, Guildford, Surrey, United Kingdom, **4** Clinical and Experimental Sciences, Faculty of Medicine, University of Southampton, University Hospital Southampton NHS Foundation Trust, Southampton, United Kingdom

Abstract

Objective: Food labelling is an important tool that assists people with peanut and tree nut allergies to avoid allergens. Nonetheless, other strategies are also developed and used in food choice decision making. In this paper, we examined the strategies that nut allergic individuals deploy to make safe food choices in addition to a reliance on food labelling.

Methods: Three qualitative methods: an accompanied shop, in-depth semi-structured interviews, and the product choice reasoning task – were used with 32 patients that had a clinical history of reactions to peanuts and/or tree nuts consistent with IgE-mediated food allergy. Thematic analysis was applied to the transcribed data.

Results: Three main strategies were identified that informed the risk assessments and food choice practices of nut allergic individuals. These pertained to: (1) qualities of product such as the product category or the country of origin, (2) past experience of consuming a food product, and (3) sensory appreciation of risk. Risk reasoning and risk management behaviours were often contingent on the context and other physiological and socio-psychological needs which often competed with risk considerations.

Conclusions: Understanding and taking into account the complexity of strategies and the influences of contextual factors will allow healthcare practitioners, allergy nutritionists, and caregivers to advise and educate patients more effectively in choosing foods safely. Governmental bodies and policy makers could also benefit from an understanding of these food choice strategies when risk management policies are designed and developed.

Editor: José César Perales, Universidad de Granada, Spain

Funding: This study was funded by the United Kingdom Food Standards Agency under project code T07058 (http://www.food.gov.uk/). The funder had no role in study design, data collection and analysis, decision to publish, or preparation of the manuscript. They provided comment on a full draft of this paper.

Competing Interests: The authors have declared that no competing interests exist.

* E-mail: Julie.Barnett@brunel.ac.uk

Introduction

Food allergy is an important public health problem [1]. Although there are difficulties in estimating prevalence, and there is some variation between countries [2], in Europe and the United States food allergies are estimated to affect up to approximately 8% of children and 2% of adults [3,4]. Peanut and tree nuts are the most common cause of severe and life-threatening food allergic reactions [5]. The prevalence of peanut allergy, tree nut allergy or both (henceforth 'nut allergies') is around 1% in North American and UK populations [6,7,8,9] and seems to be increasing [7,8,10,11]. Between 1999 and 2006, 18 out of 48 deaths which were caused by allergic reactions to foods in the UK [12], and more than 90% of fatal reactions in the US between 1994 and 1999, were provoked by peanuts or tree nuts [13]. For ease – and despite the fact that peanuts are actually legumes – the word 'nuts' is henceforth used as a convenient generic.

The quality of life of children and adolescents with a nut allergy including their families can be severely compromised [14,15] since constant vigilance about diet needs to be exercised, whilst the risk of accidental exposure and the fear of a fatal reaction cannot completely be eliminated and controlled [16]. Parents of children with a nut allergy report higher levels of impairment in their quality of life and more disruptions of familial and social relations than do parents of children with a rheumatologic disease [17]. Similarly, higher levels of disease-related anxiety were found in children with a nut allergy compared with children with diabetes [18]. Recent research in adults has revealed the difficulties and challenges that nut allergic individuals face when eating out [19] and when travelling abroad [20] where a series of often competing considerations need to be balanced.

The clinical manifestation of allergic reactions includes symptoms affecting the skin (e.g. urticarial), respiratory tract (e.g. dyspnoea, throat tightness), gastrointestinal tract (e.g. vomiting, diarrhoea), and/or the cardiovascular system (e.g. hypotensive shock) [3]. Anaphylactic reactions are life-threatening episodes involving the cardiovascular or respiratory systems, which should be treated immediately by injection of intramuscular adrenaline

[3,4]. Nut allergies are not currently curable and consequently management primarily involves effective allergen avoidance and the provision of self-injectable adrenaline for severe reactions [1,21]. However, patients do not always carry their adrenaline devices or use them appropriately [22,23], and even when correctly administered, reactions can be fatal. Therefore, recognizing and avoiding foods containing nuts remains the key self-management strategy.

Labelling on the packaging of food products is an important tool that helps nut allergic individuals to make safe purchases. Although consumers do not normally pay much regard to labels, specific dietary requirements, such as food allergies, increase their attention to food labels [24]. Nonetheless, nut allergic people often encounter a series of difficulties in identifying correctly the allergens on the labels [25,26], and in interpreting advisory labelling such as 'may contain' [27]. Moreover, an examination of 20,241 products in US revealed the ambiguities and the variety of terminologies used in advisory labelling [28] confirming the challenges that nut allergic individuals face when buying foods. Recently, qualitative research in the UK [29,30] examined the ways in which nut allergic adults used information on the packaging to inform their food choices, corroborating many of the difficulties mentioned previously in the literature. It is evident, however, that labelling was used in conjunction with a series of other decision making strategies. But, whilst food choice strategies and 'rules of thumb' have been studied extensively among consumers in general [31,32,33,34], little is known in relation to nut allergic individuals. A recent focus-group study compared the food choice behaviours and eating experiences of adults diagnosed with food allergies to those of non-allergic consumers. The results demonstrated that food allergic people usually encounter difficulties in finding safe foods; their experiences around eating are less satisfactory and spontaneous since a high level of organisation and preparation is constantly required [35].

This paper has sought to characterise the nature of strategies employed by nut allergic individuals when choosing foods that extend beyond labelling. By using a variety of qualitative methods, we aimed to examine in depth how nut allergic individuals reason about food risk and how they choose and purchase foods.

Methods

Ethics Statement

The research received ethical approval from the National Research Ethics Service (09/H1109/64) and the University of Surrey Ethics Committee.

Study Population

The study population included individuals, aged 16 or over, with a clinical history of reactions to peanuts and/or tree nuts which was compatible with IgE-mediated allergy. The participants were recruited from three sources in South England: (a) the paediatric and adult allergy clinics at University Hospital Southampton NHS Foundation Trust, (b) three General Practitioners (GP) Surgeries, and (c) the staff and students at the University of Surrey. Letters were sent to 411 individuals explaining the aim of the research and inviting them to complete a screening questionnaire. For the interested reader, the screening questionnaire is provided as File S1. Seventy-seven respondents returned this (response rate 18.73%) of which 54 were eligible to take part following examination of the information by an allergy specialist (JSL). Of the 54 eligible individuals, 32 consented to participate in the study. Participants' consent was obtained in written form.

Participants' eligibility, based on the information provided in the postal screening questionnaire, was assessed by the allergy specialist as follows: respondents were required to be aged 16 years or older with a clinical history compatible with IgE-mediated reactions to peanuts or tree nuts. Participants recruited from the specialist allergy clinic had positive skin prick tests and/or specific IgE measurements. Recruits from the University of Surrey and from primary care settings were required to have been diagnosed with peanut or tree nut allergy by a medical practitioner, and prescribed rescue medication. Individuals with allergies or intolerance to foods in addition to peanut or tree nuts were excluded because this would affect their consumer choices. The exception was inclusion of participants with oral allergy syndrome (OAS) to fruits and/or vegetables. Unlike egg or milk for example, avoidance of fruit and vegetables was unlikely to create significant dilemmas during the shopping tasks.

Of the 32 participants who took part in the study, 9 were males and 23 females, aged between 16 and 70 years old. Five participants had only peanut allergy, 9 had only tree nut allergy, and 18 had both. The severity of their worst-ever reaction was rated as mild, moderate or severe using a classification previously employed for peanut allergy [36]. Eighteen participants described severe reactions, 12 moderate and 2 mild.

Methods of Data Collection

Three different qualitative methods were used to collect data:

A. The accompanied shop (AS). Participants were followed, observed and audio-recorded in their routine weekly shop by an experienced qualitative researcher. Accompanying consumers while shopping is an established technique in consumer studies that enables direct observation of actual behaviour [37]. Participants in this research were additionally asked to think aloud about their purchase decisions, having being familiarised with and trained in the 'think aloud' method. File S2 provides the details of how participants were trained to the 'think aloud' protocol and how they were instructed to conduct the accompanied shop. To ensure that the accompanied shop was as naturalistic as possible, the researcher's input at this stage was minimal, consisting mainly of prompts such as 'what are you thinking?' when participants stopped thinking aloud.

The 'think aloud' technique allows the elicitation of a concurrent with-the-behaviour-observed verbal report. Ericsson & Simon's [38] classical work advocated the value of verbal data deriving from introspection for the examination of the cognitive processes involved in problem-solving scenarios. Since then, the 'think aloud' technique has been used extensively in several fields, including food choice research [39] usually after being adapted to serve particular research questions and in combination with other techniques [40].

B. A semi-structured interview (SSI). Issues arising during the accompanied shop were followed up in a face-to-face interview. This allowed us to examine interesting behaviours noted by the researcher during the accompanied shop that was relevant to our research questions (e.g. avoiding certain products or even parts of the supermarket). The SSI also explored the ways the participants were managing their food choices and consumption across various eating-related situations (e.g. eating-out, holidays), as well as the history of their allergies and their views on labelling.

C. The Product Choice Reasoning Task (PCRT). Participants were presented with 13 products, each of which embodied a recognized dilemma for people avoiding nuts/peanuts. These are described in detail in Barnett et al [29].

Participants were asked whether and why they would or would not consume each one of the products.

Fuller detail of the methods can be found in Barnett et al [41].

Employing this configuration of methods allowed the in-depth examination of both reported and actual food choices and the reasoning behind them. All research phases were audio recorded and fully transcribed. The accompanied shop was directly followed by the interview and the Product Choice Reasoning Task which were conducted in participants' homes.

Analytic Procedure

Thematic analysis [42,43] was used to explore the data. Given that the aim was to examine what strategies the nut allergic individuals are employing to make sense of, and manage the risk of allergic reactions when choosing food, a realist epistemological stance to participants' speeches was adopted. This means that people's accounts were considered as being reflective of their thoughts, cognitions, and reported behaviours and that language provided the means through which the researchers were able to access these.

Initially, the researchers (JB and KV) familiarised themselves with the data through repeated reading of the transcripts, and noted interesting and relevant-to-the-research-question points. Further analysis was conducted during a series of regular meetings. Codes were formed and assigned, assisted by computer software [44], to the relevant textual segments. Finally, themes and subthemes were developed by aggregating semantically identical codes; further revision and refinement of the themes took place in order to be internally homogenous, distinct from each other [45] and reflective of the data.

Results

Risk reasoning and food choice practices were located in relation to three main themes: (a) *product qualities*, (b) *past experience*, and (c) *sensory appreciation*. Food choices, however, were not exclusively defined by safety considerations; participants reported other considerations, which often competed with those pertaining to risk forming a fourth theme, named *beyond safety*.

Respondents' quotes below are identified by a. their coding number (e.g. 4015), b. their sex (M for males, F for females), c. the severity of allergy (S for severe, M for moderate and MI for mild), d. their age, and e. the corpus of data from which the quote is drawn (Accompanied shop – AS, Semi-Structured Interview – SSI, and Product Choice Reasoning Task - PCRT).

Product Qualities

Several product-related indicators were employed, sometimes in combination, to inform participants' risk assessments. These concerned the *product category*, the *brand*, the *producer and/or the provider* of the food, and the *country of origin*, and operated to provide guidance as to the desirability of purchase and consumption.

The broader *product category* was among the most salient categorisations that informed risk judgments. Certain product categories, such as bakery, chocolate, cereals, desserts, processed or ready-made meals, were considered as particularly problematic, as they were strongly associated with nuts, signalling the necessity for closer examination usually by looking the labels. Hesitation and worry around consumption of these products was often reported, while total rejection was not uncommon:

> *If it's like a savoury type thing, particularly bready stuff, for some reason, that's what freaks me out a little bit, and I'll just say…bready things, biscuits, cakes, I'll just say, "No thanks". (4015, MS34, PCRT)*

Fresh vegetables, fruits, and dairy, on the other hand, were product categories that rarely posed any safety concerns and were generally trusted immediately as safe.

The *brand* also informed risk reasoning. Well-known and reputable brand names clearly functioned to indicate safety. Notably, in some instances a trusted brand acted as such a strong indicator of safety that it could override precautionary labelling or the influence of a problematic product category:

> *Yeah, I'd eat these. Normally – oh, it says "Not suitable for peanut allergy sufferers"… I'd probably still eat them though because if they're – like [brand name] is a trusted name, and I highly doubt they actually would. I'd probably still eat them, yeah. (1011, FS18, PCRT)*

Conversely, products associated with a lesser known brand, even when they were not problematic *per se*, raised suspicions which were resolved either through avoidance or further checks of labels:

> *For a first look, I'd probably be like, "Oh yeah, I can eat them," and then I'd just be like, "Oh, hang on, it's not a main brand – I probably should have a look at it." (1008, FM16, PCRT)*

The trust accorded to well-known brands was associated with the assumed safety standards of the manufacturing processes and the perceived thoroughness and adequacy of labelling practices, although participants did not claim any knowledge of manufacturing or labelling processes:

> *That's a brand that I would be comfortable that their food labelling and their standards are adequate. (1029, FS26, PCRT)*

The *provider* of the products – which in some cases coincided with the producer – was an additional resource for risk judgments. Big companies such as supermarkets were often trusted due to the belief that they have strong interests to protect their reputation and enough resources to check the products:

> *…so if I'm buying any sort of products where it relates to nuts, I would definitely only buy them in the supermarket, because I'm pretty much trusting that someone is checking and that the risk of me finding them in the food is less. (3008, FM45, SSI)*

A smaller number of participants, however, perceived small, and usually local, producers or providers as more trustworthy than big companies.

The last product quality repeatedly articulated in risk reasoning was the *country of origin*. Foreign products were almost always treated with hesitation and were avoided compared to native products:

> *Em, anything that's foreign is a no – I just won't buy it. (4015, MS34, SSI)*

Even if the particular allergen was apparently not an ingredient the overarching designation as foreign led to rejection. Foreign products activated beliefs that in other countries there is a lower level of awareness or recognition of the problem of nut allergies and a higher tendency to use nuts in products:

They look like they're probably made somewhere else because the initial language here is not English. I have no idea how they...if they have any concept of allergies. (5009, FS38, PCRT)

Reluctance to consume foreign products was also explained in terms of unfamiliarity with the standards of production and regulation applied in other countries:

To be honest, if it was a foreign product, which had equally good labelling, I might be more reluctant because I'm not familiar with the standards that they would be obliged to comply with (1029, FS26, PCRT).

Past Experience

Past experience was a second, and particularly powerful, resource for nut allergic individuals that dictated safe food choices in an efficient and confident manner. Experiential knowledge accumulated over the course of years invited absolute trust in foods, often without reference to labels:

I could almost say yes without looking at the ingredients for these ones because I've eaten them lots of times before. (1068, FM34, PCRT)

Several participants were alert to the possibility that manufacturers may change product ingredients. Some reported that they still checked the labels for potential changes, even though past experience warranted safe consumption, but others ignored this possibility, especially when they had recently consumed the product:

If I know that it's something I've had quite recently, then I'm not bothered about it. I'll just have it straightaway, pick it up without reading it. (1016, FS18, SSI)

Importantly, uneventful past experience of consuming a product was such a powerful indicator of future safe consumption that precautionary labelling was ignored or discounted:

Yeah, I can see here it says that it's not suitable for peanut allergy sufferers and it may have traces of peanut or other nuts, but I've never ever had an allergy to [product name], and so my automatic reaction is yeah, I'd try it. (3008, FM45, PCRT)

Conversely, novel products led, at least some participants, to attend to 'contains' or 'may contain' labelling.

Positive experiences of consumption led to the routinisation of food choices and the establishment of habitual food purchase patterns. Although participants recognized that this strategy limited the trial of new foods, they were generally content since time and effort were saved:

So yes, I do tend to stick with things I know, and probably not adventurous with trying many new things [laughing]! (1042, FS26, SSI)

Negative past experiences were particularly instructive in creating an often intense aversion and rejection of the associated foods. This was often not simply restricted to the particular product that had caused the allergic reaction but was rather generalised to include other exemplars of the broader category in which the problematic food was classified, for example unrelated products within the same brand or product category, with similar ingredients, or even similar labelling:

It was a type of chocolate bar from [supermarket name] and I had a reaction to it, even though it just said "may contain", and then I never ate anything that said "may contain" again. (1112, FS21, SSI)

Sensory Appreciation

Reliance on senses such as taste, sight and smell was an additional and trusted strategy the participants employed to assess the riskiness of foods. This strategy was often used when the food was novel and there was thus some uncertainty around its safety. A sensory check provided a rapid initial assessment, yet the resulting evidence was in many cases regarded as unequivocal.

The PCRT was particularly revealing in showing that some products were directly associated with nuts simply from the way they looked. This created strong feelings of aversion to a degree that the product was ultimately rejected without further examination or seeking further validation through labelling:

It looks too much like nuts, so no. Actually, seeing – just on what it looks like, I wouldn't even, in the real world, read any ingredients. (4015, MS34, PCRT)

The texture of the product was an additional cue signifying risk. The more plain and smooth the product looked the less risky it was perceived to be. By contrast, a granular texture in the product caused concern and activated avoidance:

Well, I think it looks risky because there's lots of bits in [laughing]! That sounds simplistic, but over the years, I've learnt that means trouble. (1031, FM30, PCRT)

Olfactory evaluation was also used for risk judgments and was very much trusted as a signal of danger. Participants smelt the products and some even claimed that they had developed an acute sensitivity to detect nuts or products containing nuts with their odour even 'from a mile off'. This then provoked again avoidance and rejection of the product:

I'm just more aware, and I would trust my senses more with regards to my sense of smell, very much so...Those smells immediately send warning bells off in my head. (4015, MS34, SSI)

Finally, a sort of 'taste test' was recurrently reported. Here participants tried a little bit of the product, waited to see whether there were any adverse reactions and depending on the outcome of the trial, they then either consumed or rejected the food. The taste test was deployed when participants felt uncertain about the safety of the food or lacked previous experience. For some, this strategy was still used, even when they knew that the product was safe, thus providing further reassurance:

Even when I come to eat it, even if I know there's not actually any nuts in it, I'll taste a little bit and then wait a few minutes to see if anything happens...just to be really sure. (4001, FS24, SSI)

Beyond Safety

Arguably safety was the primary consideration in food choices. However, other factors influenced decision making. These pertained firstly to other product attributes that were taken into account in food purchases, secondly to contextual factors within which the nut allergic individuals assessed the risk of food consumption, and thirdly to their internal –physiological or psychological – states and the broader life stage. Taking into account these parameters led on occasions to a more risk adverse stance, whilst in other instances greater risk was embraced.

Much of the time participants were considering and valuing additional product attributes such as taste, cost, quality, health, convenience and ethics as well as the needs of other people for whom they were shopping. Although on many occasions these considerations were not related to problematic foods, in some instances there was evidence of how participants sought to incorporate these values alongside their risk assessments. Importantly, in the effort to balancing competing values some admitted that they were taking the risk, mainly when they liked the taste of a product:

Generally I would do, apart from in the case of the soya nuts [laughing], because I like them so I take the risk! (1042, FS26, SSI)

Assignations of risk were closely enmeshed with the context within which participants were operating. Two dimensions of the context were evaluated; firstly, respondents were more willing and relaxed to assume greater risk when they were close to medical facilities:

I mean, if I was in the centre of town in a country where I know the medical facilities are good, then I'm much more relaxed, and I'll risk certain things. If I'm up a mountain in the middle of nowhere, even if it seems safe, I would be more reluctant to eat. (1029, FS26, SSI)

Secondly, the presence of other people by whom participants and their allergy were known, and who were therefore trusted, was a further reassuring parameter that allowed people to take on greater risks:

Usually, it's with my parents, and I'm happier eating out at a restaurant with my parents because they know me, they know...like no one knows you as well as your parents do – no one ever would. So I'm happier...like when we've been on holidays and stuff, I'd be happier to risk it when they're there because they know everything. They know my medical history. (1112, FS21, SSI)

Interestingly, while the presence of others sometimes functioned as reassurance, in many instances it was a source of stress, and more particularly embarrassment, due to participants' belief that interrogating others about the content of food violated important social norms. The feelings of embarrassment and the unwillingness of people to attract attention or to offend others often obstructed the approach to managing risk:

So I did actually have a bit, even though, really, by my rules I set myself, I wouldn't have eaten that normally, but because it was my birthday cake, I felt a bit guilty! (1161, FM22, SSI)

It was evident that risk judgments made by participants were contingent upon attending to aspects of their internal state, personal characteristics or life situation. For instance, people mentioned that factors, such as hunger or tiredness, could impede a thorough risk assessment:

If you're tired, you go round the supermarket, you're really wanting to get home, you do occasionally pick things up and you haven't read it clearly. (4013, FS37, SSI)

Others related the way they managed their allergy to broader life contexts and significant transitions. A woman (1031, FM30, SSI) mentioned that she used to be much more adventurous with food choices before her baby was born as she had more time to check labels and try new foods. Another participant (1198, FM48, SSI) explained the difficulties of allergy being diagnosed as an adult as well as how a busy life with children militated against giving much attention to her own food choices. Finally, a young woman with severe allergy linked the way she managed her allergy to the general rise and fall of her stress levels:

If I'm very stressed at work or stressed for whatever reason, I'll become more paranoid about it. It's like something that I focus my energy on or relax away from, depending on everything else that's going on in my life! (1029, FS26, SSI)

Discussion

Our results indicate the complexity of risk reasoning and the variety of strategies the nut allergic individuals use to inform their decision making. Participants relied heavily on their previous experience of consuming foods and the relevant knowledge they had developed, their senses as well as their evaluations of different product characteristics, namely the product category, the brand, the provider and the country of origin. These results chime with previous research, conducted with non-allergic consumers, which demonstrates that both past experience and sensory assessments of foods constitute particularly useful rules of thumb in food choices [34]. Applying a system of categorisations and evaluating foods accordingly has also been observed with lay people when they attempt to make sense of various food risks [46,47]. Additionally, the strategies that people use to make food choices are characterised by trust, dictate confident food consumption, and provide efficiency in decision making [34]; findings which are corroborated by our results. At the same time, this study indicates the complexity of the dilemmas that nut allergic people often face when choosing food, also alluded to in recent research with food allergic consumers [35]. The current study has shed further light on the food choice practices of people with nut allergies and adds to previous research that examines the strategies of non-allergic consumers in this area [31,32,33,34].

One of the strengths of the present research is the variety of qualitative methods used that enabled a detailed insight into the complexity of risk reasoning and food management practices [48]. The accompanied shop allowed us to observe the participants while shopping. This access to their shopping practices seeks to address the challenge of obtaining relevant behavioural data and avoids a sole reliance on self-reported attitudes or behaviour.

Additionally, since participants at this stage were simply informed that the focus was on their food management strategies rather than framing this in terms of risk, the accompanied shop proved to be an ideal setting within which other product-based considerations (e.g. taste, cost) were revealed thus further reducing the likelihood of socially desirable behaviours. The interview enabled an in-depth examination of issues emerging during the accompanied shop and provided participants with the opportunity to reflect on their reasoning around their food choices and risk managing behaviour. Finally, the Product Choice Reasoning Task was particularly useful in documenting the exact risk thinking as this was being shaped as well as the, often combined, deployment of the various strategies in decision making.

Implications of the study

This study has clear implications for healthcare professionals (clinicians, allergists, allergy dieticians) that develop management plans and advise patients as to how to avoid problematic foods, while also maintaining a balanced and healthy diet. On the one hand, it is important to recognize that the strategies provide efficiency and confidence in food decision making, reducing the anxiety and thus they are likely to lead to established behaviour patterns. On the other hand, it is also crucial to acknowledge that the strategies are contingent on contextual factors and are additionally influenced by physiological and socio-psychological needs that sometimes impede thorough and extensive risk assessments and consequently lead to accidental ingestion of the allergens. Understanding and taking into account the day to day strategies that shape nut allergic individuals' food choice practices will enable healthcare professionals to advise their patients more effectively by drawing attention to potential pitfalls and by fostering the use of successful and functional strategies.

Food manufacturers, importers, distributors and retailers also have a responsibility to ensure that the foods they sell are safe for all consumers, including those with food allergies. Policy makers and governmental bodies would also benefit from an understanding of these food choice strategies when risk management policies are developed. It is notable for example that people with nut allergies are most likely to turn to labelling in the context of uncertainty when more habitual strategies do not lead to a confident decision. Under these circumstances it is vital that labelling is available, clear and trustworthy.

Supporting Information

File S1 Screening questionnaire.

File S2 Think aloud training & accompanied shop instructions.

Acknowledgments

We acknowledge the support of the Anaphylaxis Campaign and also the contribution of Jo Leftwich and Kate Muncer who collected the data on which the analysis is based.

Author Contributions

Provided advice as an allergic consumer to the project throughout: MHG. Provided clinical expertise as an allergist for the study design and analysis: JSL. Provided expertise regarding consumers' food choice strategies: MMR. Contributed to reviewing and commenting on early drafts of the paper: MHG MMR JSL. Conceived and designed the experiments: JB MHG MMR JSL. Analyzed the data: JB KV. Wrote the paper: JB KV.

References

1. Boyce JA, Assa'ad A, Burks AW, Jones SM, Sampson HA (2010) Guidelines for the diagnosis and management of food allergy in the United States: Report of the NIAID-sponsored expert panel. J Allergy Clin Immunol 126(6): S1–S58.
2. Rona RJ, Keil T, Summers C, Gislason D, Zuidmeer L, et al. (2007) The prevalence of food allergy: A meta-analysis. J Allergy Clin Immunol 120: 638–46.
3. Al-Muhsen S, Clarke AE, Kagan RS (2003) Peanut allergy: An overview. CMAJ 168(10): 1279–1285.
4. Sampson HA (2002) Clinical Practice. Peanut allergy. N Engl J Med 346(17): 1294–1299.
5. Sicherer SH, Furlong TJ, Munoz-Furlong A, Burks AW, Sampson HA (2001) A voluntary registry for peanut and tree nut allergy: Characteristics of the first 5149 registrants. J Allergy Clin Immunol 108(1): 128–132.
6. Sicherer SH, Muñoz-Furlong A, Burks AW, Sampson HA (1999) Prevalence of peanut and tree nut allergy in the US determined by a random digit dial telephone survey. J Allergy Clin Immunol 103(4): 559–562.
7. Sicherer SH, Munoz-Furlong A, Sampson HA (2003) Prevalence of peanut and tree nut allergy in the United States determined by means of a random digit dial telephone survey: A 5-year follow-up study. J Allergy Clin Immunol 112(6): 1203–1207.
8. Grundy J, Matthews S, Bateman B, Dean T, Arshad SH (2002) Rising prevalence of allergy to peanut in children: Data from 2 sequential cohorts. J Allergy Clin Immunol 110(5): 784–789.
9. Ben Shoshan M, Kagan RS, Alizadehfar R, Joseph L, Turnbull E, et al. (2009) Is the prevalence of peanut allergy increasing? A 5-year follow-up study in children in Montreal. J Allergy Clin Immunol 123(4): 783–788.
10. Sicherer SH, Munoz-Furlong A, Godbold JH, Sampson HA (2010) US prevalence of self-reported peanut, tree nut, and sesame allergy: 11-year follow-up. J Allergy Clin Immunol 125(6): 1322–1326.
11. Venter C, Arshad SH, Grundy J, Pereira B, Clayton CB, et al. (2010) Time trends in the prevalence of peanut allergy: Three cohorts of children from the same geographical location in the UK. Allergy 65: 103–108.
12. Pumphrey RS, Gowland MH (2007) Further fatal allergic reactions to food in the United Kingdom, 1999–2006 [letter to the editor]. J Allergy Clin Immunol 119(4): 1018–1019.
13. Bock SA, Muñoz-Furlong A, Sampson HA (2001) Fatalities due to anaphylactic reactions to foods. J Allergy Clin Immunol 107(1): 191–193.
14. Cummings AJ, Knibb RC, King RM, Lucas JS (2010) The psychosocial impact of food allergy and food hypersensitivity in children, adolescents and their families: A review. Allergy 65: 933–945.
15. Cummings AJ, Knibb RC, Erlewyn- Lajeunesse M, King RM, Roberts G, et al. (2010) Management of nut allergy influences quality of life and anxiety in children and their mothers. Pediatr Allergy Immunol 21: 586–594.
16. Teufel M, Biedermann T, Rapps N, Hausteiner C, Henningsen P, et al. (2007) Psychological burden of food allergy. World J Gastroenterol 13(25): 3456–3465.
17. Primeau MN, Kagan R, Joseph L, Lim H, Dufresne C, et al. (2000) The psychological burden of peanut allergy as perceived by adults with peanut allergy and the parents of peanut-allergic children. Clin Exp Allergy 30: 1135–1143.
18. Avery NJ, King RM, Knight S, Hourihane JO (2003) Assessment of quality of life in children with peanut allergy. Pediatr Allergy Immunol 14: 378–382.
19. Leftwich J, Barnett J, Muncer K, Shepherd R, Raats MM, et al. (2011) The challenges for nut-allergic consumers of eating out. Allergy 41: 243–249.
20. Barnett J, Botting N, Gowland MH, Lucas JS (2012) The strategies that peanut and nut-allergic consumers employ to remain safe when travelling abroad. Clin Transl Allergy 2: 12.
21. Sampson HA (1996) Managing peanut allergy demands aggressive intervention in prevention and treatment. BMJ 312: 1050–1051.
22. Gallagher M, Worth A, Cunningham-Burley S, Sheikh A (2011) Epinephrine auto-injector use in adolescents at risk of anaphylaxis: a qualitative study in Scotland, UK. Clin Exp Allergy 4: 869–877.
23. Macadam C, Barnett J, Roberts G, Stiefel G, King R, et al. (2012) What factors affect the carriage of epinephrine auto-injectors by teenagers? Clin Transl Allergy 2(1): 3.
24. Enright G, Good H, Williams N (2010) Qualitative research to explore people's use of food labelling information: Final report. Social Science Research Unit, Food Standards Agency.
25. Joshi P, Mofidi S, Sicherer SH (2002) Interpretation of commercial food ingredient labels by parents of food-allergic children. J Allergy Clin Immunol 109(6): 1019–1021.
26. Cornelisse-Vermaat JR, Voordouw J, Yiakoumaki V, Theodoridis G, Frewer LJ (2007) Food-allergic consumers' labelling preferences: A cross-cultural comparison. Eur J Public Health 18(2): 115–120.
27. Noimark L, Gardner J, Warner JO (2009) Parents attitudes when purchasing products for children with nut allergy: A UK perspective. Pediatr Allergy Immunol 20: 500–504.

28. Pieretti MM, Chung D, Pacenza R, Slotkin T, Sicherer SH (2009) Audit of manufactured products: Use of allergen advisory labels and identification of labeling ambiguities. J Allergy Clin Immunol 124(2): 337–341.
29. Barnett J, Leftwich J, Muncer K, Grimshaw K, Shepherd R, et al. (2011) How do peanut and nut allergic consumers use information on the packaging to avoid allergens? Allergy 66(7): 969–978.
30. Barnett J, Muncer K, Leftwich J, Shepherd R, Raats MM, et al. (2011) Using 'may contain' labelling to inform food choice: A qualitative study of nut allergic consumers. BMC Public Health 11: 734.
31. Connors M, Bisogni CA, Sobal J, Devine CM (2001) Managing values in personal food systems. Appetite 36(3): 189–200.
32. Falk LW, Bisogni CA, Sobal J (1996) Food choice processes of older adults: A qualitative investigation. J Nutr Educ 28: 257–265.
33. Furst T, Connors M, Bisogni CA, Sobal J, Falk LW (1996) Food choice: A conceptual model of the process. Appetite 26: 247–266.
34. Green J, Draper A, Dowler E (2003) Short cuts to safety: Risk and 'rules of thumb' in accounts of food choice. Health, Risk Soc 5(1): 33–52.
35. Sommer I, MacKenzie H, Venter C, Dean T (2012) Factors influencing food choices of food allergic consumers: Findings from focus groups. Allergy doi:10.1111/j.1398-9995.2012.02883.x.
36. Hourihane JO, Kilburn SA, Dean P, Warner JO (1997) Clinical characteristics of peanut allergy. Clin Exp Allergy 27: 634–639.
37. Otnes C, McGrath MA, Lowery TM (1995) Shopping with consumers: Usage as past, present, and future research technique. J Retailing Consumer Services 2(2): 97–110.
38. Ericsson KA, Simon HA (1984) Protocol analysis: Verbal reports as data. Cambridge: Massachusetts.
39. Higginson CS, Rayner MJ, Draper S, Kirk TR (2002) The nutrition label – which information is looked at? Nutr Food Sci 32(3): 92–99.
40. Nielsen J, Clemmensen T, Yssing C (2002) Getting access to what goes on in people's heads? Reflections on the think-aloud technique. Nordic Conference of Computer-Human Interaction October 19–23.
41. Barnett J, Leftwich J, Muncer K, Raats M, Shepherd R et al (2010) Understanding the food choice reasoning of nut allergic consumers. Final Technical Report T07058. Food Standards Agency. Available: http://www.food.gov.uk/science/research/allergy-research/allergy-labelling/t07058/.
42. Boyatzis RE (1998) Transforming qualitative information: Thematic analysis and code development. Thousand Oaks, CA: Sage.
43. Braun V, Clarke V (2006) Using thematic analysis in psychology. Qual Res Psychol 3: 77–101.
44. NVivo qualitative data analysis software [computer program]: Version 9 QSR International Pty Ltd.: 2008.
45. Patton MQ (1990) Qualitative evaluation and research methods. 2nd ed. Newbury Park, CA: Sage.
46. Lupton DA (2005) Lay discourses and beliefs related to food risks: an Australian perspective. Sociol Health Illn 27(4): 448–467.
47. Horlick-Jones T, Walls J, Kitzinger J (2007) Bricolage in action: learning about, making sense of, and discussing, issues about genetically modified crops and food. Health Risk Soc 9(1): 83–103.
48. Gallagher M, Worth A, Sheikh A (2009) Clinical allergy has much to gain from engagement with qualitative research. Allergy 64: 1117–1120.

Effects of Early Life Paracetamol Use on the Incidence of Allergic Disease and Sensitization: 5 Year Follow-Up of an Ethiopian Birth Cohort

Alemayehu Amberbir[1,2]*, Girmay Medhin[3], Charlotte Hanlon[4], John Britton[2], Gail Davey[5], Andrea Venn[2]

1 Department of Infectious Disease Epidemiology, London School of Hygiene and Tropical Medicine, London, United Kingdom, **2** Division of Epidemiology and Public Health, University of Nottingham, Nottingham, United Kingdom, **3** Aklilu Lemma Institute of Pathobiology, Addis Ababa University, Addis Ababa, Ethiopia, **4** Department of Psychiatry, Addis Ababa University, Addis Ababa, Ethiopia, **5** Brighton & Sussex Medical School, University of Brighton, Brighton, United Kingdom

Abstract

Introduction: The hypothesis that paracetamol, one of the most widely used medicines, may increase the risk of asthma and allergic disease is of obvious importance but prospective cohort data looking at dose and timing of exposure are lacking.

Objective: The aim of the study is to investigate the role of paracetamol use in early life on the prevalence and incidence of wheeze, eczema, rhinitis and allergic sensitization, prospectively over 5 years in an Ethiopian birth cohort.

Methods: In 2005/6 a birth cohort of 1006 newborns was established in Butajira, Ethiopia. Questionnaire data on allergic disease symptoms, paracetamol use and numerous potential confounders were collected at ages 1, 3 and 5, and allergen skin sensitivity measured at ages 3 and 5. Multivariate logistic regression was used to determine independent effects of paracetamol exposure on the incidence of each outcome between ages 3 and 5, and prevalence at age 5.

Findings: Paracetamol use in the first 3 years of life was reported in 60% of children and was associated with increased incidence of wheeze, eczema, rhinitis and allergic sensitisation between ages 3 and 5 which was statistically significant for wheeze and eczema. High exposure (reported use in the past month at age 1 and 3) was associated with a more than 3-fold increased risk of new onset wheeze (adjusted odds ratio (OR) 3.64; 95% confidence interval, 1.34 to 9.90) compared to never users. Use in the past year at age 3 but not age 1 was associated with ORs at least as large as those for use in first year of life only. Significant positive dose-response effects of early life use were seen in relation to the prevalence of all outcomes at age 5.

Conclusions: Use of paracetamol in early life is a strong risk factor for incident allergic disease in childhood.

Editor: Junji Yodoi, Institute for Virus Research, Laboratory of Infection and Prevention, Japan

Funding: The study was funded by Asthma United Kingdom project grant (07/036). The funders had no role in study design, data collection and analysis, decision to publish, or preparation of the manuscript.

Competing Interests: The authors have declared that no competing interests exist.

* E-mail: alemayehu.amberbir@lshtm.ac.uk

Introduction

A higher prevalence of asthma and allergic diseases in developed than developing countries, and in urban than rural communities, is widely reported[1–3]. Whilst genetics are likely to play some part in explaining these differences[4], most of the differences are thought to be due to environmental exposures[5]. One hypothesis which has gained much recent support from epidemiological studies in both developed and developing countries, is that paracetamol (acetaminophen) intake increases the risk of asthma and allergic diseases[6–13]. with meta-analyses of the available observational studies estimating a 63% increased risk of asthma in relation to personal paracetamol use[6], and a 21–28% increased risk of wheezing in relation to *in utero* exposure[6,7]. However the studies to date are primarily based on cross-sectional data and conducted in developed countries, and therefore alternative explanations such as aspirin avoidance, reverse causation, recall bias, and confounding, particularly by early respiratory infections, are difficult to exclude. Of the few longitudinal studies that have been conducted, only three have looked at personal use rather than *in utero* exposure, one in adults[14] and two in children [9,15], Lowe *et al* reported an adverse effect of paracetamol use on incident childhood asthma, but the effect diminished following control for confounding by early respiratory infections[15]. The other longitudinal study in children was our follow-up of an Ethiopian cohort, in which we also saw an adverse effect of paracetamol use in the first year of life on incident wheeze at age 3 which we concluded was unlikely to be due to reverse causation or confounding by indication; however no adverse effect on eczema was seen and other allergic outcomes were not available for analysis[9].

We now report findings from five year follow-up of this cohort that shed light on the relative importance of exposures at different time points and in different doses. The primary aims were to determine the association between early life paracetamol use (dose and timing) and incidence of wheeze, eczema, rhinitis and skin sensitisation between ages 3 and 5, as well as the prevalence of these outcomes at age 5.

Methods

Study setting and design

The study was a population-based prospective birth cohort of mother-child pairs followed from birth to the age of five years in Butajira, Ethiopia. The study area is predominantly rural, with a subsistence lifestyle and little motorized transport. The cohort was established in 2005 and nested in the Demographic Surveillance Site (DSS) at the Butajira Rural Health Program[16]. Details of the birth cohort, including recruitment and data collection procedures up to age 3, have been described in detail elsewhere[9,17,18]. In brief, all women aged 15–49 in their third trimester of pregnancy between July 2005 and February 2006 who lived in the DSS area were identified and 1065 (86% of eligible) were recruited. These women subsequently gave birth to 1006 singleton live babies who have been visited at regular intervals (birth, 2 months, and at or near their 1st, 3rd and 5th birthdays).

Data collection

At age 5, the children were revisited and an interview-led questionnaire administered to the mother (or other guardian) in the local language (Amharic) by the fieldworker as at previous visits. The allergic disease questions, which asked about symptoms of wheeze, eczema and rhinitis ever and in the past year, were based on the International Study of Asthma and Allergies in Children (ISAAC) questionnaire[19], and were the same as those asked at previous follow-ups[9,18]. These include: *'Has your child ever had wheezing or whistling in their chest?'* *'Has your child ever had asthma?'*, *'Has your child ever had problems with sneezing or running nose (when not affected by cold or flu), or problems with itchy watery eyes?'* and *'Has your child ever had an itchy skin rash which has affected the skin creases, eg, front of the elbow, behind the knees, the front of the ankles, around the neck, or around the eyes?'* At year 3 and 5 follow-ups, additional questions asking about symptoms in the past year were asked, and at age 5, symptoms in the past 2 years (since previous follow-up). Questions on paracetamol use were also identical to those asked at age 1 and 3, where the mothers were asked whether the child had taken or been given paracetamol in the past 12 months, and if so, were asked to quantify the dose of paracetamol consumed in the past month. At the 5 year follow-up, mothers were additionally asked to distinguish paracetamol from aspirin and about indications for use of paracetamol. The same range of potential confounders were collected at age 5 as at age 1 and 3, namely birth order and household size, immunizations, breastfeeding, maternal and paternal history of allergy, child's bed and mattress materials, housing construction materials, household water supply, soap use, method of waste disposal, antibiotic use, indoor fuel use, presence of insecticides and animals in home. To investigate confounding by indication, information on respiratory infection symptoms (cough, fast breathing and fever) were collected, as at year 1 and 3 (see Table S1, Table S2 and Table S3). In addition to the questionnaire, allergen skin tests to *D. pteronyssinus* and cockroach allergen (*Blatella germenica*) (Biodiagnostics, Upton-upon-Severn, UK) were carried out at age 5 using identical methods to those used at age 3[20]. Stool samples were taken from the children for geohelminth, *Helicobacter pylori* and selected intestinal microflora analysis.

Statistical analysis

The data were double-entered into EpiData version 3, cleaned, coded, and merged with the previous datasets using Stata 11 (Statacorp, College Station, TX). For longitudinal analysis, the primary outcome measures were incidence of new-onset wheeze, eczema, rhinitis and positive allergen sensitization between age 3 and 5. To compute the incidence of wheeze, a wheeze-free cohort comprising all children with a negative response to the wheeze questions at age 1 and 3 was selected, and children who reported wheeze at the 5 year follow-up were defined as having new onset wheeze. Incidence of eczema and rhinitis were computed in a similar way, although the rhinitis-free cohort at age 3 was based on responses given at age 3 only as the rhinitis questions were not asked at year 1. A positive skin test was defined as a corrected (allergen minus saline control) mean skin wheal diameter of 3 mm or greater, consistent with our previous work in the same birth cohort[20]. Those children who were negative to both *D. pteronyssinus* and cockroach allergens at age 3 were selected for analysis and new-onset sensitization defined as a positive result to either allergen at age 5 (see Figure 1). A variable called 'early life paracetamol use' representing paracetamol use prior to the disease outcomes was computed, with children categorised as either 'never exposed' (negative response at age 1 and 3), 'exposed at year 1 not at year 3', 'exposed at year 3 not at year 1', or 'persistently exposed' (positive response at age 1 and 3). A second variable 'early life paracetamol dose' was computed as a marker of dose during this time period, with children categorised as 'low exposure' (never reported use in the past month), 'medium exposure' (use in past month at age 1 or 3), or 'high exposure' (use in past month at both time points).

For cross-sectional analysis, the outcomes were wheeze, eczema and rhinitis in the past 12 months as reported at age 5, and sensitization to any allergens at age 5. A marker of lifetime paracetamol exposure ('lifetime paracetamol use') was computed with the categories 'never exposed' (no use in past year reported at age 1, 3 or 5), 'past exposure but not current' (use in past year reported at age 1 or 3 but not 5), 'current exposure with or without past exposure' (use in past year reported at age 5), and 'persistent exposure' (use in past year reported at age 1, 3 and 5). A variable reflecting total lifetime dose was also created by summing responses at each exposure time (year 1, 3 and 5), and categorising as 'never exposed', 'light exposure', 'medium exposure', and 'high exposure.'

For both longitudinal and cross-sectional analyses, multivariate logistic regression was used to compute adjusted odds ratios (OR) and 95% confidence intervals (CI) for each outcome in relation to the paracetamol variables, controlling for *a priori* confounders (area of residence, child's gender, and maternal education). The effect of further control for the other variables collected, including symptoms of respiratory tract infection in the first year of life (see Table S1, Table S2 and Table S3), and other demographic and lifestyle variables collected during pregnancy and birth (birth weight, initiation of breastfeeding, and pre-lacteal feeding) were also explored. These covariates were retained in the model if they altered the odds ratios for the main exposure of interest by more than 10%. Those resulting in a 10% change or above in the size of the exposure effect were retained in the final models. The significance of the association between exposure and outcome in the model was assessed using a likelihood ratio test for the association (LRT) and 95% confidence interval with the corresponding p-value. The significance of the association between exposure and outcome in the model was assessed using the P-value from LRT. Multicollinearity among the explanatory variables was

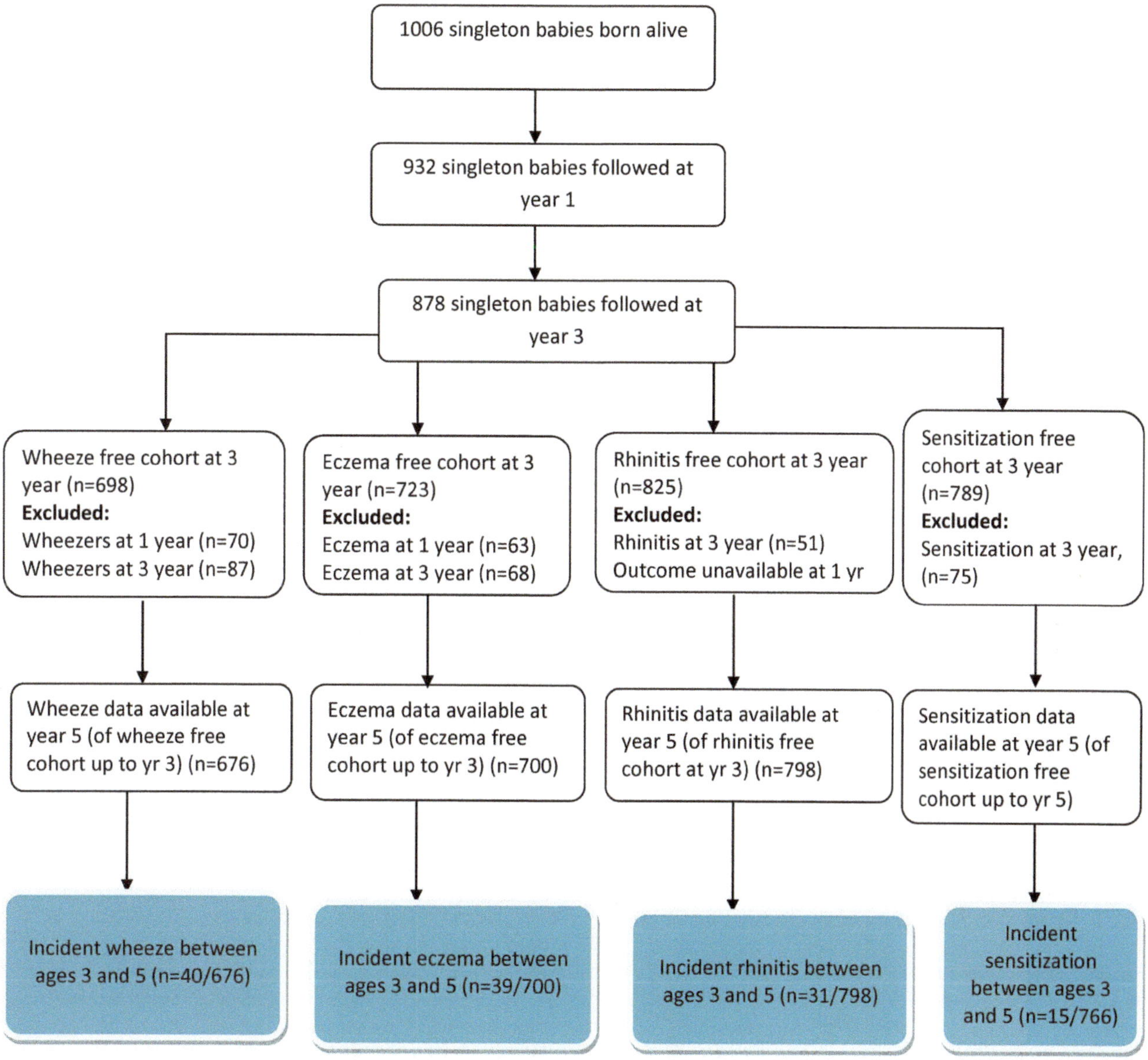

Figure 1. Flow chart showing reporting of symptom outcome measures and sensitization between 1 and 5 years.

assessed and the final model fitted in the absence of any response variable that correlated to any other.

Ethics statement

Ethical approval was granted by the National Ethical Review Committee of the Ethiopian Science and Technology Ministry and the University of Nottingham, UK. Written, informed consent was obtained from the mothers at each visit, or from the next of kin, caretakers, or guardians on behalf of the children enrolled in the study. As the majority of women or caretakers were non-literate, the information sheet and consent form was read to them and they were required to give a finger-print to signify willingness to participate. The ethics committees in Addis Ababa, Ethiopia and Nottingham, UK approved this consent procedure.

Results

Description of the cohort

At year five, 863 children were followed-up, representing 86% of the original cohort (n = 1006) and 98% of those followed-up at age 3 (n = 878) (Fig 1). Of these 863 children, 852 had reported outcome data. Children who were lost to follow up (less than 2% between ages 3 and 5) were not different to those followed in terms of paracetamol exposure or the outcomes collected.

New-onset symptoms and sensitization between ages 3 and 5

Figure 1 shows that new onset wheeze between age 3 and 5 was reported in 5.9% (40/676) of the children with no reported wheeze up to age 3. Among the eczema-free cohort, incident eczema was reported in 5.8% (39/700); in the rhinitis-free cohort, incident rhinitis was reported in 3.9% (31/798); and in children not sensitized at age 3, new sensitization to either *D. pteronyssinus* or cockroach allergen at age 5 was found in 2.0% (15/766) (Figure 1). These incidence risks did not differ by place of residence. Sensitization at age 3 significantly increased the risk of incident eczema (OR = 2.49, 95% CI 1.04 to 5.95) and rhinitis (OR = 2.54, 95% CI 1.00 to 6.45) between ages 3 and 5, but not wheeze (OR = 1.45, 95% CI 0.54 to 3.84) (data not shown).

Relation between potential confounders and allergic symptoms and sensitization

Infant symptoms of respiratory infections (cough, fever, and fast breathing) were significantly positively associated with incident wheeze between ages 3 and 5, but not eczema, whilst fever was positively associated with incident rhinitis and negatively with new onset sensitization (Table S2 and S3). Associations between other potential confounders and outcomes are shown in the (Table S2 and S3).

Paracetamol use

Paracetamol use was commonly reported in the cohort with almost 60% of the children receiving paracetamol in the first three years of life, and over 35% reporting current exposure at age 5 (Table 1, 2, 3, 4). Paracetamol was the analgesic and antipyretic drug of choice among 84% of the birth cohort mothers, and most said it was readily available (77%) and affordable (92%). The majority (78%) of mothers were able to differentiate paracetamol from aspirin. Aspirin avoidance was reported by only 1.4% of the mothers because of asthma, and 1.5% due to other allergic diseases (data not shown). The most common indications for use of paracetamol were fever (31%) and headache (23.6%), with wheeze, cough and allergy indications uncommon (<4% reported each) (see Figure S1).

Longitudinal associations between paracetamol use and incidence of allergic outcomes

Having adjusted for *a priori* confounders, early life paracetamol use was significantly associated with an increased risk of incident eczema and rhinitis between ages 3 and 5 (Table 2 and 3). For incident eczema, ORs for all exposed groups were significantly increased relative to the never exposed (overall p = 0.01), the highest OR being in relation to persistent exposure (OR = 3.96; 95% CI 1.44 to 10.89), and almost as high for exposure at year three but not at year one (OR = 3.75; 95% CI 1.39, 10.12) as for exposure at year one but not year three (OR = 3.11; 95% CI 1.05, 9.18) (Table 2). Similarly, for incident rhinitis, the ORs, all compared with never users, were higher for heavily exposed children (OR = 3.60; 95% CI 1.18, 11.03) and those exposed at age 3 but not age 1 (OR = 3.96; 95% CI 1.35, 11.65) than exposure at age 1 but not age 3 (OR = 2.75; 95% CI 0.82, 9.20; overall p = 0.04; Table 3). For incident wheeze and sensitization, no overall significant effect of the early life paracetamol use variable was seen, although adjusted ORs in relation to persistent exposure (reported use at age 1 and 3) were increased (Tables 1 and 4).

In relation to early life paracetamol dose, significant positive associations were seen for new-onset wheeze, eczema and rhinitis (Tables 1, 2, 3, 4). For wheeze, the OR was increased for high dose exposure only compared to low (adjusted OR = 4.08; 95% CI 1.51, 11.07), whereas for eczema and rhinitis, ORs were increased for medium and high exposure in a more dose dependent manner (p trend = 0.05 and 0.04, respectively; Tables 1, 2, 3). Incident sensitization was increased amongst those with high compared to low exposure (OR = 1.99; 95% CI 0.41, 9.70), but not to the point of statistical significance (Table 4).

Additional control for confounding by respiratory tract infections only marginally reduced the strength of the associations which remained statistically significant (Tables 1, 2, 3, 4). Further adjustment for other potential confounders including environmental and lifestyle factors in Table S2 and Table S3 did not materially alter the associations.

Cross-sectional associations between paracetamol and allergic outcomes at age 5

Tables 1, 2, 3, 4 show significant positive effects of 'lifetime paracetamol use' on the prevalence of all outcomes, except sensitization, at age 5. ORs, adjusted for *a priori* confounders, were increased for all exposure categories, but tended to be highest in relation to persistent use (adjusted ORs ranging from 6.1 to 12.6) and least elevated in the children exposed in the past but not currently (adjusted ORs ranging from 1.7 to 4.1). Analyses of the lifetime paracetamol dose variable revealed significant dose dependent associations for all symptom outcomes (p<0.01) and a borderline significant association for sensitization (p = 0.06). Further adjustment for potential confounders, including symptoms of current respiratory tract infections, did not materially alter these cross-sectional associations.

Discussion

We have found an adverse effect of early paracetamol use on risk of incident wheeze, with the heaviest users of paracetamol in the first three years of life having a nearly four-fold increased risk of new onset wheeze between age 3 and 5 compared to never users. We have also found strong and consistent adverse effects on incident eczema, not found at our previous follow-up[9], with increased risks not just restricted to the heaviest or most persistent users. For the first time, we were able to look at incident rhinitis and sensitization, revealing associations in the expected direction and of borderline significance for rhinitis but not reaching significance for sensitization. Our longitudinal findings are supported by significant, positive effects on all outcomes in cross-sectional analyses with clearer dose-response patterns seen and the advantage of greater statistical power.

An important strength of this study is the prospective design, with exposures measured prior to the onset of the outcomes, thereby helping to exclude reverse causation as a possible explanation. The design also allowed timing of exposures to be explored, and in particular, the relative importance of exposure in the first year of life, thought to be the important window of life in terms of immune development[21]. Contrary to this hypothesis, we observed equally large adverse effects on new onset disease amongst those exposed only in the second and third year of life; this also suggests that effects of personal exposure are not simply being driven by confounding by *in utero* exposure. Selection bias is unlikely to be important since we have used a population-based unselected birth cohort and only 6% of surviving mother-child dyads were lost to follow-up between birth and age 5. The low income rural setting of the cohort also has the advantage of reducing exposure misclassification since multiple formulations of paracetamol and other non-aspirin non-steroidal anti-inflammatory drugs (NSAIDs) are uncommon. Consistent with previous research in this setting[8], we found the mothers' ability to distinguish between paracetamol and aspirin to be high (78%), and reported aspirin avoidance due to awareness of contraindications in asthma to be very low (2%). A further strength of the study was control for multiple potential confounders including confounding by indication which can arise if children with early life respiratory tract infections, who may also be more susceptible to subsequently

Table 1. Univariate and multivariate analysis of wheeze in relation to early and lifetime use of paracetamol up to the age of 5.

Longitudinal analysis (N=676)

	Wheeze never up to age 3 (N=676)						
Exposure at age 1 and 3 yr	**Overall N (%)**	**n (%) new wheeze**	**Crude OR (95% CI)**	**Adjusted OR[*] (95% CI)**	**P-value**	**Further adjusted OR[†] (95% CI)**	**P-value**
Early life paracetamol use[£]					0.18[‡]		0.26[‡]
Never exposed	287 (42.5)	13 (4.5)	1	1		1	
Exposed at yr 1, but not at yr3	120 (17.8)	4 (3.3)	0.73 (0.23,2.78)	0.73 (0.23,2.31)		0.62 (0.20,1.96)	
Exposed at yr 3, but not at yr 1	155 (22.9)	12 (7.7)	1.77 (0.79,3.98)	1.63 (0.72,3.70)		1.49 (0.65,3.39)	
Persistently exposed	114 (16.9)	11 (9.7)	2.25 (0.98,5.18)	2.09 (0.90,4.86)		1.72 (0.74,4.03)	
Early life paracetamol dose[Σ]					0.04[‡]		0.05[‡]
Low exposure	436 (64.5)	23 (5.3)	1	1	0.05[¶]	1	0.11[¶]
Medium exposure	208 (30.8)	11 (5.3)	1.00 (0.48,2.10)	1.04 (0.50,2.19)		0.92 (0.44,1.95)	
High exposure	32 (4.7)	6 (18.8)	4.14 (1.56,11.06)	4.08 (1.51,11.07)		3.64 (1.34,9.90)	

Cross-sectional analysis (N=852)

Exposure at age 1,3 and yr 5	**Overall N (%)**	**Wheeze N (%)**	**Crude OR (95% CI)**	**Adjusted OR[*] (95% CI)**	**P-value**	**Further adjusted OR[†] (95% CI)**	**P-value**
Lifetime paracetamol use[β]					<0.01[‡]		0.01[‡]
Never exposed	258 (30.4)	4 (1.6)	1	1		1	
Past exposure but not current	285 (33.6)	10 (3.5)	2.31 (0.72,7.45)	2.38 (0.73,7.75)		2.14 (0.65,7.04)	
Current exposure ± past exposure	207 (24.4)	10 (4.8)	3.22 (1.00,10.43)	3.14 (0.97,10.20)		1.81 (0.54,6.05)	
Persistently exposed	98 (11.6)	13 (13.3)	9.71 (3.08,30.59)	10.29 (3.19,33.19)		5.87 (1.76,19.62)	
Lifetime paracetamol dose[±]					<0.01[‡]		0.01[‡]
Never exposed	258 (30.4)	4 (1.6)	1	1	<0.01[¥]	1	<0.01[¥]
Light exposure	286 (33.7)	8 (2.8)	1.83 (0.54,6.14)	1.83 (0.54,6.20)		1.50 (0.44,5.13)	
Medium exposure	190 (22.4)	11 (5.8)	3.90 (1.22,12.45)	3.90 (1.22,12.47)		2.55 (0.78,8.35)	
High exposure	114 (13.4)	14 (12.3)	8.89 (2.86,27.66)	8.96 (2.85,28.23)		5.03 (1.54,16.37)	

*ORs adjusted for child's gender, area of residence and maternal education.
[†]ORs adjusted for child's gender, area of residence and maternal education and additionally adjusted for symptoms of respiratory infections in the first year of life (and for cross-sectional analysis reported infection at year 5).
[‡]Overall p-value (likelihood ratio test).
[¶]P value for trend computed for dose of paracetamol use in the past month: low exposure (never reported use in the past month), medium exposure (use in past month at age 1 & 3), high exposure (use in past month at both time points).
[¥]P value for trend as dose of paracetamol computed using a composite score of paracetamol exposure from yr 1, 3 and 5
[£]Early life paracetamol use: refers to use prior to the disease outcomes (i.e. first three years of life).
[Σ]Early life paracetamol dose: refers to dose of exposure in past month in first three years of life prior to disease outcomes.
[β]Lifetime paracetamol use: refers to use of paracetamol up to the age of 5 (i.e. ages 1, 3 and 5).
[±]Lifetime paracetamol dose: refers to dose of paracetamol exposure up to the age of 5 (i.e. ages 1, 3 and 5).

Table 2. Univariate and multivariate analysis of eczema in relation to early and lifetime use of paracetamol up to the age of 5.

Longitudinal analysis (N = 700)

	Eczema never up to age 3 (N = 700)						
Exposure at age 1 and 3 yr	**Overall N (%)**	**n (%) new eczema**	**Crude OR (95% CI)**	**Adjusted OR[*] (95% CI)**	**P-value**	**Further adjusted OR[†] (95% CI)**	**P-value**
Early life paracetamol use[£]					0.01[‡]		0.02[‡]
Never exposed	275 (39.3)	6 (2.2)	1	1		1	
Exposed at yr 1, but not at yr3	123 (17.6)	8 (6.5)	3.12 (1.06,9.19)	3.11 (1.05,9.18)		3.01 (1.00,9.04)	
Exposed at yr 3, but not at yr 1	161 (23.0)	13 (8.1)	3.94 (1.47,10.58)	3.75 (1.39,10.12)		3.70 (1.37,10.01)	
Persistently exposed	141 (20.1)	12 (8.5)	4.17 (1.53,11.36)	3.96 (1.44,10.89)		3.82 (1.36,10.73)	
Early life paracetamol dose[Σ]					0.04[‡]		0.08[‡]
Low exposure	423 (60.4)	16 (3.8)	1	1	0.05[¶]	1	0.06[¶]
Medium exposure	230 (32.9)	20 (8.7)	2.42 (1.23,4.77)	2.39 (1.21,4.71)		2.31 (1.16,4.60)	
High exposure	47 (6.7)	3 (6.4)	1.73 (0.49,6.19)	1.65 (0.46,5.93)		1.59 (0.44,5.74)	

Cross-sectional analysis (N = 852)

Exposure at age 1,3 and yr 5	**Overall N (%)**	**Eczema n (%)**	**Crude OR (95% CI)**	**Adjusted OR[*] (95% CI)**	**P-value**	**Further adjusted OR[†] (95% CI)**	**P-value**
Lifetime paracetamol use[β]					<0.01[‡]		<0.01[‡]
Never exposed	258 (30.4)	4 (1.6)	1	1		1	
Past exposure but not current	285 (33.6)	7 (2.5)	1.60 (0.46,5.53)	1.66 (0.48,5.76)		1.61 (0.46,5.61)	
Current exposure ± past exposure	207 (24.4)	17 (8.2)	5.68 (1.88,17.16)	6.00 (1.98,18.19)		5.29 (1.67,16.80)	
Persistently exposed	98 (11.6)	8 (8.2)	5.64 (1.66,19.20)	6.12 (1.77,21.13)		5.40 (1.50,19.45)	
Lifetime paracetamol dose[†]					<0.01[‡]		0.01[‡]
Never exposed	258 (30.4)	4 (1.6)	1	1	<0.01[¥]	1	<0.01[¥]
Light exposure	286 (33.7)	11 (3.9)	2.54 (0.80,8.08)	2.71 (0.85,8.66)		2.53 (0.79,8.13)	
Medium exposure	190 (22.4)	9 (4.7)	3.16 (0.96,10.41)	3.26 (0.98,10.77)		2.78 (0.82,9.45)	
High exposure	114 (13.4)	12 (10.5)	7.47 (2.35,23.70)	8.27 (2.57,26.58)		6.70 (1.99,22.54)	

*ORs adjusted for child's gender, area of residence and maternal education.
[†]ORs adjusted for child's gender, area of residence and maternal education and additionally adjusted for symptoms of respiratory infections in the first year of life (and for cross-sectional analysis reported infection at year 5).
[‡]Overall p-value (likelihood ratio test).
[¶]P value for trend computed for dose of paracetamol use in the past month: low exposure (never reported use in the past month), medium exposure (use in past month at age 1 & 3), high exposure (use in past month at both time points).
[¥]P value for trend as dose of paracetamol computed using a composite score of paracetamol exposure from yr 1, 3 and 5.
[£]Early life paracetamol use: refers to use prior to the disease outcomes (i.e. first three years of life).
[Σ]Early life paracetamol dose: refers to dose of exposure in past month in first three years of life prior to disease outcomes.
[β]Lifetime paracetamol use: refers to use of paracetamol up to the age of 5 (i.e. ages 1, 3 and 5).
[±]Lifetime paracetamol dose: refers to dose of paracetamol exposure up to the age of 5 (i.e. ages 1, 3 and 5).

Table 3. Univariate and multivariate analysis of rhinitis in relation to early and lifetime use of paracetamol up to the age of 5.

Longitudinal analysis (N = 798)

	Rhinitis never up to age 3 (N = 798)						
Exposure at age 1 and 3 yr	**Overall N (%)**	**n (%) new rhinitis**	**Crude OR (95% CI)**	**Adjusted OR[*] (95% CI)**	**P-value**	**Further adjusted OR[†] (95% CI)**	**P-value**
Early life paracetamol use[£]					0.04[‡]		0.07[‡]
Never exposed	319 (40.0)	5 (1.6)	1	1		1	
Exposed at yr 1, but not at yr3	138 (17.3)	6 (4.4)	2.85 (0.86,9.52)	2.75 (0.82,9.20)		2.42 (0.72,8.14)	
Exposed at yr 3, but not at yr 1	182 (22.8)	11 (6.0)	4.04 (1.38,11.82)	3.96 (1.35,11.65)		3.74 (1.27,11.04)	
Persistently exposed	159 (19.9)	9 (5.7)	3.77 (1.24,11.44)	3.60 (1.18,11.03)		3.10 (1.00,9.57)	
Early life paracetamol dose[Σ]					0.10[‡]		0.18[‡]
Low exposure	485 (60.8)	13 (2.7)	1	1	0.04[¶]	1	0.07[¶]
Medium exposure	258 (32.3)	14 (5.4)	2.08 (0.96,4.50)	2.07 (0.95,4.47)		1.90 (0.87,4.12)	
High exposure	55 (6.9)	4 (7.3)	2.85 (0.90,9.06)	2.61 (0.82,8.39)		2.31 (0.72,7.46)	

Cross-sectional analysis (N = 852)

Exposure at age 1,3 and yr 5	**Overall N (%)**	**Rhinitis n (%)**	**Crude OR (95% CI)**	**Adjusted OR[*] (95% CI)**	**P-value**	**Further adjusted OR[†] (95% CI)**	**P-value**
Lifetime paracetamol use[β]					<0.01[‡]		0.07[‡]
Never exposed	258 (30.4)	2 (0.9)	1	1		1	
Past exposure but not current	285 (33.6)	9 (3.2)	4.17 (0.89,19.50)	4.10 (0.87,19.21)		3.60 (0.76,17.01)	
Current exposure ± past exposure	207 (24.4)	11 (5.3)	7.18 (1.57, 32.78)	7.09 (1.55,32.38)		3.82 (0.82,17.82)	
Persistently exposed	98 (11.6)	9 (9.2)	12.94 (2.74,61.05)	12.58 (2.63,60.02)		6.59 (1.34,32.35)	
Lifetime paracetamol dose[†]					<0.01[‡]		0.01[‡]
Never exposed	258 (30.4)	2 (0.9)	1	1	<0.01[¥]	1	<0.01[¥]
Light exposure	286 (33.7)	7 (2.5)	3.21 (0.66,15.60)	3.16 (0.65,15.38)		2.48 (0.50,12.25)	
Medium exposure	190 (22.4)	10 (5.3)	7.11 (1.54,32.84)	7.01 (1.52,32.44)		4.36 (0.93,20.55)	
High exposure	114 (13.4)	12 (10.5)	15.06 (3.31,68.47)	14.66 (3.20,67.10)		7.65 (1.63,35.97)	

*ORs adjusted for child's gender, area of residence and maternal education.
[†]ORs adjusted for child's gender, area of residence and maternal education and additionally adjusted for symptoms of respiratory infections in the first year of life (and for cross-sectional analysis reported infection at year 5).
[‡]Overall p-value (likelihood ratio test).
[¶]P value for trend computed for dose of paracetamol use in the past month: low exposure (never reported use in the past month), medium exposure (use in past month at age 1 & 3), high exposure (use in past month at both time points).
[¥]P value for trend as dose of paracetamol computed using a composite score of paracetamol exposure from yr 1, 3 and 5.
[£]Early life paracetamol use: refers to use prior to the disease outcomes (i.e. first three years of life).
[Σ]Early life paracetamol dose: refers to dose of exposure in past month in first three years of life prior to disease outcomes.
[β]Lifetime paracetamol use: refers to use of paracetamol up to the age of 5 (i.e. ages 1, 3 and 5).
[±]Lifetime paracetamol dose: refers to dose of paracetamol exposure up to the age of 5 (i.e. ages 1, 3 and 5).

Table 4. Univariate and multivariate analysis of sensitization in relation to early and lifetime use of paracetamol up to the age of 5.

Longitudinal analysis (N=766)

	Sensitization never up to age 3 (N=766)						
Exposure at age 1 and 3 yr	**Overall N (%)**	**n (%) new atopy**	**Crude OR (95% CI)**	**Adjusted OR[*] (95% CI)**	**P-value**	**Further adjusted OR[†] (95% CI)**	**P-value**
Early life paracetamol use[£]					0.78[‡]		0.59[‡]
Never exposed	290 (38.0)	5 (1.7)	1	1		1	
Exposed at yr 1, but not at yr3	133 (17.4)	2 (1.5)	0.87 (0.17,4.54)	0.85 (0.16,4.42)		1.13 (0.21,6.23)	
Exposed at yr 3, but not at yr 1	176 (23.0)	3 (1.7)	0.99 (0.23,4.19)	0.98 (0.23,4.17)		1.09 (0.25,4.70)	
Persistently exposed	165 (21.6)	5 (3.0)	1.78 (0.51,6.25)	1.73 (0.49,6.11)		2.48 (0.63,9.76)	
Early life paracetamol dose[Σ]					0.72[‡]		0.57[‡]
Low exposure	446 (58.4)	8 (1.8)	1	1	0.51[¶]	1	0.31[¶]
Medium exposure	264 (34.6)	5 (1.9)	1.06 (0.34,3.26)	1.05 (0.34,3.26)		1.26 (0.40,4.04)	
High exposure	54 (7.1)	2 (3.7)	2.11 (0.44,10.18)	1.99 (0.41,9.70)		2.59 (0.50,13.29)	

Cross-sectional analysis (N=841)

Exposure at age 1,3 and yr 5	**Overall N (%)**	**Atopy n (%)**	**Crude OR (95% CI)**	**Adjusted OR[*] (95% CI)**	**P-value**	**Further adjusted OR[†] (95% CI)**	**P-value**
Lifetime paracetamol use[β]					0.54[‡]		0.46[‡]
Never exposed	254 (30.2)	4 (1.6)	1	1		1	
Past exposure but not current	283 (33.7)	5 (1.8)	1.12 (0.30,4.23)	1.15 (0.30,4.39)		1.19 (0.31,4.53)	
Current exposure ± past exposure	206 (24.5)	4 (1.9)	1.24 (0.31, 5.01)	1.26 (0.31,5.12)		1.48 (0.34,6.44)	
Persistently exposed	98 (11.7)	4 (4.1)	2.66 (0.65,10.85)	2.83 (0.68,11.86)		3.35 (0.74,15.11)	
Lifetime paracetamol dose[†]					0.13[‡]		0.09[‡]
Never exposed	254 (30.2)	4 (1.6)	1	1	0.06[¥]	1	0.04[¥]
Light exposure	285 (33.9)	4 (1.4)	0.89 (0.22,3.59)	0.93 (0.23,3.78)		0.99 (0.24,4.06)	
Medium exposure	189 (22.5)	3 (1.6)	1.01 (0.22,4.56)	1.01 (0.22,4.58)		1.20 (0.25,5.64)	
High exposure	113 (13.4)	6 (5.3)	3.50 (0.97,12.67)	3.71 (1.01,13.68)		4.80 (1.17,19.68)	

*ORs adjusted for child's gender, area of residence and maternal education.
[†]ORs adjusted for child's gender, area of residence and maternal education and additionally adjusted for symptoms of respiratory infections in the first year of life (and for cross-sectional analysis reported infection at year 5).
[‡]Overall p-value (likelihood ratio test).
[¶]P value for trend computed for dose of paracetamol use in the past month: low exposure (never reported use in the past month), medium exposure (use in past month at age 1 3), high exposure (use in past month at both time points).
[¥]P value for trend as dose of paracetamol computed using a composite score of paracetamol exposure from yr 1, 3 and 5.
[£]Early life paracetamol use: refers to use prior to the disease outcomes (i.e. first three years of life).
[Σ]Early life paracetamol dose: refers to dose of exposure in past month in first three years of life prior to disease outcomes.
[β]Lifetime paracetamol use: refers to use of paracetamol up to the age of 5 (i.e. ages 1, 3 and 5).
[±]Lifetime paracetamol dose: refers to dose of paracetamol exposure up to the age of 5 (i.e. ages 1, 3 and 5).

develop asthma and allergic conditions[22], are given paracetamol for symptoms of these infections. We have found that our associations generally persisted after control for such symptoms in the first year of life, though the magnitudes of effect were slightly reduced.

A potential limitation of the study is that misclassification of symptom outcomes may have arisen through the use of a questionnaire. However, the increased risk of new onset symptom outcomes in relation to sensitization at the age of 3 consistent with our previous findings[18], implies the dominance of an allergic phenotype in the cohort. The questionnaire was administered by individuals known to the mothers, and used common local terms (for example '*sit sit*' for wheezing symptoms, an onomatopoeic local term) which should increase the accuracy of reporting.

Our findings fit with a recent meta-analysis of studies reporting a 63% increased risk of asthma associated with paracetamol use in children and adults[6]. Prospective evidence comes primarily from a handful of studies showing a positive relation between paracetamol exposure *in utero*, particularly in late pregnancy, and the risk of allergic diseases in childhood [13,23,24]. A recent meta-analysis of the available observational studies reporting exposure *in utero* and risk of childhood wheeze demonstrated a pooled OR of 1.21 (95% CI, 1.02, 1.44), irrespective of gestational age[7], which also fits with the previous meta-analysis that reported a pooled odds ratio of 1.50[6]. The only longitudinal study of personal intake in children reported an increased risk of wheeze in relation to paracetamol use in early life but, unlike in our study, the association did not remain after adjustment for respiratory tract infections[15]. However bias associated with over-adjustment in the model is difficult to exclude and since the children studied had parents with asthma and allergy[15], the associations may be confounded by genetic susceptibility. Randomised controlled trials (RCT) are scarce although one comparing paracetamol with ibuprofen showed children who took paracetamol had higher rates of outpatient visits for asthma than those taking ibuprofen[25]. However, the trial was not placebo-controlled and a true effect is difficult to untangle[25].

Evidence from *in vivo* and *in vitro* investigations supports these epidemiological observations. Therapeutic doses of paracetamol have been shown to reduce serum total antioxidant capacity within 14 days[26], possibly through a reduction in glutathione (GSH) levels[26,27], with the lung bearing the brunt of this depletion, which predisposes it to toxic agents[28]. Glutathione depletion may also cause a shift from Th_1 to Th_2 cytokine production favouring allergic disorders[29]. Paracetamol may also contribute to the increased risk of asthma and COPD, via its reactive metabolite NAPQI through TRPA1-dependent neurogenic inflammatory responses in the airways[30].

In conclusion, we have found that early life exposure to paracetamol increases the risks of wheeze and allergic disease in a developing country birth cohort in which alternative explanations, including reverse causation and confounding by indication, are unlikely to play a role. As most of the evidence to date comes from observational studies, an RCT is needed to generate definitive evidence before reviewing use in children. The questions that need to be addressed in RCTs are whether paracetamol causes asthma, and whether paracetamol exacerbates asthma. Designs for these might present ethical dilemmas, since the former ideally requires a controlled trial in pregnancy (or in children) and the latter a design in which the hypothesis is that active treatment makes asthma worse; the alternative might therefore be trial designs involving withdrawal of paracetamol in relevant groups using non-aspirin NSAIDs analgesics as placebo.

Supporting Information

Figure S1 Indications for child's use of paracetamol at the age of 5 year.

Table S1 Summary of relevant variables collected at different time points in the cohort.

Table S2 Distribution of potential confounders in the first year of life in relation to incident symptoms outcomes between ages 3 and 5.

Table S3 Distribution of potential confounders in the first year of life in relation to incident sensitization between ages 3 and 5.

Acknowledgments

We are grateful to the mothers and children who participated in the Butajira birth cohort, and generously provided information, and the data collectors who have followed them from pregnancy until 5 years after birth.

Author Contributions

Conceived and designed the experiments: AA AV GD JB. Performed the experiments: AA GM CH AV GD JB. Analyzed the data: AA AV GD JB. Contributed reagents/materials/analysis tools: AA GM CH AV GD JB. Wrote the paper: AA GM CH AV GD JB.

References

1. Eder W, Ege MJ, von Mutius E (2006) The Asthma Epidemic. *N Engl J Med*; 355(21):2226–2235.
2. Yemaneberhan H, Bekele Z, Venn A, Lewis S, Parry E, et al. (1997) Prevalence of wheeze and asthma and relation to atopy in urban and rural Ethiopia. *Lancet*; 350(9071):85–90.
3. Asher MI, Montefort S, Bjorksten B, Lai CKW, Strachan DP, et al. (2006) Worldwide time trends in the prevalence of symptoms of asthma, allergic rhinoconjunctivitis, and eczema in childhood: ISAAC Phases One and Three repeat multicountry cross-sectional surveys. *Lancet*; 368(9537):733–743.
4. Moffat MF, Gut IG, Demenais F, Strachan DP, Bouzigon E, et al. (2010) A Large-Scale, Consortium-Based Genome wide Association Study of Asthma. *N Engl J Med*; 363(13):1211–1221.
5. Ege MJ, Mayer M, Normand AC, Genuneit J, Cookson W, et al. (2011) Exposure to Environmental Microorganisms and Childhood Asthma. *N Engl J Med*; 364(8):701–709.
6. Etminan M., Sadatsafavi M., Jafari S, Doyle-Waters M, FitzGerald JM (2009) Acetaminophen use and the risk of asthma in children and adults. A systematic review and meta analysis. *Chest*; 136:1316–1323.
7. Eyers S, Weatherall M, Jefferies S, Beasley R (2011) Paracetamol in pregnancy and the risk of wheezing in offspring: a systematic review and meta-analysis. *Clin Exp Allergy*; 41(4):482–489.
8. Davey G, Berhane Y, Duncan P, ref-Adib G, Britton J, et al. (2005) Use of acetaminophen and the risk of self-reported allergic symptoms and skin sensitization in Butajira, Ethiopia. *J Allergy Clin Immunol*; 116(4):863–868.
9. Amberbir A, Medhin G, Alem A, Britton J, Davey G, et al. (2011) The role of acetaminophen and geohelminth infection on the incidence of wheeze and eczema: a longitudinal birth-cohort study. *Am J Respir Crit Care Med*; 183(2):165–170.
10. Farquhar H, Stewart A, Mitchell E, Crane J, Eyers S, et al. (2010) The role of paracetamol in the pathogenesis of asthma. *Clin Exp Allergy*; 40:32–41.
11. Beasley RW, Clayton TO, Crane J, Crane J, Lai CKW, et al. (2011) Acetaminophen use and risk of asthma, rhinoconjunctivitis, and eczema in adolescents: International Study of Asthma and Allergies in Childhood Phase Three. *Am J Respir Crit Care Med*; 183(2):171–178.
12. Beasley R, Clayton T, Crane J, von Mutius E, Lai CKW, et al. (2008) Association between paracetamol use in infancy and childhood, and risk of asthma, rhinoconjunctivitis, and eczema in children aged 6–7 years: analysis from Phase Three of the ISAAC programme. *Lancet*; 372(9643):1039–1048.

13. Shaheen SO, Newson RB, Sherriff A, Henderson AJ, Heron JE, et al. (2002) Paracetamol use in pregnancy and wheezing in early childhood. *Thorax*; 57(11):958–963.
14. Barr RG, Wentowski CC, Curhan GC, Somers SC, Stampfer MJ, et al. (2004) Prospective study of acetaminophen use and newly diagnosed asthma among women. *Am J Respir Crit Care Med*; 169(7):836–841.
15. Lowe AJ, Carlin JB, Bennett CM, Hosking CS, Allen KJ, et al (2010). Paracetamol use in early life and asthma: prospective birth cohort study. *BMJ*; 341(c4616).
16. Berhane Y, Wall S, Kebede D, Emmelin A, Enquselassie F, et al. (1999) Establishing an epidemiological field laboratory in rural areas-potential for public health research and interventions. Ethiop J Health Dev; 13:1–47.
17. Hanlon C, Medhin G, Alem A, Tesfaye F, Lakew Z, et al. (2009) Impact of antenatal common mental disorders upon perinatal outcomes in Ethiopia: the P-MaMiE population-based cohort study. *Trop Med Int Health*; 14(2):156–166.
18. Belyhun Y, Amberbir A, Medhin G, Erko B, Hanlon C, et al. (2010) Prevalence and risk factors of wheeze and eczema in one year old children: the Butajira birth cohort, Ethiopia. *Clin Exp Allergy*; (40):619–626.
19. Asher MI, Keil U, Anderson HR, Beasley R, Crane J, et al. (1995) International Study of Asthma and Allergies in Childhood (ISAAC): Rationale and methods. *Eur Respir J*; 8:483–491.
20. Amberbir A, Medhin G, Erku W, Alem A, Simms R, et al. (2011) Effects of Helicobacter pylori, geohelminth infection and selected commensal bacteria on the risk of allergic disease and sensitization in 3-year-old Ethiopian children. Clin Exp Allergy; 41(10):1422–1430.
21. Prescott SL, Macaubas C, Smallacombe T, Holt BJ, Sly PD, et al. (1999) Development of allergen-specific T-cell memory in atopic and normal children. *Lancet*; 353(9148):196–200.
22. Illi S, von Mutius E, Lau S, Bergmann, Niggemann B, et al. (2001) Early childhood infectious diseases and the development of asthma up to school age: a birth cohort study. *BMJ*; 322(7283):390–395.
23. Rebordosa C, Kogevinas M, Sorensen HT, Olsen J (2008) Pre-natal exposure to paracetamol and risk of wheezing and asthma in children: A birth cohort study. *Int J Epidemiol*; 37(3):583–590.
24. Perzanowski MS, Miller RL, Ali DB, Garfinkel RS, Chew GL, et al. (2008) Prenatal acetaminophen use is a risk for wheeze at age 5 years in a low income urban population with a high risk for asthma. *J Allergy Clin Immunol*; (Supp 1):S231.
25. Lesko SM, Louik C, Vezina RM, Mitchell AA (2002) Asthma morbidity after the short-term use of ibuprofen in children. *Pediatrics*; 109(2):e20.
26. Nuttall SL, Khan JN, Thorpe GH, Langford N, Kendall MJ (2003) The impact of therapeutic doses of paracetamol on serum total antioxidant capacity. *J Clin Pharm Ther*; 28(4):289–294.
27. Nuttall SL, Williams J, Kendall MJ (2003)Does paracetamol cause asthma? *J Clin Pharm Ther*; 28(4):251–257.
28. Micheli L, Cerretani D, Fiaschi A, Gioorgi G, Romeo R, et al. (1994) Effect of acetaminophen on glutathione levels in rat testis and lung. *Environ Health Perspect*; (Supp 9):63–64.
29. Peterson JD, Herzenberg LA, Vasquez K, Waltenbaugh C (1998) Glutathione levels in antigen-presenting cells modulate Th1 versus Th2 response patterns. Proceedings of the National Academy of Sciences of the United States of America; 95(6):3071–3076.
30. Nassini R, Materazzi S, Andre E, Sartiani L, Aldini G, et al. (2010) Acetaminophen, via its reactive metabolite N-acetyl-p-benzo-quinoneimine and transient receptor potential ankyrin-1 stimulation, causes neurogenic inflammation in the airways and other tissues in rodents. *FASEB J*; 24(12):4904–4916

19

The Association between Polymorphisms in the MRPL4 and TNF-α Genes and Susceptibility to Allergic Rhinitis

1

Xin Wei[1,2,3], Yuan Zhang[1,2], Zheng Fu[3], Luo Zhang[1,2]*

Department of Otolaryngology, Head and Neck Surgery, Beijing Tongren Hospital, Capital Medical University, Beijing, PR China, **2** Key Laboratory of Otolaryngology, Head and Neck Surgery (Ministry of Education of China), Beijing Institute of Otorhinolaryngology, Beijing, PR China, **3** Department of Otolaryngology, Head and Neck Surgery, People's Hospital of Hainan Province, Haikou, PR China

Abstract

Background: Allergic rhinitis (AR) is a chronic inflammatory disease of the nasal mucosa, involving a complex interaction between genetic and environmental factors. Evidence suggests that polymorphisms in the gene coding for mitochondrial ribosomal protein L4 (MRPL4), located in close proximity to intercellular adhesion molecule-1 (ICAM-1) gene on chromosome location 19p13.2, may influence the risk factor for the development of AR.

Objective: The aim of our study was to investigate any association between AR susceptibility and polymorphisms in ICAM-1 gene, as well as associations between AR risk and polymorphisms in MRPL4, nuclear factor-kappaB (NF-κB) and tumor necrosis factor alpha(TNF-α) genes, associated with ICAM-1 expression.

Methods: A cohort of 414 patients with AR and 293 healthy controls was enrolled from the Han Chinese population in Beijing, China. Blood was drawn for DNA extraction and total serum immunoglobulin E (IgE). A total of 14 single nucleotide polymorphisms (SNPs) in ICAM-1, NF-κB, TNF-α, and MRPL4 genes were selected using the CHB genotyping data from the International Haplotype Mapping (HapMap) and assessed for differences in frequencies of the alleles and genotypes between the AR patients and control subjects.

Results: TNF-α SNP rs1799964 and MRPL4 SNP rs11668618 were found to occur in significantly greater frequencies in the AR group compared to control group. There were no significant associations between SNPs in NF-κB, ICAM-1 and AR. The SNP-SNP interaction information analysis further indicated that there were no synergistic effects among the selected sets of polymorphisms.

Conclusions: Our results suggest a strong association between AR risk and polymorphisms of MRPL4 and TNF-α genes in Han Chinese population.

Editor: Andrew Dewan, Yale School of Public Health, United States of America

Funding: This work was supported by grants from the National Science Fund for Distinguished Young Scholars (81025007), the National Natural Science Foundation of China (30973282 and 81100706), the Beijing Natural Science Foundation (7102030), the Special Fund of Sanitation Elite Reconstruction of Beijing (2009-2-007), the Beijing Science and Technology program (Z111107055311040 and KZ201110025027), and the Beijing Nova Program (2010B022) to LZ, YZ and DH, and Hainan Provincial Health Department program (2011K-19) to XW. The funders had no role in study design, data collection and analysis, decision to publish, or preparation of the manuscript.

Competing Interests: The authors have declared that no competing interests exist.

* E-mail: dr.luozhang@gmail.com

These authors contributed equally to this work.

Introduction

Allergic rhinitis (AR) is a chronic inflammatory disease of the nasal mucosa, which is caused by a complex interaction between genetic and environmental factors involving allergen-IgE-mediated stimulation of a variety of immune competent cells and release or expression of a variety of proinflammatory cytokines and mediators in allergen-sensitized individuals. AR morbidity varies from10%to25% in different regions and countries; with around 11. 1% of the population in China being affected according to a telephone questionnaire survey [1].

A first genome-wide association study for atopy and AR conducted in a cohort of Chinese volunteers in Singapore has recently indicated that there may be an association between susceptibility to atopy and/or AR and polymorphisms in two candidate genes; i) the *MRPL4* gene coding for the 39S mitochondrial ribosomal protein L4 and ii) the *BCAP* gene coding for the cytosolic B-cell adapter for phosphatidylinositol 3-kinase (BCAP) [2].In this respect the MRPL4 gene is of particular interest as it is locatedonchromosomelocation19p13.2, with the gene coding for intercellular adhesion molecule-1 (ICAM-1),which plays a key role in allergic disease [3,4].One study investigated the relationship between the severity of disease and the levels of serum soluble ICAM-1 (sICAM-1) and expression of ICAM-1 in nasal mucosa of patients with persistent allergic rhinitis, and demonstrated that both serum sICAM-1 levels and nasal ICAM-1 expression were significantly higher in patients with moderate-to-severe rhinitis, compared to patients with mild rhinitis [5]. A more recent study by Li and colleagues has demonstrated that nasal saline irrigation as an adjunct treatment to tapered topical steroid treatment after 8 and 12 weeks in children with AR resulted in significantly decreased concentrations of sICAM-1 in nasal secretions accompanied by significant improvements in symptoms with lower concentrations of topical steroid.

Despite the well-documented role of ICAM-1 in AR, the mechanism/s underlying the regulation of ICAM-1 in allergic diseases is still not clear. Zhao and colleagues have shown that the expression of both the transcription factor nuclear factor-kappaB (NF-κB) and ICAM-1wassignificantly higher in patients with AR compared with non-rhinitic control subjects and that the expression of ICAM-1 mRNA was significantly correlated with the expression of NF-κB [6]. Another study has demonstrated that tumour necrosis factor alpha(TNF-α)significantly increased the expression of ICAM-1 gene expression in cultured human nasal epithelia cells *in vitro* and that the TNF-mediated-ICAM-1 mRNA and ICAM-1 surface expression at 48 h was significantly inhibited by incubation with human recombinant soluble TNF receptor I and dexamethasone [7]. To our knowledge, the association between ICAM-1 gene polymorphisms and predisposition of an individual to AR has not been reported to date. The aim of our study was therefore to investigate any associations between polymorphisms in ICAM-1 gene, in a Han Chinese cohort. Furthermore, we aimed to investigate associations between polymorphisms in MRPL4, NF-κB and TNF-α gene, which may influence ICAM-1 expression, and AR susceptibility in this cohort.

Materials and Methods

Study Subjects

414 outpatients (239 males and 175 females) with AR were recruited prospectively from the Otorhinolaryngology department of the people's hospital of Hainan province from February 2010 to February 2011. 293 healthy volunteers with ethnically similar background were also recruited from the local population as controls to determine background allele frequencies in the population.

Patients with a documented history of AR were included if they fulfilled all the criteria of the Allergic Rhinitis and its Impact on Asthma(ARIA) guidelines [8], including 1) demonstration of persistent or discontinuous symptoms of anterior rhinorrhoea, continuous sneezing, nasal obstruction and itching, 2) demonstration by nasal endoscopy of a pale and oedematous nasal mucosa, nasal discharge and swollen inferior turbinates and 3) positive serum antigen-specific IgE, as measured by the ImmunoCAP 100 system (Pharmacia, Uppsala, Sweden) or positive antigen skin prick test (SPT) (Allergopharma, Reinbeck, Germany). A diagnosis of AR was additionally confirmed by a positive skin test response to the sensitising allergen and the presence of symptoms following exposure to the same allergen. Diagnosed AR individuals were excluded from the study if they suffered from (1) hypertension, diabetes or any other chronic disease; (2) tumor in the nasal cavity; or (3) eczema or asthma.

The antigens employed for allergy tests included house dust mite (HDM) (Der f and Der p); seasonal grass pollens (Gaint Ragweed; Mugwort; Lamb's quarers; Humulus; Chenopodium album and so on); animal Hair (especially dog and cat); moulds (indoor and outdoor mustiness or floricultural environment) and cockroach. Subjects were considered to be sensitized to allergens when serum IgE was ≥0.35 kU/l. A positive SPT result was defined as a wheal size greater than or equal to one half of the diameter of the histamine control and at least 3 mm larger than the diameter of the negative control [9]. Individuals showing positive results to two or more allergens in the skin test or serum examination were defined as being poly sensitised. Serological and skin testing were performed by specialist technicians and nurses respectively, while the AR diagnoses were made by clinical rhinologists.

The healthy controls presented no clinical features, local nasal cavity signs, or a family history of allergic disease, and showed negative results for serum antigen-specific IgE.

All the subjects were of Han Chinese ethnic origin from the southern region of China and provided written informed consent prior to entry in the study. The study protocol was approved by the Ethics Committee of the People's hospital of Hainan province and performed in accordance with the guidelines of the World Medical Association's Declaration of Helsinki.

Selection of Polymorphisms in the humanicam-1, NF-κB, TNF-α and MRPL4 Genes

The majority of the tag SNPs (tSNPs) were chosen from the Hapmap database according to the following selection strategy: Firstly, the International Haplotype Mapping (HapMap) (www. hapmap. org) SNP databases were used to select tSNPs in the ICAM-1, NF-κB, TNF-α and MRPL4 genes region, and the screened region extended 10 kilobases upstream of the annotated transcription start site and downstream at the end of the last each gene exon. The tSNPs were selected to extract most of the genetic information in the region using the CHB genotyping data from the HapMap database (HapMap data rel 27 Phase II +III, Feb2009) [10]. From this dataset, genotyping data for 20 tSNPs were obtained and loaded in the Haploview software version 4.1 [11]. Secondly, tSNPs were then selected using a pairwise tagging algorithm setting the Hardy-Weinberg *p* value, minor allele frequency (MAF) and r2 thresholds at 0.01, 0.05 and 0.8, respectively. The linkage disequilibrium (LD) pattern of each gene in the CHB population exhibited strong LD in several groups of tSNPs (r2≥0.8), indicating that most common SNPs can be captured by a subset of tagging SNPs. Consequently, we choose 14 SNPs, including rs5498, rs281432, rs281428, rs1059840, rs8104608, rs11668618, rs13117745, rs230530, rs3774963, rs1598861, rs118882, rs1800629, rs3093668, and rs1799964 to represent the four genes loci for eventual genotyping.

Single nucleotide polymorphism genotyping DNA was isolated from peripheral blood leukocytes and collected in EDTA-treated tubes, using commercial DNA Isolation Kits for Mammalian Blood (Roche, Indianapolis, USA). Isolated DNA from the blood was stored at 4°C and used in further investigations within 2 days of isolation. The majority of the selected SNP genotyping was performed with the Sequenom MassARRAYiPLEX Gold platform (Sequenom, San Diego, California) according to the manufacturer's instructions. The polymerase chain reaction (PCR) and extension primers were designed using MassARRAY Assay Design 3.1 software (Table 1). Genotyping was performed without knowledge of the case or control status. A 10% random sample was tested in duplicate by different investigators to test the reproducibility of the assay; which was shown to be 100%.

Statistical Analyses

Data were initially processed for suitability for further statistical evaluation using the Haploview version 4.1 software. Hardy-Weinberg equilibrium (HWE) of each SNP was assessed in controls only and a threshold $P<0.05$ was regarded to indicate deviation from HWE. In addition, we assessed the MAF, non-missing genotype percentage and other criteria in the AR cases as well as controls to filter the data. Among them, minor allele

Table 1. Primers used in the screening of SNPs by MassArray.

Gene & position	SNP	Alleles	Primers	Extension Primers
MRPL4 (Chromosome: 19; Location: 19p13.2)	rs1059840	A/T	ACGTTGGATGAGCGGCCACCCCGTACCAC	CCCCGTACCACTGTTGA
			ACGTTGGATGAGGCTCCCAAGTCGGCCAG	
	rs8104608	A/G	ACGTTGGATGTCCTTGGCCAGAGGCTTACA	cctCTTACAGGCAACAAGC
			ACGTTGGATGTAGTGTGACTTTGTGAGCCC	
	rs11668618	C/T	ACGTTGGATGGACAAAACAGGCAAGGTCCG	ggttTGCAAGTGGCTCAGG
			ACGTTGGATGACCCACCTCAGCTTCCAGT	
ICAM-1 (Chromosome: 19; Location: 19p13.3–p13.2)	rs5498	A/G	ACGTTGGATGACTCACAGAGCACATTCACG	CATTCACGGTCACCT
			ACGTTGGATGTTGAGGGCACCTACCTCTGT	
	rs281432	C/G	ACGTTGGATGAGCTGGGACTTTCCTTCTTG	GAGTCATGGAGGGTTT
			ACGTTGGATGGCCTTCAGCTATCTAATCCC	
	rs281428	C/T	ACGTTGGATGTGGAATTACAGGCGCCCAGCA	ccccaGCCCAGCACCACGCC
			ACGTTGGATGGCCAACATGATGAAATCCCG	
NF-κB (Chromosome: 4; Location: 4q24)	rs13117745	C/T	ACGTTGGATGGACTACCCCTGATAAAGTCC	GGGGTAGTTGTTCCTATC
			ACGTTGGATGAATGAGAGGGCCCTTCTTTG	
	rs230530	C/T	ACGTTGGATGGGACATACAAGCATTCTCC	TAGCACCAAACATCTTAATTT
			ACGTTGGATGGGCATATGGTGGTTCTCATT	
	rs3774963	C/G	ACGTTGGATGATGGAAGGCATGGTGTTTGG	gggATGGTGTTTGGAATGTTC
			ACGTTGGATGGTCTATGACTGTTTCAGACT	
	rs1598861	A/C	ACGTTGGATGTTGTACCAAAACCCTGCTTC	ATGAATCCATTTAATGAAGTTTAT
			ACGTTGGATGATCCTTTTCGACTAGCCTAC	
	rs118882	A/G	ACGTTGGATGCTCTCACAAAGGCATGACAG	agggcGACAGGGTGTGAGGTTGGA
			ACGTTGGATGCTGTGCTTTTCCTCAGCTAC	
TNF-α (Chromosome: 6; Location: 6p21.3)	rs1800629	A/G	ACGTTGGATGGATTTGTGTGTAGGACCCTG	cagcGGCTGAACCCCGTCC
			ACGTTGGATGGGTCCCCAAAAGAAATGGAG	
	rs3093668	C/G	ACGTTGGATGAGGTTGCAGAGTTAGGACAG	ggggaTGATTTGAAGCCTAGACA
			ACGTTGGATGACCTGAATCACACAGCCAAG	
	rs1799964	C/T	ACGTTGGATGGGGAAGCAAAGGAGAAGCTG	cacGCAAAGGAGAAGCTGAGAAGA
			ACGTTGGATGTGTAACCCATTCCTCAGAGC	

frequency (MAF) and non-missing genotype percentage thresholds were set at <0.001 and <95%, respectively.

Differences in frequencies of the alleles and genotypes between the AR subjects and control subjects were evaluated using the chi-square test and a P-value of 0.05 was considered significant. A correction of allele distribution χ^2 test was made by using 100,000 permutation testing. The Global P values (2 degrees of freedom) were also calculated when we compared the genotype frequencies between cases and controls using a χ^2 test. Akaike's information criteria (AIC) were used to select the most parsimonious genetic model for each SNP. Odds ratios (ORs) and 95% confidence intervals (CIs) were calculated by unconditional logistic regression analysis, adjusted for age and gender. Moreover, tests for trend were done by including genotypes as an ordinal variable in regression models (df = 1) to obtain P values for trend (two-sided). These analyses were conducted using the STATA statistical package (version 11.0; Stata Corp LP, College Station, TX, USA).

A multistage strategy was employed for analysing gene–gene interactions. Firstly we first used the multifactor dimensionality reduction (MDR) method to detect and characterize locus–locus and gene–gene interaction models [12]. Interaction dendrograms and graphs based on entropy (measurement of randomness) estimates were subsequently employed to confirm, visualize, and interpret the interactions models identified by MDR.

The MDR approach [12,13,14]applies a constructive induction algorithm that creates a new attribute by pooling genotypes from multiple SNPs. This method includes a combined cross-validation/permutation-testing procedure that minimizes false-positive

Table 2. Demographic characteristics of the study population.

Characteristic	AR cases (n = 414)	Controls (n = 293)
Age Mean (Range) (years)	23.8±14.8 (4–81)	37.1±15.8 (2–81)
Sex, M/F, No. (%)	239 (57.7)/175 (42.3)	175 (59.7)/118 (40.3)
Total IgE, kU/l	312.2±560.4	74.8±152.5

results by multiple examinations of the data. Models that are true-positives are likely to be generalized to independent datasets and will have estimated testing accuracies of greater than 0.5. In addition to the testing accuracy, we also employed the cross validation consistency (CVC), a measure of how many times out of 10 divisions of the data that MDR found the same best model. Among this set of best multifactor models, the combination of genetic factors that maximized the testing accuracy and/or the highest CVC was selected and further evaluated using permutation testing. Moreover, age and gender were included as environmental factors for MDR analysis. The MDR analysis was performed by using version 1.0.0 of the open-source MDR software package freely available online (http://www.multifactordimensionalityreduction.org/).

The statistical power for the study was calculated using G*Power 2 software (http://www.psycho.uni-duesseldorf.de/aap/projects/gpower/).

Results

Population Characteristics

The characteristics of the study population are shown in Table 2. The cohort of 414 AR patients had a mean age of 23 years and consisted of 57.7% male and 42.3% female patients. The control group comprised of similar proportions of male (59.7%) and female (40.3%) subjects, although the mean age of the group was higher (37 years) compared to the AR group. The mean total serum IgE level for the case and control groups were 312.2±560.4 and 74.8±152.5 IU/ml respectively.

The statistical power of AR vs. control was 95.01%, with the sample size of 414 AR patients and 293 controls; with $\alpha = 0.05$ and the $\beta = 0.2$.

Individual SNP Association Analysis

The initial quality tests for the SNPs in the four genes selected for genotyping demonstrated that SNP (rs281428) in ICAM-1 gene and SNP (rs11882) in NF-κB gene were not suitable for study, as indicated by significant deviation from the Hardy–Weinberg equilibrium (HWE) threshold of $P<0.05$ ($P = 0.000$ and 0.005 respectively). The data for these loci were therefore excluded from further analyses, and overall a total of 12 SNPs were chosen as shown in Tables 3 and 4.

In the single-locus analyses of allele frequencies associated with increased AR risk, C allele of rs1799964 in TNF-α gene was found to be significantly different between the AR and control subjects ($P = 0.014$; $OR = 1.399$) (Table3). Moreover, age and gender adjusted logistic regression analyses, as assessed by the Akaike's information criteria (AIC) in the codominant effect model, further revealed that T allele of rs11668618 in MRPL4 gene ($P = 0.029$; $OR = 0.583$) was associated with decreased risk for AR, whereas the C allele of rs1799964 in TNF-α gene ($P = 0.049$; $OR = 1.337$) was associated with increased risk for the development of AR (Table 3). Furthermore, rs11668618 and rs1799964 remained significantly associated with AR after 100,000 permutations ($P<0.05$).

The genotype distributions of the 12 selected SNPs in AR and control subjects are summarized in Table 4. Again, rs1799964 in TNF-α gene (CT genotype, $P = 0.002$; $OR = 1.660$) was found to be significantly associated with AR susceptibility in these analyses. Age and gender adjusted logistic regression analyses again revealed that in the codominant-effect model rs11668618 in MRPL4 gene (CT genotype, $P = 0.034$; $OR = 0.564$) and rs1799964 in TNF-α gene (CT genotype, $P = 0.0059$; $OR = 1.664$) were associated with decreased and increased risk for development of AR, respectively. The rs1799964 showed significance levels ($P_{trend} = 0.011$) of the increasing trend were apparent for an indication of a dose-response relationship between the polymorphism and AR risk.

Locus–locus and Gene–gene Interactions

None of the 12SNPs in the four genes subjected to SNP-SNP synergistic analysis using the MDR function, showed any synergistic effects (Table 5).

Table 6 summarizes the best interaction models obtained for the 12 tSNPs in MRPL4, ICAM-1, NF-κB and TNF-α in the MDR analysis adjusted for age and gender as variables. The model with the lowest prediction error and the highest CVC was selected and further evaluated using the permutation test. In the one-factor model, age was the best attribute for predicting AR risk (testing accuracy = 72.57%; CVC = 10; P = 0.001). The four-factor model (i.e., age, ICAM-1 SNP2 rs281432: C/G, NF-κB SNP3 rs3774963: C/G and TNF-α SNP3 rs1799964: C/T) was the best interaction model with the highest testing accuracy of90.83%

Table 3. Allele frequencies and AR susceptibility.

Gene	SNP	Minor Allele	Case, Control Frequencies	P	OR (95% CI)	P[a]	OR (95% CI) [a]
MRPL4	rs1059840	A	0.106, 0.090	0.328	1.196 (0.836–1.712)	0.668	1.087 (0.741–1.596)
	rs8104608	A	0.117,0.122	0.794	0.957 (0.687–1.333)	0.500	0.884 (0.618–1.265)
	rs11668618	T	0.046, 0.069	0.065	1.534 (0.971–2.424)	**0.029**	**0.583 (0.358–0.947)**
ICAM-1	rs5498	G	0.232, 0.223	0.703	0.952 (0.738–1.228)	0.756	1.045 (0.794–1.375)
	rs281432	G	0.252, 0.269	0.468	1.094 (0.858–1.394)	0.386	0.891 (0.686–1.157)
NF-κB	rs13117745	T	0.064, 0.055	0.483	0.858 (0.541–1.337)	0.540	1.162 (0.719–1.879)
	rs230530	C	0.444, 0.454	0.722	0.962 (0.777–1.192)	0.649	0.948 (0.753–1.193)
	rs3774963	C	0.419, 0.444	0.350	0.902 (0.728–1.119)	0.483	0.920 (0.730–1.161)
	rs1598861	C	0.107, 0.103	0.775	0.951 (0.673–1.344)	0.808	1.047 (0.722–1.519)
TNF-α	rs1800629	A	0.107, 0.111	0.838	0.965 (0.688–1.355)	0.541	0.894 (0.623–1.282)
	rs3093668	C	0.021, 0.019	0.815	1.096 (0.509–2.357)	0.432	1.394 (0.609–3.190)
	rs1799964	C	0.230, 0.176	**0.014**	**1.399 (1.069–1.831)**	**0.049**	**1.337 (1.001–1.787)**

[a]Results from unconditional logistic regression analyses, adjusted for age and gender.

Table 4. Genotype frequencies and AR susceptibility.

Gene	SNP	Genotype	P	Global P[a]	OR (95% CI)	P[b]	OR (95% CI)	P[c]
MRPL4	rs1059840	AA	0.784	0.607	1.224 (0.290–5.169)	0.955	0.957 (0.207–4.413)	0.391
		AT	0.331		1.218 (0.818–1.814)	0.689	1.093 (0.708–1.686)	
	rs8104608	AA	0.747	0.945	0.724 (0.101–5.177)	0.842	0.813 (0.106–6.247)	0.793
		AG	0.847		0.965 (0.671–1.388)	0.655	0.913 (0.614–1.359)	
	rs11668618	CT	0.11	0.184	0.671 (0.412–1.094)	**0.034**	**0.564 (0.332–0.957)**	0.068
		TT	0.374		0.336 (0.030–3.72)	0.393	0.333 (0.027–4.150)	
ICAM-1	rs5498	AG	0.967	0.855	1.007 (0.730–1.389)	0.960	1.009 (0.709–1.437)	0.705
		GG	0.578		1.215 (0.611–2.417)	0.667	1.176 (0.562–2.463)	
	rs281432	CG	0.487	0.752	0.893 (0.649–1.228)	0.781	0.951 (0.670–1.351)	0.508
		GG	0.663		0.877 (0.486–1.582)	0.394	0.759 (0.403–1.430)	
NF-κB	rs13117745	CT	0.273	0.367	1.313 (0.806–2.139)	0.283	1.336 (0.787–2.267)	0.456
		TT	0.406		0.360 (0.033–3.997)	0.218	0.211 (0.018–2.503)	
	rs230530	CC	0.648	0.747	0.903 (0.584–1.397)	0.434	0.826 (0.512–1.333)	0.789
		CT	0.763		1.055 (0.746–1.492)	0.927	1.018 (0.697–1.485)	
	rs3774963	CC	0.234	0.185	0.772 (0.508–1.182)	0.490	0.848 (0.532–1.354)	0.359
		CG	0.496		1.126 (0.800–1.586)	0.510	1.135 (0.779–1.652)	
	rs1598861	AC	0.667	0.857	1.086 (0.745–1.583)	0.689	1.088 (0.719–1.646)	0.612
		CC	0.739		0.716 (0.100–5.117)	0.641	0.657 (0.112–3.842)	
TNF-α	rs1800629	AA	0.361	0.522	2.784 (0.309–25.072)	0.857	1.182 (0.193–7.233)	0.756
		AG	0.556		0.895 (0.618–1.296)	0.373	0.833 (0.557–1.246)	
	rs3093668	CG	0.813	0.813	1.098(0.506–2.380)	0.340	1.510 (0.648–3.519)	0.600
		CC	NA		NA	NA	NA	
	rs1799964	CC	0.823	**0.009**	1.106 (0.457–2.680)	0.840	0.911 (0.369–2.251)	**0.011**
		CT	**0.002**		**1.660(1.199–2.296)**	**0.005**	**1.664 (1.163–2.382)**	

[a]Global P values [2 degrees of freedom (df)]: genotype frequencies in cases and controls were compared using a χ^2 test with 2 df.
[b]Results from unconditional logistic regression analyses, adjusted for age and gender.
[c]P values for trend (two-sided) derived from trend tests (df = 1).
NA: not available because of the rarity of genotype.

(CVC = 9; P = 0.033). Although, the two-factor model (i.e., age and NF-κB SNP3 rs3774963: C/G) and the three-factor model (i.e., age, ICAM-1 SNP2 rs281432: C/G and NF-κB SNP3 rs3774963: C/G) also demonstrated significant interactions (P = 0.005 and 0.003, respectively), these models had lower testing accuracies (78.37% and 85.06%, respectively) than the four-factor model (Table 6).

Although the MDR analysis indicated the four-factor model to be the best model, it did not specify the presence of any synergistic relationships between the factors assessed. However, application of an interaction dendrogram and graph indicated that although the hierarchical cluster analysis placed age, NF-κB SNP3 and TNF-α SNP3 on the same branch (Figure 1), the blue line in the diagram suggested that the three-locus model may have a redundancy interaction effect on modulating risk of AR. ICAM-1 SNP2 was on another branch, revealing an interaction between them.

Discussion

Although the pathogenesis of allergic rhinitis is still not entirely clear, there is general agreement about a chronic inflammatory response of nasal mucosa dominated by Th2 immune response and characterized by migration and infiltration of a large number of eosinophils and mast cells in the lesions of the nasal mucosa; with cell adhesion molecules playing a critical role in this process.

Table 5. MDR analysis summary.

Best candidate model	Training accuracy (%)	Permutation P-value	Cross-validation Consistency
rs1799964	56.00%	0.4793	10/10
rs13117745 rs1799964	57.84%	0.5155	5/10
rs281432 rs8104608 rs3774963	60.07%	0.4678	4/10
rs5498 rs281432 rs230530 rs1799964	63.11%	0.488	5/10

Table 6. MDR analysis summary (including age).

Best candidate model	Training accuracy (%)	P-value[a]	Cross-validation Consistency
age	72.57	**0.001**	10/10
age rs3774963	78.37	**0.005**	10/10
age rs281432 rs3774963	85.06	**0.003**	7/10
age rs281432 rs3774963 rs1799964	90.83	**0.033**	9/10

[a]P values based on 1000 permutation test.

In this regardICAM-1, a member of the immunoglobulin superfamily of adhesion molecules, has been shown to be particularly important in the pathogenesis of AR because it binds to lymphocyte function-associated antigen-1 (LFA-1), aβ2 integrin ligand located on a variety of pro-inflammatory cells, which infiltrate the nasal mucosa in AR [3,4,15,16,17,18].

Similarly, nuclear factor-kappaB (NF-κB) has been shown to be important because it regulates genes of several pro-inflammatory mediators, including cytokines, chemokines, adhesion molecules, iNOS and costimulatory molecules [19,20].In the case of the ICAM-I gene located in chromosome 19, the promoter site of this gene contains binding sites for NF-κB [21]. It has been demonstrated that on activation NF-κB enters into the nucleus and combines with its lCB motif, resulting in the increased ICAM-1 mRNA transcription [22]. ICAM-1 in turn further activates NF-κB, thus creating a positive feedback loop to amplify inflammation [23]. Despite the well-documented role of ICAM-1 and NF-κB in the pathogenesis of AR, to our knowledge, this study is the first to investigate the influence of genetic polymorphisms in the genes for these mediators and to demonstrate that there does not appear to be any direct associations between the selected polymorphisms in ICAM-1 (SNP rs281428) and NF-κB (SNP rs11882) genes and susceptibility to AR. These findings, however, do not preclude the possibility that other hitherto undetected SNPs in these genes might be associated with susceptibility to AR.

Studies have shown that NF-κB also regulates the expression of TNF-α gene [24], which is of particular significance because TNF-α has also been shown to be an important mediator in the induction and maintenance of inflammation in allergic rhinitis [5,25,26]. Present study has demonstrated that, unlike ICAM-1 and NF-κB polymorphisms, a locus (rs1799964) in TNF-α gene was significantly different in the AR and healthy people, suggesting the this particular SNP polymorphism of the TNF-α gene may be associated with the risk of AR in the Han Chinese population. Moreover, we meanwhile demonstrated a genotype-dependant association pattern regarding to rs1799964_TNF-α vs AR development, i.e. only the heterozygous (CT) but not homozygous genotypes of was significantly. Although, our findings for the TNF-α gene polymorphism are contrary to those of Zhu and colleagues [27], who did not find an association between the TNF-α allele and AR, they are nevertheless in accordance with the findings of several other studies. Gentile and co-workers [28] investigated genotypes for a number of different cytokines; including TNF-α, interferon gamma (IFN-gamma), interleukin (IL)-6, IL-10, and transforming growth factor (TGF)-beta1; in 124 infants (85% white, 57% male) to determine any associations between the specific cytokine genotypes and a parental history of allergic rhinitis and/or asthma. The authors demonstrated that the frequencies of TNF-α and TGF-beta1 phenotypes were significantly associated with parental histories of AR and asthma, respectively; with no associations between IFN-gamma, IL-6, and IL-10 genotypes and any of the outcome parameters. Similarly, Minhas and colleagues [29] have shown that the frequency of the G-308A polymorphism in the promoter region of the TNF-α gene was significantly higher in AR patients compared with unrelated healthy control subjects in the Pakistani population. Moreover, assessment of genotype distribution demonstrated that the TNF2 homozygous and TNF1/2 heterozygous genotypes were significantly more common in AR patients compared with control subjects, whereas the normal TNF1 homozygous genotype was more frequent in controls. In a more recent study, Krasznai [30] and colleagues investigated the influence of TNF-α gene238A and-308G polymorphisms in Hungarian AR patients and healthy controls, and showed that in the AR patients these polymorphisms were associated with more pronounced clinical symptoms, higher cytokine and IgE levels, and low PNIF values. Indeed, another

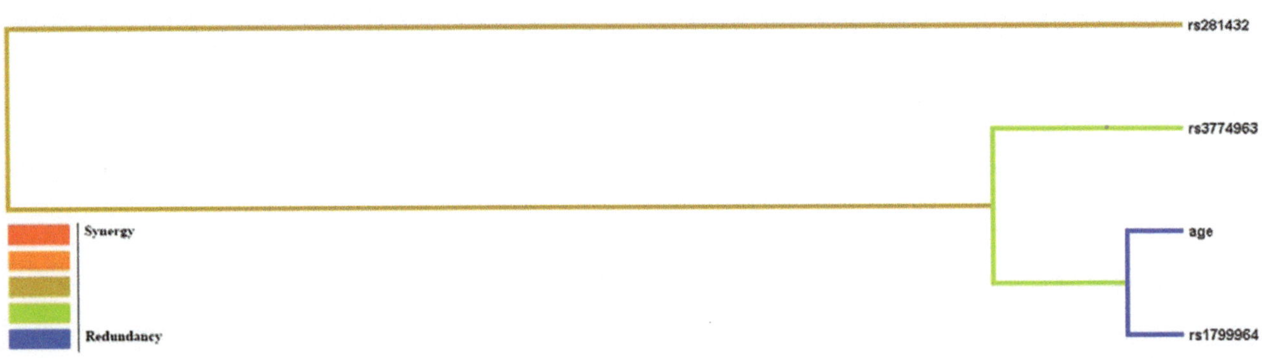

Figure 1. Dendrogram of SNP-SNP synergistic analysis by MDR. The dendrogram comprises a spectrum of colours representing a continuum from Synergy to Redundancy; with orange representing a relatively high degree of synergy (positive information gain) and blue representing redundancy (negative information gain).

recent study has indicated that the -308G polymorphism in the TNF-α gene may also be associated with nasal polyposis [31].

Although there is little information on the role of MRPL4 in the aetiology of AR, this molecule has been increasingly investigated because it has been reported to be a downstream target of hypoxia-inducible factor-1α (HIF-1α) [32], which is critical in immune and inflammatory pathways, and the inhibition of which has been shown to attenuate antigen-induced airway inflammation and hyperresponsiveness in animals [33]. Moreover, the gene encoding MRPL4 is located in close proximity to the ICAM-1 gene on chromosome location 19p13.2. Indeed, one recent study employing a genome-wide association study (GWAS) approach in an ethnic Chinese population in Singapore has indicated that MRPL4 SNP rs8111930 was significantly associated with an AR outcome in this population [2]. In accordance with these findings, here we demonstrated that another locus (rs11668618_CT genotype) of the MRPL4 gene may also be associated with AR risk in the Chinese Han population.

As AR is a polygenic inheritance disease, we have studied the gene polymorphisms associated with the ICAM-1 pathway and its upstream regulatory factors NF-κB and TNF-α, to also investigate any synergistic effects between these polymorphisms and susceptibility to AR. Using MDR software testing, our results showed that the selected sets of polymorphisms had no synergistic effect, even between MRPL4 and ICAM-1 which are located closely on the same chromosomal location. However, this conclusion is limited to present research in the Han Chinese population, and needs to be confirmed in subjects of other ethnicities. However, after adjusting for age and gender, we found that age was the best factor predicting AR risk in all four models of MDR analysis. Although we could not find a synergistic relationship among these variables when we applied the interaction dendrogram and graph, one study from Taiwan showed age and gender to be contributing differentially to different AR subtypes [34]. The risk of developing all atopic diseases is complex and the temporal pattern described in the atopic march [35,36,37] may not be a simple progression from atopic dermatitis to AR to asthma, because the development of these diseases is strongly influenced by both genetic and environmental factors. Therefore, age might be an important factor in the atopic march [38], although more research is necessary in this field to confirm the correlations between age and AR.

Last but not least, we would like to acknowledge that the number of the subjects in present study is not as substantial as can be found in other well-financed, multi-center GWAS studies, we nevertheless submit that this is a rather well-characterized population, all have been well-phenotyped according to demographic factors as well as allergen related tests, and are all ethnic Chinese in origin, ensuring a certain homogeneity to the results, which gives this population significant value nonetheless. Additionally, the statistical power of AR vs. control was 95.01%, indicating a relative ideal study sample size.

In summary, present study is the first one to investigate the interactive roles of polymorphisms in the genes coding for ICAM-1 and its upstream regulatory factors NF-κB and TNF-α, as well as MRPL4, a gene located in close vicinity of the ICAM-1 gene. Furthermore, here we investigated associations between these polymorphisms and the risk for developing AR. Our study has suggested that specific TNF-α and MRPL4 gene polymorphisms may be associated with AR susceptibility in a Han Chinese cohort, although these need to be confirmed in additional larger studies including replication in a second cohort as well as the related functional research.

Author Contributions

Conceived and designed the experiments: YZ ZF LZ. Performed the experiments: XW YZ LZ. Analyzed the data: XW YZ LZ. Contributed reagents/materials/analysis tools: YZ LZ. Wrote the paper: XW YZ LZ.

References

1. Zhang L, Han D, Huang D, Wu Y, Dong Z, et al. (2009) Prevalence of self-reported allergic rhinitis in eleven major cities in china. Int Arch Allergy Immunol 149: 47–57.
2. Andiappan AK, Wang de Y, Anantharaman R, Parate PN, Suri BK, et al. (2011) Genome-wide association study for atopy and allergic rhinitis in a Singapore Chinese population. PLoS One 6: e19719.
3. Li Y, Wang Y, Zhang Q (2006) [Expression of cell adhesion molecule and nitric oxide synthase in nasal mucosa in allergic rhinitis]. Lin Chuang Er Bi Yan Hou Ke Za Zhi 20: 315–318.
4. Canonica GW, Compalati E (2009) Minimal persistent inflammation in allergic rhinitis: implications for current treatment strategies. Clin Exp Immunol 158: 260–271.
5. Gorska-Ciebiada M, Ciebiada M, Gorska MM, Gorski P, Grzelewska-Rzymowska I (2006) Intercellular adhesion molecule 1 and tumor necrosis factor alpha in asthma and persistent allergic rhinitis: relationship with disease severity. Ann Allergy Asthma Immunol 97: 66–72.
6. Zhao J, Wang Y, Kong W (2008) [Expression and significance of nuclear factor-kappaB and ICAM-1 mRNA in nasal mucosa of allergic rhinitis]. Lin Chung Er Bi Yan Hou Tou Jing Wai Ke Za Zhi 22: 57–60.
7. Chai OH, Han EH, Lee HK, Song CH (2011) Mast cells play a key role in Th2 cytokine-dependent asthma model through production of adhesion molecules by liberation of TNF-alpha. Exp Mol Med 43: 35–43.
8. Bousquet J, Khaltaev N, Cruz AA, Denburg J, Fokkens WJ, et al. (2008) Allergic Rhinitis and its Impact on Asthma (ARIA) 2008 update (in collaboration with the World Health Organization, GA(2)LEN and AllerGen). Allergy 63 Suppl 86: 8–160.
9. The European Academy of Allergology and Clinical Immunology (1993) Position paper: Allergen standardization and skin tests. Allergy 48: 48–82.
10. The International HapMap Consortium (2005) A haplotype map of the human genome. Nature 437: 1299–1320.
11. Barrett JC, Fry B, Maller J, Daly MJ (2005) Haploview: analysis and visualization of LD and haplotype maps. Bioinformatics 21: 263–265.
12. Ritchie MD, Hahn LW, Roodi N, Bailey LR, Dupont WD, et al. (2001) Multifactor-dimensionality reduction reveals high-order interactions among estrogen-metabolism genes in sporadic breast cancer. Am J Hum Genet 69: 138–147.
13. Moore JH, Gilbert JC, Tsai CT, Chiang FT, Holden T, et al. (2006) A flexible computational framework for detecting, characterizing, and interpreting statistical patterns of epistasis in genetic studies of human disease susceptibility. J Theor Biol 241: 252–261.
14. Moore JH, Williams SM (2002) New strategies for identifying gene-gene interactions in hypertension. Ann Med 34: 88–95.
15. Asakura K, Saito H, Kataura A (1996) In vivo effects of monoclonal antibody against ICAM-1 and LFA-1 on antigen-induced nasal symptoms and eosinophilia in sensitized rats. Int Arch Allergy Immunol 111: 156–160.
16. Ciprandi G, Pronzato C, Ricca V, Bagnasco M, Canonica GW (1994) Evidence of intercellular adhesion molecule-1 expression on nasal epithelial cells in acute rhinoconjunctivitis caused by pollen exposure. J Allergy Clin Immunol 94: 738–746.
17. Gilain L, Guichard C, Beaujon G, Mom T, Monneyron E, et al. (2000) [Nasal soluble levels of ICAM-1 in allergic rhinitis]. Ann Otolaryngol Chir Cervicofac 117: 91–97.
18. Braunstahl GJ, Overbeek SE, Kleinjan A, Prins JB, Hoogsteden HC, et al. (2001) Nasal allergen provocation induces adhesion molecule expression and tissue eosinophilia in upper and lower airways. J Allergy Clin Immunol 107: 469–476.
19. Yamazaki S, Muta T, Takeshige K (2001) A novel IkappaB protein, IkappaB-zeta, induced by proinflammatory stimuli, negatively regulates nuclear factor-kappaB in the nuclei. J Biol Chem 276: 27657–27662.
20. Osada R, Takeno S, Hirakawa K, Ueda T, Furukido K, et al. (2003) Expression and localization of nuclear factor-kappa B subunits in cultured human paranasal sinus mucosal cells. Rhinology 41: 80–86.
21. Rothlein R, Dustin ML, Marlin SD, Springer TA (1986) A human intercellular adhesion molecule (ICAM-1) distinct from LFA-1. J Immunol 137: 1270–1274.
22. Yang CR, Hsieh SL, Ho FM, Lin WW (2005) Decoy receptor 3 increases monocyte adhesion to endothelial cells via NF-kappa B-dependent up-regulation of intercellular adhesion molecule-1, VCAM-1, and IL-8 expression. J Immunol 174: 1647–1656.

23. Minami T, Abid MR, Zhang J, King G, Kodama T, et al. (2003) Thrombin stimulation of vascular adhesion molecule-1 in endothelial cells is mediated by protein kinase C (PKC)-delta-NF-kappa B and PKC-zeta-GATA signaling pathways. J Biol Chem 278: 6976–6984.
24. Azzolina A, Bongiovanni A, Lampiasi N (2003) Substance P induces TNF-alpha and IL-6 production through NF kappa B in peritoneal mast cells. Biochim Biophys Acta 1643: 75–83.
25. El-Shazly AE, Moonen V, Mawet M, Begon D, Henket M, et al. (2011) IFN-gamma and TNF-alpha potentiate prostaglandin D2-induced human eosinophil chemotaxis through up-regulation of CRTH2 surface receptor. Int Immunopharmacol 11: 1864–1870.
26. Widegren H, Erjefalt J, Korsgren M, Andersson M, Greiff L (2008) Effects of intranasal TNFalpha on granulocyte recruitment and activity in healthy subjects and patients with allergic rhinitis. Respir Res 9: 15.
27. Zhu S, Chan-Yeung M, Becker AB, Dimich-Ward H, Ferguson AC, et al. (2000) Polymorphisms of the IL-4, TNF-alpha, and Fcepsilon RIbeta genes and the risk of allergic disorders in at-risk infants. Am J Respir Crit Care Med 161: 1655–1659.
28. Gentile DA, Doyle WJ, Zeevi A, Howe-Adams J, Trecki J, et al. (2004) Association between TNF-alpha and TGF-beta genotypes in infants and parental history of allergic rhinitis and asthma. Hum Immunol 65: 347–351.
29. Minhas K, Micheal S, Ahmed F, Ahmed A (2010) Strong association between the -308 TNF promoter polymorphism and allergic rhinitis in Pakistani patients. J Investig Allergol Clin Immunol 20: 563–566.
30. Krasznai M, Szaniszlo K, Kraxner H, Vargha E, Kovacs M, et al. (2011) Association of TLR-4 and TNF-alpha polymorphisms with clinical symptoms and cytokine levels in patients with allergic rhinitis. Eur Arch Otorhinolaryngol 268: 561–567.
31. Batikhan H, Gokcan MK, Beder E, Akar N, Ozturk A, et al. (2010) Association of the tumor necrosis factor-alpha -308 G/A polymorphism with nasal polyposis. Eur Arch Otorhinolaryngol 267: 903–908.
32. Benita Y, Kikuchi H, Smith AD, Zhang MQ, Chung DC, et al. (2009) An integrative genomics approach identifies Hypoxia Inducible Factor-1 (HIF-1)-target genes that form the core response to hypoxia. Nucleic Acids Res 37: 4587–4602.
33. Kim SR, Lee KS, Park HS, Park SJ, Min KH, et al. (2010) HIF-1alpha inhibition ameliorates an allergic airway disease via VEGF suppression in bronchial epithelium. Eur J Immunol 40: 2858–2869.
34. Chen BY, Chan CC, Han YY, Wu HP, Guo YL (2012) The risk factors and quality of life in children with allergic rhinitis in relation to seasonal attack patterns. Paediatr Perinat Epidemiol 26: 146–155.
35. Spergel JM (2010) From atopic dermatitis to asthma: the atopic march. Ann Allergy Asthma Immunol 105: 99–106; quiz 107–109, 117.
36. Hon KL, Wang SS, Leung TF (2012) The atopic march: from skin to the airways. Iran J Allergy Asthma Immunol 11: 73–77.
37. von Kobyletzki LB, Bornehag CG, Hasselgren M, Larsson M, Lindstrom CB, et al. (2012) Eczema in early childhood is strongly associated with the development of asthma and rhinitis in a prospective cohort. BMC Dermatol 12: 11.
38. Zheng T, Yu J, Oh MH, Zhu Z (2011) The atopic march: progression from atopic dermatitis to allergic rhinitis and asthma. Allergy Asthma Immunol Res 3: 67–73.

Targeting a Cross-Reactive Gly m 5 Soy Peptide as Responsible for Hypersensitivity Reactions in a Milk Allergy Mouse Model

Renata Curciarello[1,5], Paola L. Smaldini[1], Angela M. Candreva[1,5], Virginia González[2], Gustavo Parisi[2], Ana Cauerhff[3], Ivana Barrios[4], Luis Bruno Blanch[4], Carlos A. Fossati[1], Silvana Petruccelli[5]❡, Guillermo H. Docena[1,5]❡*

1 Laboratorio de Investigaciones del Sistema Inmune-LISIN, Departamento de Ciencias Biológicas, Facultad de Ciencias Exactas, Universidad Nacional de La Plata, La Plata, Buenos Aires, Argentina, **2** Centro de Estudios e Investigaciones, Departamento de Ciencias y Tecnología Universidad Nacional de Quilmes, Quilmes, Buenos Aires, Argentina, **3** Centro de Investigación y Desarrollo en Fermentaciones Industriales, CINDEFI (UNLP y CONICET) and Instituto de Investigaciones Bioquímicas de Buenos Aires (IIBBA-CONICET), Fundación Instituto Leloir, Buenos Aires, Argentina, **4** Cátedra de Química Medicinal, Departamento de Ciencias Biológicas, Facultad de Ciencias Exactas, Universidad Nacional de La Plata, La Plata, Buenos Aires, Argentina, **5** Centro de Investigaciones y Desarrollo en Criotecnología de Alimentos-CIDCA, Facultad de Ciencias Exactas, Universidad Nacional de La Plata, La Plata, Buenos Aires, Argentina

Abstract

Background: Cross-reactivity between soybean allergens and bovine caseins has been previously reported. In this study we aimed to map epitopes of the major soybean allergen Gly m 5 that are co-recognized by casein specific antibodies, and to identify a peptide responsible for the cross-reactivity.

Methods: Cow's milk protein (CMP)-specific antibodies were used in different immunoassays (immunoblotting, ELISA, ELISA inhibition test) to evaluate the *in vitro* recognition of soybean proteins (SP). Recombinant Gly m 5 (α), a truncated fragment containing the C-terminal domain (α-T) and peptides of α-T were obtained and epitope mapping was performed with an overlapping peptide assay. Bioinformatics tools were used for epitope prediction by sequence alignment, and for modelling the cross-recognized soy proteins and peptides. The binding of SP to a monoclonal antibody was studied by surface Plasmon resonance (SPR). Finally, the *in vivo* cross-recognition of SP was assessed in a mouse model of milk allergy.

Results: Both α and α-T reacted with the different CMP-specific antibodies. α-T contains IgG and IgE epitopes in several peptides, particularly in the peptide named PA. Besides, we found similar values of association and dissociation constants between the α-casein specific mAb and the different milk and soy components. The food allergy mouse model showed that SP and PA contain the cross-reactive B and T epitopes, which triggered hypersensitivity reactions and a Th2-mediated response on CMP-sensitized mice.

Conclusions: Gly m 5 is a cross-reactive soy allergen and the α-T portion of the molecule contains IgG and IgE immunodominant epitopes, confined to PA, a region with enough conformation to be bound by antibodies. These findings contribute to explain the intolerance to SP observed in IgE-mediated CMA patients, primarily not sensitised to SP, as well as it sets the basis to propose a mucosal immunotherapy for milk allergy using this soy peptide.

Editor: Guillermo H. Giambartolomei, National Council of Sciences (CONICET), Argentina

Funding: This work was supported by the Consejo Nacional de Investigaciones Científicas y Técnicas de Argentina (CONICET) (grant PIP 5475), by Agencia Nacional de Promoción Científica y Tecnológica (grants PICT2007-0049 and PICT 2010-2366 to SP, PICT 2008-2202 to GHD) and by Universidad Nacional de La Plata, Argentina (grants X498 to SP and X455 to CAF). The funders had no role in study design, data collection and analysis, decision to publish, or preparation of the manuscript.

Competing Interests: The authors have declared that no competing interests exist.

* E-mail: guidoc@biol.unlp.edu.ar

❡ These authors contributed equally to this work.

Introduction

Food allergy is an increasing health care concern. Cow's milk protein (CMP) is the leading cause of food allergy in children younger than 3 years in many regions, including our country [1,2]. This is reflected by most of the position papers and guidance with statements and recommendations for food allergy that are focused on CMP allergy (CMA) [3].

If symptoms were relevant and CMA were suspected, a diagnostic dietary elimination of CMP should be initiated for a certain period of time (days to 4 weeks) [4,5]. Once a diagnosis of allergy to milk proteins has been confirmed, it is important to avoid CMP and to ensure a healthy balanced diet that promotes an adequate child growth and development. Depending on the age and other food allergies a restriction or milk free diet is indicated as therapy.

Soy-based formulas have been available for almost 100 years and have been widely used as a milk substitute in children intolerant to cow's milk protein-based formula [6]. However, there are some indications and contraindications of soy formulas since gastrointestinal reactions, including hypersensitivity, have been described for more than 50 years [7], and because of the nutritional quality of soy proteins [8]. More recently, it has been reported that a small proportion of children with IgE and non IgE-mediated milk allergy develop a clinical intolerance to soy-protein-based formula during the restriction treatment, which may be explained by cross-reactivity once milk contamination has been discarded [6,9,10]. We focused our work in investigating the cross-recognition between CMP and soy components. We identified bovine caseins, the main allergens of milk [11,12], and the soybean Gly m 6 G4 as cross-reactive allergens [13–15]. The analysis of a soy variety that naturally lacks the Gly G4 led us to detect that a residual cross-reactivity may lie on Gly m 5.0101, the α subunit of the β-conglycinin. Besides, both seed proteins have been characterized as allergens in patients with IgE-mediated atopic dermatitis [16], food allergy [17,18], asthma [19] and anaphylaxis [20,21]. Therefore, we propose that the clinical intolerance observed in a restricted proportion of milk allergic patients, with documented IgE specific to milk proteins, may be due to the presence of these relevant cross-reactive allergens in soy protein-based formulas.

In this study, we immunochemically and biologically characterized the α subunit of β-conglycinin, and a C-terminal fragment called α-T, containing putative cross-reactive epitopes with bovine caseins. Using bioinformatic, immunochemical and biological tools we demonstrated the presence of B epitopes on this molecule, and we identified a polypeptide that contains critical epitopes for cross-recognition. The results presented here may shed some light to understand the concomitant soy allergy that occurs in infants with IgE-mediated CMA, and not primarily sensitised to soy proteins. However, and more challenging for us, the identification of cross-reactive B and T epitopes would set the basis to propose a soy-based immunotherapy for milk and soy allergies, taking advantage of the lower immunogenicity of soy proteins.

Methods

Protein Extracts

Cow's milk protein extract was prepared from skimmed dry milk (Svelty, Nestle). Proteins were extracted with phosphate saline buffer pH 7.4 (10 mg/ml) and filtered. Soy protein (SP) extract was prepared from *Glycine max*. L merr genotype Asgrow seeds as described previously [14]. Briefly, proteins were extracted from crushed seeds with 0.01N $NaHCO_3$ at 90°C. The extract was centrifuged (2,500×g-20 min at room temperature) and lipids were extracted with chloroform (overnight at 4°C). Finally, the extract was dialyzed against distilled water. The total protein content was quantified with the Bicinchoninic acid kit (Pierce BCA Protein Assay), using bovine serum albumin (BSA) as standard.

Production of the α Subunit of β-conglycinin and α-T Fragment in *Escherichia coli*

The cDNA coding sequence for α (GenBank: X17698) was obtained by PCR amplification of cDNA library from developing *Glycine max* L. Merr. seeds [22]. pET-mα and pET α-T [22] were transformed into *Escherichia coli* strain BL21(DE3) for protein expression of α subunit of β-conglycinin (α) and α-T, its truncated polypeptide containing three alpha helix and one cupin domain typical of the cupin superfamily [23]. Production and purification of the recombinant proteins are described elsewhere [14].

PA and PN Peptide Constructs, Expression and Purification

The oligonucleotide primers used for expression of peptides A and N (PA and PN, amino acids 357–418 and amino acids 438–499 of the pre-pro α subunit, respectively) were: F-pepA (CACCCTGTTTAGTAGAGAGGAAG) and R-pepA (TCACTTGTTGGAGTAGATGGG), F-pepN (CACCATCTTCCTCAGTATTGTGG) and R-pepN (TCATTCGGCTCTATATTTCCGC). Amplified PCR products were cloned directionally into pENTR/D TOPO (Life Technology, S.A. Buenos Aires, Argentina), and then transferred to pDEST destination vector for expression [24]. E. coli BL21 Codon Plus competent cells transformed with the construct "pDEST His-PA" and "pDEST His-PN", were induced for protein expression. Recombinant proteins were purified as described previously [14] and protein concentration was determined by BCA protein assay.

Production of Polyclonal and Monoclonal Antibodies

CMP- and SP-specific polyclonal antisera obtained in rabbit using complete or incomplete Freund's Adjuvant, and a specific α-casein monoclonal antibody (1D5 mAb) were all obtained as described in Docena et al [11]. 1D5 mAb was biotinylated for the SPR biosensor assay. Briefly, 1D5 mAb (1 mg/ml in 0.1M borate buffer, pH 8.8) was incubated with 10 mg/ml solution of N-hidroxisuccinimide-biotin in DMSO (250 µg:1 mg of biotin:mAb ratio) for 4 h at room temperature. The biotinylated mAb was desalted by dialysis against PBS and biotinylation was assessed by ELISA using alkaline phosphatase-conjugated streptavidin (Sigma Aldrich, St Louis, MO). For this assay wells were coated with CMP (1 µg/well), and after blocking, dilutions (1:100 to 1:100,000) of the biotinylated-1D5 mAb were added, followed by the alkaline phosphatase-conjugated streptavidin (1:4,000). Color was developed with *p*-nitrophenylphosphate in buffer pH 9.6, and optical density (OD) at 405 nm was measured in an ELISA reader (Sirio S SAECS, Roma, Italy).

Patient Sera Used for *In Vitro* Characterization of the Allergen Content

Sera obtained from 15 atopic children (ages ranging from 3 months to 10 years, mean age: 4.5 years) with documented IgE-mediated CMA by history, and recruited for other studies, were used. Double blind placebo-controlled food challenge was not done since it is not performed in Argentina for diagnosis. Patients showed clinical pictures of immediate reactions associated to the ingestion of milk or milk-derived products (vomiting, diarrhoea, dermatitis, bronchospasm, urticaria and rhinorrhea). Histories showed no evidence of soybean sensitization. CMP-specific IgE antibodies were detected by immunoblotting, ELISA and EAST (Class 2 or higher) as described previously [12]. Skin prick test with commercial extracts (CMP and common environmental allergens) (Alergo Pharma, Buenos Aires, Argentina) was performed. Histamine (10 µg/ml) and PBS (pH 7.4) were used as positive and negative control, respectively.

Besides, sera from 20 subjects (age- and sex-matched) with no history of food allergy, no clinical manifestations after ingestion of CM, with normal level of serum total IgE according to age, and no specific serum IgE antibodies were used as negative controls.

SDS PAGE and Immunoblotting

SDS-PAGE and immunoblotting were performed as described before [14]. Samples prepared in sample buffer were loaded on gels (10–20 μg/lane for CMP or SP, or 7–10 μg/lane for the recombinant proteins) and electrotransferred onto nitrocellulose membranes. Membranes were probed with the 1D5 mAb (1:1,500 in TBS-Tween 20), cow's milk-specific rabbit polyclonal antiserum (1:1,000 in TBS-Tween 20) for 1 h at 37°C, or with patient sera (1:4 in blocking buffer) overnight at 4°C, as primary antibody, followed by the appropriate conjugated secondary antibody which were: biotinylated goat anti-mouse immunoglobulin G (1:3,000, Chemicon Int., Temecula, CA), biotinylated mouse monoclonal antibodies specific to rabbit immunoglobulins (1:3,000, Sigma-Aldrich, St Louis, MO) and horseradish peroxidase-conjugated avidin (1:4,000, Sigma-Aldrich, St Louis, MO), or horseradish peroxidase-conjugated anti-human IgE antibodies (dilution 1:1,000, Sigma Aldrich, St Louis, MO) for 4 h at 37°C. Protein bands were visualized by enhanced chemiluminescence (ECL Plus, GE Healthcare, Bucks, UK) according to manufacturer's instructions. X-ray-sensitive films (Amersham Hypefilm^{TM} MP, GE Healthcare Limited, Pollarsd Wood, UK) were used and images were acquired with a Hewlett Packard scanner.

Indirect ELISA for IgE Reactivity

Polystyrene microtiter plates (NUNC, Maxisorp, Denmark) were coated with 1.25 μg/well of CMP, 0.05 μg/well of SP or with 0.05 μg/well of α or α-T, in 50 mM carbonate buffer (pH 9.6). Plates were blocked with 5% horse serum in PBS (pH 7.4), and the ELISA was carried out using the patient or negative control sera as primary antibody, as previously described [11,14]. Cut-off values were statistically obtained (SEM+2 SD) from the readings of the negative control sera used.

Sequential Competitive ELISA

ELISA plates were coated overnight with 1 μg/well of CMP and blocked with 5% horse serum in PBS (pH 7.4) for 1 hr at 37°C. CMP-specific rabbit antiserum diluted 1:200,000 in 3% horse serum in PBS (pH 7.4), or α-casein specific mAb diluted 1:300,000 in the same buffer, were mixed (1:1) with different concentrations of inhibitors: CMP, α α-T or bovine serum albumin (BSA) (Sigma Aldrich, St Louis, MO) for 2 h at 37°C. Then 100 μl of this pre-mixed dilution was added in triplicates to the antigen-coated wells and incubated for 30 min at 37°C. Biotinylated mouse monoclonal antibodies specific to rabbit immunoglobulins (1:3,000, Sigma-Aldrich, St Louis, MO) or biotinylated goat anti-mouse immunoglobulin G (1:3,000, Chemicon Int., Temecula, CA) were added for 1 h at 37°C. Finally, horseradish peroxidase-conjugated avidin (1:3,000, Sigma-Aldrich, MO, USA) was added (30 min at 37°C) and color was developed with *o*-phenylenediamine and 30% H_2O_2 in 0.1M citrate-phosphate buffer pH 5.0. Optical density was measured at 492 nm in an ELISA reader. Additionally, 96-well plates were coated with α or α-T (0.1 μg/well) and blocked. CMP-specific polyclonal antiserum diluted 1:6,000 was used in the inhibition mix with same inhibitors. Then, 100 μl of the pre-mixed dilution was added to the coated wells and developed as described above.

Cross-reactive Epitope Mapping on α-T

Overlapping 15-mer peptides, frame shifted by five residues, covering the entire aminoacid sequence of α-T were synthesized on a cellulose membrane (PepSpot JPT Peptide Technologies GMBH, Germany). Spots membrane-based immunoassay was carried out by incubation of the blocked membranes with different primary antibodies (pools of sera containing CMP specific IgE, CMP-specific rabbit polyclonal antiserum or 1D5 mAb), followed by the appropriate secondary antibody. Membranes were developed by chemiluminescence as described above.

Binding Kinetics Analysis Using the BIACORE Assay

Affinity sensor analysis experiments were conducted on an IAsys Plus apparatus (Affinity Sensors, Saxon Hill, Cambridge, U.K.). Streptavidin (Sigma Aldrich, USA) (100 μg/ml in acetate buffer, pH 5.0) was covalently coupled to carboxymethyl dextran sensor chips (Affinity Sensors, Saxon Hill, Cambridge, U.K.) (5 ng of protein per cuvette). Then, a solution of 20 μg/ml in saline buffer of the biotinylated 1D5 mAb (the ligand) was added to the cuvette during 10 minutes, the antibody excess was removed by adding 1M NaCl and 10 mM acetate buffer at pH 4.5. Binding reactions with the ligate were carried out in PBS, 0.05% Tween 20 at 25°C, with constant stirring set up at 90%. Data were collected at intervals of 0.3 sec. Ligate binding to the immobilized ligand was monitored at multiple ligate concentrations, ranging 10-fold below to at least 10-fold above preliminary estimates of equilibrium dissociation constants (K_D) for each reaction. Kinetic and Scatchard analysis were performed by using the FAST FIT software (Affinity Sensors, Saxon Hill, Cambridge, U.K.).

Bioinformatics Analysis

Caseins and subunits of soybean β-conglycinin were compared using bioinformatics tools. The sequences of α (gi:9967357: 543 aa), α′ (gi:15425631: 621 aa) and β (gi: 9967359: 416 aa) subunits of β-conglycinin, and αs1- (gi:162792: 214 aa), αs2- (gi:27806963:222 aa), β- (gi:162931:224 aa) and κ- (gi:1228078: 190 aa) caseins were retrieved from the GenBank database. Several epitope prediction methods available in the B Cell Epitope Prediction Tools at the Immune Epitope Database (IEDB) [25] (http://www.immuneepitope.org) were applied. These methods included Chou & Fasman Beta-Turn Prediction [26], Emini Surface Accessibility Prediction [27], Karplus & Schulz Flexibility Prediction [28], Kolaskar & Tongaonkar Antigenicity [29], and Parker Hydrophilicity Prediction [30]. Peptides identified as putative epitopes based on these predictions were collected in a database. A second database was built using overlapping peptides (15 residues long) of the cow milk and soybean proteins mentioned above. Both databases were aligned with the BLASTP program using parameters fixed to short peptides (Expect Value = 20,000, Score Matrix = PAM30, Word Size = 2, SEG Filter = off) [31] and a shorter region of α located on the α-T segment, containing most amino acid coincidences with bovine caseins epitopes, and named "Peptide A (PA)", was selected. We have used MODELLER [32] to build structural models of α protein based on templates found with FFAS03 fold assignment method [33]. Three-D models were assessed using ProsaII [34] and the PyMOL (http://www.pymol.org) was employed to map α-T and PA on the best 3D models obtained. Calculation of the electrostatic potential surface was made with the web-based graphical user interface PBEQ-Solver [35] and the electrostatic map was visualized in PyMOL.

The hit distribution graph was done to represent those similar amino acid positions shared by soybean α, α-T, and bovine casein peptides. The amino acid sequence of 73 peptides of αS1-, αs2-, β- and κ-casein, described as T and/or B epitopes (IEDB, (http://www.immuneepitope.org/), were aligned with α-T sequence by the ClustalW2 server (http://www.ebi.ac.uk/Tools/msa/clustalw2/). The hits represent the accumulation of consensus amino acid in every position of the sequence analyzed. A score of "3" was assigned for conserved aminoacid (identity), "2" for similar, but not identical amino acids (punctuation over 0.5 on

Gonnet or PAM 250 matrixes), and "1" for slightly similar amino acids (punctuation below 0.5 on Gonnet or PAM 250 matrixes).

Secondary Structure Prediction

Bioinformatics studies described above allowed us to find out that the PA fragment has a primary structure alignment with a fragment of bovine α-casein. Different secondary structure prediction servers and softwares were used to analyze both fragments. Prediction programs belong to the Network Protein Sequence Analysis server [36], which contains SOPM, SOPMA, Hierarchical Neural Network, GOR I, GOR III, GOR IV, DPM, DSC, PHD, PREDATOR, SIMPA 96 and Secondary consensus prediction. Other programs such as CFSSP [37], Jpred [38], JUFO 3D [39], NetSurfP and Multivariate Linear Regression Combination were also used. The final secondary structure prediction was the average of all structures obtained with those prediction programs. Besides, the alignments were performed using the BLAST program.

Mice and Experimental Model of IgE-mediated Food Allergy

Sensitization and Antigenic Challenge. Male 6- to 8-week old Balb/c mice were purchased from the School of Animal Sciences, University of La Plata, and kept under pathogen-free conditions with water and commercial diet provided *ad libitum.* Cow's milk sensitization protocol was carried out as previously described [15]. Briefly, mice received 6 weekly intragastric (ig) doses of CMP (20 mg/dose) plus cholera toxin (10 μg/dose) (Sigma Aldrich, St Louis, MO, USA) in a final volume of 200 μl of bicarbonate buffer (sensitization group), or CMP (20 mg/dose) without cholera toxin (control group). Mice were fasted for 2 h before sensitization, and 3% sodium bicarbonate solution was given 30 min before the immunization. Ten days following the last boost mice were ig challenged with different proteins: 20 mg of CMP, 5 mg of SP or 10 mg of OVA (Sigma-Aldrich, St Louis, MO, USA) as an unrelated antigen. Additionally, some animals were sublingual (sl) challenged with 10 μg of purified proteins [β-lactoglobulin (β-lg), α, α-T, PA or OVA]. Symptoms immediately triggered after the oral challenge were scored in a blinded manner by two independent observers.

In vivo evaluation of the allergic state

Assessment of Clinical Signs. Symptoms were observed 30–60 min following the oral challenge, in a blinded fashion by 2 independent researchers, and scored on a scale from 0 to 5. Some animals received sl 10 μg of recombinant soybean proteins, β-lg (positive control), or OVA (unrelated negative control), and elicited symptoms were scored.

Cutaneous Tests. Mice were shaved on both flanks and subcutaneously injected with 200 μg of CMP, 400 μg of SP, 10 μg of α, α-T or PA in 50 μl of sterile saline in one flank, and 10 μg of saline in the other flank, as a negative control. Mice were also intravenous injected in the tail vein with 100 μl of 0.1% Evans blue dye (Anedra, Buenos Aires, Argentina). The presence of blue color in the skin 15 to 30 min following the injection was considered a positive cutaneous test.

In vitro evaluation of the allergic state

Specific IgE Detection. Serum specific IgE antibodies were measured by EAST using the method described by Ceska et al [40]. Briefly, cyanogen bromide -activated cellulose paper discs were coupled with CMP (1.75 mg/ml), SP (0.5 mg/ml), or the recombinant proteins (0.2 mg/ml). Discs were blocked with 0.5 mM ethanolamine, and incubated overnight at 4°C with 50 μl of undiluted serum samples. Then, the assay was developed as described by Smaldini et al [15].

Specific IgG1 and IgG2a Detection. serum CMP- or SP-specific IgG1 and IgG2a were measured by ELISA as described by Smaldini et al [15]. Briefly, microtitre plates were coated with 1 μg/100 μl of either CMP, SP, α, α-T or PA in carbonate-bicarbonate buffer, pH 9.6. The assay was developed as indicated [15].

Cytokine Response of Antigen-stimulated Splenocytes. 24 h following the oral challenge mice were killed, spleens were removed and cells were isolated. Splenocytes (4×10^6 cells/well) were plated in complete medium (RPMI-1640 supplemented with 10% FBS, 100 U/ml penicillin and 100 mg/ml streptomycin), and stimulated for 72 h with CMP (350 μg/ml), SP (200 μg/ml), ConA (5 μg/ml), α (15 μg/100 μl), α-T (15 μg/100 μl) or PA (15 μg/100 μl). Supernatants were collected, and cytokines were quantified by ELISA: IL-5, IFN-γ (Invitrogen, Invitrogen Corporation, USA).

Ethics Statement

All experimental protocols of this study were conducted in strict agreement with international ethical standards for animal experimentation (Helsinki Declaration and its amendments, Amsterdam Protocol of welfare and animal protection and National Institutes of Health, USA NIH, guidelines: Guide for the Care and Use of Laboratory Animals) and were approved by the local Institutional Animal Care and Use Committee at the School of Animal Science (University of La Plata). Anesthetized mice (intraperitoneal injection of 100 mg/kg ketamine and 5 mg/kg xylacine) were killed by cervical dislocation by experienced research personnel, which performed it humanely and effectively. All efforts were made to alleviate suffering during the whole experiment.

For the human sample analysis a written informed consent was obtained from parents of patients and the project was approved by the Ethics Committee of the Argentinean Association of Allergy and Clinical Immunology (February 2012). Sera were obtained from patients assisted at Hospital San Juan de Dios de La Plata.

Statistical Analysis

All statistical analyses were carried out using GraphPad Prism 5 software. The significance of the difference was determined using an independent-sample t-test or ANOVA test. A p-value$<$0.05 was regarded as statistically significant.

Results

Beta conglycinin Alpha Subunit and the Polypeptide Fragment α-T are Specifically recognized by Different CMP specific Antibodies

We previously showed that although the soybean variety Raiden lacks the cross-reactive G4 glycinin, a residual cross-reactivity, probably due to the 7S seed globulin α-subunit of β-conglycinin (Gly m 5.0101), was detected [14]. In this work, recombinant Gly m 5.0101 (α) and a 235 amino acid residue polypeptide fragment (~27 kDa) containing the three helix and one cupin domain, α-T, were immunochemically evaluated. Different CMP-specific antibodies were used to assess the cross-reactivity of these soy components (Figure 1). The amount of different coated antigens was adjusted in the indirect ELISA to have the same molar relationship. We found that all sera recognized CMP (100%), while most of the milk allergic patient sera presented IgE antibodies that recognized α (86.6%) and α-T (93.3%) (Figure 1A). The pattern reactivity obtained by immunoblotting revealed that human and rabbit polyclonal sera recognized caseins

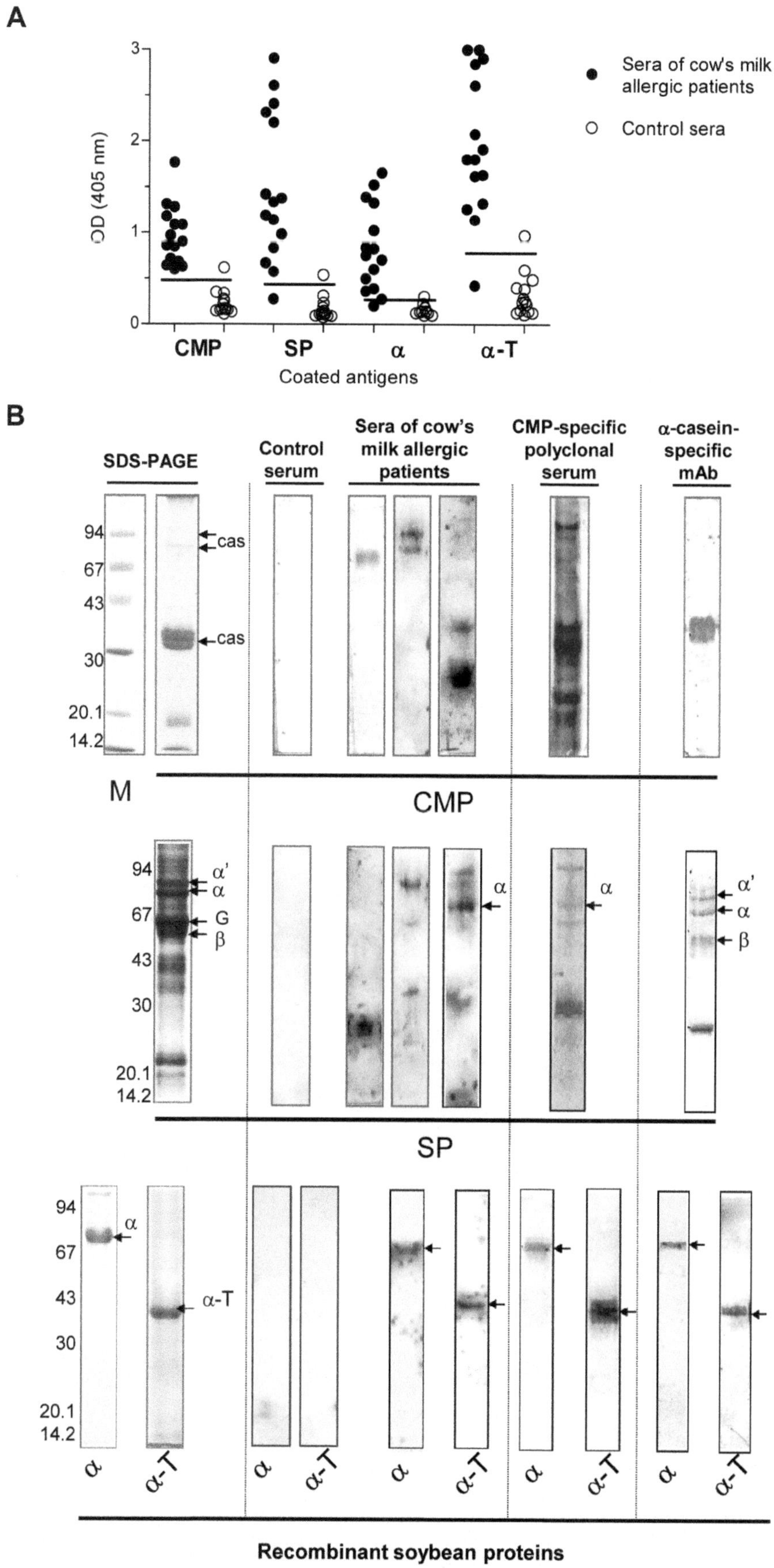
A
OD (405 nm)
3
2
1
0
Sera of cow's milk allergic patients
Control sera
CMP
SP
α
α-T
Coated antigens
B
SDS-PAGE
Control serum
Sera of cow's milk allergic patients
CMP-specific polyclonal serum
α-casein-specific mAb
94
67
43
30
20.1
14.2
cas
cas
M
CMP
α'
α
G
β
SP
α-T
Recombinant soybean proteins

Figure 1. Immunochemical cross-reactivity. A) Detection of specific human serum IgE antibodies by indirect ELISA. Microtiter plates were coated with CMP, SP, recombinant α-subunit of β-conglycinin "α" or α-T, and sequentially incubated with sera of CMA patients and anti-human IgE specific conjugate. 15/15 sera contained IgE antibodies specific for CMP, 13/15 sera contained IgE antibodies specific for α and 14/15 sera contained IgE antibodies for α-T. **B) SDS-PAGE and immunoblotting of CMP and SP.** SDS-PAGE was performed under non reducing conditions for CMP (**upper panel**), SP (**middle panel**), and purified recombinant α and the α-T fraction (**lower panel**). Immunoblottings were developed with patient sera containing milk-specific IgE antibodies or control sera (from non-allergic patients) (1:4), CMP-specific rabbit polyclonal antiserum (1:1,000), and α-casein-specific monoclonal antibody (1D5 mAb 1:1,500). *CMP: Cow's milk protein, cas: caseins, SP: soybean protein, G: 11S glycinin subunits; β-conglycinin subunits are indicated as α, α' and β. M: Molecular masses are given on the left in kilo Daltons (kDa).*

as monomers or aggregates (Figure 1B upper panel), whereas the 1D5 mAb bound α- casein. As it can be seen in the medium panel, these sera recognized soy components of 30 kDa and higher MW, corresponding to α, α', and β subunit of β-conglycinin. The 30 kDa-band may correspond to the processed polypeptide A5A4B3 of G4 glycinin, previously described as cross-reactive protein [13,14]. The lower panel shows that recombinant α and α-T were recognized by the different milk specific antibodies.

We next investigated the specificity of the antigen-antibody interaction with a sequential competitive ELISA. To enhance the sensitivity and the detection capacity of the assay, the CMP-specific antiserum or the mAb were pre-incubated with different concentrations of soluble inhibitors (reactant proteins). Then, soluble unbound CMP-specific antibodies were allowed to react with the coated antigen. The sigmoid shape of the dose-response curve obtained confirmed the specificity of the Ag-Ab binding (Figure 2). The binding of the CMP-specific polyclonal antiserum to the immobilized CMP was 100% inhibited with 3 mg/ml of soluble CMP, while 50% of inhibition (IC50) was achieved with 0.002 mg/ml CMP and 0.2 mg/ml α (Figure 2A). On the other hand, when any of the recombinant polypeptides was coated to the solid phase, sigmoid curves were obtained with a lower dilution of the polyclonal antiserum (1:6,000), as compared with that used when CMP was coated to the solid phase. This assay rendered an IC50 of 0.1 mg/ml for CMP (Figure 2B). Taken together, and not surprisingly, CMP binding to milk-specific antibodies was more efficiently inhibited with CMP than with soybean components. However, the recombinant soy polypeptides could specifically inhibit the binding of the milk-specific antibodies to the coated homologous antigen. Figure 2C shows the sigmoid curves obtained with the α-casein-specific mAb used in the immunoblottings depicted in figure 1B. More than 95% of inhibition was achieved with a minimum of 0.01 mg/ml CMP as soluble inhibitor, while none of the other proteins could achieve such values at the range of the concentration assessed. The IC50 was 0.0015 mg/ml for CMP, 0.019 mg/ml for α-T and 0.13 mg/ml for α. A non-related control protein (BSA) rendered a constant basal inhibition of less than 10% in all assays (Figures 2A and C).

Kinetic and Equilibrium Constants between α-casein-specific mAb 1D5 and Bovine α-casein and the Recombinant Soybean Proteins

The 1D5 mAb was employed to analyse the kinetic, equilibrium and affinity constants with α-casein and soy components (Table 1). According to the affinity constant (K_A) value of 1.18×10^7 M^{-1} for α-casein we consider that this antibody recognizes with a medium affinity its identity antigen. Interestingly, similar values were found for α and α-T. However, a lower K_A (4.06×10^6 M^{-1}) was measured for PA, which may be due to the smaller size of this fragment, and hence to fewer contacts with the antibody, as compared to α and α-T. Besides, a discrete increase in association constant (k_{ass}) was observed for α as compared with its specific antigen, α-casein. This result may be explained by a different conformation or a different charge on the surface of the epitope in α, which produced more productive contacts with the 1D5 mAb.

Peptides containing Cross-reactive Epitopes were identified in α-T

Once we have detected that α-T contained B epitopes, 24 overlapping 15-mer peptides with 5 amino acid overlaps were synthesized on modified cellulose paper covering the whole sequence of α-T. Spots were probed with different CMP-specific antibodies to identify IgE and IgG cross-recognized zones (Figure 3). We observed similar reactivity patterns with the rabbit polyclonal antiserum and human sera: spots 1, 2 and 9 exhibited strong human IgE binding, while spots 1 and 2 showed a strong reactivity with the rabbit antiserum. We observed a faint reactivity on spots 16 and 22 with the pooled sera, and, on spots 9 and 12 with the rabbit antiserum. Peptides on spots 14 and 23 were only recognized by the rabbit antiserum. On the other hand, the α-casein-specific monoclonal antibody recognized peptides on spots 1, 2, 9, 12, 16 and 22 with high or middle intensity, and, unlike human IgE and rabbit IgG, it also recognized peptides on spots 4, 10 and 14. In summary, 10 peptides along the aminoacidic sequence of α-T were recognized by the different CMP-specific antibodies, indicating that cross-reactivity is not due to a single epitope (spots marked with grey boxes).

Furthermore, we calculated the net charge of the peptides and remarkably we found that reactive peptides are all positive, but peptide 14 (charge −2.2), whereas non reactive peptides are all negatively charged at pH 7.5 (Figure S1 A).

In Silico Analysis showed that Conformational and Linear Epitopes are implicated in Cross-reactivity

In agreement with the epitope mapping of α-T done *in vitro* (Figure 3), sequence alignment analysis in figure 4A and figure S2 showed a high aminoacidic similitude (hits) in those positions where positive spots were obtained in the overlapping assay. High hit values along the α-T sequence where observed around amino acid positions 20 and 40 (region corresponding to positive spots 2 and 4), 77 and 90–100 (spots 9 and 10), 150 (spot 16), and 220 (spots 22 and 23). In figure 4B the sequence of α-T is depicted along with the peptides analyzed in the overlapping assay and the secondary structure predicted with different bioinformatics tools. As it can be observed, the selected PA peptide contains the region with the highest hits (peptides 9, 10 and 12).

The *in silico* predicted secondary structure (Figure 4B) showed that PA contains α-helix and β-sheet conformations. PN peptide was proposed as a control peptide since no secondary structure was predicted in this sequence and it contains low hit regions.

In addition, the amino acid composition was analyzed and we found hydrophilic (serine, asparagine, alanine and lysine) and hydrophobic amino acids (phenylalanine, isoleucine and leucine) as the most frequent amino acids in the different positive peptides in the overlapping assay of α-T. PA contains a compositional bias to hydrophilic amino acids such as glutamic acid (E), serine (S),

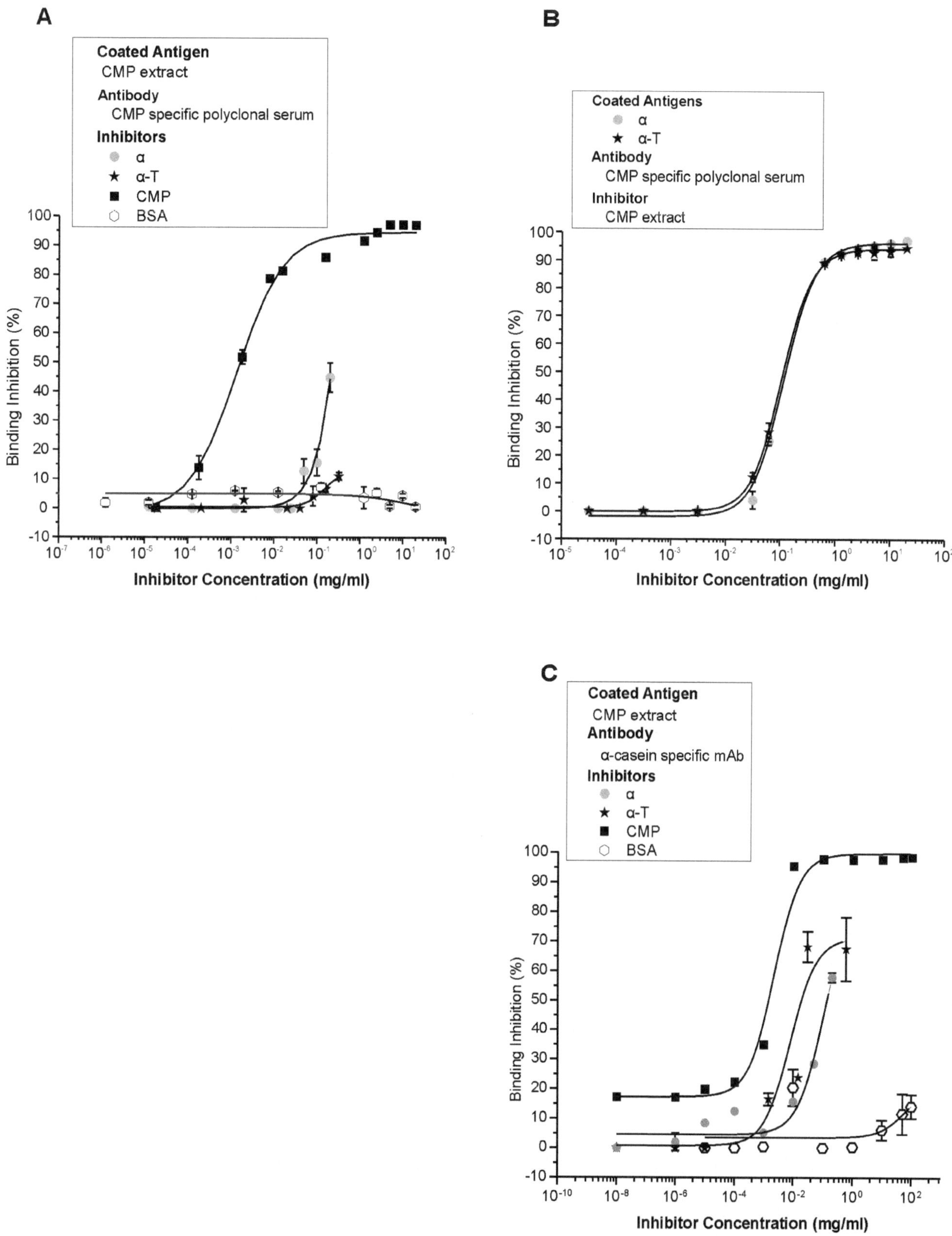

Figure 2. Sequential competitive ELISA with the CMP-specific rabbit polyclonal antiserum and 1D5 mAb. Microtiter plates were coated with CMP (1 μg/well) (**A** and **C**), α (0.1 μg/well) or α-T (0.1 μg/well) (**B**). CMP-specific polyclonal antiserum (**A**: 1:200,000; **B**: 1:6,000) or α-casein-specific mAb (**C**: 1:300,000) were pre-incubated with different inhibitors at several concentrations and then added to Ag-coated wells. Then the appropriate conjugated secondary antibodies were added and the color was developed.

Table 1. Kinetic and equilibrium constants for complexes formed by α-casein, α subunit of β-conglycinin (α), α-T and PA with the 1D5 mAb, specific for α-casein.

	k_{ass} (M^{-1} s^{-1})	k_{diss} (s^{-1})	K_A (M^{-1})	K_D (M^{-1})
Bovine α-casein	$1.05\times10^4\pm0.14\times10^4$	$8.88\times10^{-4}\pm0.22\times10^{-4}$	$1.18\times10^7\pm0.13\times10^7$	$8.44\times10^{-8}\pm1.48\times10^{-8}$
α	$1.89\times10^4\pm0.18\times10^4$	$9.79\times10^{-4}\pm1.47\times10^{-4}$	$1.93\times10^7\pm0.22\times10^7$	$5.18\times10^{-8}\pm0.60\times10^{-8}$
α-T	$3.14\times10^4\pm0.44\times10^4$	$2.70\times10^{-3}\pm0.40\times10^{-3}$	$1.16\times10^7\pm0.06\times10^7$	$8.60\times10^{-8}\pm0.44\times10^{-8}$
PA	$6.92\times10^3\pm0,48\times10^3$	$1.70\times10^{-3}\pm1.15\times10^{-3}$	$4.06\times10^6\pm2.75\times10^6$	$2.46\times10^{-7}\pm1.67\times10^{-7}$

k_{ass}: Association constant, k_{diss}: Dissociation constant, K_A: Affinity constant, K_D: Equilibrium Dissociation constant.

lysine (K) and arginine (R) in the α-helix secondary structures (Figure S2).

Since conformational epitopes may be involved in this cross-recognition, homology models of α, α-T and PA were built (Figure 5A). As it can be seen in figure 5A the α-helix and β-sheet conformations are highly critical for the spatial distribution of all components. It became evident that peptides containing the cross-reactive domains are surface exposed and accessible to the solvent (Figure 5B).

The 3D models obtained were built using the structure of the soy α′ subunit of β-conglycinin from soybean (PDB 1UIK), which shows 90% identity with α subunit of β-conglycinin, as derived from fold assignment. The best structural model was evaluated using ProsaII and a Z-score = −7, indicating a high reliability.

According to the peptide reactivity and localization on the surface of the α subunit of β-conglycinin, three putative epitopes can be proposed (Figures 5B I and II). The region 1 would be contained in the PA fragment, while regions 2 and 3 could be structurally close, but on the opposite side of PA in the molecule.

Analyzing the secondary structure of the three immune reactive regions, and taking into account homology modeling results (Modeller) and the superficial residues visualized by PyMol, we found that α-helices, β-strands and connecting loops are relevant for the region 1-containing PA, which includes the positive spots 9, 10 and 12 of the overlapping assay. Instead, region 2 (contains P16, P22 and P23) and region 3 (contains P1, P2 and P4) would be mainly composed of superficial connecting loops. Furthermore, we studied the electrostatic potential on the surface of the three reactive regions using the PBEQ-Solver interface [35] on the web. The surface charge of the region 1 is positive (Figure S1B I) suggesting the predominance of electrostatic interactions with antibodies. On the other hand, the analysis of the electrostatic potential of the accessible solvent surface of region 2 and 3 (located on the opposite side of the molecule) (Figure S1B II) showed different features which may imply different interactions with antibodies. As judge for the electrostatic potential, surface epitopes contained in region 2 may be recognized by antibodies through hydrophobic or non-ionic interactions, while for the region 3 hydrophobic forces may be mainly involved, with a component of electrostatic bonds.

Immunoassays showed the Presence of Linear and Conformational Epitopes on PA

Immunoblotting with different cow's milk-specific antibodies was assessed to validate the cross-reactivity of recombinant PA and PN. The immunoblotting pattern reactivity observed for PA indicates the presence of IgG- and IgE-binding epitopes, whereas PN showed no reactivity (Figure 5C). Elucidation of conformational epitopes involved in the cross-recognition of PA was assessed by dot-blot under different denaturing conditions (Figure 5D). Peptides heated or treated with urea and SDS showed a lower intensity when membranes were revealed with the CMP-specific antibodies (human sera containing IgE, the rabbit polyclonal antiserum and the mAb specific for α-casein), as compared to untreated PA. However, the reactivity observed with the rabbit polyclonal antiserum with DTT- and urea-treated PA led us to speculate that this antiserum also contains milk-specific antibodies capable of recognizing linear IgG epitopes.

In Vivo and *In Vitro* Cross-reactivity of Soybean Components was confirmed with a CMA Murine Model

To further investigate the clinical relevance of the immunochemical cross-reactivity described, orally sensitized Balb/c mice with CMP were challenged with soy proteins (Figure 6A). Signs and symptoms were observed and scored on a scale from 0 to 5 according to the criteria shown in Table 2. We found that milk sensitized mice developed hypersensitivity symptoms immediately following the oral exposure to soy (SP, α, α-T and PA) or milk components (CMP and β-lg) (Figure 6A and B). No symptoms were observed in sensitized mice exposed to OVA, or in sham mice exposed to the different antigens. Remarkably, the sl challenge with individual proteins triggered immediate clinical signs (Figure 6B), thus reflecting the compromise of the mouth mucosa in animals that were intragastrically sensitized. These findings correlated with the high serum specific IgE levels (Figure 6C) and positive skin tests (Figure 6D) found in milk allergic mice injected with α, α-T and PA. Positive skin tests were also obtained with CMP and SP (pictures not shown). In addition, control mice rendered negative skin tests when injected with CMP, SP or soy recombinant components (pictures not showed). Every mice were injected with saline as control in the contra-lateral side and in all cases the reaction was negative (one is showed in Figure 6D). Moreover, Th2-associated IgG1 antibodies that were induced during the sensitization phase with cholera toxin, also recognized the different soy components. Specific IgG2a remained undetectable during the experiment (data not showed), indicating no Th1 induction during the sensitization phase.

Finally, we found an increased secretion of IL-5 by spleen cells stimulated with CMP, SP, α and α-T (Figure 6E). PA showed a slight increase in the production of this Th2-associated cytokine, while IFN-γ remained low, as expected. These findings clearly indicate that CMP-specific T cells elicited during the sensitization phase can be *in vitro* stimulated with soy components.

Discussion

The characterization of the cross-reactivity between milk and soy allergens may shed light on the structural and immunologic

Spot #	Sequence
1	**LITLAIPVNKPGRFE**
2	**IPVNKPGRFE**SFFLS
3	SFFLSSTEAQQSYLQ
4	QSYLQ**GFSRN**ILEAS
5	ILEASYDTKFEEINK
6	EEINKVLFSREEGQQ
7	EEGQQQGEQRLQESV
8	LQESVIVEISKEQIR
9	KEQIR**ALSKRAKSSS**
10	**AKSSSRKTIS**SEDKP
11	SEDKPFNLRSRDPI
12	SRDPI**YSNKL**GKFFE
13	GKFFEITPEKNPQLRD
14	NPQLRD**LDIFL**SIVD
15	LSIVDMNEGALLLPH
16	LLLPH**FNSKA**IVILV
17	IVILVINEGDANIEL
18	ANIELVGLKEQQQEQ
19	QQQEQQQEEQPLEVR
20	PLEVRKYRAELSEQD
21	LSEQDIFVIPAGYPV
22	AGYPV**VVNATSNLNF**
23	**SNLNFFAIGI**NAENN
24	NAENNQRNFL

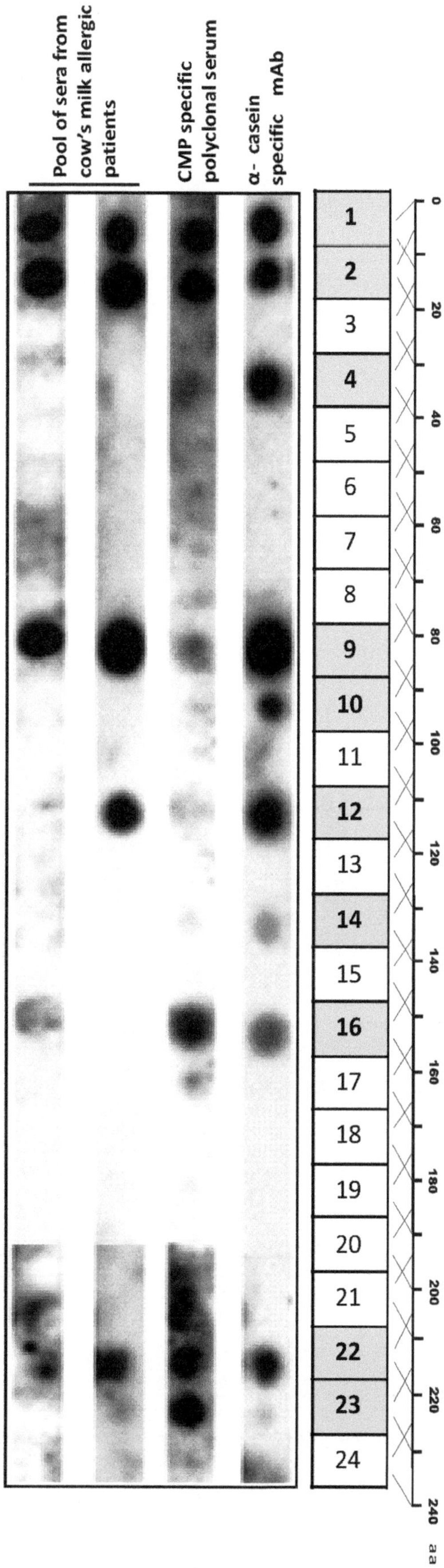

Figure 3. Epitope mapping of α-T. SPOTs array depicting the overlapping 15-aminoacid peptides covering the complete sequence of α-T, and probed with two different pools of serum from cow's milk allergic patients, a rabbit CMP-specific polyclonal serum and the 1D5 α-casein-specific mAb, followed with the appropriate conjugated secondary antibodies. Positive spots are shaded in grey boxes and recognized amino acids are bolded in the sequence depicted for spotted peptides.

relationships between phylogenetically unrelated allergens. Our recent studies show that members of the 11S (Gly m 6) and 7S (Gly m 5) globulin storage soy proteins are cross-reactive allergens with bovine caseins [13–15]. The immunochemical cross-reactivity described has been biologically confirmed using an IgE-mediated mouse model of food allergy with mice exclusively sensitized to CMP [15]. This finding highlights the potential clinical relevance of this phenomenon in allergic patients, although limitations are obvious with conclusions extrapolated from animal models. However, we consider they provide a useful biological tool when ethics is concerning, and in situations in which co-sensitization in patients is almost impossible to disprove. There are some studies reporting the occurrence of clinical intolerance to soy-based formula in milk allergic patients without previous sensitization to soy allergens [9,10]. Although they show that it occurs in a small proportion of patients (<15%), this intolerance is a clinical common concern in our population. Milk allergic patients may develop hypersensitivity reactions following accidental exposure to soy after the ingestion of soy-containing foods, or during the restrictive treatment with soy-based formula.

In this study, we have focused on investigating shared B and T epitopes of Gly m 5 with bovine caseins, which are relevant allergens of soy and milk respectively [11,20]. Of note, the soy recombinant components were recognized as soluble antigens by a rabbit CMP-specific polyclonal antiserum and the α-casein specific monoclonal antibody in a competitive ELISA. These findings discard the possibility of neo epitopes created during the coating of antigens to the solid phase as responsible for this cross-reactivity

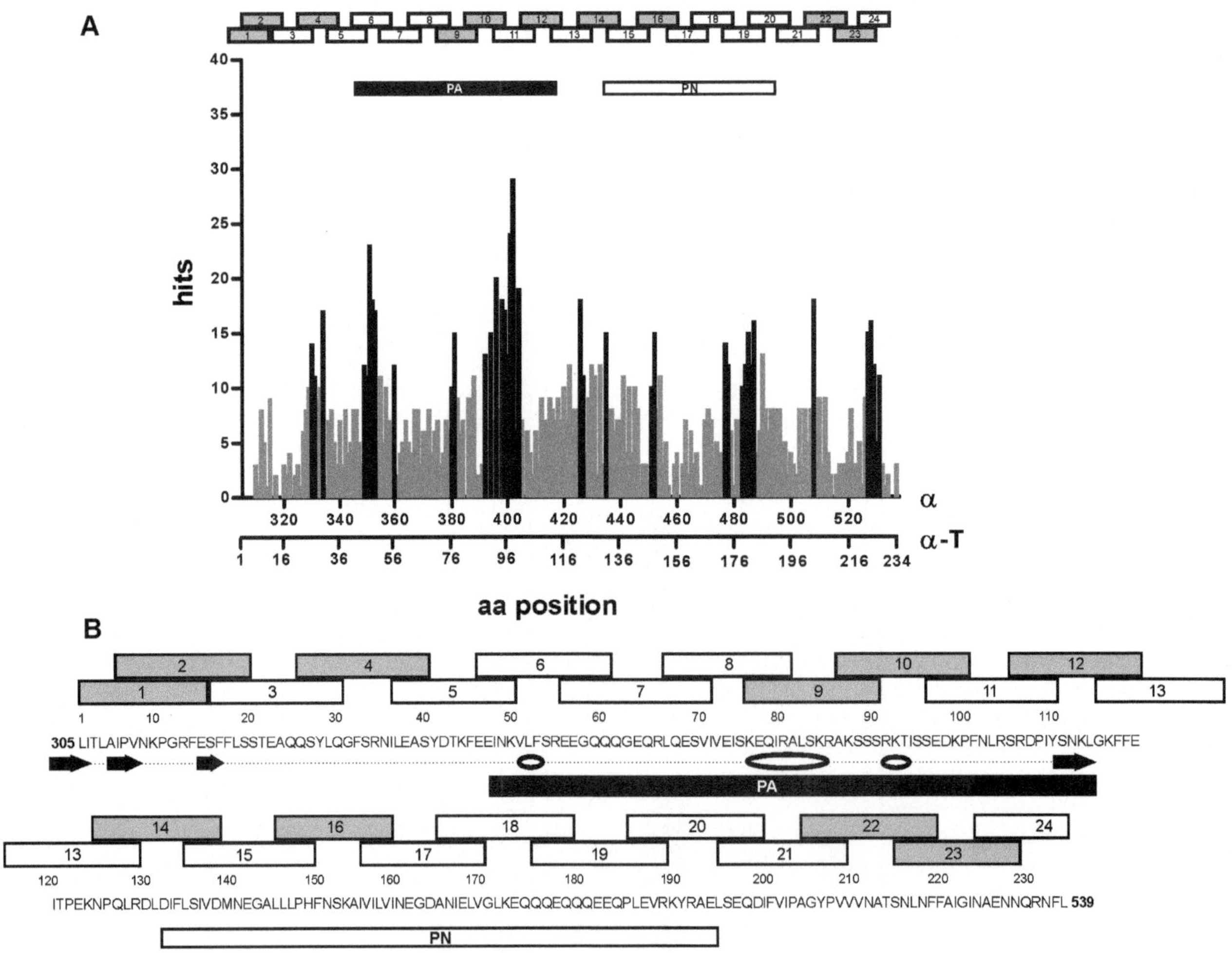

Figure 4. Schematic localization of the identified spots along the α-T sequence and sequence alignment analysis. A) Analysis of the sequence alignment of α-T with IgE epitopes in bovine caseins (IEDB) shown as hit distribution of amino acid similitude per position along the sequence of α-T. Positions of α-T with high hit values (black columns) correlate with positive spots of the overlapping assay (spots 9, 10 and12); **B**) The sequence of α-T (1–234 aa) is depicted along with overlapped peptides, PA and PN (305–539 aa correspond to α). *In silico* predicted alpha-helix (white ovals) and beta-sheet (black arrows) zones are indicated. PA contains the amino acid positions with the highest hits and the α-helix and β strand secondary structures.

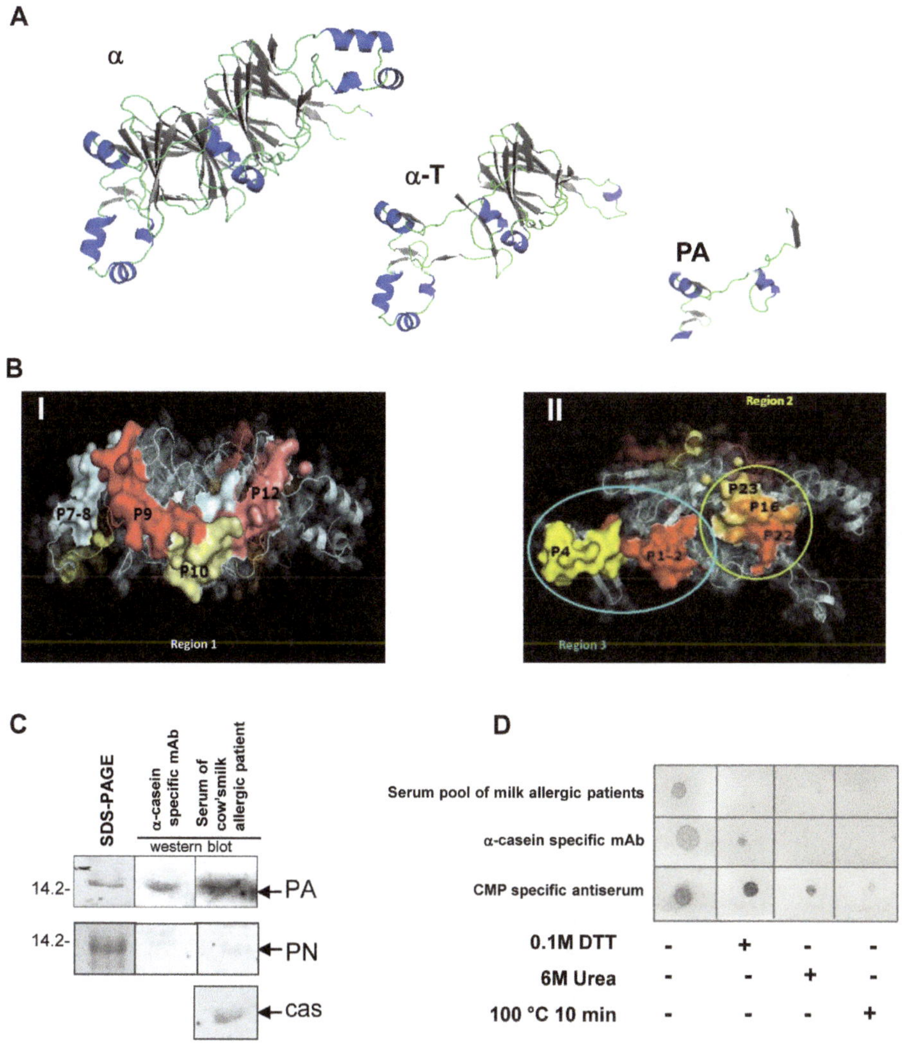

Figure 5. ***In silico* and *in vitro* analysis of α, α-T and PA. A)** Homology model obtained using the Modeller and visualized by PyMOL of α-subunit of β-conglycinin, α-T and PA, based on NCBI Conserved Domain Search results with α′ subunit as template (α-helices are shown in blue and β-sheets as dark grey arrows on the structure). **B)** Surface representation of positive overlapped peptides marked in different colors according to the intensity of the reaction (from pale yellow to red); I and II correspond to opposite sides of the α molecule. Positive peptides localized on the surface of the molecule seem to converge in three regions or putative epitopes. The remaining part of the molecule is represented in transparent spheres showing the secondary structure. **C)** SDS-PAGE of recombinant PA and PN and immunoblotting developed with 1D5 α-casein-specific mAb and a representative serum of CMA patients. Alpha-s1 casein was used as positive control (Molecular masses are shown on the left as kDa). **D)** Dot-blot of recombinant treated and untreated PA revealed with a pool of CMA patient sera, α-casein-specific mAb and CMP-specific polyclonal rabbit antiserum. Denaturing conditions consisted on: 0.1M DTT solution, 6M urea or 100°C for 10 minutes. *Cas: Alpha-s1 casein.*

and confirm that α and α-T contain cross-reactive B epitopes. This assay rendered a higher IC50 for α than that for CMP with the polyclonal and monoclonal antibodies (150 and 86 times respectively), which is reasonable since these antibodies are primary specific for milk components. These results and the shape of the dose-response curves indicate that the antigen-antibody interaction is specific, that the α protein and its fraction α-T bear cross-reactive epitopes with bovine α-casein, and that a restricted population of CMP-specific antibodies specifically recognized B epitopes in α and α-T polypeptides. These findings were further characterized with the biosensor binding assay, which showed that α-casein, α and α-T present similar affinity constant to the α-casein-specific mAb. The higher k_{ass} value found for α-T as compared with that for α and α-casein can be due to stronger favourable contacts in the interface formed between mAb 1D5 and α-T. However, the k_{diss} value means that this complex is more unstable than those formed with α and α-casein. Likewise, the smaller k_{ass} value found for PA as compared to the other components analyzed can be explained by lower contacts with 1D5, which may be due to its smaller size and conformational changes. As expected, we found medium affinities for this monoclonal antibody with different cross-reactive antigens, which may reflect an overall approach to understand the cross-reactivity implicated in a hypersensitivity reaction. Recently, and using synthetic allergens, it has been shown that IgE antibodies do not necessarily need to have a high affinity with its specific antigen to trigger mast cell degranulation [41]. In this study we have shown that even a 64 amino acid residue peptide of moderate affinity triggers a specific allergic response in milk allergic mice, thus indicating that it can activate sensitized cells.

To gain more insight into the molecular feature of this cross-reactivity we next characterized B epitopes (IgG and IgE) on

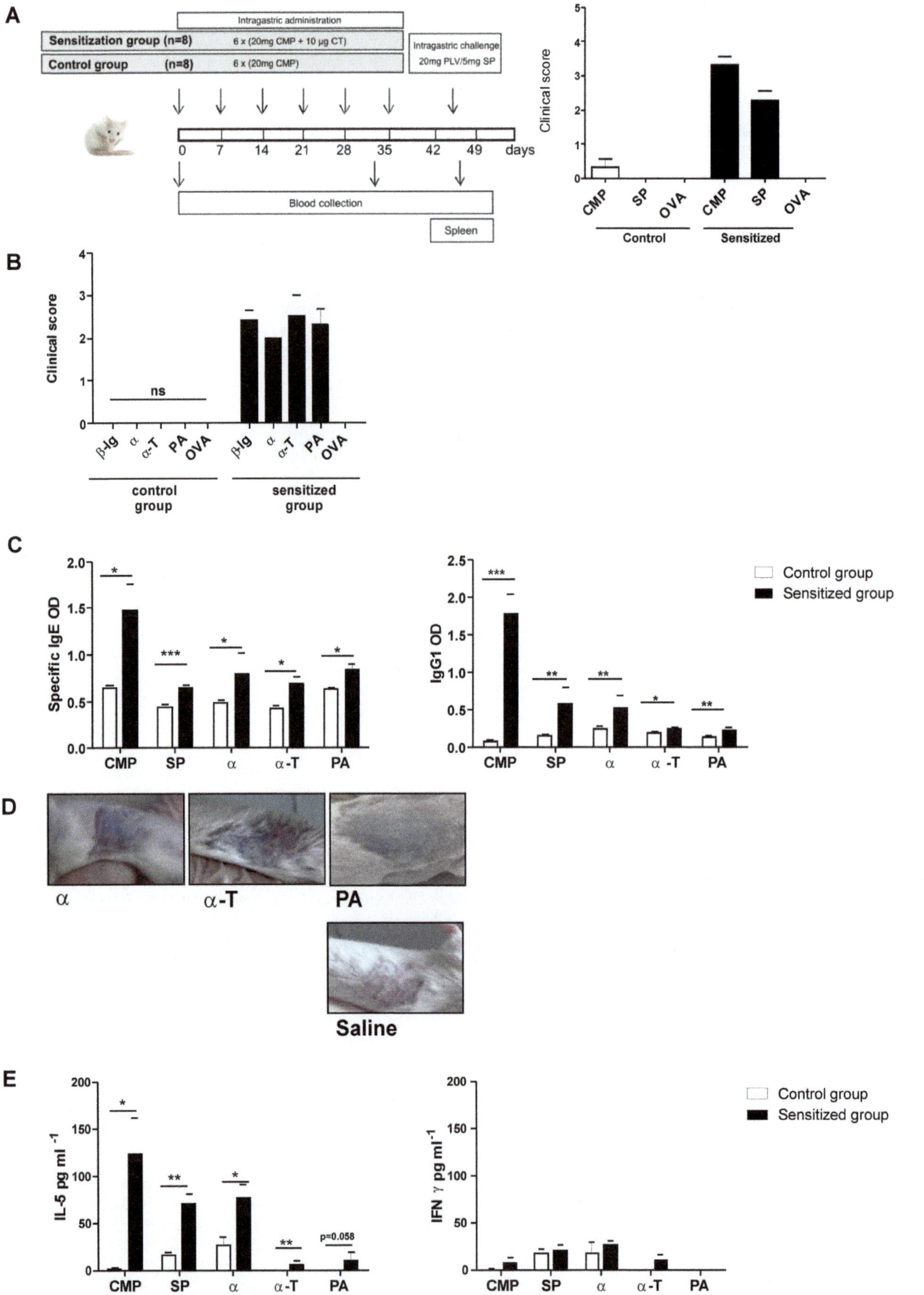
A
Intragastric administration
Sensitization group (n=8) 6 x (20mg CMP + 10 µg CT)
Control group (n=8) 6 x (20mg CMP)
Intragastric challenge 20mg PLV/5mg SP
0 7 14 21 28 35 42 49 days
Blood collection
Spleen
Clinical score
CMP SP OVA CMP SP OVA
Control
Sensitized
B
Clinical score
ns
β-lg α α-T PA OVA β-lg α α-T PA OVA
control group
sensitized group
C
Specific IgE OD
IgG1 OD
CMP SP α α-T PA
Control group
Sensitized group
D
α
α-T
PA
Saline
E
IL-5 pg ml -1
IFN γ pg ml -1
p=0.058
CMP SP α α-T PA
Control group
Sensitized group

Figure 6. ***In vivo*** **cross-reactivity assessed in a food allergy mouse model. A)** Schematic representation of the experimental protocol: BALB/c mice were subjected to weekly intragastric sensitization with cholera toxin and CMP from day 0 through day 35. Challenge was performed at day 45 by ig administration of proteins (CMP, SP or OVA). Control mice only received CMP and then they were challenged with the different antigens. Symptoms were observed 30 min following the oral challenge and scored according to Table 2. **B)** Clinical scores assigned to symptoms observed 30 min following the sublingual challenge with 10 μg of β-lg, α, α-T, PA or OVA. **C)** Specific IgE and IgG1 in serum of milk-sensitized and control mice were assessed by EAST or indirect ELISA at day 45, respectively (mean values ± SEM). **D)** Cutaneous test performed in sensitized mice subcutaneously injected with 10 μg of antigens (α, α-T or PA) in the right flank and with saline in the left flank. The presence of blue color in the skin within minutes was considered a positive cutaneous test. **E)** Levels of IL-5 and IFN-γ assayed on stimulated splenocyte supernatants by ELISA (mean values ± SEM). Results correspond to a single experiment with five mice per condition, representative of three separate experiments that gave similar results. Statistically significant differences are denoted as starred values (*) ***p<0.005, **p<0.01, *p<0.05.

different peptides of α (α-T and PA) using overlapping synthetic peptides, recombinant allergenic fragments and unfolded fragments. Besides, the overlapped peptide scanning revealed that cross-reactivity is not due to a unique shared epitope. The overlapping peptide assay showed that the epitope-bearing 15-mer peptides contain 33.8% of hydrophobic (A: alanine, F: phenylalanine and L: leucine), 29% of neutral hydrophilic (S: serine and N: asparagine) and 9.6% of charged hydrophilic aminoacids (K: lysine, E: glutamic acid) with a positive net charge, suggesting that different ways of antibody-antigen recognition may be possible in this type of cross-reactivity (Figure S1). Since the combining site of an antibody may present different zones with different charges, and furthermore, different conformers of the paratope can be found in unbound antibodies exhibiting different surfaces of interaction with antigens in this regard, a single antibody can interact with different epitopes even on the same antigen. In the particular case of the PA, which is mainly positively charged, the interactions with antibodies are expected to be electrostatic with a net negatively charged paratope. Regarding epitopes present in the region 2, the type of interactions are mainly hydrophobic, but analyzing epitopes in the region 3 those interaction could be a combination of hydrophobic and electrostatic ones. Thus, the studied cross-reactivity implies a more complex interpretation than just considering the presence of a unique and shared epitope.

The *in silico* analysis for prediction of cross-reactive epitopes, secondary structure and modeling of Gly m 5 indicated that PA contains cross-recognized conformational and linear epitopes that are exposed on the surface of the allergen to interact with antibodies. Then, IgG and IgE cross-reactive epitopes were confirmed in PA using different milk-specific antibodies and immunoassays. It has been described that the feature of the epitope in caseins is critical for the history of milk allergy in allergic patients [42–44], and the recognition of conformational epitopes is a predictive factor for a later acquisition of tolerance to CMP. Therefore, monitoring the reactivity of serum antibodies against PA might constitute an additional prognostic tool for achievement of immune tolerance in patients. Although the disruption of dominant epitopes in PA using chaotropic agents provided preliminary data, further investigations with structural biology techniques such as X-ray crystallography and nuclear magnetic resonance are necessary to visualize these conformational cross-reactive epitopes. In this sense, the combination of different mapping techniques with the visualization of the 3D models is needed to assess the structural integrity of allergens. Food antigens, which have mainly linear epitopes following food processing or digestion, also contain conformational epitopes that can be affected by food processing, thus interfering with the conformation, IgE binding activity and hence the allergenicity.

The use of different sequence databases of caseins allergenic epitopes provided no information of shared sequences with the soy component studied here. However, the sequence database obtained by us, using the describe techniques above, provided of several peptides of α-subunit of β-conglycinin that presented homology with milk caseins and their cross-reactivity was *in vitro* confirmed. Therefore, based on *in silico* and experimental data we have selected a peptide from the sequence of α-T (PA) that matched the identified IgE-binding epitopes in caseins [42,45,46]. Fu et al [47] identified IgG sequential and solvent-exposed epitopes (185–231) in the N-terminus domain of the α-subunit of the β-conglycinin, which is not coincident with the epitope here described in the C-terminus domain. Therefore this peptide of Gly m 5 represents a new IgE-binding epitope that occurs in a conformational region of the protein exposed to the solvent.

In this study, the combination of bioinformatics tools for prediction of epitopes, secondary structure, surface electrostatic charge, sequence alignment, molecular modeling and visualization of immunodominant regions in 3D modeled molecules, with immunochemical techniques (immunoblotting, indirect ELISA and competitive ELISA), SPR biosensor and *in vivo* experiments, allowed us to strongly demonstrate the existence of cross-reactivity between Gly m 5 and caseins. Besides, we have selected a candidate peptide that contains linear and conformational B, and T epitopes, which could be easily rendered hypoallergenic for a potential and safe therapeutic treatment.

The clinical symptoms elicited after the sublingual challenge with α, α-T and PA, and the positive skin prick tests confirmed the presence of at least two IgE-binding epitopes on the Gly m 5.0101 soy fractions. Of note, the presence of linear T epitopes could be evidenced when

Table 2. Clinical scores assigned to symptoms triggered following the oral or sublingual challenge.

Score	Symptoms
0	No symptoms
1	Scratching and rubbing around the snout and head
2	Puffiness around the eyes and mouth, pilar-erecti, diarrhea, reduced activity and/or decreased activity with increased respiratory rate
3	Respiratory distress, cyanosis around snout and tail
4	No activity upon stimuli, convulsion
5	Death

spleen cells were stimulated with these fractions, with the secretion of IL-5. The ability of α, α-T and mainly PA for T cell activation encourage us to propose them in a potential mucosal therapy for tolerance induction in patients with milk and/or soy allergy.

As a conclusion, using *in vitro*, *in vivo* and *in silico* approaches we have identified a peptide of Gly m 5 that contains B and T cross-reactive epitopes with bovine casein. This information sheds light on the characterization of this relevant soybean allergen, and may provide a molecular explanation for the complex IgE cross-reactivity between the phylogenetically unrelated milk and soy allergens. This phenomenon may explain the secondary soy allergy elicited during the treatment of some cow's milk allergic patients. Finally, this knowledge may be exploited to develop a mucosal tolerizing immunotherapy using PA for intervention in soy and milk allergy.

Supporting Information

Figure S1 Electrostatic and charge analysis of α-T. **A**) pI and charge at pH = 7.5 for peptides of the overlapping assay estimated with the Protein Calculator v3.3 (http://www.scripps.edu/~cdputnam/protcalc.html). **B**) Electrostatic potential surface on the α subunit of β-conglycinin showing **I**) region 1, which contains the PA fragment, and **II**) regions 2 and 3. Note that the region 1 is mostly positively charged, region 2 is mostly hydrophobic and region 3 is hydrophobic and slightly positively charged.

Figure S2 Multiple sequence alignment between sequences of α-T and epitopes on bovine casein peptides. A total of 73 peptides of α-S1 (1–55), α-S2 (56–63), β (64–67) and κ (68–73) bovine caseins, described as T and/or B epitopes (IEDB, (http://www.immuneepitope.org/) were aligned with α-T sequence using the ClustalW2 server (http://www.ebi.ac.uk/Tools/msa/clustalw2/). Common amino acids are shaded in red on casein peptide sequences, or in grey in the α-T sequence. Blue rectangles delimit the highest frequencies of similitude observed (which correspond to the high hit values in Figure 4 A). Green and yellow boxes underneath the α-T sequence correspond to PA and PN respectively.

Acknowledgments

GP, AC, CAF, SP and GHD are scientists' members of the CONICET; AMC is a post-doctoral fellow of CONICET.

Author Contributions

Conceived and designed the experiments: AC LBB GP AMC RC PLS SP GHD. Performed the experiments: RC AMC PLS AC IB VG. Analyzed the data: RC AMC PLS VG GP AC SP GHD. Contributed reagents/materials/analysis tools: CAF LBB AC GP SP GHD. Wrote the paper: RC SP AC GHD. Performed bioinfomatic analysis: VG GP AC SP AMC RC.

References

1. Rona RJ, Keil T, Summers C, Gislason D, Zuidmeer L, et al. (2007) The prevalence of food allergy: a meta-analysis. J Allergy Clin Immunol 120: 638–646. doi:10.1016/j.jaci.2007.05.026.
2. Sicherer SH (2011) Food allergy. Mt Sinai J Med New York 78: 683–696. doi:10.1002/msj.20292.
3. Fiocchi A, Brozek J, Schünemann H, Bahna SL, von Berg A, et al. (2010) World Allergy Organization (WAO) Diagnosis and Rationale for Action against Cow's Milk Allergy (DRACMA) Guidelines. World Allergy Organ J 3: 57–161. doi:10.1097/WOX.0b013e3181defeb9.
4. Koletzko S, Niggemann B, Arato A, Dias JA, Heuschkel R, et al. (2012) Diagnostic approach and management of cow's-milk protein allergy in infants and children: ESPGHAN GI Committee practical guidelines. J Pediatr Gastroenterol Nutr 55: 221–229. doi:10.1097/MPG.0b013e31825c9482.
5. Dupont C (2011) Food allergy: recent advances in pathophysiology and diagnosis. Ann Nutr Metab 59 Suppl 1: 8–18. doi:10.1159/000334145.
6. Bhatia J, Greer F (2008) Use of soy protein-based formulas in infant feeding. Pediatrics 121: 1062–1068. doi:10.1542/peds.2008-0564.
7. COOK CD (1960) Probable gastrointestinal reaction to soybean. N Engl J Med 263: 1076–1077. doi:10.1056/NEJM196011242632109.
8. Agostoni C, Axelsson I, Goulet O, Koletzko B, Michaelsen KF, et al. (2006) Soy protein infant formulae and follow-on formulae: a commentary by the ESPGHAN Committee on Nutrition. J Pediatr Gastroenterol Nutr 42: 352–361. doi:10.1097/01.mpg.0000189358.38427.cd.
9. Zeiger RS, Sampson HA, Bock SA, Burks AW Jr, Harden K, et al. (1999) Soy allergy in infants and children with IgE-associated cow's milk allergy. J Pediatr 134: 614–622.
10. Klemola T, Vanto T, Juntunen-Backman K, Kalimo K, Korpela R, et al. (2002) Allergy to soy formula and to extensively hydrolyzed whey formula in infants with cow's milk allergy: a prospective, randomized study with a follow-up to the age of 2 years. J Pediatr 140: 219–224. doi:10.1067/mpd.2002.121935.
11. Docena GH, Fernandez R, Chirdo FG, Fossati CA (1996) Identification of casein as the major allergenic and antigenic protein of cow's milk. Allergy 51: 412–416.
12. Docena G, Rozenfeld P, Fernández R, Fossati CA (2002) Evaluation of the residual antigenicity and allergenicity of cow's milk substitutes by in vitro tests. Allergy 57: 83–91.
13. Rozenfeld P, Docena GH, Añón MC, Fossati CA (2002) Detection and identification of a soy protein component that cross-reacts with caseins from cow's milk. Clin Exp Immunol 130: 49–58.
14. Curciarello R, Lareu JF, Fossati CA, Docena GH, Petruccelli S (2008) Immunochemical characterization of Glycine max L. Merr. var Raiden, as a possible hypoallergenic substitute for cow's milk-allergic patients. Clin Exp Allergy J Br Soc Allergy Clin Immunol 38: 1559–1565. doi:10.1111/j.1365-2222.2008.03062.x.
15. Smaldini P, Curciarello R, Candreva A, Rey MA, Fossati CA, et al. (2012) In vivo evidence of cross-reactivity between cow's milk and soybean proteins in a mouse model of food allergy. Int Arch Allergy Immunol 158: 335–346. doi:10.1159/000333562.
16. Ogawa T, Bando N, Tsuji H, Nishikawa K, Kitamura K (1995) Alpha-subunit of beta-conglycinin, an allergenic protein recognized by IgE antibodies of soybean-sensitive patients with atopic dermatitis. Biosci Biotechnol Biochem 59: 831–833.
17. Ballmer-Weber BK, Holzhauser T, Scibilia J, Mittag D, Zisa G, et al. (2007) Clinical characteristics of soybean allergy in Europe: a double-blind, placebo-controlled food challenge study. J Allergy Clin Immunol 119: 1489–1496. doi:10.1016/j.jaci.2007.01.049.
18. Krishnan HB, Kim W-S, Jang S, Kerley MS (2009) All three subunits of soybean beta-conglycinin are potential food allergens. J Agric Food Chem 57: 938–943. doi:10.1021/jf802451g.
19. Codina R, Ardusso L, Lockey RF, Crisci CD, Jaén C, et al. (2002) Identification of the soybean hull allergens involved in sensitization to soybean dust in a rural population from Argentina and N-terminal sequence of a major 50 KD allergen. Clin Exp Allergy J Br Soc Allergy Clin Immunol 32: 1059–1063.
20. Holzhauser T, Wackermann O, Ballmer-Weber BK, Bindslev-Jensen C, Scibilia J, et al. (2009) Soybean (Glycine max) allergy in Europe: Gly m 5 (beta-conglycinin) and Gly m 6 (glycinin) are potential diagnostic markers for severe allergic reactions to soy. J Allergy Clin Immunol 123: 452–458. doi:10.1016/j.jaci.2008.09.034.
21. Ogawa A, Samoto M, Takahashi K (2000) Soybean allergens and hypoallergenic soybean products. J Nutr Sci Vitaminol (Tokyo) 46: 271–279.
22. Petrucelli S, Chirdo FG, Añón MC (n.d.) Immunochemical reactivity of soybean b-conglycinin subunits. Food Agric Immunol 16: 17–28.
23. Mills EN, Jenkins J, Marigheto N, Belton PS, Gunning AP, et al. (2002) Allergens of the cupin superfamily. Biochem Soc Trans 30: 925–929. doi:10.1042/.
24. Nallamsetty S, Austin BP, Penrose KJ, Waugh DS (2005) Gateway vectors for the production of combinatorially-tagged His6-MBP fusion proteins in the cytoplasm and periplasm of Escherichia coli. Protein Sci Publ Protein Soc 14: 2964–2971. doi:10.1110/ps.051718605.
25. Peters B, Sidney J, Bourne P, Bui H-H, Buus S, et al. (2005) The immune epitope database and analysis resource: from vision to blueprint. PLoS Biol 3: e91. doi:10.1371/journal.pbio.0030091.
26. Chou PY, Fasman GD (1978) Prediction of the secondary structure of proteins from their amino acid sequence. Adv Enzymol Relat Areas Mol Biol 47: 45–148.
27. Emini EA, Hughes JV, Perlow DS, Boger J (1985) Induction of hepatitis A virus-neutralizing antibody by a virus-specific synthetic peptide. J Virol 55: 836–839.
28. Karplus PA, Schulz GE (1985) Prediction of chain flexibility in proteins. Naturwissenschaften 72: 212–213.
29. Kolaskar AS, Tongaonkar PC (1990) A semi-empirical method for prediction of antigenic determinants on protein antigens. FEBS Lett 276: 172–174.
30. Parker JM, Guo D, Hodges RS (1986) New hydrophilicity scale derived from high-performance liquid chromatography peptide retention data: correlation of

predicted surface residues with antigenicity and X-ray-derived accessible sites. Biochemistry (Mosc) 25: 5425–5432.
31. Altschul SF, Madden TL, Schäffer AA, Zhang J, Zhang Z, et al. (1997) Gapped BLAST and PSI-BLAST: a new generation of protein database search programs. Nucleic Acids Res 25: 3389–3402.
32. Marti-Renom MA, Madhusudhan MS, Fiser A, Rost B, Sali A (2002) Reliability of assessment of protein structure prediction methods. Struct Lond Engl 1993 10: 435–440.
33. Jaroszewski L, Rychlewski L, Li Z, Li W, Godzik A (2005) FFAS03: a server for profile–profile sequence alignments. Nucleic Acids Res 33: W284–288. doi:10.1093/nar/gki418.
34. Wiederstein M, Sippl MJ (2007) ProSA-web: interactive web service for the recognition of errors in three-dimensional structures of proteins. Nucleic Acids Res 35: W407–410. doi:10.1093/nar/gkm290.
35. Jo S, Vargyas M, Vasko-Szedlar J, Roux B, Im W (2008) PBEQ-Solver for online visualization of electrostatic potential of biomolecules. Nucleic Acids Res 36: W270–275. doi:10.1093/nar/gkn314.
36. Combet C, Blanchet C, Geourjon C, Deléage G (2000) NPS@: network protein sequence analysis. Trends Biochem Sci 25: 147–150.
37. Chou PY, Fasman GD (1974) Prediction of protein conformation. Biochemistry (Mosc) 13: 222–245.
38. Cole C, Barber JD, Barton GJ (2008) The Jpred 3 secondary structure prediction server. Nucleic Acids Res 36: W197–201. doi:10.1093/nar/gkn238.
39. Jones DT (1999) Protein secondary structure prediction based on position-specific scoring matrices. J Mol Biol 292: 195–202. doi:10.1006/jmbi.1999.3091.
40. Ceska M (1981) Radioimmunoassay of IgE using paper disks. Methods Enzymol 73: 646–656.
41. Handlogten MW, Kiziltepe T, Alves NJ, Bilgicer B (2012) Synthetic allergen design reveals the significance of moderate affinity epitopes in mast cell degranulation. ACS Chem Biol 7: 1796–1801. doi:10.1021/cb300193f.
42. Chatchatee P, Järvinen KM, Bardina L, Vila L, Beyer K, et al. (2001) Identification of IgE and IgG binding epitopes on beta- and kappa-casein in cow's milk allergic patients. Clin Exp Allergy J Br Soc Allergy Clin Immunol 31: 1256–1262.
43. Chatchatee P, Järvinen KM, Bardina L, Beyer K, Sampson HA (2001) Identification of IgE- and IgG-binding epitopes on alpha(s1)-casein: differences in patients with persistent and transient cow's milk allergy. J Allergy Clin Immunol 107: 379–383. doi:10.1067/mai.2001.112372.
44. Vila L, Beyer K, Järvinen KM, Chatchatee P, Bardina L, et al. (2001) Role of conformational and linear epitopes in the achievement of tolerance in cow's milk allergy. Clin Exp Allergy J Br Soc Allergy Clin Immunol 31: 1599–1606.
45. Cerecedo I, Zamora J, Shreffler WG, Lin J, Bardina L, et al. (2008) Mapping of the IgE and IgG4 sequential epitopes of milk allergens with a peptide microarray-based immunoassay. J Allergy Clin Immunol 122: 589–594. doi:10.1016/j.jaci.2008.06.040.
46. Cocco RR, Järvinen K-M, Sampson HA, Beyer K (2003) Mutational analysis of major, sequential IgE-binding epitopes in alpha s1-casein, a major cow's milk allergen. J Allergy Clin Immunol 112: 433–437.
47. Fu CJ, Jez JM, Kerley MS, Allee GL, Krishnan HB (2007) Identification, characterization, epitope mapping, and three-dimensional modeling of the alpha-subunit of beta-conglycinin of soybean, a potential allergen for young pigs. J Agric Food Chem 55: 4014–4020. doi:10.1021/jf070211o.

21

Suppression of Cytokine Release by Fluticasone Furoate vs. Mometasone Furoate in Human Nasal Tissue *Ex-Vivo*

Nan Zhang[1]*, Koen Van Crombruggen[1], Gabriele Holtappels[1], Feng Lan[1], Michail Katotomichelakis[2], Luo Zhang[3], Petra Högger[4], Claus Bachert[1,5]

1 Upper Airway Research Laboratory, Ghent University Hospital, Ghent, Belgium, **2** Department of Otorhinolaryngology, Medical School, Democritus University of Thrace, Alexandroupolis, Greece, **3** Department of Otolaryngology Head and Neck Surgery, Beijing TongRen Hospital, Capital Medical University, Beijing, P.R.China, **4** Institute for Pharmacy and Food Chemistry, Julius-Maximilians-Universitity, Würzburg, Germany, **5** Division of ENT Diseases, Clintec, Karolinska Institutet, Stockholm, Sweden

Abstract

Background: Topical glucocorticosteroids are the first line therapy for airway inflammation. Modern compounds with higher efficacy have been developed, but head-to-head comparison studies are sparse.

Objective: To compare the activity of two intranasal glucocorticoids, fluticasone furoate (FF) and mometasone furoate (MF) with respect to the inhibition of T helper (Th)1, Th2 and Th17 cytokine release in airway mucosa.

Methods: We used an ex-vivo human nasal mucosal tissue model and employed pre- and post- Staphylococcus aureus enterotoxin B (SEB)-challenge incubations with various time intervals and drug concentrations to mimic typical clinical situations of preventive or therapeutic use.

Results: At a fixed concentration of 10^{-10} M, FF had significantly higher suppressive effects on interferon (IFN)-γ, interleukin (IL)-2 and IL-17 release, but not IL-5 or tumor necrosis factor (TNF)-α, vs. MF. While the maximal suppressive activity was maintained when FF was added before or after tissue stimulation, the cytokine suppression capacity of MF appeared to be compromised when SEB-induced cell activation preceded the addition of the drug. In a pre-challenge incubation setting with removal of excess drug concentrations, MF approached inhibition of IL-5 and TNF-α after 6 and 24 hours while FF maximally blocked the release of these cytokines right after pre-incubation. Furthermore, FF suppressed a wider range of T helper cytokines compared to MF.

Conclusion: The study demonstrates the potential of our human mucosal model and shows marked differences in the ability to suppress the release of various cytokines in pre- and post-challenge settings between FF and MF mimicking typical clinical situations of preventive or therapeutic use.

Editor: Christian Taube, Leiden University Medical Center, Netherlands

Funding: This work was supported by an investigator initiated grant from GlaxoSmithKline Belgium and by grants to Claus Bachert from the Flemish Scientific Research Board, FWO, projects G.0436.04, 3G.048.09, G.0642.10N, G.0641.10; by the Global Allergy and Asthma European Network (GA2LEN), the European Commission's Seventh Framework programme under grant agreement N° 260895 (PREDICTA), and the Interuniversity Attraction Poles Program - Belgian State Belgian Science Policy, Nr. IAP P7/30. The funders had no role in study design, data collection and analysis, decision to publish, or preparation of the manuscript.

Competing Interests: Claus Bachert has received a grant from GlaxoSmithKline, Belgium, supporting the experiment and cytokine measurements.

* E-mail: nan.zhang@ugent.be

Introduction

Topical glucocorticosteroids (GCS) are the first line therapy for allergic rhinitis, sinusitis and nasal polyposis [1,2]. Over the last decades, GCS compounds with higher efficacy and less systemic bioavailability have been developed, with fluticasone furoate (FF) as the latest compound being introduced to the market [3,4]. FF has the molecular backbone of fluticasone that is also present in fluticasone propionate (FP) but the properties of both molecules are distinctly different [5]. Although FF has a higher receptor affinity and better tissue retention compared to mometasone furoate (MF) [6,7], the clinical advantage of FF over MF has not been demonstrated yet in rigorous clinical trials. In absence of head-to-head comparison studies for both drugs, such comparison may also be extrapolated from ex-vivo human nasal mucosal models using diseased and control mucosa with different stimuli.

To optimally respond to the expectations of the patients, a nasal topical corticosteroid should have a fast onset of action, which requires a fast uptake and strong binding to the glucocorticoid receptor, translocation of the glucocorticoid receptor complex into the nucleus and interaction with glucocorticoid response elements (GREs), resulting in a long duration of action allowing for once daily application, and a high efficacy in suppressing the local inflammation with a broad panel of cytokines from Th1, Th2 and Th17 cells included [8].

We have developed an ex-vivo human mucosal tissue model for Staphylococcus aureus enterotoxin (SEB) induced T-effector cell activation [9,10], in which we can interfere with glucocorticoster-

Table 1. Nasal polyp tissue (n = 9) was incubated with FF or MF at different concentrations for 1 hour and subsequently stimulated with SEB for 24 hours (pre-challenge incubation).

Cytokine	Fluticasone furoate			p- value for max. inhibition	Mometasone furoate		
	Max. inhibition (median (Interquartile range) in %	*Concentr. of max. inhibition*	*Lowest concentr. with significant inhibition*		*Max. inhibition (median (Interquartile range) in %*	*Concentr. of max. inhibition*	*Lowest concentr. with significant inhibition*
IFN-γ	66 (56.5-77.5)	10^{-8} M	10^{-10} M	P = 0.7040	69 (62.8-78.)	10^{-8} M	10^{-9} M
IL-2	67.5 (52-75.6)	10^{-8} M	10^{-10} M	P = 0.7223	75 (46.5-79)	10^{-8} M	10^{-9} M
IL-5	81.5 (72-88)	10^{-8} M	10^{-11} M	P = 0.3606	89 (80.5-91)	10^{-8} M	10^{-10} M
IL-17	76 (68-82.5)	10^{-9} M	10^{-10} M	P = 0.7223	77 (65.8-79)	10^{-8} M	10^{-9} M
TNF-α	65.5 (46-75.5)	10^{-8} M	10^{-10} M	P = 0.2008	42 (32.5-69)	10^{-8} M	10^{-9} M

There was no significant difference in the maximal inhibition of cytokine release over 24 h; however, FF induced a comparable inhibition for all cytokines at lower molar concentrations.

oids and other therapeutic compounds. The model is very robust and reproducible, but sensitive to demonstrate differences in the efficacy of compounds. At the same time, it is very close to the real-life situation and may thus predict the clinical outcome. We here used this model for a comparative study of FF vs MF in their efficacy, duration of their effect and onset of action. The inhibition of the release of a pattern of Th1, Th2 and Th17 cytokines was studied in three groups of experiments.

The experiments were designed to reflect optimal conditions for the drugs with incubation prior to and together with the stimulus, or real life conditions, with application of the drugs after initiation of disease exacerbation by a stimulus, and finally to study onset and duration of action after a defined exposure to the drug.

Methods

Human specimen

Nasal polyp samples were collected during functional endoscopic sinus surgery from 9 patients (median age, 52 years; range, 28-72 years; 5 men and 4 women). Nasal polyposis was diagnosed on the basis of symptoms, clinical examination, nasal endoscopy, and sinus computed tomography scan according to the European Position Paper on Rhinosinusitis and Nasal Polyps guidelines [1]. The atopic status of patients was evaluated by skin prick tests (SPTs) with the European standard panel of 14 inhalant allergens. Negative and positive controls (10 mg/mL histamine solution) were included with each SPT. 5 nasal polyp patients with positive SPT for at least 1 of the most common aeroallergens, 4 negative. Three patients reported mild asthma in their history, and one patient reported aspirin intolerance.

All patients were asked to refrain from topical or oral corticosteroids or antibiotics 4 weeks preoperatively and gave their written informed consent and the ethics committee of the Ghent University Hospital approved the study.

Mechanical disruption of human nasal tissue

The nasal tissue was cut thoroughly as described before [9,10] in tissue culture medium (TCM) of RPMI 1640 (Sigma-Aldrich, Bornem, Belgium) containing 2 mmol/L L-glutamine (Invitrogen, Merelbeke, Belgium), antibiotics (50 IU/mL penicillin and 50 mg/mL streptomycin; Invitrogen), and 0.1% BSA (Sigma). The tissue was passed through a mesh ($\pm$0.9 mm^2) to achieve comparable fragments. The fragments ($\pm$0.9 mm^3) were weighed, suspended as 0.04 g tissue/mL TCM and incubated for 1 hour at 37°C, 5% CO_2. In a following step tissue fragments were washed, resuspended in the appropriate amount of TCM, and distributed into a 48-well plate (BD Falcon, VWR International, Belgium) with 0.5 mL tissue fragment suspension in each well.

Pre-challenge incubation - the experiment to compare the effect of compounds under optimal conditions

The polyp tissue fragments were pre-incubated with TCM (RPMI+DMSO), 10^{-8} M, 10^{-9} M, 10^{-10} M and 10^{-11} M fluticasone furoate (FF; GSK Stevenage, UK) (29,6 mg FF dissolved in 5500 µl DMSO made a stock solution of 10 mM (10^{-2} M)) or mometasone furoate (MF; Schering Plough) (52,14 mg in 10 ml DMSO made a stock solution of 10 mM (10^{-2} M)) for 1 hour at 37°C/5% CO_2 and then stimulated with TCM (negative control) or 0.5 µg/mL SEB (# S4881; Sigma) for 24 hours. The final concentration of DMSO was 0.1% in each well. Aliquots of the supernatants were stored immediately at −20°C until analysis of cytokines.

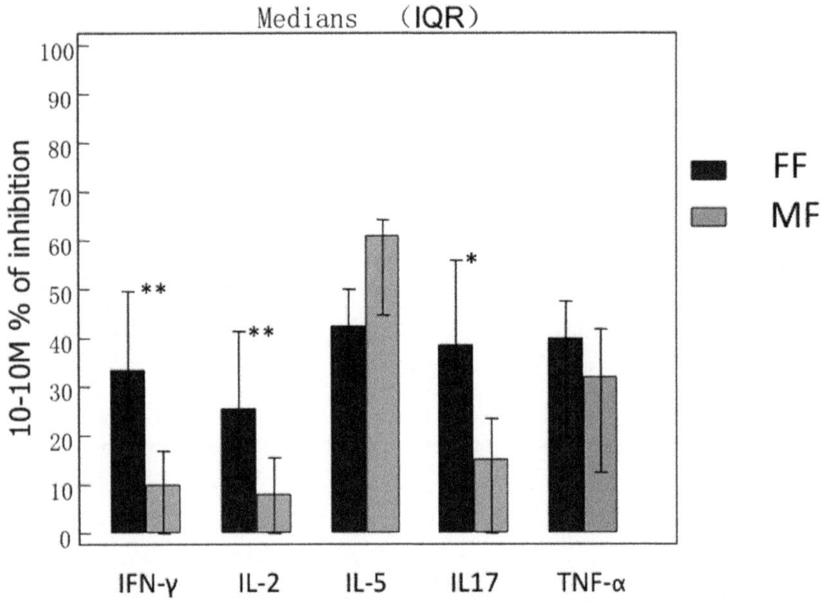

Figure 1. Nasal polyp tissue (n = 9) was pre-incubated with FF or MF at different concentrations for 1 hour and consequently stimulated with SEB for 24 hours (pre-challenge incubation). % inhibition of cytokine release was calculated at a fixed concentration of 10^{-10} M; FF had a significantly higher suppressive effect on IFN-γ, IL-2 and IL-17 release vs. MF.

Post challenge incubation - the experiment to compare the effect of drugs on a running stimulation

The polyp tissue fragments were stimulated with TCM (negative control) or 0.5 μg/mL SEB 1 hour or 2 hours or 4 hours then followed with TCM, 10^{-8} M, 10^{-9} M, 10^{-10} M and 10^{-11} M FF or MF for 24 hour at 37°C/5% CO_2. Aliquots of the supernatants were stored immediately at −20°C until analysis of cytokines.

Pre-challenge incubation with time interval - the experiment to compare the uptake and translocation of compounds

The polyp tissue fragments were pre-incubated with TCM, 10^{-8} M, 10^{-9} M, 10^{-10} M and 10^{-11} M FF or MF for 1 hour at 37°C/5% CO_2, washed 2 times with TCM, and after 0 hour, 6 hours and 24 hours stimulated with TCM (negative control) or 0.5 μg/mL SEB for 24 hours. Aliquots of the supernatants were stored immediately at −20°C until analysis of cytokines.

Measurements of T effector cell cytokines in supernatants of stimulated tissue fragments

Concentrations of the cytokines IFN-γ, IL-5 and IL-17, IL-1β, TNF-α, IL-2, IL-4, IL-8, IL-6, IL-10, IL-12p70, and IL-13 were measured in tissue supernatants obtained after the ex vivo stimulations using Multi-spot assays (Meso Scale Discovery, Gaithersburg, Maryland, USA) following the instructions of the manufacture. The plates were analyzed by using a Sector Imager 6000 (Meso Scale Discovery). Calculations of maximum percentage of inhibition for the different compounds, time points and cytokines were done.

Statistical analysis

Statistical analysis was performed by using the Wilcoxon test (for paired comparisons). The Mann-Whitney U test was used for between-group (unpaired) comparisons. P values of less than .05 were considered statistically significant.

Results

Under optimal conditions, the suppressive effect of FF is superior to MF

FF and MF showed a dose-dependent suppressive effect on the release of IFN-γ, IL-2, IL-5, IL-17, and TNF-α upon stimulation. There were no significant differences in maximum percentage of inhibition of major cytokines between FF and MF after pre-challenge incubation conditions (Table 1). However, FF reached a significant suppressive effect at a 1-molar or lower concentration for all cytokines. We further calculated the percentage of inhibition at a fixed concentration of 10^{-10} M; FF had a significantly higher suppressive effect on IFN-γ, IL-2 and IL-17 release vs. MF (Figure 1).

Upon challenge with SEB, FF has a stronger effect at lower concentrations compared to MF

SEB stimulation resulted in a strong inflammation with the release of all cytokines, which was reduced with both drugs. Added an hour after SEB, FF showed a higher max. % inhibition on the release of IFN-γ, IL-2, IL-5, IL17, and TNF-α over 24 hours compared to MF (Table 2 and Figure 2). The maximum % inhibition was similar when drugs were added after 1, 2 or 4 h after SEB stimulation (data not provided).

Onset of action is significantly faster with FF vs. MF, and the suppressive effects of FF are superior to MF for IFN-γ, IL-2 and IL-17

Polyp tissue fragments were incubated with FF or MF for 1 hour, then washed to remove drug not bound to the tissue, and stimulated with SEB immediately or after 6 or 24 hours. Both drugs showed a time dependent dynamic suppression of IFN-γ, IL-2, IL-17 and TNF-α release. FF showed a much faster uptake and suppressive effect after 1-hour incubation compare to MF, the max % inhibition was significantly superior for FF vs. MF ($P<0.05$).

Table 2. Nasal polyp tissue (n = 9) was stimulated with SEB for 1 hour before incubation with FF and MP at different concentrations for further 24 hours (post-challenge incubation).

Cytokine	Fluticasone furoate			p- value for max. inhibition	Mometasone furoate		
	Max. inhibition (median (Interquartile range) in %	*Concentr. of max. inhibition*	*Lowest concentr. with significant inhibition*		*Max. inhibition (median (Interquartile range) in %*	*Concentr. of max. inhibition*	*Lowest concentr. with significant inhibition*
IFN-γ	77 (71.8–78.5)	10^{-8} M	10^{-11} M	P = 0.0005	41 (33.8–56)	10^{-8} M	N
IL-2	64 (55–67)	10^{-8} M	10^{-10} M	P = 0.0027	33 (20–46)	10^{-8} M	N
IL-5	73 (67.5–87)	10^{-8} M	10^{-11} M	P = 0.0340	58 (31.8–73.3)	10^{-8} M	10^{-8} M
IL-17	80 (72.5–82.8)	10^{-8} M	10-11 M	P = 0.0092	58 (42–63	10-8 M	10-9 M
TNF-α	46 (40.8–63.8)	10^{-9} M	10-11 M	P = 0.0047	29 (12.8–38.5)	10-8 M	N

We observed a significantly better maximal inhibition for all cytokines with FF compared to MF. Furthermore, a significant inhibition was reached for all cytokines with FF, whereas MF failed to significantly suppress IFN-γ, IL-2 and TNF-α. For IL-5 and IL-17, a significant inhibition was reached with FF at one order of magnitude lower molar concentrations compared to MF.
N = no significant reduction reached at any concentration tested.

Especially for IL-5, 1-hour incubation of the tissue with FF resulted in an immediate maximum % inhibition, whereas an inhibitory effect in the same range needed at least 6 hours with MF (Table 3 and Figure 3). For other cytokines, the inhibitory activity of FF always remained superior to MF even when stimulated after 6 or 24 hours.

Stimulation with SEB after 24 hours revealed a true 24 hours effect of FF on cytokine release in the range of 74 to 94% for all cytokines, after just one hour of incubation with the compound.

Discussion

In the current investigation we compared the effects of fluticasone furoate (FF) and mometasone furoate (MF) on the release of a pattern of Th1, Th2 and Th17 cytokines from human nasal polyp tissue. We simulated three possible real-life drug-use patterns including pre- and post-challenge exposure with FF or MF. In all experimental settings we observed stronger effects of FF compared to MF in terms of concentrations necessary to suppress cytokine release, onset of action, maximal inhibition of release and range of cytokines that could be suppressed.

A typical clinical situation would be the initiation of drug therapy after allergen exposure or onset of symptoms. This setting was mimicked by a post-challenge incubation with a concentration range of 10^{-8} to 10^{-11} M FF and MF. We observed a concentration-dependent inhibition of cytokine release, which was stronger for FF compared to MF. The maximal inhibition achieved by FF was statistically significantly higher than for MF, which did not suppress IFN-γ and TNF-α. The experimental setting can be reversed to a pre-challenge exposure resembling a prophylactic use of drugs. In this setup the corticosteroids were pre-incubated with the nasal polyp tissue fragments for one hour before SEB was supplemented. Under these conditions, the maximal cytokine inhibition was not significantly different between FF and MF, but FF consistently inhibited cytokine release at lower concentrations compared to MF. At concentrations as low as 10^{-10} M, FF showed a significantly higher suppressive effect versus IL-2, IL-17 and IFN-γ secretion compared to MF. Interestingly, when the extent of inhibitory effects in this pre- versus the post-challenge exposure setting are compared, it is striking that FF produced maximal inhibition of IL-2, IL-5, IL-17, IFN-γ and TNF-α in comparable magnitudes in both experimental setups. In contrast, the maximal inhibition of cytokine release by MF was compromised in the post-challenge incubation setting.

The third experimental setting we designed to mimic a preventive use of intranasal glucocorticoids. In a clinical context, any excess drug that is not taken up into the nasal tissue cells will be rapidly removed by mucociliary clearance within about 30 min [11]. This was mimicked by washing the tissue in our setup. Subsequently, exposure with SEB was either performed immediately after washing off excess glucocorticoids (t = 0), or after another 6 or 24 hours, respectively. Generally, FF inhibited the cytokine release significantly stronger and at earlier time points than MF. Especially the release of IL-5 and TNF-α was most effectively suppressed even by low concentrations of FF and irrespectively of the time interval between removal of the drug excess and exposure with SEB. Thus, the inhibitory activity of FF fully unfolded after only one hour incubation with the drug and was not attenuated over the evaluated time interval. The observation that FF still yielded a very potent suppression in cytokine production by SEB after 24 hours, while the tissue fragments were only exposed to the drug for one hour, is consistent with our previous results that showed a fast uptake and a high

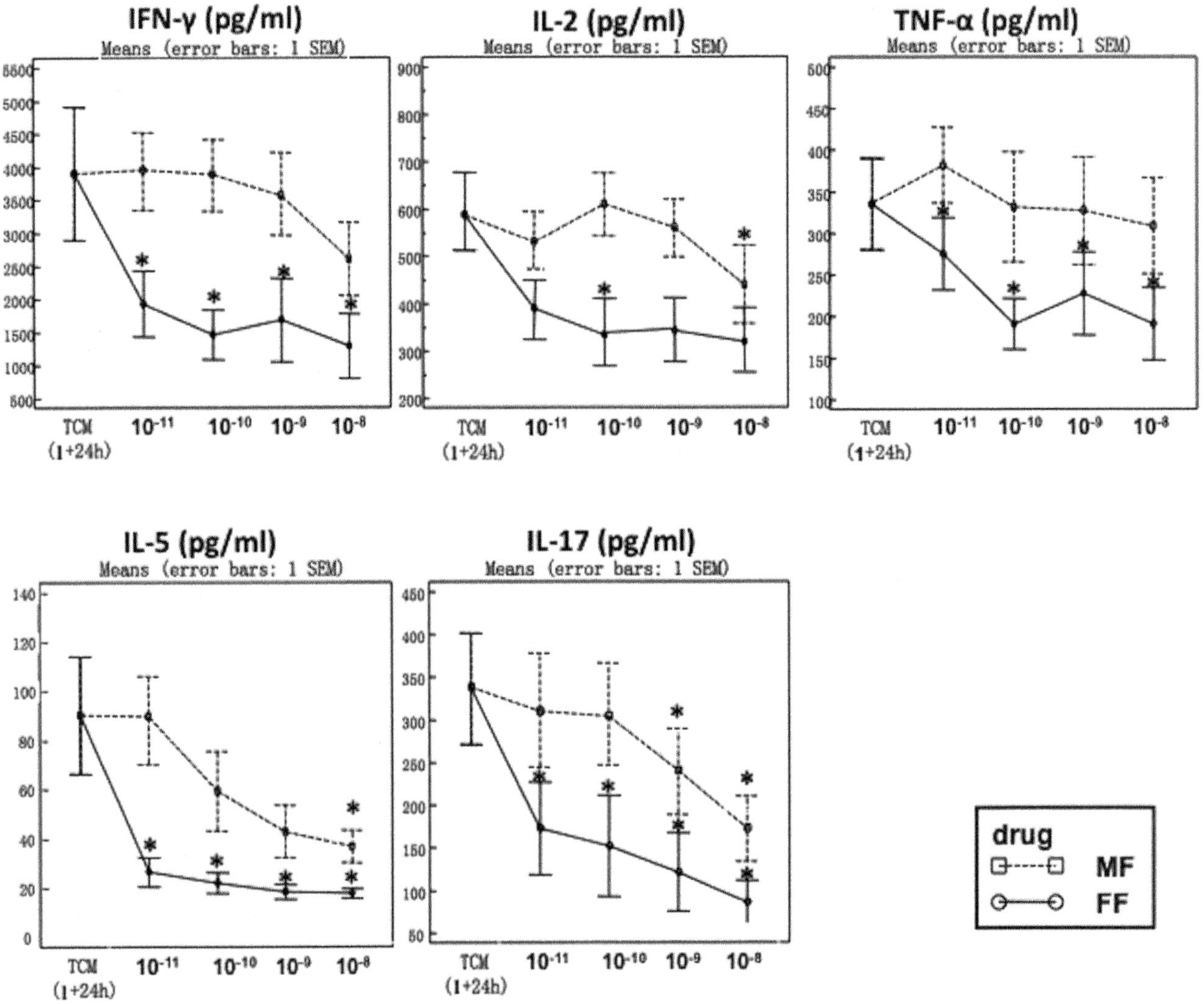

Figure 2. Nasal polyp tissue (n = 9) was stimulated with SEB for 1 hour before incubation with FF and MP at 10^{-11} to 10^{-8} molar concentrations for further 24 hours (post-challenge incubation). The figures show a concentration-dependent inhibition of cytokine release, reaching significance at different concentrations per drug and cytokine. Significance is indicated vs. baseline (* $p<0.05$). Please refer to table 2 for a comparison between drugs.

binding of FF to human nasal tissue [7] and with the report that FF was still detectable in cell nuclei 30 hours after treatment with this drug [12,13]. Moreover, FF revealed a longer duration of action, characterized by inhibition of GM-CSF release compared to fluticasone propionate and budesonide.

However, in this pre-challenge incubation with subsequent drug removal not all cytokines were influenced to the same extent by the two corticosteroids. Specifically, the maximal inhibition of release of IL-5 and TNF-α was similar for FF and MF when the human nasal polyp tissue was challenged with SEB 6 and 24 hours after incubation with the glucocorticoids. In contrast, this was not observed for IL-2, IL-17 and IFN-γ, the release of which was significantly more inhibited by FF compared to MF over all analyzed time intervals. Furthermore, the release of IL-5 and TNF-α was already almost completely blocked by lowest concentrations of FF right after pre-incubation ($t = 0$), indicating a fast translocation of the drug and a fast onset of action. The observation that the influence of the glucocorticoids was distinct for certain cytokines might reflect differences in the regulation and/or mechanisms of cytokine secretion [14]. Cytokines are typically produced as response to T-cell receptor stimulations either by upregulation of their transcription or by translation of pre-existing mRNA transcripts [15].

The overall more pronounced anti-inflammatory activity of FF compared to MF is highly consistent with the higher relative receptor affinity (RRA) of FF compared to MF [6,16].

In our experimental setting the nasal mucosal cells were in contact with the glucocorticoids typically for one hour, with the readout performed 24–48 hours later; it can be assumed that classical effects on transcription and translation of genes encoding inflammatory mediators were responsible for the observations [17]. Rapid effects or nongenomic actions also have been described within seconds to a few minutes [18–23].

Although an inhibition of inflammatory mediators is the prerequisite for clinical symptom management in allergic rhinitis, the required magnitude and temporal relation of cytokine suppression and the improvement of symptoms is not definite. Lately, both the FDA and the EMA issued recommendations for

Table 3. Nasal polyp tissue (n = 9) was incubated with FF and MF at different concentrations for 1 hour, and then washed and SEB was added immediately (0 hour), after 6 or 24 hours (pre-challenge incubation with time interval).

Cytokine		Fluticasone furoate				Mometasone furoate		
	time	*Max. inhibition (median (Interquart. range) in %*	*Concentr. of max. inhibition*	*Lowest concentr. with significant inhibition*	*p-value for max. inhibition*	*Max. inhibition (median (Interquart. range) in %*	*Concentr. of max. inhibition*	*Lowest concentr. with significant inhibition*
IFN-γ	0 h	63 (58.3–78)	10^{-8} M	10^{-11} M	**P = 0.0054**	34 (9,5–43.5)	10^{-8} M	10^{-8} M
	6 h	86 (82.5–90)	10^{-8} M	10^{-11} M	**P = 0.007**	71 (36.8–81.3)	10^{-9} M	10^{-9} M
	24 h	94 (91.3–96)	10^{-9} M	10^{-11} M	**P = 0.0033**	70 (55.5–73.5)	10^{-8} M	10^{-9} M
IL-2	0 h	65 (50–73.8)	10^{-8} M	10^{-11} M	**P = 0.0092**	39 (13.5–43.8)	10^{-9} M	10^{-9} M
	6 h	90 (79.591.5)	10^{-9} M	10^{-11} M	**P = 0.0041**	74 (37.5–76.3)	10^{-9} M	10^{-11} M
	24 h	93 (87.5–95)	10^{-10} M	10^{-11} M	**P = 0.0297**	64 (60.8–86)	10^{-8} M	10^{-11} M
IL-5	0 h	90 (80.8–94.3)	10^{-8} M	10^{-11} M	**P = 0.0118**	51 (27.8–73.3)	10^{-8} M	10^{-8} M
	6 h	90 (81.5–97.3)	10^{-9} M	10^{-11} M	P = 0.1022	76 (63.5–90.3)	10^{-9} M	10^{-9} M
	24 h	85 (84.3–95.8)	10^{-11} M	10^{-11} M	P = 0.1599	82 (67.5–92.5)	10^{-8} M	10^{-11} M
IL-17	0 h	78 (72.3–85)	10^{-8} M	10^{-11} M	**P = 0.0027**	47 (28.5–70.3)	10^{-8} M	10^{-8} M
	6 h	83 (77.8–92.3)	10^{-8} M	10^{-11} M	**P = 0.038**	72 (49–79.5)	10^{-9} M	10^{-11} M
	24 h	90 (84.8–94.8)	10^{-10} M	10^{-11} M	**P = 0.0181**	70 (60.8–79.5)	10^{-8} M	10^{-10} M
TNF-α	0 h	70 (64–78)	10^{-11} M	10^{-11} M	**P = 0.0054**	38 (25.3–54.5)	N	N
	6 h	70 (58.3–76)	10^{-11} M	10^{-11} M	P = 0.112	63 (23–66.3)	10^{-9} M	10^{-10} M
	24 h	74 (60.5–81.8)	10^{-10} M	10^{-11} M	P = 0.2248	61 (55.3–69.5)	10^{-8} M	10^{-11} M

Cells were then incubated for another 24 hours. When SEB stimulation was performed immediately, FF demonstrated a faster onset of action with a significantly higher maximal inhibition of all cytokines vs. MF. For most cytokines and time points, FF reached a significant reduction at a lower concentration; however, when the time interval between pre-incubation and challenge was minimally 6 hours, the suppression capacity of MF reached the same levels as FF for IL-5 and TNF-α.

N = no significant reduction reached at any concentration tested.

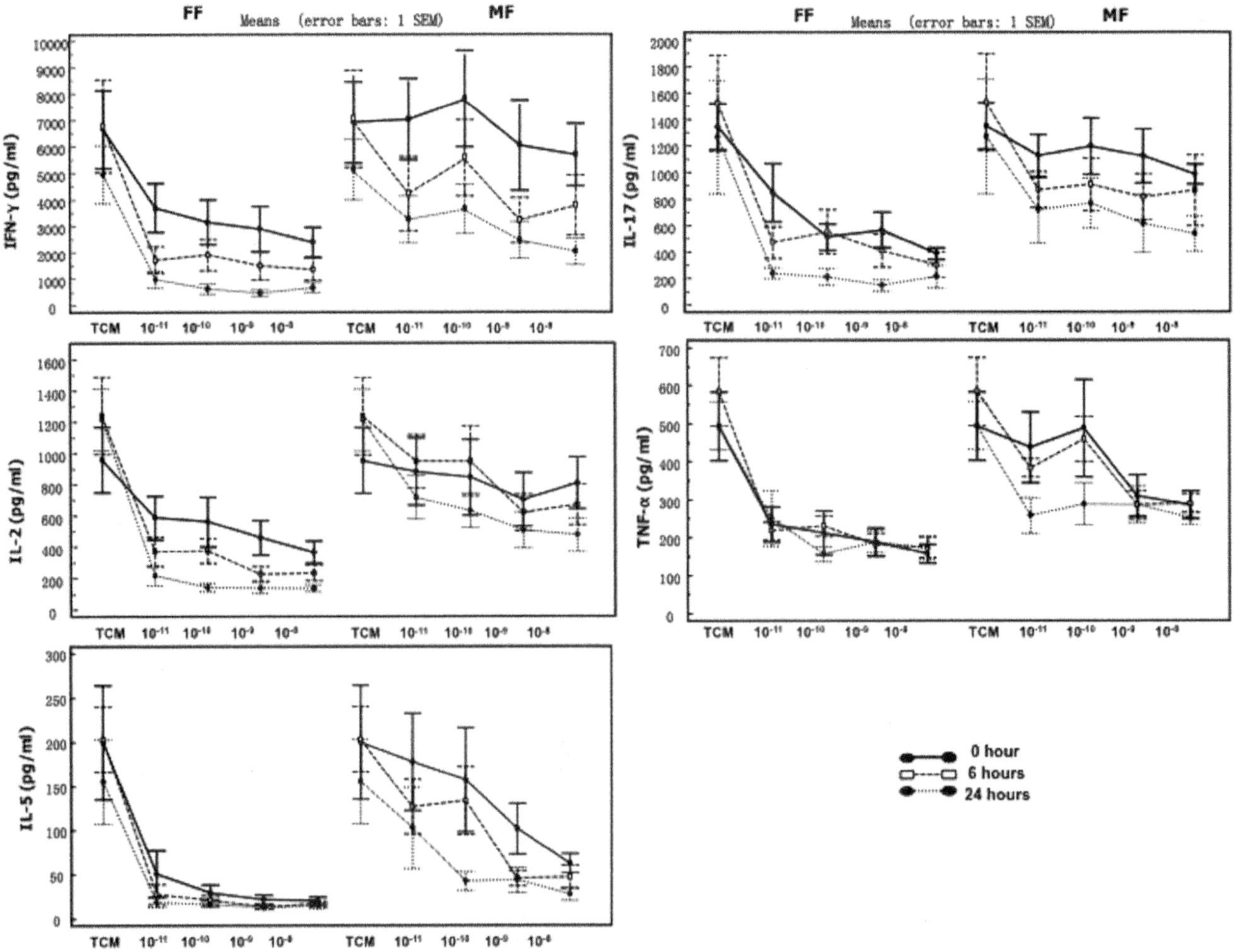

Figure 3. Nasal polyp tissue (n = 9) was incubated with FF and MF at different concentrations for 1 hour, then washed and SEB was added either immediately (0 hour), after 6 or 24 hours (pre-challenge incubation with time interval) Cells were then incubated for another 24 hours. When SEB stimulation was performed immediately, FF demonstrated a faster onset of action with a significantly higher maximal inhibition of all cytokines vs. MF. For most cytokines and time points, FF reaches a significant reduction at a lower concentration; however, when the time interval between pre-incubation and challenge was minimally 6 hours, the suppression capacity of MF reached the same levels as FF for IL-5 and TNF-α.

including the onset of action into the evaluation of drugs for allergic rhinitis [24,25] which confer with the proposal of an EAACI workshop group [26]. Efficacy of intranasal corticosteroids can be expected after 7–8 hours of dosing, but some patients appear to benefit more rapidly, e.g. within the first two hours [2,27]. In case of rapid improvement of clinical symptoms nongenomic glucocorticoid effects may play a role as well.

Limitations to this study include the fact that the clinical importance of these observations is unknown, and that the mechanisms underlying the observations are not identified. The study also uses whole tissue fragments and is thus not suitable to study effects on single cell components, but rather was aimed to resemble the in vivo situation in humans as much as possible.

To summarize, in the present study we demonstrated the potential of our human mucosal model and compared for the first time the activity of two modern intranasal glucocorticoids regarding inhibition of Th1, Th2 and Th17 cytokine release from human nasal polyp tissue. Thereby, we employed pre- and post-challenge incubations with FF or MF to mimic typical clinical situations of preventive use or therapy after exposure to allergens. All results revealed an uptake, receptor activation and prolonged binding of the drugs in the mucosal tissue with a rapid uptake and sustained suppression of cytokine release that was stronger for FF compared to MF. While the maximal suppressive activity was not different when FF was added before or after tissue stimulation with SEB, the cytokine suppression capacity of MF appeared to be compromised if the SEB induced cell activation preceded the drug addition. In a pre-challenge incubation with removal of excess drug concentrations MF approached inhibition of IL-5 and TNF-α comparable to FF. However, this was only observed after 6 and 24 hours while FF maximally blocked the release of these cytokines already right after pre-incubation and at concentrations up to four degrees of magnitude lower than for MF. Furthermore, there was a difference in the cytokines that were suppressed, with a wider range of T helper signatures for FF compared to MF. These data underline the high efficacy of FF in allergic and other inflammatory diseases and indicate the necessity of head-to-head comparison studies *vs.* MF and other corticosteroids in adequate clinical settings using appropriate concentrations.

Author Contributions

Conceived and designed the experiments: NZ PH CB. Performed the experiments: NZ GH FL KVC. Analyzed the data: NZ GH FL KVC MK LZ. Contributed reagents/materials/analysis tools: MK LZ. Wrote the paper: NZ PH CB.

References

1. Fokkens WJ, Lund VJ, Mullol J, Bachert C, Alobid I, et al. (2012) EPOS 2012: European position paper on rhinosinusitis and nasal polyps 2012. A summary for otorhinolaryngologists. Rhinology 50(1):1–12.
2. Hellings PW, Fokkens WJ, Akdis C, Bachert C, Cingi C, et al. (2013) Uncontrolled allergic rhinitis and chronic rhinosinusitis: where do we stand today? Allergy 68(1):1–7.
3. Rodrigo GJ, Neffen H (2011) Efficacy of fluticasone furoate nasal spray vs. placebo for the treatment of ocular and nasal symptoms of allergic rhinitis: a systematic review. Clin Exp Allergy 41(2):160–70.
4. Carr W, Bernstein J, Lieberman P, Meltzer E, Bachert C, et al. (2012) A novel intranasal therapy of azelastine with fluticasone for the treatment of allergic rhinitis. J Allergy Clin Immunol 129(5): 1282–1289.
5. Biggadike K (2011) Fluticasone furoate/fluticasone propionate - different drugs with different properties. Clin Respir J 5: 183–4.
6. Valotis A, Högger P (2007) Human receptor kinetics and lung tissue retention of the enhanced-affinity glucocorticoid fluticasone furoate. Respir Res 8: 54.
7. Baumann D, Bachert C, Högger P (2009) Dissolution in nasal fluid, retention and anti-inflammatory activity of fluticasone furoate in human nasal tissue ex vivo. Clin Exp Allergy 39: 1540–50.
8. Zhang N, Van Zele T, Perez-Novo C, Van Bruaene N, Holtappels G, et al. (2008) Different types of T-effector cells orchestrate mucosal inflammation in chronic sinus disease. J Allergy Clin Immunol 122:961–968.
9. Patou J, Gevaert P, Van Zele T, Holtappels G, van Cauwenberge P, et al. (2008) Staphylococcus aureus enterotoxin B, protein A, and lipoteichoic acid stimulations in nasal polyps. J Allergy Clin Immunol 121: 110–5.
10. Van Crombruggen K, Holtappels G, De Ruyck N, Derycke L, Tomassen P, et al. (2012) RAGE processing in chronic airway conditions: involvement of Staphylococcus aureus and ECP. J Allergy Clin Immunol 129 (6):1515–1521.
11. Marttin E, Schipper NG, Verhoef JC, Merkus FW (1998) Nasal mucociliary clearance as a factor in nasal drug delivery. Adv Drug Deliv Rev 29: 13–38.
12. Rossios C, To Y, To M, Ito M, Barnes PJ, et al. (2011) Long-acting fluticasone furoate has a superior pharmacological profile to fluticasone propionate in human respiratory cells. Eur J Pharmacol 670: 244–51.
13. Jankowski R, Klossek JM, Attali V, Coste A, Serrano E (2009) Long-term study of fluticasone propionate aqueous nasal spray in acute and maintenance therapy of nasal polyposis. Allergy 64(6):944–50.
14. Duitman EH, Orinska Z, Bulfone-Paus S (2011) Mechanisms of cytokine secretion: a portfolio of distinct pathways allows flexibility in cytokine activity. Eur J Cell Biol 90: 476–83.
15. Huse M, Quann EJ, Davis MM (2008) Shouts, whispers and the kiss of death: directional secretion in T cells. Nat Immunol 9: 1105–11.
16. Valotis A, Neukam K, Elert O, Högger P (2004) Human receptor kinetics, tissue binding affinity, and stability of mometasone furoate. J Pharm Sci 93: 1337–50.
17. Munck A, Holbrook NJ (1984) Glucocorticoid-receptor complexes in rat thymus cells. Rapid kinetic behavior and a cyclic model. J Biol Chem 259: 820–31.
18. Cato AC, Nestl A, Mink S (2002) Rapid actions of steroid receptors in cellular signaling pathways. Sci STKE 2002: re9.
19. Croxtall JD, Choudhury Q, Flower RJ (2000) Glucocorticoids act within minutes to inhibit recruitment of signalling factors to activated EGF receptors through a receptor-dependent, transcription-independent mechanism. Br J Pharmacol 130: 289–98.
20. Löwenberg M, Tuynman J, Bilderbeek J, Gaber T, Buttgereit F, et al. (2005) Rapid immunosuppressive effects of glucocorticoids mediated through Lck and Fyn. Blood 106: 1703–10.
21. Löwenberg M, Verhaar AP, Bilderbeek J, Marle J, Buttgereit F, et al. (2006) Glucocorticoids cause rapid dissociation of a T-cell-receptor-associated protein complex containing LCK and FYN. EMBO Rep 7: 1023–9.
22. Derendorf H, Meltzer EO (2008) Molecular and clinical pharmacology of intranasal corticosteroids: clinical and therapeutic implications. Allergy. 63(10): 1292–300.
23. Brattsand R (2002) Drug development of inhaled steroids. In: Schleimer RP, O'Byrne PM, Szefler SJ, Brattsand R eds. Inhaled steroids in asthma - optimizing the effects in the airways. New York: Marcel Dekker, Inc 3–32.
24. Food and Drug Administration (2000) FDA draft guidance for industry - Allergic rhinitis: clinical development programs for drug products. In: US Department of Health and Human Services Food and Drug Administration and Center for Drug Evaluation and Research (CDER). Available: http://www.fda.gov/downloads/Drugs/GuidanceComplianceRegulatoryInformation/Guidances/ucm071293.pdf. Accessed 2014 Mar 12.
25. European Medicines Agency (2004) Guideline on the clinical development of medicianl products for the treatment of allergic rhino-conjunctivitis: European Medicines Agency and Committee for Medicinal Products for Human Use (CHMP). Available: http://www.ema.europa.eu/docs/en_GB/document_library/Scientific_guideline/2009/09/WC500003554.pdf. Accessed 2014 Mar 12.
26. Bousquet J, Van Cauwenberge P, Bachert C, Canonica GW, Demoly P, et al. (2003) Requirements for medications commonly used in the treatment of allergic rhinitis. European Academy of Allergy and Clinical Immunology (EAACI), Allergic Rhinitis and its Impact on Asthma (ARIA). Allergy 58: 192–7.
27. Katial RK, Salapatek AM, Patel P (2009) Establishing the onset of action of intranasal corticosteroids: is there an ideal study design? Allergy Asthma Proc 30: 595–604.

22

Consumption of Artificially-Sweetened Soft Drinks in Pregnancy and Risk of Child Asthma and Allergic Rhinitis

Ekaterina Maslova[1,2]*, Marin Strøm[1], Sjurdur F. Olsen[1,2], Thorhallur I. Halldorsson[1,3,4]

1 Centre for Fetal Programming, Department of Epidemiology, Statens Serum Institut, Copenhagen, Denmark, **2** Department of Nutrition, Harvard School of Public Health, Boston, Massachusetts, United States of America, **3** Faculty of Food Science and Nutrition, School of Health Sciences, University of Iceland, Reykjavik, Iceland, **4** Unit for Nutrition Research, Landspitali University Hospital, Reykjavik, Iceland

Abstract

Background: Past evidence has suggested a role of artificial sweeteners in allergic disease; yet, the evidence has been inconsistent and unclear.

Objective: To examine relation of intake of artificially-sweetened beverages during pregnancy with child asthma and allergic rhinitis at 18 months and 7 years.

Methods: We analyzed data from 60,466 women enrolled during pregnancy in the prospective longitudinal Danish National Birth Cohort between 1996 and 2003. At the 25th week of gestation we administered a validated Food Frequency Questionnaire which asked in detail about intake of artificially-sweetened soft drinks. At 18 months, we evaluated child asthma using interview data. We also assessed asthma and allergic rhinitis through a questionnaire at age 7 and by using national registries. Current asthma was defined as self-reported asthma diagnosis and wheeze in the past 12 months. We examined the relation between intake of artificially-sweetened soft drinks and child allergic disease outcomes and present here odds ratios with 95% CI comparing daily vs. no intake.

Results: At 18 months, we found that mothers who consumed more artificially-sweetened non-carbonated soft drinks were 1.23 (95% CI: 1.13, 1.33) times more likely to report a child asthma diagnosis compared to non-consumers. Similar results were found for child wheeze. Consumers of artificially-sweetened carbonated drinks were more likely to have a child asthma diagnosis in the patient (1.30, 95% CI: 1.01, 1.66) and medication (1.13, 95% CI: 0.98, 1.29) registry, as well as self-reported allergic rhinitis (1.31, 95% CI: 0.98, 1.74) during the first 7 years of follow-up. We found no associations for sugar-sweetened soft drinks.

Conclusion: Carbonated artificially-sweetened soft drinks were associated with registry-based asthma and self-reported allergic rhinitis, while early childhood outcomes were related to non-carbonated soft drinks. These results suggest that consumption of artificially-sweetened soft drinks during pregnancy may play a role in offspring allergic disease development.

Editor: Susanne Krauss-Etschmann, Ludwig-Maximilians-University Munich, Germany

Funding: Declaration of all sources of funding: the study was supported by the Danish Council for Stra-tegic Research (09-067124); the Danish Council for Independent Research | Medical Sciences, Danish Agency for Science, Technology and Innovation (09-063410); the Lundbeck foundation (R13-A907); and the European Union (EU) Integrated Research Project EARNEST (FOOD-CT-2005-007036). The EU project EARNEST (http://www.metabolic-programming.org) receives financial support from the Commission of the European Communities under the FP 6 priority 5: food quality and safety. The Danish National Birth Cohort has been financed by the March of Dimes Birth Defects Foundation, the Danish Heart Association, the Danish Medical Research Council, and the Sygekassernes Helsefond, Danish National Research Foundation, Danish Pharmaceutical Association, Ministry of Health, National Board of Health, Statens Serum Institut. The funders had no role in study design, data collection and analysis, decision to publish, or preparation of the manuscript.

Competing Interests: The authors have declared that no competing interests exist.

* E-mail: emaslova@post.harvard.edu

Introduction

It has been hypothesized that diet during pregnancy may modulate child immune system development and later allergic disease. Past studies have examined numerous dietary factors during pregnancy, including fruits and vegetables [1–6], fish [1–5,7–12] and fish oil [13], butter and margarine [2,3,5,7], nut and peanuts [2,4,14], and dairy and milk intake [2–5,14,15] in relation to allergic disease in the child. We recently conducted an analysis of the relation between milk and yoghurt consumption during pregnancy and wheeze, asthma, and allergic rhinitis in the Danish National Birth Cohort (DNBC) [16]. We found that the strongest and most consistent association was between maternal low-fat yoghurt intake and child asthma and allergic rhinitis. These results suggested a causal agent specific to low-fat yoghurt. We hypothesized that artificial sweeteners could be a plausible candidate as these compounds are often added to low-fat/'light' products to compensate for flavour or reduce sugar content [17]. The current state of knowledge on the role of artificial sweeteners in allergic disease development is at best limited. A few studies have examined aspartame in relation to inflammation; yet, these results have been inconsistent [18–20]. A study from the 1980s [21] examined *in vitro* immunological properties and found small inhibitory effects on antigen-induced histamine release from cultured mouse mast cells. However, the authors could not explain the origin or meaning of this effect. Other studies have shown improvements in dermatitis with aspartame avoidance [22,23], while yet others found no elicit allergic reactions [24,25]. This suggests that improvement in dermatitis is most likely a relatively rare side effect of aspartame avoidance. To our knowledge, there are no epidemiological studies assessing the relation between intake of artificial sweeteners during pregnancy and asthma or other allergic diseases.

We therefore decided to examine whether artificially-sweetened soft drinks during pregnancy modify offspring risk of wheeze, asthma, and allergic rhinitis in the DNBC. We chose soft drink as the exposure because these have been identified as a primary source of artificial sweeteners [26]. We included intake of sugar-sweetened beverages as a control for potential activity of other nutritional components and additives in soft drinks [26].

Methods

Ethics Statement

Mothers provided written informed consent on behalf of their children. The Regional Scientific Ethics Committee for the municipalities of Copenhagen and Frederiksberg approved all study protocols, and all procedures were in accordance with the Declaration of Helsinki.

Population and Study Design

Participants in the DNBC, a large prospective cohort study, were enrolled between January 1996 and October 2002 during their first antenatal visit between weeks 6 and 10 of gestation [27]. All women living in Denmark were eligible if they could speak Danish and were planning to carry to term. About 60% of all eligible women received an invitation from their general practitioner; of those 60% chose to enrol. Women participated in four telephone interviews, twice during pregnancy and twice postpartum, at 6 and 18 months. They also filled out a food frequency questionnaire (FFQ) around the 25th week of gestation. We have followed the mother-child pairs through national registries, linked by the unique identity number given to all Danish citizens. A questionnaire regarding the child was sent to the mothers when the child was 7 years.

A total of 101,045 pregnancies were enrolled into the study. To avoid dependency among correlated observations, we included only the first liveborn singleton child enrolled for each woman (n = 89,333). We further excluded multiple births (n = 87,056). After eliminating women with missing exposure data, 60,466 women had information on artificially-sweetened carbonated beverage consumption.

Exposure Variables

Maternal diet assessment was based on a validated 360-item semi-quantitative FFQ completed around gestation week 25 and covered intake during the previous four weeks [28]. Intake of individual food items were estimated in grams per day based on standard portion sizes; total energy and nutrients were quantified using Danish food tables [29]. Women were asked a number of questions on beverage consumption with response categories ranging from never to >= 8 servings/d. One serving was equivalent to one glass. We used four beverage items in our analyses: carbonated soft drinks/cola (sugar sweetened), carbonated soft drinks/cola (sugar-free, light), noncarbonated soft drinks (sugar sweetened), and noncarbonated soft drinks (sugar-free, light). The wording of the responses used the words sugar-free and light to refer to products that contained artificial sweeteners. We distinguished between carbonated and non-carbonated beverages as they contain different types of artificial sweeteners [26]. These beverages were subject to a repeatability study where 103 women filled in the FFQ twice during pregnancy (in week 25 and 35 of gestation). For these women the observed Spearman correlation coefficient for all four types of soft drink consumption was around 0.7 [30].

Outcome Measurements

Asthma at 18 months. Women were telephone interviewed when the child was 18 months (N~45,000). The women answered questions about child health and diagnoses since birth. We defined *asthma at 18 months* as self-reported doctor asthma diagnosis.

Asthma and allergic rhinitis at 7 years. We evaluated asthma and allergic rhinitis diagnosis at the 7 year follow-up by numerous sources. *Current asthma at age 7* (N~38,000) by self-report was defined as a positive response to standardized International Study of Asthma and Allergies in Childhood questions on doctor-diagnosed asthma and wheezing symptoms in the past 12 months [31,32]. *Ever allergic rhinitis* (N~38,000) by self-report was based on a reported doctor-diagnosis of hay fever.

We further used data on hospital admissions collected by the mandatory Danish National Patient Registry (DNPR). Admission information has been collected since 1977, and emergency room and outpatient contacts since 1995. The registry has been validated against asthma diagnosis from hospital records [33]. We extracted data from the DNPR in Aug 2010 and linked it to our data using the CPR number. We identified *ever admitted asthma* (N~38,000) cases using the International Classification of Disease 10 (ICD-10) for asthma (J45, J45.0, J45.1, J45.8, J45.9, J46, and J46.9).

We also used the Register of Medicinal Product Statistics (RMPS) that was initiated in 1995 and contains detailed individual-level dispensary information [34]. Based on a previous validation study [35] we combined Anatomical Therapeutic Chemical codes for the classification of *ever medication-related asthma* (N~38,000) cases. The outcome was defined as at least two prescriptions of drugs for obstructive airway disease, except for beta-2-agonists as liquid, inhaled beta-2-agonists only once, or inhaled steroid only once.

Both registry outcomes were limited to children with self-reported data to avoid discordance in findings due to differences in study populations.

Covariates

We collected information of a number of covariates. These included socioeconomic status by parental education level and occupation (SES: high level proficiency, medium level proficiency, skilled, unskilled, student, unemployment), maternal age at birth of child (< = 20 years, 21–39 years, > = 40 years), parity (nulli- and multiparous), maternal prepregnancy Body Mass Index (BMI in kg/m^2) (< = 18.5, 18.6–24.9, 25.0–29.9, 30–34.9, > = 35.0), maternal smoking during pregnancy (nonsmoker, occasional smoker, current smoker), maternal exercise during pregnancy (yes/no), gestational weight gain (g/week), breastfeeding duration (none, 0–1, 2–3, 4–6, 7–9, > = 10 months), birth weight (in grams), gestational age (in days since the last menstrual period), child sex, maternal and paternal history of asthma and allergies, and total energy intake. We also examined, in stability analyses, dietary variables (fruits, vegetables, alcohol, vitamin A, D, E, selenium, and zinc intake from diet and supplements); and mode

Table 1. Age-standardized covariate distribution across categories of maternal consumption of artificially-sweetened carbonated soft drinks during pregnancy, N = 60,465.

Frequency of intake	N[1] (%)	Never N = 40,523% or means (SD)	<1 serv/week N = 7,588% or means (SD)	Weekly N = 9,971% or means (SD)	>= 1 serv/day N = 2,383% or means (SD)
Maternal age (years)*					
≤20	586 (1)	1	1	1	1
21–39	59,311 (98)	98	98	98	98
≥40	567 (1)	1	1	1	1
Prepregnancy BMI (kg/m^2)					
≤18.5	2,476 (4)	5	3	2	2
18.6–24.9	38,212 (68)	71	68	61	54
25.0–29.9	10,885 (19)	18	20	24	27
30.0–34.9	3,299 (6)	5	6	9	11
≥35.0	1,219 (2)	2	3	3	5
Physical activity					
Yes	22,399 (39)	37	43	41	37
Smoking in pregnancy					
Current smokers	7,470 (12)	13	9	10	17
Parity					
Nullipara	30,590 (53)	51	58	56	52
Socioeconomic position					
High level proficiencies	12,449 (23)	23	23	22	22
Medium level proficiencies	16,692 (31)	30	32	32	30
Skilled	14,601 (27)	26	27	28	29
Unskilled	6,810 (13)	13	12	12	14
Students	2,425 (4)	5	4	4	4
Unemployed	1,462 (3)	3	2	2	2
Breastfeeding duration					
No breastfeeding	862 (2)	2	2	2	4
0–1 months	3,988 (9)	9	8	11	13
2–3 months	4,424 (10)	10	9	11	14
4–6 months	8,004 (19)	18	18	20	21
7–9 months	11,636 (27)	27	29	28	22
≥10 months	14,078 (33)	34	33	28	26
Maternal asthma					
Yes	5,289 (9)	9	9	9	10
Maternal allergies					
Yes	18,404 (32)	32	31	32	33
Paternal asthma					
Yes	4,720 (8)	8	8	9	9
Paternal allergies					
Yes	13,739 (24)	24	24	24	24
Child gender					
Male	30,754 (51)	51	52	51	52
Gestational weight gain (g/week)	41,681	468 (213)	465 (211)	465 (223)	460 (241)
Birth weight (g)	57,403	3,572 (571)	3,593 (573)	3,596 (577)	3,595 (588)
Gestational age (days)	60,454	280 (14)	280 (15)	280 (13)	279 (16)
Dietary intake					
Energy intake (kJ/day)	60,227	10,208 (2,706)	9,707 (2,570)	9,787 (2,588)	9,945 (2,809)
Fruit intake (g/day)	60,461	320 (267)	327 (270)	329 (258)	335 (327)
Vegetable intake (g/day)	60,461	129 (99)	130 (95)	128 (96)	132 (129)
Alcohol (g/day)	60,227	1.5 (2.3)	1.6 (2.1)	1.7 (2.3)	1.7 (2.8)

Table 1. Cont.

Frequency of intake	N[1] (%)	Never N=40,523% or means (SD)	<1 serv/week N=7,588% or means (SD)	Weekly N=9,971% or means (SD)	>=1 serv/day N=2,383% or means (SD)
Total vitamin A (RE/day)	60,227	1,500 (24,090)	1,297 (569)	2,125 (50,352)	2,672 (68,549)
Total vitamin D (μg/day)	60,227	8.9 (5.5)	9.2 (5.5)	9.2 (5.6)	8.9 (5.6)
Total vitamin E (α-TE/day)	60,227	16.4 (19.7)	16.3 (19.9)	15.8 (15.6)	15.4 (14.7)
Total selenium (μg/day)	60,227	70.1 (27.9)	72.8 (27.4)	72.6 (26.9)	70.9 (26.6)
Total zinc (mg/day)	60,227	19.6 (7.7)	20.2 (7.7)	20.1 (7.4)	19.7 (7.4)

Values are standardized to the age distribution of the study population.
*Value not age-adjusted.
[1]Total may be <N due to missing values.

of delivery (cesarean section, vaginal), pets at home, exposure do smoking during infancy (no, occasional, yes), daycare attendance during infancy, and use of antibiotics and paracetamol during pregnancy and child use of antibiotics (against ear infections) at 6 month.

Statistical Analysis

We evaluated the distribution of covariates across categories of beverage intake for potential confounding factors. We age-standardized the distributions using direct standardization as there was a significant difference in intake across maternal age categories. Final set of covariates were determined by chi-square and partial F-tests with a P<0.10 as well as *a priori* considerations based on the current literature. We excluded covariates suspected to be intermediates on the causal pathways, such as birth weight, gestational age, and gestational weight gain, to avoid over-adjusting the model. The importance of these variables was instead assessed using stratification. In the final logistic regression model, we adjusted for maternal age, smoking, parity, prepregnancy BMI, physical activity, breastfeeding duration, socio-economic status, child sex, maternal history of asthma, maternal history of allergies, paternal history of asthma, paternal history of allergies, and energy (in quintiles). Soft drinks intake was entered as an indicator variable and individual exposure categories compared to the lowest category. We collapsed categories at the higher end due to scarce data on high-consumers and to increase power. We therefore ended up with four intake categories (never, <1serving/week, weekly (2–6 times/week), >=1serving/day). When comparing results to the non-collapsed variables, there was a slight change in effect estimates and confidence intervals, but directionality remained the same. We estimated odds ratios (ORs) and 95% CI for the final models. Only exposures with strongest and most consistent results are presented in the main text; the reader is referred to the **Supporting Materials** for additional details. Median values (0, 0.5, 3.5, and 7) for the intake categories were modelled as a continuous variable to evaluate P-value for trend. We evaluated the independent associations for each outcome by entering all beverage variables into the same model. We also collapsed intake of artificially-sweetened beverage (carbonated and non-carbonated) to assess the full effect of the sweeteners. Since the same frequency number could be obtained across two different individual intake categories we ended up with the following combined categories ('never to <1serv/week', '<1serv/week', '<1serv/week to weekly', 'weekly to >=1serv/day').

All tests were two-sided and statistical significance was considered at P<0.05. The analyses were performed using the Statistical Analyses System software (release 9.2; SAS Institute, Cary, NC).

Results

Study Cohort

A total of 60,466 women had information on artificially-sweetened carbonated beverage intake. Majority of women were between the ages 21 and 39 years (98%), of higher socioeconomic position (high level proficiencies: 23%), and nulliparous (53%) (**Table 1**). More than 68% of all women reported a prepregnancy BMI within 18.6–24.9 kg/m^2. Nearly 25% of participants reported having smoked during pregnancy with 12% being daily smokers. Prevalence of maternal history of asthma and allergies was 9% and 32% respectively. Among the exposure variables, intake of sugar-sweetened non-carbonated soft drinks was highest with 22% consuming >=1 servings/day, followed by artificially-sweetened non-carbonated soft drinks at 13%.

When comparing women with and without self-reported child asthma data at 18 months and 7 years we found that, at 18 months, the 45,604 participants (vs. 16,269 non-participants) in the analyses were of higher sociodemographic status (54% vs. 51%), were multiparous (48% vs. 44%), did not smoke during pregnancy (76% vs. 72%), and had slightly lower gestational weight gain (464 vs. 475 g/week). At 7 years, compared to women without data on current child asthma (N=22,947), the 38,926 women with data on child asthma were of higher sociodemographic status (55% vs. 50%), were more like to have a BMI within 18.6–24.9 kg/m^2 (70% vs. 65%), exercise (40% vs. 36%), and not smoke during pregnancy (77% vs. 72%). No differences were found for maternal age, parental asthma and allergies, or intake of selected micronutrients during pregnancy.

Exposure Associations

We assessed intake of artificially-sweetened carbonated beverages across age-standardized study participant characteristics (**Table 1**). Compared to never consumers, women with daily intake of artificially-sweetened carbonated soda drinks tended to be of a skilled and unskilled level proficiency, have lower parity, and a prepregnancy BMI >=25 kg/m^2. They also smoked more during pregnancy and breastfed <7 months. They reported lower energy intake and higher intake of fruit, vegetables, and alcohol, but lower intake of vitamin E. Trends were similar for artificially-sweetened non-carbonated beverages.

Table 2. Associations between artificially-sweetened non-carbonated soft drinks consumption during pregnancy and child asthma in the Danish National Birth Cohort.

Frequency of intake		Cases/N	Asthma (18 months)	*P* for trend**	Cases/N	Asthma (7 years - ISAAC)	*P* for trend**	Cases/N	Ever asthma (DNPR)	*P* for trend**	Cases/N	Ever asthma (RMPS)	*P* for trend**
			N = 44,650			N = 38,165			N = 38,272			N = 38,272	
			OR (95% CI)			OR (95% CI)			OR (95% CI)			OR (95% CI)	
Never	Crude	4,632/29,392	1.00 (ref.)	<0.0001	1,018/25,508	1.00 (ref.)	0.20	1,443/25,584	1.00 (ref.)	0.001	7,78725,586	1.00 (ref.)	<0.0001
	Adjusted*			<0.0001			0.84			0.08			0.001
<1 serv/week	Crude	606/3,258	1.22 (1.11, 1.34)		97/2,685	0.90 (0.73, 1.12)		172/2,692	1.14 (0.97, 1.34)		851/2,690	1.06 (0.97, 1.15)	
	Adjusted*		1.22 (1.09, 1.36)			0.98 (0.76, 1.27)			1.20 (0.98, 1.48)			1.06 (0.95, 1.18)	
Weekly	Crude	1,179/6,137	1.27 (1.18, 1.36)		216/5,087	1.07 (0.92, 1.24)		326/5,102	1.14 (1.01, 1.29)		1,750/5,102	1.19 (1.12, 1.27)	
	Adjusted*		1.21 (1.11, 1.31)			0.94 (0.77, 1.14)			1.13 (0.97, 1.33)			1.07 (0.99, 1.16)	
>=1 serv/day	Crude	1,202/5,863	1.38 (1.28, 1.48)		210/4,885	1.08 (0.93, 1.26)		333/4,894	1.22 (1.08, 1.38)		1,765/4,894	1.29 (1.21, 1.38)	
	Adjusted*		1.23 (1.13, 1.33)			1.00 (0.82, 1.22)			1.14 (0.98, 1.34)			1.15 (1.06, 1.25)	

*Adjusted for maternal age, smoking, parity, prepregnancy BMI, physical activity, breastfeeding, socioeconomic position, child sex, maternal history of asthma, maternal history of allergies, paternal history of asthma, paternal history of allergies, and energy (in quintiles).
**Median values (0, 0.5, 3.5, and 7) for each intake group entered as a continuous variable into the model.
ISAAC: International Study of Asthma and Allergies in Childhood.
DNPR: Danish National Patient Registry.
RMPS: Register of Medicinal Products Statistics.

Table 3. Associations between artificially-sweetened carbonated soft drink consumption during pregnancy and child asthma in the Danish National Birth Cohort.

Frequency of intake		Cases/N	Asthma (18 months)	*P* for trend**	Cases/N	Asthma (7 years - ISAAC)	*P* for trend**	Cases/N	Ever asthma (DNPR)	*P* for trend**	Cases/N	Ever asthma (RMPS)	*P* for trend**
			N = 44,638			N = 38,149			N = 38,258			N = N = 38,258	
			OR (95% CI)			OR (95% CI)			OR (95% CI)			OR (95% CI)	
Never	Crude	4,942/29,896	1.00 (ref.)	<0.0001	1,018/25,661	1.00 (ref.)	0.09	1,509/25,733	1.00 (ref.)	0.04	7,944/25,731	1.00 (ref.)	<0.0001
	Adjusted*			0.14			0.27			0.19			0.01
<1 serv/week	Crude	1,013/5,620	1.11 (1.03, 1.20)		185/4,856	0.96 (0.82, 1.13)		287/4,866	1.01 (0.88, 1.15)		1,606/4,868	1.10 (1.03, 1.18)	
	Adjusted*		1.17 (1.07, 1.27)			0.91 (0.74, 1.12)			1.01 (0.85, 1.19)			1.11 (1.02, 1.20)	
Weekly	Crude	1,327/7,399	1.10 (1.03, 1.18)		267/6,189	1.09 (0.95, 1.25)		351/6,212	0.96 (0.85, 1.08)		2,092/6,211	1.14 (1.07, 1.21)	
	Adjusted*		1.06 (0.98, 1.15)			1.04 (0.87, 1.23)			0.98 (0.84, 1.14)			1.10 (1.02, 1.19)	
>=1 serv/day	Crude	346/1,723	1.27 (1.12, 1.43)		66/1,443	1.16 (0.90, 1.50)		118/1,447	1.43 (1.17, 1.73)		511/1,448	1.22 (1.09, 1.36)	
	Adjusted*		1.10 (0.95, 1.27)			1.18 (0.87, 1.59)			1.30 (1.01, 1.66)			1.13 (0.98, 1.29)	

*Adjusted for maternal age, smoking, parity, prepregnancy BMI, physical activity, breastfeeding, socioeconomic position, child sex, maternal history of asthma, maternal history of allergies, paternal history of asthma, paternal history of allergies, and energy (in quintiles).

**Median values (0, 0.5, 3.5, and 7) for each intake group entered as a continuous variable into the model.

ISAAC: International Study of Asthma and Allergies in Childhood.

DNPR: Danish National Patient Registry.

RMPS: Register of Medicinal Products Statistics.

Multivariate Analysis

Child asthma at 18 months follow-up. The prevalence of child asthma was 17% (N = 7,628/44,638). At the 18 month follow-up, only intake of artificially-sweetened non-carbonated soft drinks were associated with higher risk of self-reported child asthma diagnosis (> = 1serving/day vs. never: 1.23, 95% CI: 1.13, 1.33) (**Table 2**). No associations were found for sugar-sweetened beverages (**Tables S1–2**). Combining intake of artificially-sweetened beverages generated effect estimates between the two sub-categories and was strongest for child asthma (> = 1serving/day vs. never: 1.14, 95% CI: 1.00, 1.28) (data not shown).

Ever asthma and current child asthma at the 7 year follow-up. The prevalence of ever asthma by DNPR was 6% (2,265/38,258) and 32% (12,153/38,258) by RMPS. About 4% (1,536/38,149) of children were classified with current asthma. Both carbonated and non-carbonated artificially-sweetened soft drinks were associated with a DNPR and RMPS diagnosis (**Tables 2–3**). Mothers who drank at least 1 serving of artificially-sweetened carbonated soft drink serving per day were 1.30 (95% CI: 1.01, 1.66) times more likely to have a child with an asthma diagnosis in the DNPR, and 1.13 (95% CI: 0.98, 1.29) times more likely to have a child RMPS asthma diagnosis. For artificially-sweetened non-carbonated soft drinks these odds ratios were 1.14 (95% CI: 0.98, 1.34) and 1.15 (95% CI: 1.06, 1.25) for a DNPR and RMPS asthma diagnosis respectively. No associations were found between maternal intake of sugar-sweetened beverages and child asthma (**Tables S1–2**). Combining artificially-sweetened beverage intake categories strengthened the associations for RMPS asthma diagnosis only (weekly to > = 1serving/day vs. never to < 1serving/week: 1.20, 95% CI: 1.07, 1.35). We further excluded the first 3 years of life for the registry diagnoses and found that results strengthened with the DNPR diagnosis for both artificially-sweetened carbonated (> = 1serving/day vs. never: 1.44, 95% CI: 1.00, 2.09) and non-carbonated (> = 1serving/day vs. never: 1.31, 95% CI: 1.03, 1.66) soft drinks.

Ever child allergic rhinitis at the 7 year follow-up. Close to 5% (1,855/37,971) of mothers reported an ever child allergic rhinitis doctor diagnosis on the 7 year questionnaire. Artificially-sweetened carbonated beverages were directly related to ever allergic rhinitis (> = 1serving/day vs. never: 1.31, 95% CI: 0.98, 1.74) (**Table 4**). No associations were found for the other types of beverages (**Tables S3**). Combining the artificially-sweetened beverage intake generated results in between the carbonated and non-carbonated intake categories (> = 1serving/day vs. never: 1.11, 95% CI: 0.86, 1.43).

Sensitivity Analyses

The difference between crude and adjusted effect estimates was primarily accounted for by maternal prepregnancy BMI, socio-economic position, and breastfeeding duration. However, most examined covariates were weak confounders and rarely accounted for more than 10% change in the effect estimates. We further adjusted the models for other foods and nutrient intake; however, this did not change the results. When sugar- and artificially-sweetened beverages were mutually adjusted for, some associations weakened (e.g. artificially-sweetened carbonated beverages and child asthma at 18 months), while others strengthened (e.g. artificially-sweetened carbonated beverages and ever allergic rhinitis), but the general direction of the associations and the conclusions did not change. The most notable change was a strengthening of the effect estimate for artificially-sweetened carbonated beverages and ever allergic rhinitis (> = 1serving/day vs. never: 1.42, 95% CI: 1.05, 1.91). Further adjustment for other potential confounders of child asthma and allergies (mode of

Table 4. Associations between artificially-sweetened carbonated and non-carbonated soft drink consumption during pregnancy and self-reported ever child allergic rhinitis in the Danish National Birth Cohort.

Frequency of intake		Cases/N	Artificially-sweetened carbonated soft drinks	*P* for trend**	Cases/N	Artificially-sweetened non-carbonated soft drinks	*P* for trend**
			N = 37,971			N = 37,984	
			OR (95% CI)			OR (95% CI)	
Never	Crude	1,210/25,539	1.00 (ref.)	0.16	1,248/25,384	1.00 (ref.)	0.59
	Adjusted*			0.01			0.83
<1 serv/week	Crude	251/4,835	1.10 (0.96, 1.27)		128/2,666	0.98 (0.81, 1.18)	
	Adjusted*		0.97 (0.80, 1.16)			0.96 (0.75, 1.21)	
Weekly	Crude	319/6,160	1.10 (0.97, 1.25)		243/5,071	0.97 (0.85, 1.12)	
	Adjusted*		1.15 (0.98, 1.35)			0.86 (0.71, 1.04)	
> = 1 serv/day	Crude	75/1,437	1.11 (0.87, 1.41)		231/4,863	0.97 (0.84, 1.11)	
	Adjusted*		1.31 (0.98, 1.74)			1.03 (0.86, 1.24)	

*Adjusted for maternal age, smoking, parity, prepregnancy BMI, physical activity, breastfeeding, socioeconomic position, child sex, maternal history of asthma, maternal history of allergies, paternal history of asthma, paternal history of allergies, and energy (in quintiles).

**Median values (0, 0.5, 3.5, and 7) for each intake group entered as a continuous variable into the model.

delivery, pets at home, exposure do smoking during infancy, daycare attendance during infancy, and use of antibiotics and paracetamol during pregnancy and child use of antibiotics at 6 months as suggested in a recent review by Nurmatov et al [36]) did not alter the effect estimates. For example, effect estimates for artificially-sweetened carbonated beverages and asthma at 18 months were 1.07 (95% CI: 0.93, 1.24) (vs. 1.10, 95% CI: 0.95, 1.27) and for artificially-sweetened carbonated beverages and asthma at 7 years 1.17 (95% CI: 0.87, 1.59) (vs. 1.18, 95% CI: 0.87, 1.59). This analysis was performed to examine the stability of the estimates but we are cautious about adding these seven covariates, some of which are conditioning on future conditions, since we might be imposing overadjustment and bias in our analyses [37,38].

Based on a previous study from our cohort [16] where we found a direct association between low-fat yoghurt intake, and asthma and allergic rhinitis, we examined the relation between intake of artificially-sweetened beverages and low-fat yoghurt. The strongest Spearman correlation was with low-fat yoghurt with fruit ($r = 0.07$–0.09, $P < 0.0001$) for both carbonated and non-carbonated beverages. When we adjusted for low-fat yoghurt with fruit, there was no change in effect estimates.

To exclude the possibility that our results were mediated by preterm birth [30], we restricted the analyses to term births (>37 and $<=42$ weeks of gestation), which did not substantially alter the results. The results for artificially-sweetened carbonated beverages and self-reported allergic rhinitis strengthened ($>=1$ serving/day vs. never: 1.44, 95% CI: 1.07, 1.94 vs. 1.31, 95% CI: 0.98, 1.74), while the association between artificially-sweetened non-carbonated beverages and asthma diagnosis by DNPR weakened ($>=1$ serving/day vs. never: 1.06, 95% CI: 0.89, 1.27 vs. 1.14, 95% CI: 0.98, 1.34).

Discussion

In our prospective study of the relation between maternal intake of artificially-sweetened beverages during pregnancy and development of child allergic disease, we found that artificially-sweetened beverages moderately increased risk of asthma and allergic rhinitis both in early and later childhood. These results appeared stronger for carbonated beverages. We did not find similar results for sugar-sweetened beverages, suggesting that artificial sweeteners, rather than other additives and aromatic compounds in soft drinks, may play a role in the development of allergic diseases.

Little is currently know about artificial sweeteners in relation to allergic disease development. Artificial sweeteners, and particularly aspartame, have, however, been studied more broadly in the context of inflammation [18–20]. One study examined the effect of aspartame on oxidation in mice brain and liver and found an increase in tumour-necrosis factor-α and lipid peroxidation in the brain, while reducing glutathione [18]. Another study in zebra fish found increased infiltration of inflammatory cells and production of radical oxygen species in the liver and brain after exposure to aspartame [19]. In contrast, they did not find anti-inflammatory properties of aspartame, but found that it did reduce mechanical allodynia in arthritic rats [20]. Aspartame has also been implicated in alleviation of autoimmune disease [20,39]. One early study examined aspartame in relation to allergic activity, specifically the ability of aspartame to generate 'allergic' reactions by inducing histamine release from mast cells and basophils by a pharmacological mechanism or by an IgE-dependent process of mast cell activation [21]. The authors found that aspartame did not act as a direct mast cell secretagogue, and did not cause degranulation of cultured mouse mast cells or human basophils *in vitro*. Aspartame did decrease antigen-induced histamine release from cultured mouse mast cells after long-term exposure only. The authors could not fully explain the origin of this effect but speculated that by increasing mast cell proliferation, it made mast cells less responsive to anaphylactic stimulation.

Among human studies, a randomized, double-blind, cross-over trial among patients with a history of headaches did not find any difference in histamine levels according to aspartame exposure [40]. Aspartame has also shown not to cause allergic reaction in adults when compared to placebo in randomized, double-blinded studies administering aspartame doses at one time point [24,25]. A number of smaller studies have shown improvement in dermatitis with aspartame avoidance [22,23,41]. No human study has specifically investigated the relation between artificial sweeteners and the prevention of allergic disease; and it is unclear whether results from animal experimental and *in vitro* studies can be transposed to the human condition in pregnancy. Furthermore, while majority of these studies involved aspartame; other artificial sweeteners, such as acesulfame-K, sucralose, or saccharine, need to be considered as potential active agents. Soft drinks often contain a mixture of different sweeteners. The predominant sweeteners in soft drinks appearing on the Danish market are aspartame and acesulfame-K [26]. Their average concentration is approximately 2–3-fold higher in carbonated versus noncarbonated soft drinks, which is why we examined them separately. This could explain the slightly stronger effect size we found for carbonated soft drink, and furthermore suggests that less frequently used sweeteners found in non-carbonated beverages, such as cyclamate and saccharine [26], may not be associated with allergic disease outcomes. We were not, however, able to distinguish between intake of specific artificial sweeteners.

It is possible that other additives may account for the observed findings. The role of food additives in allergic disease is well known. However, as these are rare events, establishing a causal link is complex and most of the current knowledge is based on case reports [42]. As food additives may cause allergic reaction, exposing subjects to a group of food additives, including sweeteners, has been recommended in screening for food allergy [43]. The word "food additives" covers a broad range of chemically unrelated substances and this approach highlights the general absence of mechanistic insight for several suspected allergens.

There were several strengths to our study. These included examining detailed dietary data collected in pregnancy in a large, prospective study in relation to several allergic outcomes. We used outcomes both in early and later childhood in order to differentiate potential etiologically pathways between outcomes in infancy that may later resolve and later outcomes that are more likely to capture clinically relevant asthma and allergic rhinitis. Furthermore, we took advantage of both registry-based and self-reported outcome assessment. These allowed us to better identify clinical asthma in the patient registry, particularly after exclusion of early registry diagnoses, an outcome that may not be as well reported by questionnaire. The previous paper comparing different assessment methods of asthma in the DNBC [44] indicated higher specificities (but lower sensitivities) for the registry based outcomes. If the registries are more likely to capture the true asthma cases, while the self-reported outcomes represent a less valid outcome, then this could explain why we observe associations mainly for the registry based outcomes. In further analysis we found that the results strengthened somewhat for ever asthma diagnosed during inpatient visits, suggesting that disease severity may be an important mediating factor. Questionnaires may be better for assessing outcomes such as allergic rhinitis as these are less likely to end up in registries due to more moderate symptom manifestation and more prevalent use of over-the-counter medication. Self-reported asthma may capture mild to moderate disease and can be used for more direct comparison with other studies using the International Study of Asthma and Allergies in Childhood questionnaire.

We found that results differed by outcome with early life outcomes being associated with artificially-sweetened non-carbonated beverages and registry outcomes more strongly associated with higher intake of artificially-sweetened carbonated beverages. This suggests that different sweeteners or other additives may be accounting for some of the relations. Other plausible explanations include a difference in timing of outcome or etiological pathways. For example, the latter may be more governed by T helper (Th) 2 mechanisms while the former by a mixture of Th1- and Th2-driven pathways [45,46]. As mentioned in the results section, our results strengthened somewhat after we excluded the first 3 years of diagnoses from the hospital registry, influence of artificial sweeteners on pathways in early vs. later childhood may be different. In an attempt to limit residual confounding, in our statistical models we adjusted for numerous covariates covering anthropometry, lifestyle, breastfeeding and familial history of asthma and other known predictors of asthma. However, we may have failed to identify all relevant confounders and thus our findings may be due to residual confounding by unmeasured or unidentified covariates.

Our study was limited primarily by self-reported assessment of diet and outcomes. Although there is always some concern with misclassification when using FFQs for dietary assessment, we expect it to have differentiated well between low and high beverage consumers. We therefore expect any misclassification to have been non-differential and therefore underestimated the true effect estimates. Furthermore, due to the complex mixtures used in different beverages we cannot quantify accurately the amount consumed of individual sweeteners from soft drinks. This may lead to less precise estimation of effect size and contribute to divergent conclusions when comparing the results for carbonated and non-carbonated beverages. Our definition of current asthma has shown high agreement among cases (>60%) and non-cases (>90%) in a recent study from our cohort [44] when compared to the DNPR; yet, the results for the self-reported outcome did not track those of the registry asthma diagnoses. This could have been due to failure to capture clinically-relevant asthma. Finally, potential for selection bias is plausible in a longitudinal study with loss to follow-up. When we compared participants of this study with non-participants, participants tended to display healthier life-style habits. We do however not believe these differences to be large enough to change our findings.

To conclude, our results from a large prospective cohort study are indicative of a weak to moderate association between consumption of artificially-sweetened beverages during pregnancy and offspring risk of asthma and allergic rhinitis. While this could be due to residual confounding, we hypothesize that artificial sweeteners may be the plausible causal agent since no similar associations were found for sugar-sweetened beverages. We do not claim our results to be affirmative, but rather they are suggestive and hypothesis generating. These findings need to be further explored at a mechanistic level and examined with more detailed assessment of exposure to artificial sweeteners.

Supporting Information

Table S1 Associations between sugar-sweetened non-carbonated soft drinks consumption during pregnancy and child asthma in the Danish National Birth Cohort.

Table S2 Associations between sugar-sweetened carbonated soft drink consumption during pregnancy and child asthma in the Danish National Birth Cohort.

Table S3 Associations between sugar-sweetened carbonated and non-carbonated soft drinks consumption during pregnancy and self-reported ever child allergic rhinitis in the Danish National Birth Cohort.

Author Contributions

Conceived and designed the experiments: EM TIH. Analyzed the data: EM. Wrote the paper: EM TIH MS SFO.

References

1. Chatzi L, Apostolaki G, Bibakis I, Skypala I, Bibaki-Liakou V, et al. (2007) Protective effect of fruits, vegetables and the Mediterranean diet on asthma and allergies among children in Crete. Thorax 62: 677–683.
2. Nwaru BI, Ahonen S, Kaila M, Erkkola M, Haapala A-M, et al. (2009) Maternal diet during pregnancy and allergic sensitization in the offspring by 5 yrs of age: a prospective cohort study. Pediatr Allergy Immunol 21: 29–37.
3. Sausenthaler S, Koletzko S, Schaaf B, Lehmann I, Borte M, et al. (2007) Maternal diet during pregnancy in relation to eczema and allergic sensitization in the offspring at 2 y of age. Am J Clin Nutr 85: 530–537.
4. Willers S, Wijga A, Brunekreef B, Kerkhof M, Gerritsen J, et al. (2008) Maternal food consumption during pregnancy and the longitudinal development of childhood asthma. Am J Respir Crit Care Med 178: 124–131.
5. Willers SM, Devereux G, Craig LCA, McNeill G, Wijga AH, et al. (2007) Maternal food consumption during pregnancy and asthma, respiratory and atopic symptoms in 5-year-old children. Thorax 62: 773–779.
6. Miyake Y, Sasaki S, Tanaka K, Hirota Y (2010) Consumption of vegetables, fruit, and antioxidants during pregnancy and wheeze and eczema in infants. Allergy 65: 758–765.
7. Calvani M, Alessandri C, Sopo S, Panetta V, Pingitore G, et al. (2006) Consumption of fish, butter and margarine during pregnancy and development of allergic sensitizations in the offspring: role of maternal atopy. Pediatr Allergy Immunol 17: 94–102.
8. Jedrychowski W, Perera F, Maugeri U, Mrozek-Budzyn D, Miller RL, et al. (2011) Effects of prenatal and perinatal exposure to fine air pollutants and maternal fish consumption on the occurrence of infantile eczema. Int Arch Allergy Immunol 155: 275–281.
9. Miyake Y, Sasaki S, Tanaka K, Ohfuji S, Hirota Y (2009) Maternal fat consumption during pregnancy and risk of wheeze and eczema in Japanese infants aged 16–24 months: the Osaka Maternal and Child Health Study. Thorax 64: 815–821.
10. Romieu I, Torrent M, Garcia-Esteban R, Ferrer C, Ribas-Fitó N, et al. (2007) Maternal fish intake during pregnancy and atopy and asthma in infancy. Clin Exp Allergy 37: 518–525.
11. Salam M, Li Y, Langholz B, Gilliland F (2005) Maternal fish consumption during pregnancy and risk of early childhood asthma. J Asthma 42: 513–518.
12. Øien T, Storrø O, Johnsen R (2011) Do early intake of fish and fish oil protect against eczema and doctor-diagnosed asthma at 2 years of age? A cohort study. J Epidemiol Community Health 64: 124–129.
13. Olsen SF, Osterdal ML, Salvig JD, Mortensen LM, Rytter D, et al. (2008) Fish oil intake compared with olive oil intake in late pregnancy and asthma in the offspring: 16 y of registry-based follow-up from a randomized controlled trial. Am J Clin Nutr 88: 167–175.
14. Chatzi L, Torrent M, Romieu I, Garcia-Esteban R, Ferrer C, et al. (2008) Mediterranean diet in pregnancy is protective for wheeze and atopy in childhood. Thorax 63: 507–513.
15. Miyake Y, Sasaki S, Tanaka K, Hirota Y (2010) Dairy food, calcium and vitamin D intake in pregnancy, and wheeze and eczema in infants. Eur Respir J 35: 1228–1234.
16. Maslova E, Halldorsson TI, Strøm M, Olsen SF (2012) Low-fat yoghurt intake in pregnancy associated with increased child asthma and allergic rhinitis risk: a prospective cohort study. Journal of Nutritional Science 1: 1–11.
17. Association AD (2004) Position of the American Dietetic Association: Use of Nutritive and Nonnutritive Sweeteners. J Am Diet Assoc 104: 255–275.

18. Abdel-Salam OME, Salem NA, Hussein JS (2011) Effect of Aspartame on Oxidative Stress and Monoamine Neurotransmitter Levels in Lipopolysaccharide-Treated Mice. Neurotox Res.
19. Kim J-Y, Seo J, Cho K-H (2011) Aspartame-fed zebrafish exhibit acute deaths with swimming defects and saccharin-fed zebrafish have elevation of cholesteryl ester transfer protein activity in hypercholesterolemia. Food and Chemical Toxicology 49: 2899–2905.
20. LaBuda CJ, Fuchs PN (2001) A comparison of chronic aspartame exposure to aspirin on inflammation, hyperalgesia and open field activity following carrageenan-induced monoarthritis. Life Sciences 69: 443–454.
21. Szucs EF, Barrett KE, Metcalfe DD (1986) The effects of aspartame on mast cells and basophils. Fd Chem Toxic 24: 171–174.
22. Hill AM, Belsito DV (2003) Systemic contact dermatitis of the eyelids caused by formaldehyde derived from aspartame? Contact Dermatitis 49: 258–272.
23. Jacob SE, Stechschulte S (2008) Formaldehyde, aspartame, and migraines: a possible connection. Dermatitis 19: E10–11.
24. Garriga MM, Berkebile C, Metcalfe DD (1991) A combined single-blind, double-blind, placebo-controlled study to determine the reproducibility of hypersensitivity reactions to aspartame. J Allergy Clin Immunol 87: 821–827.
25. Geha R, Buckley CEI, Greenberger P, Patterson R, Polmar S, et al. (1993) Aspartame is no more likely than placebo to cause urticaria/angioedema: Results of a multicenter, randomized, double-blind, placebo-controlled, crossover study. J Allergy Clin Immunol 93: 513–520.
26. Leth T, Jensen U, Fagt S, Andersen R (2008) Estimated intake of intense sweeteners from non-alcoholic beverages in Denmark, 2005. Food Addit Contam Part A Chem Anal Control Expo Risk Assess 25: 662–668.
27. Olsen J, Melbye M, Olsen SF, Sorensen TI, Aaby P, et al. (2001) The Danish National Birth Cohort–its background, structure and aim. Scand J Public Health 29: 300–307.
28. Mikkelsen TB, Osler M, Olsen SF (2005) Validity of protein, retinol, folic acid and n–3 fatty acid intakes estimated from the food-frequency questionnaire used in the Danish National Birth Cohort. Public Health Nutrition 9: 771–778.
29. Saxholt E, Christensen AT, Møller A, Hartkopp HB, Hess Ygil K, et al. (2008) Danish Food Composition Databank, revision 7.: Department of Nutrition, National Food Institute, Technical University of Denmark.
30. Halldorsson TI, Strom M, Petersen SB, Olsen SF (2010) Intake of artificially sweetened soft drinks and risk of preterm delivery: a prospective cohort study in 59,334 Danish pregnant women. Am J Clin Nutr 92: 626–633.
31. Asher MI, Keil U, Anderson HR, Beasley R, Crane J, et al. (1995) International study of asthma and allergies in childhood (ISAAC): rationale and methods. Eur Respir J 8: 483–491.
32. Hederos CA, Hasselgren M, Hedlin G, Bornehag CG (2007) Comparison of clinically diagnosed asthma with parental assessment of children's asthma in a questionnaire. Pediatr Allergy Immunol 18: 135–141.
33. Moth G, Vedsted P, Schiøtz PO (2007) National registry diagnoses agree with medical records on hospitalized asthmatic children. Acta Pædiatrica 96: 1470–1473.
34. Forskningsdatabaser (2002) Databeredskab i Danmarks Statistik. (In Danish). Copenhagen, Denmark: Danmarks Statistik.
35. Moth G, Vedsted P, Schiøtz PO (2007) Identification of asthmatic children using prescription data and diagnosis. Eur J Clin Pharmacol 63: 605–611.
36. Nurmatov U, Nwaru BI, Devereux G, Sheikh A (2012) Confounding and effect modification in studies of diet and childhood asthma and allergies. Allergy 67: 1041–1059.
37. Hernandez-Diaz S, Schisterman EF, Hernan MA (2006) The birth weight "paradox" uncovered? Am J Epidemiol 164: 1115–1120.
38. Schisterman EF, Cole SR, Platt RW (2009) Overadjustment bias and unnecessary adjustment in epidemiologic studies. Epidemiology 20: 488–495.
39. Ramsland PA, Movafagh BF, Reichlin M, Edmundson AB (1999) Interference of rheumatoid factor activity by aspartame, a dipeptide methyl ester. J Mol Recognit 12: 249–257.
40. Schiffman SS, Buckley CEI, Sampson HA, Massey EW, Baraniuk JN, et al. (1987) Aspartame and Susceptibility to Headache. N Engl J Med 317: 1181–1185.
41. Veien NK, Lomholt HB (2012) Systemic allergic dermatitis presumably caused by formaldehyde derived from aspartame. Contact Dermatitis 67: 315–316.
42. Gultekin F, Doguc DK (2012) Allergic and Immunologic Reactions to Food Additives. Clin Rev Allergy Immunol.
43. Reese I, Zuberbier T, Bunselmeyer B, Erdmann S, Henzgen M, et al. (2009) Diagnostic approach for suspected pseudoallergic reaction to food ingredients. J Dtsch Dermatol Ges 7: 70–77.
44. Hansen S, Strom M, Maslova E, Mortensen EL, Granstrom C, et al. (2012) A comparison of three methods to measure asthma in epidemiologic studies: results from the danish national birth cohort. PLoS One 7: e36328.
45. Pitrez PMC, Machado DC, Jones MH, Andrade F, Camozzato C, et al. (2005) Th-1 and Th-2 cytokine production in infants with virus-associated wheezing. Braz J Med Biol Res 38: 51–54.
46. Psarras S, Papadopoulos NG, Johnston SL (2004) Pathogenesis of respiratory syncytial virus bronchiolitis-related wheezing. Paediatric Respiratory Reviews 5: S179–S184.

23

Rhinitis Symptoms and Asthma among Parents of Preschool Children in Relation to the Home Environment in Chongqing, China

Juan Wang[1,2], Baizhan Li[2]*, Wei Yu[2], Qin Yang[2], Han Wang[2], Duchai Huang[2], Jan Sundell[2,3], Dan Norbäck[1]

1 Department of Medical Sciences, Uppsala University and University Hospital, Uppsala, Sweden, **2** Key Laboratory of Three Gorges Reservoir Region's Eco-Environment, Ministry of Education, Chongqing University, Chongqing, China, **3** Department of Building Science, Tsinghua University, Beijing, China

Abstract

Risk factors for rhinitis and asthma in the home environment were studied by a questionnaire survey. Parents of 4530 1–8 year old children (one parent per child) from randomly selected kindergartens in Chongqing, China participated. 70.4% were females; 47.1% had rhinitis symptoms in the last three months (current rhinitis, CR); 1.6% reported a history of allergic asthma (AA); 2.7% reported a history of allergic rhinitis (AR); 16.4% were current smokers; 50.8% males and 2.4% females were current smokers. Stuffy odor, unpleasant odor, tobacco smoke odor and dry air were associated with CR (adjustment for gender, current smoking and other perceptions of odor or humidity). Associations between home environment and CR, AR, and AA were studied by multiple logistic regression analyses, adjusting for gender, current smoking and other significant home factors. Living near a main road or highway was a risk factor for both CR (OR(95%CI): 1.31(1.13,1.52)) and AR (OR(95%CI): 2.44(1.48,4.03)). Other risk factors for CR included living in rural areas (OR(95%CI): 1.43(1.10,1.85)), new furniture (OR(95%CI): 1.28(1.11,1.49)), water damage (OR(95%CI): 1.68(1.29,2.18)), cockroaches (OR(95%CI): 1.46(1.23,1.73)), and keeping pets (OR(95%CI): 1.24(1.04,1.49)). Other risk factors for AR included redecoration (OR(95%CI): 2.14(1.34,3.41)), mold spots (OR(95%CI): 2.23(1.06,4.68)), window pane condensation (OR(95%CI): 2.04(1.28,3.26)). Water damage was the only home factor associated with AA (2.56(1.34,4.86)). Frequently put bedding to sunshine was protective for CR (OR(95%CI): 0.79(0.68,0.92); cleaning every day was protective for AR (OR(95%CI): 0.40(0.22,0.71)). In conclusion, parents' CR and AR were related to a number of factors of the home environment.

Editor: Oliver Schildgen, Kliniken der Stadt Köln gGmbH, Germany

Funding: This study was supported by the Key National Project of Physical Science (Theory and Method for Control and Dynamic Regulation of Building Thermal Environment, 50838009) and National Technology Support Project (Technology for Monitoring and Operation of Building Indoor Air Pollution, 2012BAJ02B06). The funders had no role in study design, data collection and analysis, decision to publish, or preparation of the manuscript.

Competing Interests: The authors have declared that no competing interests exist.

* E-mail: baizhanli@cqu.edu.cn

Introduction

Rhinitis is a worldwide health problem that generates a significant healthcare burden among people in all ages. Although it is not a life threatening condition, its negative impact on human's quality of life has been reported in studies from different countries [1–4].

Rhinitis can be divided into allergic rhinitis (AR) and non-allergic rhinitis (NAR). It is considered to be allergic rhinitis (AR) when these symptoms are accompanied by allergen-specific IgE production. The absence of outdoor symptoms in the spring, no parental history of allergy, no symptoms around cats, the presence of symptoms around perfumes and fragrances, are predictive of NAR [5]. Pollen, allergens from certain pets, house dust mites and molds are common causes of allergic rhinitis. Moreover, indoor air pollution, lifestyle factors (ownership of pets, infant feeding, childhood infections, nutrient intake, family and sibship size, hygiene standard, food, vaccination, stress) and socioeconomic conditions, are quoted as adjuvant factors for allergic sensitization and possible causes of the increased prevalence [6]. NAR is when obstruction and rhinorrhea occurs in relation to non-allergic, noninfectious triggers such as change in the weather, exposure to caustic odors or cigarette smoke, barometric pressure differences, etc [7].

Females [8,9], young adults [9–11], and those with allergic heredity [12] are at higher risk of having AR. Home exposures may contribute to the development of AR. Allergen sources from home, such as having pets [13] and the presence of cockroaches [11,14] are important risk factors for AR. Chinese studies has shown that house dust mite allergy was the most common allergy in AR patients [15,16]. Building dampness can be another risk factor for AR [17,18]. Few studies have reported associations between levels of microbiologic agents and AR [19]. Cooking fumes exposure [11] and using wood as heating and wood or biomass as cooking material are other risk factors for AR [17]. Moreover, environment tobacco smoke (ETS) can induce nasal obstruction and decreased muco-ciliary clearance in NAR [20,21].

During past decades, the prevalence of allergic rhinitis has increased, especially in developed countries. The prevalence of adults' rhinitis seems to still be increasing but the prevalence is different in different countries [22,23]. The increased diagnostic activity and observance may have contributed to the increase. AR is a common manifestation of allergic disease affecting approximately 10%–25% of the world population [24], and has been reported to be one of the top ten reasons for visits to primary care clinics [25]. One cross-sectional study in Turkey in parents of primary school children showed that the prevalence of AR was: 17.5% for males and 21.2% for females in rural areas; 11.7% for males and 17.0% for females in urban areas [17]. The prevalence of AR increased from 22% to 31% from 1990 to 2008 in Swedish young adults [26]. Although the prevalence and epidemiologic features of AR are well defined, less information is available on the prevalence of NAR in the general population. It is estimated that NAR affects as many as 17 million Americans [27]. One study on 975 patients reported that 43% of them had only AR, 23% had only NAR, and 34% had mixed rhinitis [27]. Many people with rhinitis have both AR and NAR, which makes it difficult to study pure AR or NAR [28]. One study has shown that a substantial subset of individuals with AR were in addition hyperreactive to non-allergic triggers [29].

Rhinitis and asthma commonly coexist. A recent study found that 64% of asthmatic patients had AR and 20% of AR patients had asthma [30]. Another study showed that 60% of asthmatics reported AR [31]. Rhinitis is a significant risk factor for asthma incidence [32]. Not only the intensity, but also the duration of rhinitis is correlated with the development of asthma [33]. A survey in Chinese patients with asthma and/or rhinitis found that patients with both asthma and rhinitis had higher prevalence of positive skin-prick tests (SPT) and specific IgE positivity to most allergens as compared to those with asthma or rhinitis alone [34]. Rhinitis and asthma may be manifestations of the same disease and share common pathologic and physiologic characteristics, as proposed by the 'united airways' hypothesis [35].

There is a lack of epidemiological studies on environmental risk factors for rhinitis in China, and we have found no previous study about the home environment and rhinitis in Chinese adults. In this cross-sectional study the main aim is to estimate cumulative incidence of allergic asthma and allergic rhinitis, and prevalence of current rhinitis in Chongqing adults with young children, and to identify domestic environmental factors associated with these health variables. In addition, we studied the association between perceptions of odors and air humidity and rhinitis and asthma.

Methods

Ethics Statement

The study and the consent procedure were approved by the Medical Research Ethics Committee of School of Public Health, Fudan University. The participants gave informed consent.

Selection of the study subjects

The present study is a part of an epidemiological multi-center study of asthma and allergies among children and their relation to the home environment in China (China, Children, Homes,Health, CCHH) [36–38]. The study is using the same study protocol and questionnaire as earlier studies [39,40], starting with a cross-sectional questionnaire survey followed by a nested case-control study. The survey was carried out from December 2010 to April 2011.

The questionnaires were distributed to children's parents through teachers in kindergartens in three districts (Shapingba, Jiulongpo, Yubei) that were randomly selected from 9 districts of Chongqing city. From the 54 randomly selected kindergartens (15 from Shapingba, 21 from Jiulongpo and 18 from Yubei), 7117 subjects (one parent per child aged from 1–8 years old) were selected and invited for the questionnaire survey. Completed questionnaires were collected one week later by the teachers.

Questionnaire

A modified version of a self-administered questionnaire previously used in Sweden, and among Chinese university students [39,40] has been used in this study. The questionnaire was slightly modified to be more appropriate for Chinese culture, lifestyle, building structure and interior characteristics.

Questions on subjects' gender, own current smoking habit, current smoking of the spouse, rhinitis symptoms in the last three months (current rhinitis), history of allergic rhinitis (cumulative incidence of allergic rhinitis), history of allergic asthma (cumulative incidence of allergic asthma), and perceptions of odors and air humidity were collected by a self-reported questionnaire.

Question about current rhinitis followed the Northern Swedish Office Illness study [41]. "During the last three months, have you had irritating, stuffy or runny nose?" There were three options: often (every week); sometimes; never. Any current rhinitis was defined as those who reported often or sometimes; weekly current rhinitis was defined as those reported often; less common current rhinitis was defined as those who reported sometimes.

Questions about odor and air humidity perceptions were: during the last three months, have you had any of the following perceptions: Stuffy odor; Unpleasant odor; Pungent odor; Mold odor; Tobacco smoke odor; Humid air; Dry air. There were three options: weekly; sometimes; never. For each odor or humidity perception, "Yes" was defined as those who reported weekly or sometimes; "No" was defined as those who only reported never.

Questions about exposure indicators and building characteristics contained in present paper are:

(1) House site (urban/suburban/rural);
(2) * Whether current residence is near a main road or highway with a distance of 200 m (yes/no);
(3) Building construction year (before 1980/1980–1990/1991–2000/2001–2005/after 2005);
(4) Residence area (<=40 m^2/41–60 m^2/61–75 m^2/76–100 m^2/101–150 m^2/>150 m^2);
(5) Wall materials on children's bedroom (wall paper/cement/lime/paint/emulsion paint/other);
(6) Floor materials (wood/cement/ceramic tile or stone/laminated floor/other);
(7) Whether any redecoration has been done since one year before pregnancy (yes/no);
(8) * Whether any new furniture has been bought since one year before pregnancy (yes/no);
(9) * Whether subject has reported any mold spots in child bedroom (yes/no);
(10) * Whether subject has reported any damp stains in child bedroom (yes/no);
(11) * Whether subject has reported any water damage in child bedroom (yes/no);
(12) * Whether subject has reported window pane condensation during winter in child bedroom (yes/no);
(13) * Whether subject has seen cockroaches in home before (yes/no);
(14) * Whether subject has seen rats in home before (yes/no);
(15) * Whether subject has seen mosquitoes/flies in home before (yes/no);

(16) * Whether subject has used mosquito-repellent incense in home before (yes/no);

(17) * Whether subject has used incense in home before (yes/no);

(18) * Whether subject has pets in home currently (yes/no); if yes, it is (cat/dog/rodent (rabbit/rat)/bird/aquarium fishes or reptiles/other);

(19) The frequency of cleaning child's bedroom (every day/Less or equal twice a week);

(20) * The frequency of putting child's bedding to sunshine (frequently/never or rarely);

(21) The frequency of opening window in child's bedroom in winter (frequently/never or rarely).

"*" included in a risk factor score.

Indoor environment nasal risk factors score

From twenty one questions about exposure indicators and building characteristics above, an indoor environment risk factors score (0–13) was constructed (Continuous Score, range from 0–13), by adding the number of yes response to 13 exposure indicators of home environment significantly associated with current rhinitis (which marked with "*", question 20 was changed by asking if put bedding to sunshine frequently (yes/no), "yes" was coded as "0" and "no" was coded as "1").

The Continuous Score was then classified in five categories to make another Categorized Score: by adding number of indoor environment risk factors, separately as score category 0 (0, 1, 2, 3 and 4 risk factors out of 13), score category 1 (5 risk factors out of 13), score category 2 (6 out of 13), score category 3 (7 out of 13) and score category 4 (8 or more out of 13).

From four questions about indoor dampness above, an indoor dampness score (0–4) was constructed (Continuous Dampness Score, range from 0–4), by adding the number of yes response to four dampness indicators of home environment (question 9–12). The Continuous Dampness Score was then classified in three categories to make another Categorized Dampness Score: by adding different numbers dampness indicators, separately as score category 0 (0 dampness indicators out of 4), score category 1 (1 dampness indicator out of 4), score category 2 (2 or more out of 4).

Statistical analysis

All statistical analyses were conducted with SPSS 17.0. Initially, factor analysis was applied to all exposure indicators and building characteristics questions except question 3 which is about building construction year (question 5 was changed to five separate questions by given yes and no answers to each type of wall material; question 6 was changed to four separate questions by given yes and no answers to each type of floor material). Principal component analysis and rotated component matrix (varimax with Kaiser normalisation) was used.

Then, the association between gender and current rhinitis, history of allergic rhinitis, history of allergic asthma were analyzed by multiple logistic regression with adjustment of current smoking. The association between current smoking and current rhinitis, history of allergic rhinitis, history of allergic asthma were analyzed by multiple logistic regression with adjustment of gender.

Initially, associations between building characteristics and exposure indicators and current rhinitis, history of allergic rhinitis, history of allergic asthma were evaluated in multiple logistic regression by analyzing one factor each time with adjustment of gender and current smoking.

Since the number of variables analyzed in the models was relatively large, stepwise multiple logistic regression models (forward elimination, condition method) were used to find the most significant variables for current rhinitis, history of allergic rhinitis and history of allergic asthma. Then, reduced multiple logistic regression models were applied by adding gender, current smoking and all significant factors from stepwise regression models. Multi-nominal regression models were applied for weekly and less common current rhinitis by adding the same factors as in the reduced multiple logistic regression models. Results achieved by the reduced multiple models and multi-nominal models were compared with initial logistic regression models.

As a next step, associations between current rhinitis and Continuous Score, Categorized Score (score 0–4), Categorized Dampness Score were calculated by multiple logistic regression adjusting for gender and current smoking. Odds Ratios (OR) for Continuous Score were calculated by one unit increase on the 13 steps.

Associations between each odor and humidity perception and current rhinitis, history of allergic rhinitis, history of allergic asthma were calculated by multiple logistic regression with mutual adjustment including gender, current smoking and other six types of odors or humidity perceptions.

Percentages given for each question are for valid data. The reference category for logistic and multi-nominal regression were subjects never having the particular symptom. Associations were expressed as odds ratios (OR) with a 95% confidence interval (CI) for logistic regression but relative risk ratios (RRR) with a 95% confidence interval (CI) for multi-nominal regression. Analyses were considered to be statistically significant if the p-value is less than 0.05. In all statistical analysis, two-tailed tests and a 5% level of significance were applied.

Results

Totally, 5299 parents out of 7117 who were invited to answer the questionnaire (one parent per child) participated, total response rate is 74.5%. The fluctuation of different kindergartens' response rate was small. In this analysis, 4530 complete questionnaires answered by children' parents were included, excluding 769 questionnaires answered by children's grandparents or other persons.

The prevalence of history of allergic asthma, history of allergic rhinitis, current rhinitis and current smoking is shown in Table 1. In total, missing values for history of allergic asthma, history of allergic rhinitis, current rhinitis and current smoking and were 311, 311, 564 and 222, respectively. Men had less history of allergic rhinitis and were more often current smokers. Among those with history of allergic rhinitis, 12.1% did not have current rhinitis, 60.7% had less common current rhinitis and 27.1% had weekly current rhinitis. Among those without any current rhinitis, 0.6% reported history of allergic rhinitis; among those with less common current rhinitis, 3.9% reported history of allergic rhinitis and among those with weekly current rhinitis, 24.8% reported history of allergic rhinitis.

Perceptions of odor and humidity were risk factors for rhinitis but not for asthma. Tobacco smoke odor was a risk factor for current rhinitis and history of allergic rhinitis in logistic regression with mutual adjustment of gender, current smoking and other odors and humidity perceptions. Stuffy odor, unpleasant odor and the perception of dry air were all associated with current rhinitis in logistic regression with mutual adjustment of other odors and humidity perceptions, gender and current smoking (Table 2).

The prevalence of home environmental characteristics is shown in Table 3. The majority of the homes were from urban areas.

Table 1. The prevalence of history of allergic asthma, history of allergic rhinitis, current rhinitis and current smokers among participating parents (%) (n = 4530).

Demographic information		Total	Male	Female	*p*-value
		100	29.6	70.4	
History of allergic asthma		1.6	1.6	1.6	0.934[a]
History of allergic rhinitis		2.7	1.6	3.2	0.005[a]
Current rhinitis	Weekly	3.1	2.9	3.2	
	Less common	44.0	43.0	44.5	
	Never	52.9	54.1	52.3	0.533[b]
Current smoker[c]		16.4	50.8	2.4	<0.001[a]

[a]*p*-value Chi-square test for 2×2 contingency table.
[b]*p*-value Chi-square test for 2×3 contingency table.
[c]Subjects who are current smokers.

Subjects with current rhinitis associated with more report of home risk factors than others.

There was no significant association between gender and current rhinitis, history of allergic rhinitis, history of allergic asthma in logistic regression models with adjustment of current smoking. Current smoking was not associated with current rhinitis, history of allergic rhinitis in logistic regression with adjustment of gender, but current smoking was negatively associated with history of allergic asthma (OR(95%CI): 0.39(0.15,0.99), P = 0.047). Spouses' current smoking (passive smoking) was a risk factor for non-smoking females' current rhinitis (OR(95%CI): 1.17(1.004,1.36), P = 0.044), however, no association was found between passive smoking among non-smoking females and history of allergic rhinitis, history of allergic asthma. When adjusting for gender and current smoking, history of allergic asthma was associated with current rhinitis and history of allergic rhinitis (Table 4); history of allergic rhinitis was associated with current rhinitis (OR(95%CI): 9.09(4.96,16.7), P<0.001).

Factor analysis was applied to identify environmental characteristics patterns by including all questions except building construction year. Question 5 was changed to five separate questions by given yes and no answers to each type of wall material, and question 6 was changed to 4 separate questions by given yes and no answers to each type of floor material. Out of a total of 27 variables, eleven different factors were identified:

(1) area, lime wall and cement floor (area >= 75 m^2 was associated with lime wall and cement floor);
(2) house site (urban/suburban/rural), cement wall and cement floor (there was a trend of increasing presence of cement walls and cement floors from urban to suburban and rural areas);
(3) wall paper and wood floor;
(4) ceramic/stone floor and laminated floor (negative association);
(5) paint and emulsion paint (negative association);
(6) redecoration and new furniture;
(7) mold spots and damp stains;
(8) window pane condensation and frequently open window in winter (negative association).
(9) cockroaches and rats;
(10) mosquitoes/flies and mosquito repellent incense;
(11) cleaning every day and frequently put bedding to sunshine;

Four variables were not included in any factor: living near a main road or highway, water damage, current pets and use of incense.

Associations between house site, construction year, area, history of allergic asthma, and current rhinitis, history of allergic rhinitis calculated by logistic regression adjusting for gender and current smoking, are shown in Table 4. Subjects living in rural areas had more current rhinitis, but those living in suburban and rural areas had less history of allergic rhinitis.

Table 2. Associations between current rhinitis, history of allergic rhinitis, history of allergic asthma and odors and humidity perceptions OR(95%CI)[a].

Type of odor	Current rhinitis	*p*-value	History of allergic rhinitis	*p*-value	History of allergic asthma	*p*-value
Stuffy odor	1.51(1.28,1.79)	<0.001	1.12(0.69,1.80)	0.653	0.78(0.41,1.51)	0.465
Unpleasant odor	1.41(1.17,1.69)	<0.001	1.38(0.84,2.27)	0.209	1.83(0.96,3.51)	0.069
Pungent odor	1.18(0.96,1.45)	0.125	1.37(0.81,2.34)	0.241	0.70(0.31,1.56)	0.378
Mold odor	1.02(0.80,1.30)	0.876	0.49(0.22,1.07)	0.072	1.53(0.65,3.60)	0.327
Tobacco smoke odor	1.38(1.19,1.61)	<0.001	1.73(1.12,2.69)	0.014	1.68(0.94,3.00)	0.081
Humid air	1.17(0.99,1.38)	0.061	0.94(0.59,1.52)	0.813	0.57(0.29,1.13)	0.107
Dry air	1.27(1.09,1.49)	0.003	1.58(1.004,2.50)	0.048	1.60(0.88,2.89)	0.121

[a]Calculated by logistic regression with mutual adjustment, odds ratios were adjusted for gender and current smoking.

Table 3. Home environmental characteristics of participating parents (n = 4530).

		Current rhinitis		Total
		Yes(%)	No(%)	%
House site	Urban	70.4	72.4	71.3
	Suburban	18.0	19.0	18.6
	Rural	11.6	8.6*	10.1
Living near a main road or highway[a]	Yes	48.3	40.5***	44.2
Construction year	Before 1980	3.5	3.6	3.6
	1980–1990	9.5	8.4	9.1
	1991–2000	22.6	21.7	22.6
	2001–2005	35.1	35.3	34.7
	After 2005	29.2	31.0	29.9
Area	<= 40 m^2	14.8	13.4	14.4
	41–60 m^2	13.0	13.4	13.3
	61–75 m^2	18.5	18.2	18.4
	76–100 m^2	26.0	26.4	26.1
	101–150 m^2	22.6	23.6	22.9
	>150 m^2	5.1	4.9	4.9
Wall material	Wall paper	11.8	11.9	12.0
	Paint	8.7	8.9	8.8
	Lime	19.5	18.3	19.0
	Cement	8.9	7.1	8.1
	Emulsion paint	46.2	49.1	47.1
	other	8.0	6.1	7.5
Floor material	Wood floor	15.4	19.5	17.7
	Cement	19.2	15.2	17.5
	Ceramic tile/Stone	35.0	33.3	34.2
	Laminated	28.5	29.0	28.1
	Other	2.0	2.2***	2.2
Redecoration[b]	Yes	34.8	33.0	34.1
New furniture[c]	Yes	60.4	54.3***	57.4
Dampness[d]	Yes	53.0	42.8***	47.3
Mold spots	Yes	6.9	4.0***	5.4
Damp stains	Yes	10.6	6.5***	8.4
Water damage	Yes	12.0	6.5***	9.2
Window pane condensation	Yes	36.7	31.9**	33.5
Cockroaches[e]	Yes	79.4	71.6***	76.1
Rats[e]	Yes	46.1	40.6**	44.3
Mosquitoes/flies[e]	Yes	88.6	82.5***	85.5
Current pets	Yes	22.8	18.5**	20.8
Mosquito-repellent incense[f]	Yes	88.7	85.1**	86.7
Incense[f]	Yes	19.4	15.3**	17.1
Cleaning every day	Yes	39.4	41.9	41.1
Frequently put bedding to sunshine	Yes	37.5	43.5**	40.6
Frequently open window in winter	Yes	34.0	36.0	35.7

[a]Subject's home located within a distance of 200 meters of a main road or highway.
[b]Subject's home has been redecorated/renovated since 1 year before pregnancy.
[c]Subject's home has acquired new furniture since 1 year before pregnancy.
[d]Subject has reported any of the four dampness signs at home: mold spots, damp stains, water damage or window pane condensation during winter in child's bedroom.
[e]Subject has seen cockroaches/rats/mosquitoes/flies in home.
[f]Subject has used mosquito-repellent incense/incense in home.
*$p<0.05$;
**$p<0.01$;
***$p<0.001$.

Associations between home environmental characteristics and current rhinitis, history of allergic rhinitis calculated by logistic regression adjusting for gender and smoking are shown in Table 5. Living near a main road or highway, new furniture, having pets and indicators of an impaired indoor environment, such as with dampness problems, cockroaches, rats, mosquitoes/flies, current pets, using mosquito-repellent incense and incense, were all risk factors for current rhinitis. For history of allergic rhinitis, risk factors included living near a main road or highway, redecoration, new furniture, mold spots, window pane condensation and current pets. Compared with ceramic tile/stone floor, those living in homes with wood floor had less current rhinitis. Frequently put bedding to sunshine was protective for current rhinitis. Cleaning every day was protective for history of allergic rhinitis.

Stepwise logistic regression was applied to reduce the models (Table 5). House site, living near a main road or highway, new furniture, water damage, cockroaches, current pets and frequently open window in winter were significant factors in the stepwise regression for current rhinitis. Reduced multiple logistic and multi-nominal models were applied by adding gender, current smoking and all significant factors from stepwise regression for current rhinitis (Table 6). Living near a main road or highway, redecoration, mold spots, window pane condensation, cleaning every day and frequently open window in winter were significant factors in the stepwise regression for history of allergic rhinitis. Reduced multiple logistic and multi-nominal model was applied for history of allergic rhinitis (Table 7). Water damage was the only significant factor for history of allergic asthma in the stepwise regression. When adjusting for gender and current smoking in reduced multiple models, water damage was still associated with history of allergic asthma (OR(95%CI): 2.56(1.34,4.86), $p = 0.004$).

Logistic regression models for the association between current rhinitis and Continuous Score (range from 0-13) were calculated, adjusted for gender and current smoking. There were significant associations between each unit increase of risk factors and current rhinitis (OR(95%CI): 1.17(1.12,1.23), $P<0.001$). Logistic regression models for the association between current rhinitis and Categorized Score (0–4) were calculated (Table 8). Results shows that more risk factors were related with higher risk of having current rhinitis, with stratified analysis.

Logistic regression models for the association between current rhinitis and Categorized Dampness Score (0–4) were calculated. 58.7% reported 0 dampness indicators (which is the reference group, score 0); 32.8% reported 1 dampness indicators (score category 1); 8.5% reported 2 or more dampness indicators (score category 2). Compared with score category 0, OR(95%CI) (when adjusting for gender and current smoking) for score category 1 was 1.28(1.09, 1.50) and for score category 2 was 1.91(1.46, 2.49), showed that more dampness indicators were related with higher risk of having current rhinitis.

Discussions

The prevalence of weekly current rhinitis, history of allergic rhinitis and history of allergic asthma among parents of young children (3–6 years old) in Chongqing were low but current rhinitis occurring less than once a week was common. A number of indoor environmental risk factors were associated with adults' current rhinitis and a history of allergic rhinitis: the most important risk factors were living near a main road or highway, redecoration, new furniture, mold spots, water damage, window pane condensation, the presence of cockroaches, current pets; protective factors were cleaning every day and frequently put bedding to sunshine. Subjects living in rural areas reported more current rhinitis than those in urban areas. Water damage was a risk factor for adults' history of allergic asthma.

Epidemiological studies can be affected by selection bias. In this study, we included all parents from a large cross-sectional study among children in random daycare centers, with no prior information on parents' health status. The sample size was reasonably large, and the response rate was relatively high (74.5%). Thus, a selection bias is fairly unlikely. However, the study population is representative of parents, especially mothers and does not include all ages of adults in Chongqing.

Recall bias is another potential problem. Subjects may overestimate or underestimate their personal symptoms or reports on indoor environment risk factors. Recall bias for rhinitis symptoms should not be a big issue in this study, since questions about rhinitis symptoms are for the last three months. Information bias, in which subjects are aware that certain factors have previously been identified as risks, is another potential problem. However, the risk factors studied in this paper (e.g. wall and floor materials, dampness, and lifestyle), are likely not well known among the Chinese population.

In this study, questions on mold spots, damp stains, window pane condensation and cleaning frequency are based on child's bedroom. This could lead to some miss-classification of parents' exposure. However, we still found strong associations between dampness and parents' rhinitis symptoms. Usually, Chinese homes

Table 4. Associations between house site, construction year, area, history of allergic asthma and current rhinitis, history of allergic rhinitis calculated by logistic regression OR(95%CI)[a].

		Current rhinitis	p-value	History of allergic rhinitis	p-value
House site	Urban	1.00		1.00	
	Suburban	1.00(0.85,1.18)	0.991	0.47(0.25,0.87)	0.017
	Rural	1.36(1.10,1.69)	0.005	0.38(0.15,0.94)	0.037
Construction year	After 2001	1.00		1.00	
	Before 2000	1.08(0.94,1.23)	0.274	0.75(0.50,1.14)	0.183
Area	>75 m^2	1.00		1.00	
	<=75 m^2	1.05(0.92,1.19)	0.452	0.69(0.46,1.02)	0.062
Cumulative incidence of allergic asthma		3.40(1.89,6.14)	<0.001	7.51(3.81,14.8)	<0.001

[a]Odds ratios were adjusted for gender and current smoking.

Table 5. Associations between building characteristics and exposure indicators and current rhinitis, history of allergic rhinitis calculated by logistic regression OR (95%CI)[a].

		Current rhinitis	*p*-value	History of allergic rhinitis	*p*-value
Living near a main road or highway		1.36(1.20,1.55)	<0.001	2.24(1.50,3.34)	<0.001
Wall materials	Wall paper	1.00		1.00	
	Cement	1.24(0.91,1.68)	0.168	0.36(0.12,1.07)	0.067
	Lime	1.08(0.85,1.37)	0.547	0.48(0.24,0.97)	0.041
	Paint	0.94(0.70,1.26)	0.692	0.85(0.41,1.77)	0.661
	Emulsion paint	0.96(0.78,1.18)	0.677	0.71(0.42,1.21)	0.211
Floor type	Ceramic tile/stone	1.00		1.00	
	Cement	1.20(0.99,1.45)	0.058	0.35(0.15,0.84)	0.018
	Wood floor	0.74(0.62,0.89)	0.002	0.90(0.49,1.60)	0.696
	Laminated floor	0.93(0.80,1.10)	0.406	1.77(1.14,2.73)	0.011
Redecoration		1.09(0.94,1.25)	0.257	2.26(1.51,3.37)	<0.001
New furniture		1.26(1.11,1.44)	<0.001	2.42(1.54,3.81)	<0.001
Mold spots		1.78(1.33,2.39)	<0.001	2.19(1.15,4.16)	0.017
Damp stains		1.67(1.32,2.11)	<0.001	1.62(0.90,2.94)	0.110
Water damage		1.93(1.52,2.44)	<0.001	1.62(0.91,2.88)	0.101
Window pane condensation		1.22(1.06,1.41)	0.006	2.53 (1.69,3.79)	<0.001
Cockroaches		1.54(1.32,1.79)	<0.001	1.47(0.89,2.43)	0.131
Rats		1.26(1.11,1.44)	0.001	0.68(0.45,1.03)	0.068
Mosquitoes/flies		1.62(1.34,1.95)	<0.001	1.90(0.95,3.77)	0.069
Current pets		1.29(1.11,1.51)	0.001	1.80(1.20,2.71)	0.005
Mosquito-repellent incense		1.39(1.15,1.68)	0.001	0.87(0.52,1.47)	0.606
Incense		1.31(1.11,1.56)	0.002	1.54(0.97,2.42)	0.065
Cleaning every day		0.91(0.80,1.03)	0.130	0.44(0.28,0.69)	<0.001
Frequently put bedding to sunshine		0.78(0.69,0.89)	<0.001	0.78(0.52,1.16)	0.220
Frequently open window in winter		0.91(0.79,1.04)	0.154	1.03(0.70,1.53)	0.870

[a]Odds ratios were adjusted for gender and current smoking habit.

are not very big and bedrooms are close to each other. Thus, dampness and other impaired factors could influence the whole family members.

While statistical models can affect results, consistent results have been obtained from different tests, and good agreement was found between multiple logistic regression models and logistic regression models using stepwise method.

Previous studies have shown that the most frequent sensitization sources are both perennial allergens (house dust mites) and seasonal allergens (spring pollens and autumn pollens) [42]. The peak seasons for pollen in Chongqing is in March in spring and in autumn from September to October. Spring pollens accounting for 65.8% of the annual pollen spreading, and the main airborne pollens are from pinus, moraceae and cupressaceae [43]. Allergen testing allergy patients shows that the main pollen allergen is in Autumn in Chongqing [43]. Another study in Chongqing showed that there were two peaks of AR, one in early-spring and another mid-autumn [44]. Our questionnaire study was performed from December 2010 to April 2011, and parents were asked about their rhinitis symptoms in the last three months (current rhinitis) which was about the time of the pollen and infection peak season. The prevalence of current rhinitis in our study is comparable with another cross-sectional, population-based study in Chongqing from 2008 [44] using the ISAAC questionnaire [45] for rhinitis which showed a prevalence of 32.3% self-reported AR in the last 12 months. The majority of subjects who had a history of allergic rhinitis reported current rhinitis in our study indicating that they could exposed to the allergens during the study recall period.

We found that current smokers reported less history of allergic asthma. This negative association has been shown in studies about allergic sensitization and smoking habit [46,47]. Selection could be the reason for this finding, as the awareness of smoking is harmful for asthmatic people, those with asthma choose to avoid smoking. However, we have found that passive smoking (spouses' current smoking) was a risk factor for non-smoking females' current rhinitis. Our finding that history of allergic asthma was associated with more reports of rhinitis symptoms is in line with other studies [7,12].

Associations between tobacco smoke odor and current rhinitis as well as history of allergic rhinitis were found in our study. Moreover, stuffy odor, unpleasant odor and the perception of dry air were all significantly associated with current rhinitis. Mold odor was not a risk factor in our study, however, it was the largest risk observed in one review article on dampness and molds with rhinitis risk [48]. Perception of strong odors has been shown to be a predisposing factor for NAR patients [49]. These perceptions could be indicators of a lack of ventilation as well as emissions from indoor sources.

A noteworthy finding in our study is that people living near a main road or highway reported more rhinitis symptoms. One

Table 6. Significant variables identified in reduced multiple models for current rhinitis.

		Any		Less common		Weekly	
		OR(95%CI)[a]	*p*-value	RRR(95%CI)[b]	*p*-value	RRR(95%CI)[b]	*p*-value
Male gender		0.92(0.75,1.12)	0.400	0.92(0.75,1.13)	0.418	0.89(0.49,1.63)	0.714
Current smoker		1.05(0.83,1.34)	0.675	1.04(0.82,1.33)	0.741	1.24(0.61,2.52)	0.559
House site	Urban	1.00		1.00		1.00	
	Suburban	1.13(0.93,1.37)	0.221	1.13(0.93,1.38)	0.225	1.12(0.63,1.98)	0.707
	Rural	1.43(1.10,1.85)	0.007	1.45(1.11,1.88)	0.006	1.10(0.48,2.50)	0.827
Living near a main road or highway		1.31(1.13,1.52)	$<$0.001	1.29(1.11,1.50)	0.001	1.71(1.10,2.67)	0.018
New furniture		1.28(1.11,1.49)	0.001	1.30(1.12,1.51)	0.001	1.10(0.71,1.72)	0.674
Water damage		1.68(1.29,2.18)	$<$0.001	1.54(1.18,2.01)	0.002	4.21(2.47,7.16)	$<$0.001
Cockroaches		1.46(1.23,1.73)	$<$0.001	1.46(1.22,1.73)	$<$0.001	1.55(0.89,2.73)	0.125
Current pets		1.24(1.04,1.49)	0.020	1.22(1.01,1.47)	0.036	1.61(0.98,2.65)	0.058
Frequently put bedding to sunshine		0.79(0.68,0.92)	0.002	0.79(0.68,0.92)	0.002	0.74(0.47,1.18)	0.205

[a]Gender, current smoking and factors significant in stepwise regression (enter model *p*-value level is $p<0.10$).
[b]Same factors in [a] but analyzed by multi-nominal regression.

Table 7. Significant variables identified in reduced multiple models for history of allergic rhinitis.

	OR(95%CI)[a]	*p*-value
Male gender	0.66(0.33,1.31)	0.235
Current smoker	0.19(0.04,0.84)	0.029
Living near a main road or highway	2.44(1.48,4.03)	<0.001
Redecoration	2.14(1.34,3.41)	0.001
Mold spots	2.23(1.06,4.68)	0.035
Window pane condensation	2.04(1.28,3.26)	0.003
Cleaning every day	0.40(0.22,0.71)	0.002
Frequently open window in winter	0.84(0.52,1.37)	0.488

[a]Gender, current smoking and factors significant in stepwise regression (enter model *p*-value level is $p<0.10$).

Chinese study has shown that living or working place near the traffic artery had 1.94-fold increased risk for development of NAR compared with AR [49]. One Swedish study found that living within 100 m from a road with high traffic intensity was associated with a higher prevalence of allergic rhinitis for adults, but not with rhinitis triggered by non-allergic factors [50]. An Italian study in adults found that outdoor traffic related NO_2 exposure was associated with increased prevalence of allergic rhinitis [51]. Traffic pollutions may potentiate allergic reactions in different ways [52]: firstly, by attaching to the surface of e.g. pollen grains, air pollutants can change their morphology and enhance allergenic potential; secondly, by inducing inflammation; thirdly, diesel exhaust emissions can have an adjuvant effects in atopic subjects. We did not measure outdoor pollutants, but one study on the air pollutants at the highway toll gates in Chongqing showed that the indoor and outdoor average concentrations of CO, NO_2 and PM_{10} exceeded indoor air quality standards [53]. Moreover, a recent study on air fine particles pollution in Chongqing showed that $PM_{2.5}$ exposure in the city came mainly from vehicle emission [54].

The present study confirms the findings of many previous studies that indoor dampness and mold are risk factors for rhinitis and asthma. Excess moisture in buildings becomes a critical factor for mold (fungal) proliferation in nutrient-rich environments, as well as for house Dust Mites. As a result, building occupants may be exposed to increased levels of microbial agents. Consistent positive associations between dampness and multiple allergic, respiratory effects have been shown [55]. The risk of rhinitis is significantly increased in relation to home dampness and mold exposures [48]. The risk of current asthma, current asthma symptoms, allergic rhinitis, and atopic dermatitis was higher in homes with self-reported dampness in the past year among 18–25 years Finish students [18]. Another Finish study found that self-reported mold in homes was associated with rhinitis among adults [56]. One American study found that water stains was associated with students' nasal symptoms in college buildings [57]. The association between dampness in dwellings and wheeze, asthma among adults has been well studied [58]. Even if the mechanisms of the effects of dampness on health are unknown, there is sufficient evidence to find out and remediate the reasons for the dampness problem and take preventive measures against dampness in buildings [48,58–60]. The result of our study could guide practical prevention and remediation for Chongqing, as it has a humid subtropical monsoon climate. An annual outdoor average relative humidity was around 78% [44].

This study showed that the presence of cockroaches was associated with an elevated risk of rhinitis symptoms. One Chinese study has found that cockroach allergens were detected in 93% of the household samples [61]. Exposure to cockroaches was also found to be associated with wheeze in Chinese ninth grade students [62]. 25.7% of the patients with allergic rhinitis and asthma had positive cockroach sensitization in mainland China in one Chinese study [63].

We found that pet keeping was associated with an elevated risk of having rhinitis symptoms, this is in agreement with another study reported that the prevalence of rhinitis was more common in families with animals than in those without [13]. The association between pet allergens (such as allergens from cats and dogs) and allergic symptoms has been widely discussed in epidemiological studies. Cats and dogs were the most common pets in our study (5.1% of the parents reported having cats and 6.9% reported having dogs). In rural areas in China, cat and dog epithelium in rural areas were the most common allergens [64].

Our study found that redecoration and new furniture at home were risk factors for parents' rhinitis symptoms. Redecoration and new furniture could be a source of chemical emissions. Factor analysis showed that these two exposures were associated with each other. Buying new furniture is usually done the same time as redecoration in China. Although this study did not measure indoor pollutants, chemical emissions, such as formaldehyde and volatile organic compounds (VOC) from furniture and decorating process has been studied [65–67]. We have not found any study on the association between renovation, new furniture or new materials and rhinitis. However, the association between renovation or new materials and asthma-related and lower respiratory symptoms have been studied: recent painting was associated with wheezing in the last 12 months and any allergy in Russia schoolchildren [66]; new wall covering and new furniture were associated with any allergy [66]; new synthetic carpet was associated with current asthma and any allergy [66]. The presence of particleboard (formaldehyde-emitting materials) was associated with current asthma and any allergy [66]. Plastic-containing or other materials (possible VOC emitting materials), such as new linoleum floor, PVC flooring, textile wall covering, synthetic bedding, were found to be associated with history of asthma, asthma-related or bronchial obstruction in children [66,68,69]. One home study found exposed to higher formaldehyde levels in the bedroom were associated with atopy and increasing severity of sensitization among children [70]. Expose to high level of formaldehyde increased nasal mucosal hypersensitivity to histamine in medical students during cadaver dissection [71]. One toxicological

Table 8. Associations between current rhinitis and Categorized Score identified in reduced multiple models.

		Any		Less common		Weekly	
Score category 0–4[c]	**%**	**OR(95%CI)**[a]	***p*-value**	**RRR(95%CI)**[b]	***p*-value**	**RRR(95%CI)**[b]	***p*-value**
Score category 0	33.6	1.00		1.00		1.00	
Score category 1	23.4	1.36(1.10,1.69)	0.005	1.42(1.14,1.77)	0.002	0.54(0.23,1.28)	0.159
Score category 2	20.0	1.62(1.29,2.04)	<0.001	1.65(1.30,2.08)	<0.001	1.33(0.65,2.70)	0.432
Score category 3	14.0	1.69(1.31,2.17)	<0.001	1.65(1.27,2.14)	<0.001	2.15(1.09,4.27)	0.028
Score category 4	9.0	2.17(1.60,2.94)	<0.001	2.10(1.53,2.86)	<0.001	3.15(1.50,6.63)	0.003

[a]Calculated by multiple logistic regression, odds ratios were adjusted for gender and current smoking.
[b]Calculated by multi-nominal regression, odds ratios were adjusted for gender and current smoking.
[c]Categorized Score: by adding numbers of indoor environment risk factors, separately as score category 0 (0, 1, 2, 3 or 4 risk factors out of 13), score category 1 (5 out of 13), score category 2 (6 out of 13), score category 3 (7 out of 13) and score category 4 (8 or more out of 13).

chamber study found provocation with formaldehyde at a dose of 0.5 mg/m3 over 2 hours caused transient rhinitis symptoms in both patients with skin sensitization and healthy subjects [72]. One French study found that high concentrations of VOC in homes were associated with an increasing prevalence of asthma and rhinitis in adults [73].

Cleaning every day and frequently put bedding to sunshine were protective factors for rhinitis in our study. Factor analyses showed that cleaning every day and frequently put bedding to sunshine were associated with each other as one factor. Frequently cleaning and putting bedding to sunshine could be associated with reduced risk of impaired indoor environment. We found no other study about the association between the frequency of cleaning, putting bedding to sunshine and rhinitis symptoms among adults in the home environment. However, an intervention study found that comprehensive cleaning reduced the airborne dust and also reduced nonsmokers' mucosal symptoms and nasal congestion in offices [74]. House dust mites are commonly found in beds. One Chinese survey found that the most common allergen was house dust mites in urban homes [64]. Another Chinese study found that house dust mite allergen levels were detectable in 99% of the bedding samples [61]. Frequently putting bedding to sunshine could reduce house dust mite allergens.

Conclusions

Factors in the home environment, especially living near a main road or highway, redecoration, new furniture, mold spots, water damage, window pane condensation in winter, having pets may increase the risk of having current rhinitis and history of allergic rhinitis in Chinese residents. The results of this study indicate a need to reduce dampness and indoor mold growth, use low emission furniture and paints in homes and encourage frequent cleaning and putting bedding to sunshine to decrease occupants' risk of having rhinitis symptoms in indoor environment.

Acknowledgments

The authors would like to give thanks to the support of the CCHH workgroup in Chongqing. Thank you to all the parents who filled out questionnaires, and teachers from kindergartens who provided assistance for our survey.

Author Contributions

Conceived and designed the experiments: JW BL WY QY HW JS. Performed the experiments: JW QY HW DH. Analyzed the data: JW JS DN. Contributed reagents/materials/analysis tools: BL JS DN. Wrote the paper: JW DN.

References

1. Bousquet J, Khaltaev N, Cruz AA, Denburg J, Fokkens WJ, et al. (2008) Allergic Rhinitis and its Impact on Asthma (ARIA) 2008 update (in collaboration with the World Health Organization, GA(2)LEN and AllerGen). Allergy 86: 8–160.
2. Shariat M, Pourpak Z, Khalesi M, Kazemnejad A, Sharifi L, et al. (2012) Quality of life in the Iranian adults with allergic rhinitis. Iran J Allergy Asthma Immunol 11: 324–328.
3. Maspero J, Lee BW, Katelaris CH, Potter PC, Cingi C, et al. (2012) Quality of life and control of allergic rhinitis in patients from regions beyond western Europe and the United States. Clin Exp Allergy 42: 1684–1696.
4. Ke X, Qian D, Zhu L, Hong S. (2010) Analysis on quality of life and personality characteristics of allergic rhinitis. Lin Chung Er Bi Yan Hou Tou Jing Wai Ke Za Zhi 24: 200–202.
5. Brandt D, Bernstein JA. (2006) Questionnaire evaluation and risk factor identification for nonallergic vasomotor rhinitis. Ann Allergy Asthma Immunol 96: 526–532.
6. Wang DY. (2005) Risk factors of allergic rhinitis: genetic or environmental? Ther Clin Risk Manag 1: 115–123.
7. Tran NP, Vickery J, Blaiss MS. (2011) Management of rhinitis: allergic and non-allergic. Allergy Asthma Immunol Res 3: 148–156.

8. Eriksson J, Ekerljung L, Rönmark E, Dahlén B, Ahlstedt S, et al. (2012) Update of prevalence of self-reported allergic rhinitis and chronic nasal symptoms among adults in Sweden. Clin Respir J 6: 159–168.
9. Nihlén U, Greiff L, Montnémery P, Löfdahl CG, Johannisson A, et al. (2006) Incidence and remission of self-reported allergic rhinitis symptoms in adults. Allergy 61: 1299–1304.
10. Warm K, Backman H, Lindberg A, Lundbäck B, Rönmark E. (2012) Low incidence and high remission of allergic sensitization among adults. J Allergy Clin Immunol 129: 136–142.
11. Ng TP, Tan WC. (1994) Epidemiology of allergic rhinitis and its associated risk factors in Singapore. Int J Epidemiol 23: 553–558.
12. Radon K, Gerhardinger U, Schulze A, Zock JP, Norbäck D, et al. (2008) Occupation and adult onset of rhinitis in the general population. Occup Environ Med 65: 38–43.
13. Bener A, Mobayed H, Sattar HA, Al-Mohammed AA, Ibrahimi AS, et al. (2004) Pet ownership: its effect on allergy and respiratory symptoms. Eur Ann Allergy Clin Immunol 36: 306–310.
14. Nyembue TD, Jorissen M, Hellings PW, Muyunga C, Kayembe JM. (2012) Prevalence and determinants of allergic diseases in a Congolese population. Int Forum Allergy Rhinol 2: 285–293.
15. Lü Y, Xie Z, Zhao S, Zhang H, Liu Y, et al. (2011) Prevalence of allergens for Changsha patients with allergic rhinitis. Lin Chung Er Bi Yan Hou Tou Jing Wai Ke Za Zhi 25: 491–494.
16. Li J, Sun B, Huang Y, Lin X, Zhao D, et al. (2009) A multicentre study assessing the prevalence of sensitizations in patients with asthma and/or rhinitis in China. Allergy 64: 1083–1092.
17. Kurt E, Metintas S, Basyigit I, Bulut I, Coskun E, et al. (2009) Prevalence and Risk Factors of Allergies in Turkey (PARFAIT): results of a multicentre cross-sectional study in adults. Eur Respir J 33: 724–733.
18. Kilpeläinen M, Terho EO, Helenius H, Koskenvuo M. (2001) Home dampness, current allergic diseases, and respiratory infections among young adults. Thorax 56: 462–467.
19. Araki A, Kanazawa A, Kawai T, Eitaki Y, Morimoto K, et al. (2012) The relationship between exposure to microbial volatile organic compound and allergy prevalence in single-family homes. Sci Total Environ 423: 18–26.
20. Baena-Cagnani CE, Gómez RM, Baena-Cagnani R, Canonica GW. (2009) Impact of environmental tobacco smoke and active tobacco smoking on the development and outcomes of asthma and rhinitis. Curr Opin Allergy Clin Immunol 9: 136–140.
21. Shusterman D. (2007) Environmental non allergic rhinitis. Clin Allergy Immunol 19: 249–266.
22. De Marco R, Cappa V, Accordini S, Rava M, Antonicelli L, et al. (2012) Trends in the prevalence of asthma and allergic rhinitis in Italy between 1991 and 2010. Eur Respir J 39: 883–892.
23. Gíslason D, Bjœrnsdóttir US, Blœndal T, Gíslason T. (2002) European Community Respiratory Health Survey: The main results so far with special reference to Iceland. Laeknabladid 88: 891–907.
24. Bousquet J, Van Cauwenberge P, Khaltaev N, Aria Workshop Group, World Health Organization. (2001) Allergic rhinitis and its impact on asthma. J Allergy Clin Immunol 108: S147–334.
25. Weiss KB, Sullivan SD. (2001) The health economics of asthma and rhinitis. I. Assessing the economic impact. J Allergy Clin Immunol 107: 3–8.
26. Bjerg A, Ekerljung L, Middelveld R, Dahlén SE, Forsberg B, et al. (2011) Increased prevalence of symptoms of rhinitis but not of asthma between 1990 and 2008 in Swedish adults: comparisons of the ECRHS and GA^2LEN surveys. PLoS One 6: e16082.
27. Settipane RA, Lieberman P. (2001) Update on non-allergic rhinitis. Ann Allergy Asthma Immunol 86: 494–507.
28. Settipane RA, Charnock DR. (2007) Epidemiology of rhinitis: allergic and nonallergic. Clin Allergy Immunol 19: 23–34.
29. Shusterman D, Murphy MA. (2007) Nasal hyperreactivity in allergic and non-allergic rhinitis: a potential risk factor for non-specific building-related illness. Indoor Air 17: 328–333.
30. Eriksson J, Bjerg A, Lötvall J, Wennergren G, Rönmark E, et al. (2011) Rhinitis phenotypes correlate with different symptom presentation and risk factor patterns of asthma. Respir Med 105: 1611–1621.
31. Bugiani M, Carosso A, Migliore E, Piccioni P, Corsico A, et al. (2005) Allergic rhinitis and asthma comorbidity in a survey of young adults in Italy. Allergy 60: 165–170.
32. Mahesh PA, Vedanthan PK, Holla AD, Jayaraj BS, Prabhakar AK. (2009) Time interval and the factors associated with the development of asthma in patients with allergic rhinitis. Lung 187: 393–400.
33. Boulay ME, Morin A, Laprise C, Boulet LP. (2012) Asthma and rhinitis: what is the relationship? Curr Opin Allergy Clin Immunol 12: 449–454.
34. Li J, Huang Y, Lin X, Zhao D, Tan G, et al. (2012) Factors associated with allergen sensitizations in patients with asthma and/or rhinitis in China. Am J Rhinol Allergy 26: 85–91.
35. Togias A. (2003) Rhinitis and asthma: evidence for respiratory system integration. J Allergy Clin Immunol 111: 1171–1183.
36. Wang J, Li B, Yang Q, Yu W, Wang H, et al. (2013) Odors and Sensations of Humidity and Dryness in Relation to Sick Building Syndrome and Home Environment in Chongqing, China. PLoS One 8:e72385.
37. Wang J, Li BZ, Yang Q, Wang H, Sundell J. (2013) Sick building syndrome among parents of preschool children in relation to home environment in Chongqing, China. Chin Sci Bull 58: 4267–4276.
38. Zhang YP, Li BZ, Huang C, Yang X, Qian H, et al. (2013) Ten cities cross-sectional questionnaire survey of children asthma and other allergies in China. Chin Sci Bull 58: 4182–4189.
39. Bornehag CG, Sundell J, Hagerhed-Engman L, Sigsggard T, Janson S, et al. (2005) 'Dampness' at home and its association with airway, nose and skin symptoms among 10851 preschool children in Sweden: a cross-sectional study. Indoor Air 15: 48–55.
40. Sun Y, Sundell J, Zhang Y. (2007) Validity of building characteristics and dorm dampness obtained in a self-administrated questionnaire. Sci Total Environ 387: 276–282.
41. Sundell J. (1994) On the association between building ventilation characteristics, some indoor environmental exposures, some allergic manifestations and subjective symptom reports. Indoor Air 4: 7–49.
42. Qian D, Hong SL. (2008) Prevalence of allergens for Chongqing patients with allergic rhinitis. J Chongqing Med Univ 33: 531–535.
43. Hong S, Huang J, Bai Y. (2001) A survey of pollens in Chongqing. Lin Chuang Er Bi Yan Hou Ke Za Zhi 15: 558–560.
44. Shen J, Ke X, Hong S, Zeng Q, Liang C, et al. (2011) Epidemiological features of allergic rhinitis in four major cities in Western China. J Huazhong Univ Sci Technolog Med Sci 31: 433–440.
45. Worldwide variation in prevalence of symptoms of asthma, allergic rhinoconjunctivitis, and atopic eczema: ISAAC. The International Study of Asthma and Allergies in Childhood (ISAAC) Steering Committee. Lancet 1998; 351:1225–1232.
46. Hancox RJ, Welch D, Poulton R, Taylor DR, McLachlan CR, et al. (2008) Cigarette smoking and allergic sensitization: a 32-year population-based cohort study. J Allergy Clin Immunol 121: 38–42.
47. Linneberg A, Nielsen NH, Madsen F, Frølund L, Dirksen A, et al. (2001) Smoking and the development of allergic sensitization to aeroallergens in adults: a prospective population-based study. The Copenhagen Allergy Study. Allergy 56: 328–332.
48. Jaakkola MS, Quansah R, Hugg TT, Heikkinen SA, Jaakkola JJ. (2013) Association of indoor dampness and molds with rhinitis risk: A systematic review and meta-analysis. J Allergy Clin Immunol 132: 1099–1110.
49. Zhu LP, Wang F, Sun XQ, Chen RX, Lu MP, et al. (2010) Comparison of risk factors between patients with non-allergic rhinitis and allergic rhinitis. Zhonghua Er Bi Yan Hou Tou Jing Wai Ke Za Zhi 45: 993–998.
50. Lindgren A, Stroh E, Nihlén U, Montnémery P, Axmon A, et al. (2009) Traffic exposure associated with allergic asthma and allergic rhinitis in adults. A cross-sectional study in southern Sweden. Int J Health Geogr 8: 25.
51. De Marco R, Poli A, Ferrari M, Accordini S, Giammanco G, et al. (2002) The impact of climate and traffic-related NO2 on the prevalence of asthma and allergic rhinitis in Italy. Clin Exp Allergy 32: 1405–1412.
52. Salvi S. (2001) Pollution and allergic airways disease. Curr Opin Allergy Clin Immunol 1: 35–41.
53. Chen KJ, Chen KL, Zhang LJ, Leng GY. (2007) Characteristics and influencing factors of air pollution in and out of the highway tollgates. Environ Sci 28: 1847–1853.
54. Fang MJ, Zhu GC, Zheng XX, Yin Zhongyi. (2011) Study on air fine particles pollution prediction of main traffic route using artificial neural network. In: Proceedings of 2011 International Conference on Computer Distributed Control and Intelligent Environmental Monitoring Changsha, Hunan, China 2011; 1346–1349.
55. Mendell MJ, Mirer AG, Cheung K, Tong M, Douwes J. (2011) Respiratory and allergic health effects of dampness, mold, and dampness-related agents: a review of the epidemiologic evidence. Environ Health Perspect 119: 748–756.
56. Koskinen OM, Husman TM, Meklin TM, Nevalainen AI. (1999) The relationship between moisture or mould observations in houses and the state of health of their occupants. Eur Respir J 14: 1363–1367.
57. Park JH, Schleiff PL, Attfield MD, Cox-Ganser JM, Kreiss K. (2004) Building-related respiratory symptoms can be predicted with semi-quantitative indices of exposure to dampness and mold. Indoor Air 14: 425–433.
58. WHO. (2009) WHO Guidelines for Indoor Air Quality: Dampness and Mould. Geneva: World Health Organization; 2009.
59. Bornehag CG, Blomquist G, Gyntelberg F, Järvholm B, Malmberg P, et al. (2001) Dampness in buildings and health. Nordic interdisciplinary review of the scientific evidence on associations between exposure to "dampness" in buildings and health effects (NORDDAMP). Indoor Air 11: 72–86.
60. Bornehag CG, Sundell J, Bonini S, Custovic A, Malmberg P, et al. (2004) Dampness in buildings as a risk factor for health effects, EUROEXPO: a multidisciplinary review of the literature (1998–2000) on dampness and mite exposure in buildings and health effects. Indoor Air 14: 243–257.
61. Zhang C, Gjesing B, Lai X, Li J, Spangfort MD, et al. (2011) Indoor allergen levels in Guangzhou city, southern China. Allergy 66: 186–191.
62. Salo PM, Xia J, Johnson CA, Li Y, Avol EL, et al. (2004) Indoor allergens, asthma, and asthma-related symptoms among adolescents in Wuhan, China. Ann Epidemiol 14: 543–550.
63. Sun BQ, Lai XX, Gjesing B, Spangfort MD, Zhong NS. (2010) Prevalence of sensitivity to cockroach allergens and IgE cross-reactivity between cockroach and house dust mite allergens in Chinese patients with allergic rhinitis and asthma. Chin Med J 123: 3540–3544.

64. Wang ZH, Lin WS, Li SY, Zhao SC, Wang L, et al. (2011) Research on prevalence and related factors in allergic rhinitis. Zhonghua Er Bi Yan Hou Tou Jing Wai Ke Za Zhi 46: 225–231.
65. Reitzig M, Mohr S, Heinzow B, Knoppel H. (1998) VOC emissions after building renovations: Traditional and less common indoor air contaminants, potential sources, and reported health complaints. Indoor Air 8: 91–102.
66. Jaakkola JJ, Parise H, Kislitsin V, Lebedeva NI, Spengler JD. (2004) Asthma, wheezing, and allergies in Russian schoolchildren in relation to new surface materials in the home. Am J Public Health 94: 560–562.
67. Choi H, Schmidbauer N, Spengler J, Bornehag CG. (2010) Sources of propylene glycol and glycol ethers in air at home. Int J Environ Res Public Health 7: 4213–4237.
68. Jaakkola JJ, Oie L, Nafstad P, Botten G, Samuelsen SO, et al. (1999) Interior surface materials in the home and the development of bronchial obstruction in young children in Oslo, Norway. Am J Public Health 89: 188–192.
69. Trevillian LF, Ponsonby AL, Dwyer T, Kemp A, Cochrane J, et al. (2005) Infant sleeping environment and asthma at 7 years: a prospective cohort study. Am J Public Health 95: 2238–2245.
70. Garrett MH, Hooper MA, Hooper BM, Rayment PR, Abramson MJ. (1999) Increased risk of allergy in children due to formaldehyde exposure in homes. Allergy 54: 330–337.
71. Hisamitsu M, Okamoto Y, Chazono H, Yonekura S, Sakurai D, et al. (2011) The influence of environmental exposure to formaldehyde in nasal mucosa of medical students during cadaver dissection. Allergol Int 60: 373–379.
72. Pazdrak K, Górski P, Krakowiak A, Ruta U. (1993) Changes in nasal lavage fluid due to formaldehyde inhalation. Int Arch Occup Environ Health 64: 515–519.
73. Billionnet C, Gay E, Kirchner S, Leynaert B, Annesi-Maesano I. (2011) Quantitative assessments of indoor air pollution and respiratory health in a population-based sample of French dwellings. Environ Res 111: 425–434.
74. Skulberg KR, Skyberg K, Kruse K, Eduard W, Djupesland P, et al. (2004) The effect of cleaning on dust and the health of office workers: an intervention study. Epidemiology 15: 71–78.

Obstructive Sleep Apnea and the Risk of Atopic Dermatitis: A Population-Based Case Control Study

Kai-Jen Tien[1,2], Chien-Wen Chou[1], Shang-Yu Lee[1], Nai-Cheng Yeh[1], Chwen-Yi Yang[1], Feng-Chieh Yen[1], Jhi-Joung Wang[3], Shih-Feng Weng[3,4]*

1 Division of Endocrinology and Metabolism, Department of Internal Medicine, Chi Mei Medical Center, Tainan, Taiwan, **2** Center of General Education, Chia Nan University of Pharmacy and Science, Tainan, Taiwan, **3** Department of Medical Research, Chi Mei Medical Center, Tainan, Taiwan, **4** Department of Hospital and Health Care Administration, Chia Nan University of Pharmacy and Science, Tainan, Taiwan

Abstract

Background: Obstructive sleep apnea (OSA) is associated with systemic inflammation and induces various comorbid medical diseases. To date, no study has explored the relationship between OSA and atopic dermatitis (AD), an inflammatory and autoimmune skin disorder. This study investigated the longitudinal risk for AD in patients with OSA.

Methods: A random sample of 1,000,000 individuals from Taiwan's National Health Insurance database was collected. From this sample, 1222 patients with newly-diagnosed OSA between 2000 and 2005 were identified and compared with a matched cohort of 18330 patients without OSA. All patients were tracked for 5.5 years from the index date in order to identify which patients subsequently developed AD.

Results: During the 5.5-year follow-up period, the incidence rates of AD in the OSA cohort and comparison groups were 9.81 and 6.21 per 1000 person-years, respectively. After adjustment for age, gender, diabetes, hypertension, coronary heart disease, obesity, allergy, allergic rhinitis, asthma, monthly income, and geographic location, patients with OSA were 1.5-times more likely to develop AD than patients without OSA (95% CI = 1.15–1.95, $p = 0.0025$). The hazard risk for AD was greater in male OSA patients and young OSA patients (0–18 and 19–34 years), adjusted HRs being 1.53 (95% CI = 1.14–2.06, $p = 0.005$), 4.01(95% CI = 1.57–10.26, $p = 0.0038$) and 1.75(95% CI = 1.00–3.04, $p = 0.0483$), respectively. The log-rank test indicated that OSA patients <35-years-old had significantly higher cumulative incidence rates of AD than those patient of the same age in the comparison group ($p = 0.0001$).

Conclusion: Patients with OSA, especially male patients and younger patients, are at an increased risk for AD later in life.

Editor: Tesfaye Mersha Baye, Cincinnati Children's Hospital Medical center, United States of America

Funding: The authors have no support or funding to report.

Competing Interests: The authors have declared that no competing interests exist.

* E-mail: cacmmc@gmail.com

Introduction

Atopy is defined as a condition that involves hyperreactivity to allergic triggers. The prevalence of atopic dermatitis (AD), a chronic inflammatory and pruritic skin disease [1], appears to be increasing, especially in industrialized counties. Although not a life-threatening disease, AD negatively impacts health and quality of life and increases the medical burden. The cause of AD is poorly understood; however, theories include an impaired epidermal barrier, immune system dysregulation, and an inflammatory reaction of the skin [2]. Increasing evidence suggests that AD is more than a local inflammatory disease and may be the result of systemic inflammation. Chemokines, cytokines, T-cells and other inflammatory cells appear to contribute to the initiation and maintenance of this disease [3].

Obstructive sleep apnea (OSA) is a sleep disorder caused by recurrent episodes of upper airway collapse and is characterized by repetitive episodes of apnea/hypopnea and oxygen desaturation during sleep [4]. Recurring arousal from sleep, daytime sleepiness, and fatigue are signs of disturbed sleep. The prevalence of OSA in the general population is approximately 20% [5]. OSA is recognized as a potential cause of many debilitating medical problems, including ischemic heart disease, hypertension, insulin resistance, type 2 diabetes, and mental illness [6–8]. Although the underlying pathogenesis linking OSA to these comorbidities is not fully understood, more and more evidence suggests that the systemic inflammation and the procoagulant and thrombotic activity in OSA can lead to endothelial dysfunction, atherosclerosis, and cardiovascular events [9].

OSA has been extensively studied in relation to metabolic and cardiovascular disease (CVD) but rarely in relation to dermatologic disease. Psoriasis, a chronic immune-mediated inflammatory skin disease, is thought to be associated with OSA, metabolic syndrome, and CVD [10–12]. The interaction between OSA and psoriasis is very complex and likely linked via systemic inflammation [10,13,14]. Few reports have investigated the association between OSA and AD. Some cross-sectional studies have suggested that some OSA features might be associated with atopy, although longitudinal studies are lacking. Chng et al. found atopy to be associated with snoring and other features of OSA [15]. One questionnaire study of children showed an association between snoring and eczema. A case study suggested that continuous positive airway pressure for OSA might resolve dyshidrotic eczema by reducing pro-inflammatory cytokines [16]. Marsell et al. reported that risk factors for snoring were similar to those for allergic disorders [17]. Because both OSA and AD are considered systemic inflammatory diseases, it is reasonable to hypothesize that there might be a relationship between one condition and the development of the other condition. The current study used a national population-based cohort in Taiwan to investigate the risk for the development of AD in patients with OSA over a 5.5-year period.

Methods

Data sources

Taiwan launched a single-payer National Health Insurance (NHI) program on March 1, 1995, and as of 2009, the NHI has collected one of the largest and most complete population-based datasets in the world. Data used in this study came from a subset of the NHI database, the Longitudinal Health Insurance Database 2000 (LHID2000), which contains all claims data between 1996 and 2009 from one million beneficiaries randomly selected in 2000 for follow-up study. There are no significant differences in age, gender, and healthcare costs between the sample group and all enrollees. The LHID2000 provides encrypted patient identification numbers, gender, date of birth, dates of admission and discharge, the International Classification of Diseases, Ninth Revision, Clinical Modification (ICD-9-CM) codes of diagnoses and procedures, details of prescriptions, registry of Catastrophic Illness Patient Database, and costs covered by Taiwan's NHI. The institutional review board of Chi Mei Medical Center approved the protocol of this study. The requirement of informed consent was waived because the datasets were devoid of identifiable personal information.

Study sample

A retrospective cohort study was conducted with two study groups: a new-onset OSA group and a matched non-OSA (comparison) group recruited from 2000-2006. OSA was defined in a patient if (1) he or she had at least two outpatient service claims with the codes of OSA (ICD-9-CM code 78051, 78053, 78057, 32723) at any hospital or local medical clinic and received a polysomnography test or (2) he or she had a single hospitalization for OSA among the 5 claims diagnosis codes. AD was defined in patients if they had been diagnosed on two occasions with AD by dermatologists. Patients diagnosed with OSA before 2000 were excluded, and patients who were diagnosed with AD (ICD-9-CM code 691) before OSA was diagnosed were also excluded. Sex, age, and date of first registration into the NHI program were recorded. Patients not diagnosed with OSA were randomly selected from the dataset and matched with the OSA group by sex, age (±30 days), and index date of first registration into the NHI program and then categorized into the non-OSA group at a ratio of 15 non-OSA for each OSA patient.

For both groups, the geographic area of residence and monthly income (record as NT$) as well as baseline co-morbidities, including diabetes mellitus (ICD-9-CM code: 250), hypertension (ICD-9-CM code: 401-405), coronary heart disease (ICD-9-CM code: 410-414), obesity (ICD-9-CM code: 278), allergy (ICD-9-CM code: 9953, 7080, V150 and V196), allergic rhinitis (ICD-9-CM code: 477) and asthma (ICD-9-CM code: 493) were recorded. These represent critical factors that can affect the risk of AD (ICD-9-CM code: 691). AD might be mediated by oxidative stress and circulating inflammatory cytokines [2,18]. Since diabetes, hypertension, and coronary heart disease are well-established with increasing inflammatory factors and oxidative stress, these factors were taken in consideration and adjusted for [19,20]. Obesity was thought to be associated with AD and could represent a trigger for AD [21,22]. Allergy, allergic rhinitis, and asthma are associated with adaptive immune system dysfunction and are thought to be associated with AD [23]. These comorbidities were included if they presented in an inpatient setting or in three or more ambulatory care claims coded one year before the index medical care date. Person-years (PY) of the follow-up time were calculated for each person until AD diagnosis, death, or the end of the follow-up period in 2009.

Statistical analyses

All statistical operations were performed using the SAS 9.3 statistical package (SAS Institute, Inc., Cary, North Carolina, USA). Pearson's $\chi2$ tests were used to compare differences in the baseline characteristics, comorbid medical disorders, and socio-demographic status between the two groups. The incidence rate was calculated as the number of AD cases during the follow-up divided by the total person-years for each group by sex and age. Stratified Cox proportional hazard regression, stratified by gender and age group (0–18, 19–34, 35–49, and >50 yr), was performed to calculate the risk for AD between patients with OSA compared to those patients without OSA during the follow-up period. A Kaplan-Meier analysis was used to calculate the cumulative incidence rates for AD between the two cohorts, and the log-rank test was used to analyze the differences between survival curves. A two-sided P value <0.05 was considered significant.

Results

A summary of the baseline characteristics and comorbid conditions of the two groups is shown in Table 1. A total of 1222 OSA patients and 18330 age-, gender-, and index date-matched non-OSA patients were followed for 5.5 years. Approximately 3% of the group was 0–18 years old, 21% was 19–34 years old, 39% was 35–49 years old, and 37% was ≥50 years old. Eighty percent were males. Patients with OSA had a higher prevalence of diabetes mellitus (DM), hypertension (HTN), coronary heart disease (CHD), obesity, allergy, allergic rhinitis, and asthma. Additionally, patients with OSA had a higher economic status and were more likely to live in central and northern Taiwan than the comparison group.

Table 2 shows the risk for AD for OSA patients stratified by age and gender. During the 5.5-year follow-up period, the incidence rates for AD for the OSA and non-OSA cohorts were 9.81 and 6.21 per 1000 person-years, respectively. Patients with OSA were at significantly higher risk for AD than those without OSA (crude HR = 1.58, 95% CI = 1.23–2.04, P = 0.0004). After adjusting for age, gender, DM, HTN, CHD, obesity, allergy, allergic rhinitis, asthma, monthly income, and geographic location, OSA patients were 1.5-fold more likely to develop AD (adjusted HR = 1.5, 95% CI = 1.15–1.95, P = 0.0025). The adjusted HRs were most pronounced in the younger age groups 0–18 years and 19–34 years (adjusted HR = 4.01, 95% CI = 1.57–10.26, P = 0.0038 and adjusted HR = 1.75, 95% CI = 1.00–3.04, P = 0.0483, respectively). There were no group differences in risk for AD in the age groups 35–49 years and ≥50 years. Males with OSA were 1.53-times more likely to develop AD than males without OSA after adjusting for confounders (adjusted HR = 1.53, 95% CI = 1.14–

Table 1. Demographic Characteristics and Comorbid Medical Disorders for OSA patients and comparison group patients.

Category	Subcategory	Patients with obstructive sleep apnea (N = 1222)	Comparison patients (N = 18330)	P-value
Age (yr)	0–18	42(3.44%)	630(3.44%)	1.0000
	19–34	258(21.11%)	3882(21.18%)	
	35–49	471(38.54%)	7056(38.49%)	
	≥50	451(36.91%)	6762(36.89%)	
Gender	Female	240(19.64%)	3600(19.64%)	1.0000
	Male	982(80.36%)	14730(80.36%)	
Follow-up years (Mean±SD)		5.50±2.06	5.52±2.05	0.7432
Diabetes	Yes	91(7.45%)	945(5.16%)	0.0005
	No	1131(92.55%)	17385(94.84%)	
Hypertension	Yes	292(23.90%)	1824(9.95%)	<0.0001
	No	930(76.10%)	16506(90.05%)	
Coronary heart disease	Yes	106(8.67%)	498(2.72%)	<0.0001
	No	1116(91.33%)	17832(97.28%)	
Obesity	Yes	11(0.90%)	17(0.09%)	<0.0001
	No	1211(99.10%)	18313(99.91%)	
Allergy	Yes	24(1.96%)	93(0.51%)	<0.0001
	No	1198(98.04%)	18237(99.49%)	
Allergic rhinitis	Yes	94(7.69%)	308(1.68%)	<0.0001
	No	1128(92.31%)	18022(98.32%)	
Asthma	Yes	53(4.34%)	188(1.03%)	<0.0001
	No	1169(95.66%)	18142(98.97%)	
Geographic area	North	751(61.46%)	9247(50.45%)	<0.0001
	Central	277(22.67%)	3206(17.49%)	
	South	191(15.63%)	5472(29.85%)	
	East	3(0.25%)	405(2.21%)	
Income	NT<15840	410(33.55%)	6921(37.76%)	<0.0001
	NT 15841~25000	268(21.93%)	6008(32.78%)	
	NT>25001	544(44.52%)	5401(29.47%)	

2.06, P = 0.0050). No difference in risk for AD was identified among women with and without OSA (adjusted HR = 1.39, 95% CI = 0.79–2.46, P = 0.2522). Kaplan-Meier analysis revealed that OSA patients <35 years of age had a higher cumulative incidence rate for AD than those patients of the same age in the comparison cohort (log-rank test P<0.0001) (Figure 1). In patients >35 years of age, there was no significant difference in cumulative incidence rate for AD between the two groups (log-rank test P = 0.0519) (Figure 2).

Discussion

Many studies have reported OSA to be comorbid with cardiovascular disease, HTN, type 2 DM, and insulin resistance, but few have investigated the possible relationship between OSA and dermatologic diseases. To the best of our knowledge, this is the first study to investigate the relationship between the OSA and risk for AD. The incidence rate for AD in patients with OSA was 9.81 per 1000 person-years. This study also showed that the incidence for AD was 1.5-times higher in patients with OSA than it was in the age- and gender-matched comparison groups during a 5.5-year follow-up period, after adjusting for age, gender, medical comorbidities, geographic area, and monthly income. The medical comorbidities that were adjusted for have been noted in the literature as risk factors for AD. Although the HR decreased after adjustment, OSA patients still had a significantly higher risk for AD. Subgroup analysis found the risk for developing AD was greater in men with OSA (adjusted HR: 1.53) and younger OSA patients age 0–18years and 19–35 years (adjusted HRs 4.01 and 1.75, respectively).

The prevalence of AD is estimated at 2% to 10% in adults in Europe, where the incidence has grown 2- to 3-fold [24,25]. One community-based survey in Taiwan by Chen et al. reported the prevalence of AD to be 4.33%, higher than a previous report [26]. Although the prevalence of AD varies from country to country, its incidence appears to be increasing. AD is a very common, pruritic, relapsing inflammatory skin disorder associated with a poor quality of sleep [27]. AD may further aggravate the severity of daytime hypersomnolence in patients with OSA. The wide range of prevalence worldwide seems to suggest expression of this disease may be influenced by racial, environmental, and many other unidentified factors [25]. Although the pathomechanisms underlying AD are not fully understood, the chronic relapsing nature of this disease requires careful monitoring both for the disease itself as well as its associated risk factors. OSA and AD may share similar

Table 2. Risk for atopic dermatitis (AD) in patients with and without obstructive sleep apnea (OSA).

		Patients with OSA				Patients without OSA				Crude HR		Adjusted HR	
		N	AD	PY#	Rate*	N	AD	PY#	Rate*	95%CI	P value	95%CI	P value
All		1222	66	6724.62	9.81	18330	629	101232.86	6.21	1.58(1.23–2.04)	0.0004	1.50(1.15–1.95)	0.0025
Age (yr)	0–18	42	6	213.43	28.11	630	26	3473.78	7.48	3.78(1.51–8.93)	0.0041	4.01(1.57–10.26)	0.0038
	19–34	258	16	1394.12	11.48	3882	118	21275.30	5.55	2.07(1.23–3.48)	0.0065	1.75(1.00–3.04)	0.0483
	35–49	471	22	2637.58	8.34	7056	216	39505.95	5.47	1.53(0.98–2.37)	0.0589	1.40(0.88–2.22)	0.1559
	≥50	451	22	2479.49	8.87	6762	269	36977.83	7.27	1.22(0.79–1.88)	0.3716	1.22(0.78–1.90)	0.3927
Gender	Male	982	52	5456.56	9.53	14730	474	81904.02	5.79	1.65(1.24–2.19)	0.0006	1.53(1.14–2.06)	0.0050
	Female	240	14	1268.07	11.04	3600	155	19328.84	8.02	1.38(0.80–2.38)	0.2519	1.39(0.79–2.46)	0.2522

#PY, person-years.
*Rate: per 1000 person-years.
Adjusted by age, gender, diabetes, hypertension, coronary heart disease, obesity, allergy, allergic rhinitis, asthma, monthly income, and geographic location.

pathogenic pathways [28]. One study by Al Lawati et al. reported that ethnicity was a risk factor for OSA and that Asians appeared to be at greater risk for OSA at a given body mass index [29]. These findings along with the results of the current study suggest that clinicians in Asia should be aware of the increased risk for AD among patients with OSA.

Although the underlying mechanism contributing to the association between OSA and AD is likely complex, some possible explanations for our findings should be considered. First, obesity is a strong risk factor for OSA, and OSA is a major complication of obesity [30,31]. According to a study by Hersoug and Linneberg, there is increasing epidemiologic evidence that obesity also increases the risk for AD [21]. This study suggested that obesity might induce decreased immune tolerance and result in atopy [21]. In obese subjects, increases in the circulating levels of interleukin-6 (IL-6) and leptin, and decreases in IL-10 have been reported to down-regulate the immunologic activity of regulatory T-lymphocytes [32–35]. Additionally, Vieira et al. reported that obese subjects had a higher frequency of specific IgE positivity than non-obese subjects [36]. These changes could possibly decrease the immunologic tolerance to antigen and possibly result in atopic disease. AD is a disease of altered skin barrier and immune system dysregulation. A defect in filaggrin (FLG) may induce skin barrier dysfunction [37]. One study by Silverberg et al. showed that obesity might act as a trigger in disease associated with FLG mutations and suggested that obesity can be a trigger for AD or exacerbate it [22]. The association between OSA and AD may be in part due to obesity, and this issue merits further investigation. Since obesity was controlled in the present study, the relationship between OSA and AD survived. Obesity alone does not explain the relationship between OSA and AD.

A population-based study by Chung et al investigating the risk factors for AD in Taiwan found DM, CHD, and HTN to be significantly associated with AD (OR = 1.54, P<0.001; OR = 1.36, P<0.001; and OR = 1.22, P<0.001, respectively) [38]. DM increases the expression of pro-inflammatory factors and induces both oxidative stress and endothelial dysfunction [20]. HTN can contribute to oxidative stress, which is an important molecular mechanism associated with cardiovascular disease and tissue injury [19]. One review study by Okayama showed that inflammatory skin diseases like AD are mediated by oxidative stress [18]. Since DM, HTN, and CHD are associated with increasing systemic inflammatory factors and oxidative stress, the association among DM, HTN, and CHD, and AD observed by Chung et al in Taiwan is not surprising [38].Although the true mechanisms contributing to the associations between these comorbidities and AD remain unknown, oxidative stress and systemic inflammation might play substantial roles in this relationship. Therefore, our study examined DM, CHD, and HTN as confounders for AD.

Repeated episodes of hypoxemia during sleep are characteristic of OSA. Periodic hypoxia can lead to activation of sympathetic tone and stimulate the rennin-angiotensin-aldosterone system [39]. Angiotensin II stimulates the release of reactive oxygen species (ROS) and pro-inflammatory cytokines, which initiate and perpetuate oxidative stress and systemic inflammation [40]. The cytokines and chemokines in the circulation and skin cells orchestrate the inflammation reaction in atopic skin [2]. One review study by Okayama showed that inflammatory skin diseases like AD are mediated by oxidative stress [18]. Therefore, one link between OSA and AD might be related to the oxidative stress and systemic inflammation. Furthermore, AD is characterized as a T-helper-$_2$ (TH_2) mediated inflammatory skin disease. The sympathetic activation in OSA increases the release of catecholamine which might induce TH_2 [41].

A neurocognitive disorder associated with OSA may result from frequent arousals and fragmented sleep. Patients may suffer from psychological problems including daytime sleepiness, poor memory and concentration, irritable mood, anxiety, and emotional stress [29,42,43]. Clinical observations have found that psychological stress might act not only as a trigger for but also aggravate the presence of AD [41,44]. A complete psychological evaluation and specialized care may help alleviate the symptoms of AD and even prevent outbreaks [44,45].

Age and gender may play a role in modifying the occurrence of AD in patients with OSA. We found a clear relationship between our younger population of OSA patients and increased likelihood of developing AD. Individuals who were diagnosed with OSA later in life were at much less risk for AD. We also found male patients were at higher risk for AD. One prospective clinical epidemiologic study in eastern India showed the prevalence of AD in children to have a slight female-to-male preponderance [46]. Montnemery et al., who conducted a questionnaire study of 12071 adults in Sweden ranging in age from 20 to 59 years [24], found AD to be more frequently reported by women. One previous 8-year national study in Taiwan reported the prevalence of AD to be higher in younger populations and reported that the prevalence decreased with age [47]. That same study reported the prevalence of AD to be lower in females than in males before the age of 8 years, but to

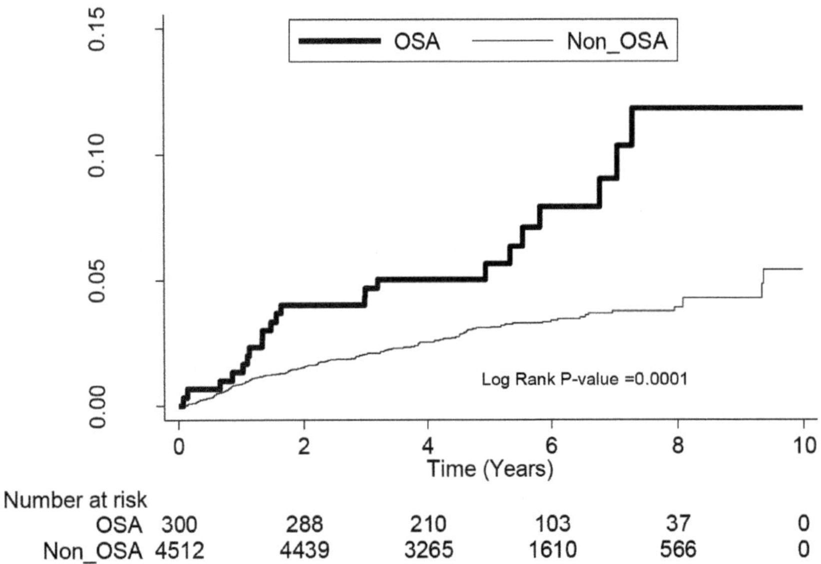

Figure 1. The cumulative incidence rate for atopic dermatitis for patients <35 years of age with obstructive sleep apnea (OSA) and without OSA (log-rank P value =0.0001).

increase in females beyond 8 years of age [47]. The underlying reason for the relationship between gender and incidence of AD in OSA patients is unclear. Sex hormones might influence mast cell activation and allergic sensitization. Estradiol promotes sensitization and IgE production, and testosterone suppresses IgE production [48,49]. AD may, in part, be a consequence of low testosterone in male patients [50]. There is a variable degree of hypogonadism associated with OSA. Male OSA patients may have low testosterone levels, and female OSA patients may have low estradiol levels [31]. Any possible association would be conjecture at this point and would need further investigation.

This study has some limitations. The diagnoses of OSA and AD were based on diagnostic codes recorded by the physician in the NHI claims database; therefore, some registration bias might be involved. To ensure the accuracy of these diagnostic codes, only the OSA patients diagnosed by polysomnography or by two patient claims records citing OSA a primary diagnosis were recorded. The AD patients were those patients who had been diagnosed on 2 occasions with AD by dermatologists. Disease severity could not be assessed from our dataset, and it was not possible to report the association between the severity of OSA and the occurrence of AD. Furthermore, individual information including occupation, mental health, environmental factors, and family history were not available. Further study to investigate the effects of these factors is needed. The strength of this study, however, is that it has a longitudinal, large population-based

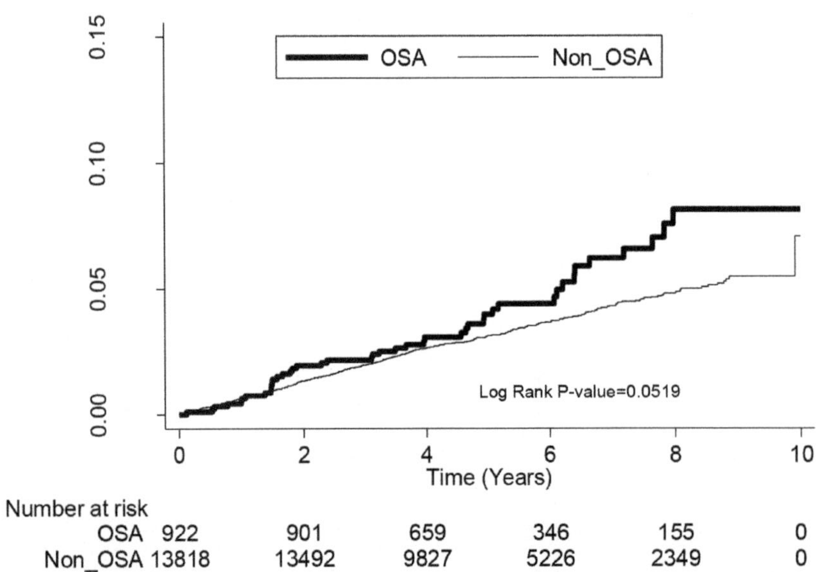

Figure 2. The cumulative incidence rate for atopic dermatitis for patients >35 years of age with obstructive sleep apnea (OSA) and without OSA (log-rank P value =0.0519).

design. The database covers nearly all of Taiwan's residents, so referral and selection biases were minimized.

In conclusion, we found that patients with OSA are at higher risk for developing AD. The risk was more pronounced in the younger age groups and in men. Further studies are needed to explore the mechanisms underlying these relationships.

Acknowledgments

This study is based in part on data from the National Health Insurance Research Database provided by the Bureau of National Health Insurance, Department of Health and managed by the National Health Research Institutes (Registered number 100057). The interpretation and conclusions contained herein do not represent those of the Bureau of National Health Insurance, Department of Health, or the National Health Research Institutes.

Author Contributions

Conceived and designed the experiments: KJT CWC JJW SFW. Performed the experiments: SYL NCY CYY FCY. Analyzed the data: KJT JJW SFW. Contributed reagents/materials/analysis tools: CWC SYL NCY CYY. Wrote the paper: KJT SFW.

References

1. Spergel JM, Paller AS (2003) Atopic dermatitis and the atopic march. J Allergy Clin Immunol 112: S118–127.
2. Homey B, Steinhoff M, Ruzicka T, Leung DY (2006) Cytokines and chemokines orchestrate atopic skin inflammation. J Allergy Clin Immunol 118: 178–189.
3. Chan LS (2008) Atopic dermatitis in 2008. Curr Dir Autoimmun 10: 76–118.
4. Rosario IC (2011) Obstructive sleep apnea: a review and update. Minn Med 94: 44–48.
5. Young T, Palta M, Dempsey J, Peppard PE, Nieto FJ, et al. (2009) Burden of sleep apnea: rationale, design, and major findings of the Wisconsin Sleep Cohort study. WMJ 108: 246–249.
6. Monahan K, Redline S (2011) Role of obstructive sleep apnea in cardiovascular disease. Curr Opin Cardiol 26: 541–547.
7. Ioja S, Weir ID, Rennert NJ (2012) Relationship between sleep disorders and the risk for developing type 2 diabetes mellitus. Postgrad Med 124: 119–129.
8. Lin WC, Winkelman JW (2012) Obstructive sleep apnea and severe mental illness: evolution and consequences. Curr Psychiatry Rep 14: 503–510.
9. Lurie A (2011) Inflammation, oxidative stress, and procoagulant and thrombotic activity in adults with obstructive sleep apnea. Adv Cardiol 46: 43–66.
10. Dalamaga M, Papadavid E, Vlami K (2013) Unmasking the Janus face of the association between psoriasis, metabolic syndrome and obstructive sleep apnea. Sleep Breath 17: 449–450.
11. Karaca S, Fidan F, Erkan F, Nural S, Pinarcı T, et al. (2013) Might psoriasis be a risk factor for obstructive sleep apnea syndrome? Sleep Breath 17: 275–280.
12. Yang YW, Kang JH, Lin HC (2012) Increased risk of psoriasis following obstructive sleep apnea: a longitudinal population-based study. Sleep Med 13: 285–289.
13. Buslau M, Benotmane K (1999) Cardiovascular complications of psoriasis: does obstructive sleep apnoea play a role? Acta Derm Venereolo 79: 234.
14. Papadavid E, Vlami K, Dalamaga M, Giatrakou S, Theodoropoulos K, et al. (2012) Sleep apnea as a comorbidity in obese psoriasis patients: a cross-sectional study. Do psoriasis characteristics and metabolic parameters play a role? J Eur Acad Dermatol Venereolo 27: 820–826.
15. Chng SY, Goh DY, Wang XS, Tan TN, Ong NB (2004) Snoring and atopic disease: a strong association. Pediatr Pulmonol 38: 210–216.
16. Matin A, Bliwise DL, Wellman JJ, Ewing HA, Rasmuson P (2002) Resolution of dyshidrotic dermatitis of the hand after treatment with continuous positive airway pressure for obstructive sleep apnea. South Med J 95: 253–254.
17. Marshall NS, Almqvist C, Grunstein RR, Marks GB, Childhood Asthma Prevention Study (2007) Predictors for snoring in children with rhinitis at age 5. Pediatr Pulmonol 42: 584–591.
18. Okayama Y (2005) Oxidative stress in allergic and inflammatory skin diseases. Curr Drug Targets Inflamm Allergy 4: 517–519.
19. Montezano AC, Touyz RM (2012) Oxidative stress, Noxs, and hypertension: experimental evidence and clinical controversies. Ann Med 44: S2–S16.
20. Fiorentino T, Prioletta A, Zuo P, Folli F (2013) Hyperglycemia-induced oxidative stress and its role in diabetes mellitus related cardiovascular diseases. Curr Pharm Des 19: 5695–5703.
21. Hersoug LG, Linneberg A (2007) The link between the epidemics of obesity and allergic diseases: does obesity induce decreased immune tolerance? Allergy 62: 1205–1213.
22. Silverberg JI, Silverberg NB (2012) Atopic Dermatitis: Update on Pathogenesis and Comorbidities. Current Dermatology Reports 1: 168–178.
23. Zheng T, Yu J, Oh MH, Zhu Z (2011) The atopic march: progression from atopic dermatitis to allergic rhinitis and asthma. Allergy Asthma Immunol Res 3: 67–73.
24. Montnemery P, Nihlén U, Göran Löfdahl C, Nyberg P, Svensson A (2003) Prevalence of self-reported eczema in relation to living environment, socio-economic status and respiratory symptoms assessed in a questionnaire study. BMC Dermatol 3: 4.
25. Bieber T (2010) Atopic dermatitis. Ann Dermatol 22: 125–137.
26. Chen GY, Cheng YW, Wang CY, Hsu TJ, Hsu MM, et al. (2008) Prevalence of skin diseases among schoolchildren in Magong, Penghu, Taiwan: a community-based clinical survey. J Formos Med Assoc 107: 21–29.
27. Beattie PE, Lewis-Jones MS (2006) A comparative study of impairment of quality of life in children with skin disease and children with other chronic childhood diseases. Br J Dermatol 155: 145–151.
28. Mannarino MR, Di Filippo F, Pirro M (2012) Obstructive sleep apnea syndrome. Eur J Intern Med 23: 586–593.
29. Al Lawati NM, Patel SR, Ayas NT (2009) Epidemiology, risk factors, and consequences of obstructive sleep apnea and short sleep duration. Prog Cardiovasc Dis 51: 285–293.
30. Shochat T, Pillar G (2003) Sleep apnoea in the older adult: pathophysiology, epidemiology, consequences and management. Drugs Aging 20: 551–560.
31. Attal P, Chanson P (2010) Endocrine aspects of obstructive sleep apnea. J Clin Endocrinol Metab 95: 483–495.
32. Kershaw EE, Flier JS (2004) Adipose tissue as an endocrine organ. J Clin Endocrinol Metab 89: 2548–2556.
33. Manigrasso MR, Ferroni P, Santilli F, Taraborelli T, Guagnano MT, et al. (2005) Association between circulating adiponectin and interleukin-10 levels in android obesity: effects of weight loss. J Clin Endocrinol Metab 90: 5876–5879.
34. De Rosa V, Procaccini C, Calì G, Pirozzi G, Fontana S, et al. (2007) A key role of leptin in the control of regulatory T cell proliferation. Immunity 26: 241–255.
35. Bulló M, García-Lorda P, Megias I, Salas-Salvadó J (2012) Systemic inflammation, adipose tissue tumor necrosis factor, and leptin expression. Obes Res 11: 525–531.
36. Vieira VJ, Ronan AM, Windt MR, Tagliaferro AR (2005) Elevated atopy in healthy obese women. Am J Clin Nutr 82: 504–509.
37. Boguniewicz M, Leung DY (2011) Atopic dermatitis: a disease of altered skin barrier and immune dysregulation. Immunol Rev 242: 233–246.
38. Chung SD, Keller JJ, Lin HC (2012) Association of erectile dysfunction with atopic dermatitis: a population-based case-control study. J Sex Med 9: 679–685.
39. Pratt-Ubunama MN, Nishizaka MK, Boedefeld RL, Cofield SS, Harding SM, et al. (2007) Plasma aldosterone is related to severity of obstructive sleep apnea in subjects with resistant hypertension. Chest 131: 453–459.
40. Das U (2005) Angiotensin-II behaves as an endogenous pro-inflammatory molecule. J Assoc Physicians India 53: 472–476.
41. Buske-Kirschbaum A, Geiben A, Höllig H, Morschhäuser E, Hellhammer D (2002) Altered responsiveness of the hypothalamus-pituitary-adrenal axis and the sympathetic adrenomedullary system to stress in patients with atopic dermatitis. J Clin Endocrinol Metab 87: 4245–4251.
42. Malhotra A, White DP (2002) Obstructive sleep apnoea. Lancet 360: 237–245.
43. Akmal MK, Ezat M, Raafat O, Hamed H, Bediwy A (2013) Association of depression, anxiety, and impairment in executive functions in patients with obstructive sleep apnea. Middle East Current Psychiatry 20: 30–34.
44. Morren M-A, Przybilla B, Bamelis M, Heykants B, Reynaers A, et al. (1994) Atopic dermatitis: triggering factors. J Am Acad Dermatol 31: 467–473.
45. Schut C, Weik U, Tews N, Gieler U, Deinzer R, et al. (2012) Psychophysiological effects of stress management in patients with atopic dermatitis: a randomized controlled trial. Acta Derm Venereol 93: 57–61.
46. Kumar MK, Singh PK, Tahir MMA (2012) The clinico-epidemiological profile and the risk factors associated with the severity of atopic dermatitis (AD) in eastern Indian children. Journal of Clinical and Diagnostic Research [serial online] 6: 1162–1166.
47. Hwang CY, Chen YJ, Lin MW, Chen TJ, Chu SY, et al. (2010) Prevalence of atopic dermatitis, allergic rhinitis and asthma in Taiwan: a national study 2000 to 2007. Acta Derm Venereol 90: 589–594.
48. Chen W, Mempel M, Schober W, Behrendt H, Ring J (2008) Gender difference, sex hormones, and immediate type hypersensitivity reactions. Allergy 63: 1418–1427.
49. Cho S, Kim HJ, Oh SH, Park CO, Jung JY, et al. (2010) The influence of pregnancy and menstruation on the deterioration of atopic dermatitis symptoms. Ann Dermatol 22: 180–185.
50. Canguven O (2013) The role of low testosterone associated with erectile dysfunction with atopic dermatitis. J Sex Med 10: 618.

Is the Determination of Specific IgE against Components Using ISAC 112 a Reproducible Technique?

Rubén Martínez-Aranguren[1], María T. Lizaso[2], María J. Goikoetxea[1], Blanca E. García[2], Paula Cabrera-Freitag[1], Oswaldo Trellez[3], María L. Sanz[1]*

1 Department of Allergology and Clinical Immunology, Clínica Universidad de Navarra, Pamplona, Spain, **2** Allergology Service, Complejo Hospitalario de Navarra, Pamplona, Spain, **3** Department of Computer Architecture, Universidad de Málaga, Málaga, Spain

Abstract

Background: The ImmunoCAP ISAC 112 is a fluoro-immunoassay that allows detection of specific IgE to 112 molecular components from 51 allergenic sources. We studied the reliability of this technique intra- and inter- assay, as well as inter-batch- and inter-laboratory-assay.

Methods: Twenty samples were studied, nineteen sera from polysensitized allergic patients, and the technique calibrator provided by the manufacturer (CTR02). We measured the sIgE from CTR02 and three patients' sera ten times in the same and in different assays. Furthermore, all samples were tested in two laboratories and with two batches of ISAC kit. To evaluate the accuracy of ISAC 112, we contrasted the determinations of CTR02 calibrator with their expected values by T Student test. To analyse the precision, we calculated the coefficient of variation (CV) of the 15 allergens that generate the calibration curve, and to analyse the repeatability and the reproducibility, we calculated the intraclass coefficient correlation (ICC) to each allergen.

Results: The results obtained for CTR02 were similar to those expected in 7 of 15 allergens that generate the calibration curve, whereas in 8 allergens the results showed significant differences. The mean CV obtained in the CTR02 determinations was of 9.4%, and the variability of sera from patients was of 22.9%. The agreement in the intra- and inter-assay analysis was very good to 94 allergens and good to one. In the inter-batch analyse, we obtained a very good agreement to 82 allergens, good to 14, moderate to 5 allergens, poor to one, and bad to 1 allergen. In the inter-laboratory analyse, we obtained a very good agreement to 73 allergens, good to 22, moderate to 6 and poor to two allergens.

Conclusion: The allergen microarray immunoassay, ISAC 112, is a repeatable and reproducible in vitro diagnostic tool for determination of sIgE beyond the own laboratory.

Editor: Vladimir N. Uversky, University of South Florida College of Medicine, United States of America

Funding: RM is supported by a grant from the Spanish Research Network on Adverse Reactions to Allergens and Drugs (RIRAAF RD12 00130010: Red de Investigación de Reacciones Adversas a Alérgenos y Fármacos) of the Carlos III Health Institute, Madrid, Spain. All the authors (except PCF) belong to RIRAAF RD12 00130010. This study has been partly funded by a grant FIS 11/01634 from the Carlos III Health Institute. The funders had no role in study design, data collection and analysis, decision to publish, or preparation of the manuscript.

Competing Interests: Thermofisher supplies part of the material (ISAC CRD 112 kits) required for this study.

* E-mail: mlsanzlar@unav.es

Introduction

Component-based allergological diagnosis has opened up a new era in the study of allergies. It allows the identification of specific sensitization against proteins or specific molecular components [1–4]. This new approach helps to clarify the molecular bases of primary sensitization and cross-reactivity phenomena [5–11]. It also helps to rationalize the indication for immunotherapy based on the administration of allergenic components [12–14] and constitutes a necessary tool in the choice of a diet free from allergens in food-allergic patients [12,15].

The technique of the commercially available protein microarray ImmunoCAP ISAC® specific IgE (sIgE) 112 offers the possibility of analyzing sIgE against 112 components of purified natural proteins and recombinant proteins from 51 different allergenic sources. Since its launch onto the market, this platform has generated great expectations [16–19], and its use is being introduced into clinical practice because, at least from the conceptual point of view, it could be an aid to the clinician in the diagnosis or treatment indication of certain patients, especially those polysensitized ones [6,20]. However, clinical and technical validations and comparative studies are still needed [21–23]. In fact, previous version of this platform (ISAC 103) showed high variability for certain allergens [21], and even low efficiency in diagnosing sensitizations to certain proteins [24]. Thus, data assessing reliability of this technique, now for version ISAC 112, are required even beyond each laboratory.

The objective of this study was to assess the accuracy, precision, repeatability and reproducibility of this platform. To this aim we carried out assays with the technique's calibrating sample and sera from polysensitized patients under different conditions including determinations performed both in the same assay and in different assays and considering as possible sources of additional variability the use of different batches of reagents and the performance of the technique in different laboratories.

Materials and Methods

Samples

A total of 20 samples were analyzed: the calibrator sample (CTR02), provided by the manufacturer and 19 sera from polysensitized patients. The research ethical committee from the Universidad de Navarra approved the study "Technical and clinical validation of the diagnostic capacity of microarrays of allergenic molecules in allergy to pollens and/or vegetable foods" in which this work has been done. Patients provided their written informed consent to participate in this study. After inclusion for this work, the data from the patients' sera were analyzed anonymously.

The CTR02 calibrator, according to information provided by the manufacturer, is composed of known amounts of chimeric monoclonal antibodies humanized against 15 molecular components (Amb a 1, Art v 1, Bet v 1, Can f 1, Can f 2, Can f 5, Der p 1, Der p 2, Fel d 1, Gal d 1, Gal d 2, Ole e 1, Phl p 1, Phl p 5, and Pru p 3). The antibodies against these 15 allergenic components are found in the calibrator in a range of 4 different concentrations expressed in ISAC Standardized Units (ISU) values for sIgE (1, 4, 15 and 50 ISU). This allows a calibration curve to be plotted from

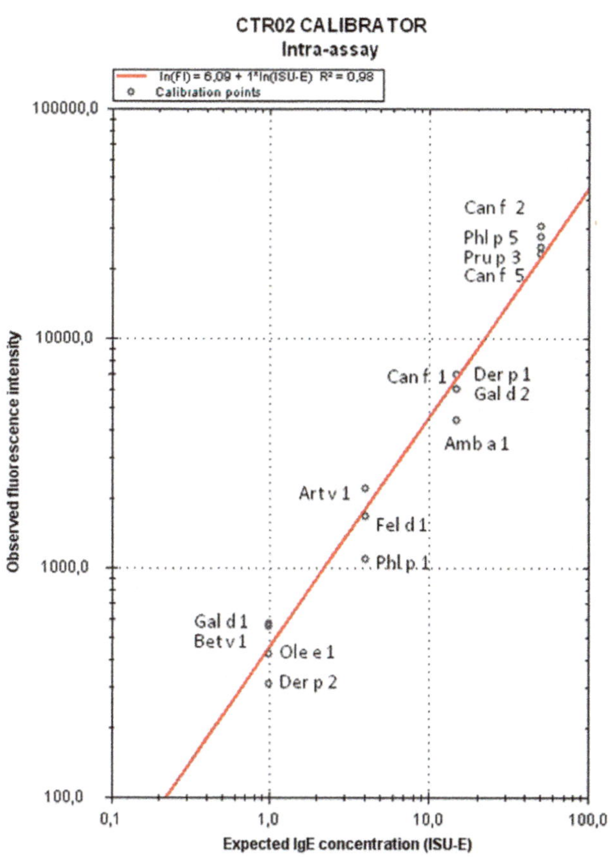

Figure 1. Calibration curve. Example of calibration curve used for the intra-assay analysis.

the 4 points of fluorescence intensity corresponding to the different ISU (figure 1).

Of the 19 sera from the polysensitized patients, sera 1, 2, and 3, contained as a group detectable amounts of sIgE against the 15 allergens making up the calibration curve and against another 80 allergens (of the 112 represented in the microarray). Sixteen additional sera, numbered 4–19, showing a broad variety of sensitizations were also included in the study.

Patients' sera were frozen at −20°C after the blood collection until the immunoassays were performed and, among the different assays, samples were conserved at 4°C.

InmunoCAP ISAC 112 microarray

The microarray ISAC 112 (ThermoFisher, Uppsala, Sweden) is a solid phase fluoro immunoassay that detects IgE antibodies against the proteins fixed on ISAC surface. One slide contains 4 microarray and one kit 5 slides, 20 microarrays in total. The technique was performed following the manufacturer's instructions. Each microarray is incubated with a serum in order to label sIgE to each protein and subsequently it is incubated with a human anti IgE detection antibody conjugated with fluorescence.

Finally the fluorescence intensity of each microarray is measured by the scanner (LuxScan 10K/A, CapitalBio, Beijing, China) using following parameters: laser power (LP = 60) and photo-multiplier tube (PMT = 600).

The analysis of the digitalized images is performed with the software Phadia Microarray Image Analyzer (ThermoFisher). This software allows transforming the images fluorescence intensity in numerical data according to the calibration curve built with the calibrator CTR02 sample included in each assay, as previously described (figure 1). An acceptable calibration curve needs to show slope parameters (Y) between 5.5 and 6.8, and $R^2 > 0.85$ according to the information provided by ThermoFisher.

The sIgE values are expressed semiquantitatively as ISU. Results equal or greater than 0.30 ISU are considered positive, according to the indications of the manufacturer.

Intra-assay analysis

The repeatability of the ISAC 112 technique was assessed by analyzing the sIgE from the CTR02 calibrator and sera 1 to 3 obtained in 10 determinations performed in the same assay with 2 ISAC 112 kits from the same production batch. The calibration curve was obtained with the first determination of the CTR02 calibrator in the first kit in the first slide, first microarray.

Inter-assay analysis

The reproducibility of the technique was assessed by analyzing the sIgE results from the CTR02 calibrator and sera 1 to 3 obtained in 10 assays performed on 10 different days using 2 ISAC 112 kits from the same production batch. For each assay a calibration curve was plotted with the calibration curve performed in its own assay.

Inter-laboratory analysis

The reproducibility of the ISAC 112 technique was assessed by analyzing the levels of sIgE obtained from the 20 samples studied with 2 kits from the same batch. The analyses were performed in two different laboratories i.e.: Clínica Universidad de Navarra, and the Complejo Hospitalario de Navarra, both in Pamplona, Navarra, Spain. The reading of the chips was performed with the same conditions in each laboratory. The calibration curve was plotted with the determination of the CTR02 calibrator performed

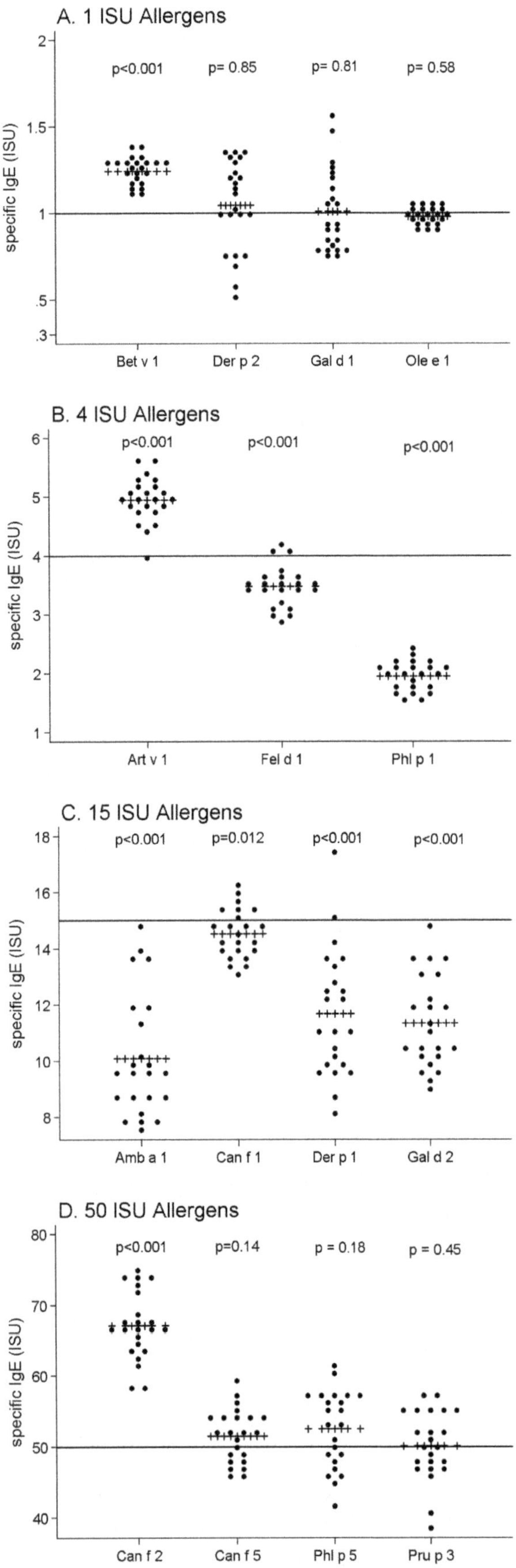

Figure 2. Accuracy of ISAC 112. Results obtained for the allergens that form the calibration curve with the intra-assay, inter-assay, inter-laboratory and inter-batch determinations performed with the calibrator CTR02, composed by chimeric antibodies. Expected ISU results are depicted by red line and the observed mean ISU results are depicted by red +++. Student T test was used for statistical analysis.

in each laboratory. Both scanners had been calibrated similarly by the same technician, the same day.

Inter-batch analysis

The reproducibility of the ISAC 112 technique was also assessed by analyzing sIgE levels from the 20 samples under study obtained from two kits from different production batch.

Statistical analysis of the data

We studied the *accuracy* of ISAC 112, understood as the similarity between the values obtained and those expected, and its *precision*, understood as the dispersion of the group of results obtained.

We evaluated the *accuracy* by the analysis of the determinations performed in all the assays with the sample CTR02, after comparison of the results expected and those obtained for each one of the 15 allergens that constitute the calibration curve by means of the Student's T test.

Furthermore, the *precision* of the allergens from the calibration curve was analyzed by calculating the coefficient of variation (CV) in all the assays, as the percentage of the standard deviation of the determinations divided by the mean. We calculated the CV from the results obtained from the CTR02 calibrator.

We analyzed the strength of agreement of the determinations under the same conditions, *repeatability*, and different conditions, *reproducibility*, of the results obtained in the different assays by calculating the intraclass coefficient correlation (ICC) for each allergen [25,26]. The level of agreement using the ICC was expressed using the classification of Fleiss [27] as: very good (ICC>0.90), good (0.71–0.90), moderate (0.51–070), mediocre (0.31–0.50) or poor (ICC<0.30).

Also, we analysed the *reliability* of the semiquantitative character of the technique comparing the number of allergens that modified the category of the IgE according to the range established by the manufacturer (<0.3 ISU, not detectable; ≥0.3–<1 ISU, low; ≥1–<15 moderated or high; and ≥15, very high), in the interassay determinations for each serum.

The Student's T test and the ICC for each allergen were performed using the statistical software package SPSS (Statistical Packaged for social science) for Windows, version 15.0 (Chicago, Illinois, USA). The CV was calculated using the program Excel version 12.0, Microsoft Office 2007.

Results

Accuracy

The average values obtained in the sIgE determinations against the allergens of the calibration curve Der p 2, Gal d 1, Ole e 1, Can f 1, Can f 5, Phl p 5 and Pru p 3 by ISAC resulted to be similar to those expected (figure 2). Nevertheless, the determinations of the remaining 8 allergens showed statistically significant differences ($p<0.05$) between the observed levels and those expected. Of these 8 allergens, six allergens (Art v 1, Fel d 1, Phl p 1, Amb a 1, Can f 1, Der p 1 and Gal d 2) are in the intermediate points of the calibration curve (4 and 15 ISU), whereas the Bet v 1 belongs to a 1 ISU calibration point and the

Can f 2 belongs to the 50 ISU calibration point. Despite these differences, all the calibrator CTR02 determinations gave place to a calibration curve within the slope parameters and R^2 considered by the manufacturer as acceptable (Y and R^2 maximum and minimum obtained at the assays 6.52–5.8 and 0.99–0.95, respectively)

Precision

When we analyzed the global variability in the results from the different determinations of the CTR02 calibrator, we obtained a mean CV of 9.42%.

The individual data of the calibrating sera allergens are expressed in figure 3.

Repeatability and reproducibility

Repeatability and reproducibility calculated using the ICC are summarised in table 1.

The analysis of the repeatability (intra-assay analysis) was very good for 94 of the 112 allergens represented in the microarray and good for the Bos d lactoferrin allergen. For the remaining 17 allergens the ICC could not be calculated as all the determinations were equal to 0 ISU.

The analysis of the inter-assay reproducibility was very good for 94 of the 112 allergens and good for the Pol d 5 allergen.

The reproducibility between the analyses of the determinations in two laboratories was very good for 73 allergens and good for 22 of the allergens represented in the microarray. The allergens Ara h 9, Art v 1, Bla g 5, Bos d 8, Bos d lactoferrin, and Phl p 12, showed a moderate agreement whereas in Jug r 2 and Alt a 6 agreement was mediocre. The ICC values could not be calculated for 9 allergens in inter-laboratories analysis because all the determinations for them were equal to 0 ISU.

Finally, in the analysis of the reproducibility between the two kits from different production batches we obtained a very good agreement for 82 allergens and good for 14 allergens. For the allergens Bos d 8, Lep d 2, Pen m 1, Ses i 1 and Ves v 5 we obtained a moderate ICC while for Bos d lactoferrin and Alt a 6 gave a mediocre and poor agreement respectively. The ICC values could not be calculated for 9 allergens in inter-batch analysis because all the determinations for them were equal to 0 ISU.

Disagreements in the IgE level

When analysing the number of disagreements in the interassay analysis determinations in patients' sera, we obtained the following results. The results of sIgE obtained modified from "not detectable" level to "low" level for 7 allergens when analysing sera 1 and 2, and for 9 allergens when analysing sera 3. The specific IgE levels modified from "low" to "moderate-high" for 7 allergens when analysing sera 1 and 2, and for 13 when analysing sera 3. The specific IgE level change from "moderate-high" to "very high" happened in 16 occasions when analysing sera 1, and in 15 occasions when analysing sera 2. Finally, the IgE level change from "not detectable" to "high" was observed for 4 and 5 allergens when using sera 1 and 2 respectively. This allergens were Act d 1, Asp f 1, Ara h 8, Ber e 1, Cor a 9, Mal d 1, Phl p 5, Phl p 12 and Pla l 1. The allergens that showed a greater number of disagreements were Jug r 2, Jug r 3 and Ses i 1, which had disagreements on the IgE level in the three sera studied.

Discussion

The technique of protein microarrays has been accepted as a useful method for the detection of sIgE against molecular components [28,29]. Thus, it has been shown its usefulness for the diagnosis of food allergies, to determine cross-reactivity phenomena or sensitization patterns in specific geographical areas [14,20]. Previously, several comparative studies between ISAC and other conventional techniques of sIgE detection, such as ImmunoCAP have been performed. These studies state that although the results obtained between both methods are not comparable, a good agreement between them was found [13,20,30].

However, few studies have been carried out into the variability and accuracy of this technique showing improvable results in previous versions of this microarray [17,21]. In the present study, we analyzed accuracy, variability and reproducibility in the new version, ImmunoCAP ISAC 112. The results obtained in the study show good reproducibility of the technique not only for one assay but even considering changes of the assays in different days, and using different batches and in different laboratories.

When analysing the accuracy of the technique, 8 of the 15 allergens that form the calibration curve showed statistically significant differences between the values obtained and those expected. Despite this fact, all the calibration lines were within

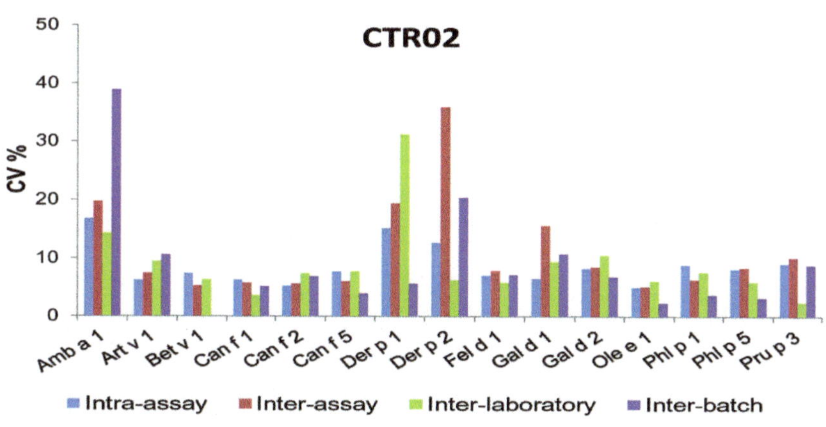

Figure 3. Variability of the ISAC 112 technique in the calibrator sample. Coefficient of Variation (CV) obtained to allergens of calibration curve. The results are the mean CV of 10 determinations intra- and inter-assay, and 2 determinations inter-laboratory and inter-batches of the calibrator sample.

Table 1. Intraclass Correlation Coefficient (ICC) of ISAC 112 results obtained from 10 determinations of 4 sera intra- and inter-assay and two determinations of 20 sera inter-laboratory and inter-batch.

ALLERGEN	INTRA-ASSAY	INTER-ASSAY	INTER-LAB	INTER-BATCH	ALLERGEN	INTRA-ASSAY	INTER-ASSAY	INTER-LAB	INTER-BATCH
Act d 1	0.983	0.978	0.950	0.995	Equ c 1	0.998	0.983	0.914	0.914
Act d 2	0.999	0.985	0.851	0.879	Equ c 3	0.999	0.996	0.948	0.954
Act d 5	0.978	0.955	0.834	*	Fag e 2	0.998	0.980	0.986	0.996
Act d 8	0.987	0.848	0.907	0.970	Fel d 1 †	0.994	0.987	0.981	0.993
Aln g 1	0.977	0.956	0.867	0.707	Fel d 2	0.996	0.996	0.987	0.775
Alt a 1	0.999	0.993	0.897	0.878	Fel d 4	0.997	0.966	0.970	0.925
Alt a 6	0.988	0.977	0.497	0.267	Gad c 1	0.999	0.986	0.995	0.988
Amb a 1 †	0.996	0.994	0.981	0.900	Gal d 1 †	1.000	0.918	0.970	0.993
Ana o 2	0.998	0.986	0.945	*	Gal d 2 †	0.998	0.969	0.987	0.986
Ani s 1	*	0.994	0.984	0.987	Gal d 3	1.000	0.993	0.998	0.999
Ani s 3	*	*	0.988	0.998	Gal d 5	0.998	0.986	0.997	0.922
Api g 1	0.998	0.978	0.986	0.980	Gly m 4	0.998	0.983	0.998	0.961
Api m 1	*	*	0.973	0.998	Gly m 5	0.997	0.990	0.838	0.944
Api m 4	*	*	*	*	Gly m 6	0.997	0.989	0.955	0.960
Ara h 1	0.997	0.990	0.979	0.963	Hev b 1	*	*	0.945	*
Ara h 2	0.997	0.993	0.937	0.991	Hev b 3	*	*	0.973	0.991
Ara h 3	*	*	0.991	0.928	Hev b 5	1.000	0.995	0.998	0.997
Ara h 6	0.990	0.983	0.868	0.960	Hev b 6.01	0.993	*	0.990	0.995
Ara h 8	0.994	0.980	0.853	0.850	Hev b 8	1.000	0.997	0.999	0.997
Ara h 9	0.997	0.971	0.680	0.992	Jug r 1	0.996	0.986	0.880	0.974
Art v 1†	1.000	0.996	0.703	0.997	Jug r 2	0.994	0.979	0.446	0.881
Art v 3	0.999	0.998	0.986	0.996	Jug r 3	0.999	0.984	0.921	0.983
Asp f 1	0.995	0.984	0.938	0.859	Lep d 2	0.999	0.977	0.941	0.697
Asp f 3	0.999	0.994	0.955	0.998	Mal d 1	0.998	0.994	0.992	0.998
Asp f 6	0.991	0.997	*	*	Mer a 1	1.000	0.996	0.991	0.984
Ber e 1	0.996	0.983	0.779	0.715	Mus m 1	0.992	0.994	0.813	0.997
Bet v 1†	0.999	0.994	0.984	0.973	MUXF3	1.000	0.989	0.923	0.998
Bet v 2	0.999	0.992	0.951	0.946	Ole e 1†	1.000	0.995	0.992	0.990
Bet v 4	0.998	0.990	0.885	0.846	Ole e 7	0.999	0.989	0.831	0.907
Bla g 1	*	*	*	*	Ole e 9	0.999	0.993	0.980	0.995
Bla g 2	*	*	*	*	Par j 2	0.998	0.985	0.998	0.996
Bla g 5	0.992	0.980	0.646	0.776	Pen m 1	*	*	0.994	0.663
Bla g 7	*	*	0.959	0.955	Pen m 2	*	*	*	*
Blo t 5	*	*	0.924	0.993	Pen m 4	0.999	0.995	0.911	0.973
Bos d 4	*	*	0.998	0.969	Phl p 1†	1.000	0.996	0.991	0.989
Bos d 5	0.998	0.995	0.882	0.883	Phl p 11	0.997	0.989	0.994	0.968
Bos d 6	0.999	0.986	0.988	0.983	Phl p 12	0.998	0.979	0.586	0.725
Bos d 8	0.996	0.966	0.566	0.670	Phl p 2	0.998	0.981	0.944	0.886
Bos d Lact	0.865	0.981	0.596	0.464	Phl p 4	0.997	0.993	0.891	0.969
Can f 1 †	0.998	0.993	0.973	0.983	Phl p 5†	1.000	0.992	0.952	0.990
Can f 2 †	1.000	0.999	0.977	0.998	Phl p 6	0.993	0.974	0.829	0.920
Can f 3	0.919	0.981	0.994	0.991	Phl p 7	0.999	0.987	0.784	0.995
Can f 5 †	0.999	0.998	0.996	0.999	Pla a 1	1.000	0.991	0.839	0.818
Che a 1	0.999	0.989	0.940	0.944	Pla a 2	1.000	0.988	0.733	0.904
Cla h 8	*	*	*	*	Pla a 3	0.986	0.964	0.821	0.984
Cor a 1.0101	0.998	0.991	0.998	0.988	Pla l 1	0.990	0.933	0.951	0.994
Cor a 1.0401	0.992	0.984	0.986	0.993	Pol d 5	0.983	0.891	0.996	0.998
Cor a 8	0.999	0.988	0.931	0.990	Pru p 1	0.994	0.944	0.972	0.969

Table 1. Cont.

ALLERGEN	INTRA-ASSAY	INTER-ASSAY	INTER-LAB	INTER-BATCH	ALLERGEN	INTRA-ASSAY	INTER-ASSAY	INTER-LAB	INTER-BATCH
Cor a 9	0.997	0.991	0.827	0.987	Pru p 3†	0.999	0.997	0.985	0.994
Cry j 1	1.000	0.988	0.751	0.839	Sal k 1	1.000	0.997	0.985	1.000
Cup a 1	0.999	0.990	0.981	0.990	Ses i 1	0.990	0.994	0.986	<u>0.533</u>
Cyn d 1	0.999	0.985	0.950	0.909	Tri a 14	0.999	0.993	0.985	0.993
Der f 1	0.999	0.997	0.988	0.944	Tri a 19.0101	1.000	0.994	1.000	0.999
Der f 2	0.991	0.989	0.951	0.955	Tri a aA_TI	0.999	0.994	0.979	0.995
Der p 1 †	0.997	0.994	0.931	0.983	Ves v 5	*	*	0.996	0.634
Der p 10	*	*	0.932	0.994					
Der p 2†	0.993	0.972	0.874	0.961					

*The ICC could not be calculated as all the determinations were equal to 0 ISU.
†Allergens detected by the calibration curve.
ICC ranges: very good (>0.9), good (0.71–0.90), moderate (0.51–0.70), mediocre (0.31–0.50) and poor (<0.30). Underlined are showed ICC values below 0.7.

acceptable limits of slope and R2 established by the technique's supplier. The fact that most allergens keep their category, even at low sIgE levels, supports the reliability of the results offered by the technique. Nevertheless, it should be highlighted that this is a semiquantitative technique and the IgE levels close to the cut off points between categories can fluctuate in different assays.

Regarding the technique's precision, the results obtained show a low variability when we analyse the determinations of the control sample CTR02, which is under 10% in most allergens. Also, the CV is similar both in the analysis performed in the same assay and in those performed in different assays. It is worth noting that the capacity of the allergen to attach itself to the surface of the ISAC array is lower than in quantitative techniques such as ImmunoCAP, in which the allergen is fixed under excess molarity conditions. This fact could make more clear differences in the allergen ability to bind to the microarray leading into differences in variability of specific IgE binding. Differences in reliability of some allergens from the microarray (like Amb a 1, Der p 1 or Der p 2) and considering that ISAC microarray is a semiquantitative technique suggest that ISAC 112 is not the best method to monitor sensitizations and patient's follow-up.

However, in our opinion these analyses demonstrated an evident improvement in the new version of the ISAC microarray. This improvement can be, among others, due to the calibration curve consisting in chimeric antibodies (sIgE) in contrast to the serum with known sIgE concentration from previous versions ISAC 103 [21]. This might be due to a good characterization of chimeric antibodies and the absence of other isotypes able to bind to the spotted allergens.

Finally, we studied the repeatability and reproducibility of the technique, analysing the ICC in the different assays. The results obtained in the intra-assay analysis show a good repeatability, obtaining good agreement strength for almost all the allergens present in microarray. Also, the reproducibility of the interassay analysis showed good concordance strength for these allergens. The reproducibility in the inter-laboratory and inter-batch analysis still has good agreement strength for most allergens. Nevertheless, this agreement strength was lower for 8 allergens in the inter-laboratory analysis and for 7 allergens in the inter-batch agreement. This slight decrease in the results' agreement strength could be due to the fact that only two determinations were performed in each analysis instead of 10 repetitions like in the interassay analysis. Also, the performance of analysis in different laboratories and with different batches means a greater source of variability.

In conclusion, ISAC 112 yields good reliability results taking into account that ISAC 112 gives semi-quantitative results. However, due to the low accuracy obtained in some of the studied allergens, the application of this semi-quantitative technique for diagnosis in clinical situations where results may have a major impact on the therapy prescribed may not be advisable. Even more, this study suggests that neither laboratory specific condition neither the change from one batch to another affect substantially microarray reliability.

Acknowledgments

All the authors of this article belong to the Research network in Adverse Reactions to Foods and Drugs (Red de Investigacion de Reacciones Adversas a Alimentos y Fármacos (RIRAAF)) RD12/0013/0010 at the Instituto Carlos III. ML Sanz and BE García belongs to the Committees of Immunology and Food Allergy of the Spanish Society of Allergy and Clinical Immunology (SEAIC).

Author Contributions

Conceived and designed the experiments: MTL MJG BEG MLS. Performed the experiments: RMMA MTL PCF. Analyzed the data: RMMA MTL MJG OT. Contributed reagents/materials/analysis tools: MTL BEG OT MLS. Wrote the paper: RMMA MJG BEG PCF MLS.

References

1. Valenta R, Lidholm J, Niederberger V, Hayek B, Kraft D, et al. (1999) The recombinant allergen-based concept of component-resolved diagnostics and immunotherapy (CRD and CRIT). Clin Exp Allergy 29: 896–904.
2. Asero R, Jimeno L, Barber D (2008) Component-resolved diagnosis of plant food allergy by SPT. Eur Ann Allergy Clin Immunol 40: 115–21.
3. Barber D, de la Torre F, Lombardero M, Antépara I, Colas C, et al. (2009) Component-resolved diagnosis of pollen allergy based on skin testing with profilin, polcalcin and lipid transfer protein pan-allergens. Clin Exp Allergy 39: 1764–73.

4. Lin J, Bardina L, Shreffler WG, Andreae DA, Ge Y, et al. (2009) Development of a novel peptide microarray for large-scale epitope mapping of food allergens. J Allergy Clin Immunol 124: 315–22.
5. Gamboa PM, Sanz ML, Lombardero M, Barber D, Sánchez-Monje R, et al. (2009) Component-resolved in vitro diagnosis in peach-allergic patients. J Investig Allergol Clin Immunol 19: 13–20.
6. Goikoetxea MJ, Cabrera-Freitag P, Sanz ML, Fernández-Benítez M (2010) The importance of in vitro component-resolved diagnosis in paediatric patients. Allergol Immunopathol 38: 37–40.
7. Palacin A, Quirce S, Armentia A, Fernández-Nieto M, Pacios LF, et al. (2007) Wheat lipid transfer protein is a major allergen associated with baker's asthma. J Allergy Clin Immunol 120: 1132–8.
8. Barber D, de la Torre F, Feo F, Florido F, Guardia P, et al. (2008) Understanding patient sensitization profiles in complex pollen areas: a molecular epidemiological study. Allergy 63: 1550–8.
9. Twardosz-Kropfmüller A, Singh MB, Niederberger V, Horak F, Kraft D, et al. (2010) Association of allergic patients' phenotypes with IgE reactivity to recombinant pollen marker allergens. Allergy 65: 296–303.
10. Díaz-Perales A, Lombardero M, Sánchez-Monge R, García-Selles FJ, Pernas M, et al. (2000) Lipid-transfer proteins as potential plant panallergens: cross-reactivity among proteins of Artemisia pollen, Castanea nut and Rosaceae fruits, with different IgE-binding capacities. Clin Exp Allergy 30: 1403–10.
11. Ebo DG, Bridts CH, Verweij MM, De Knop KJ, Hagendorens MM, et al. (2010) Sensitization profiles in birch pollen-allergic patients with and without oral allergy syndrome to apple: lessons from multiplexed component-resolved allergy diagnosis. Clin Exp Allergy 40: 339–47.
12. Ferrer M, Sanz ML, Sastre J, Bartra J, del Cuvillo A, et al. (2009) Molecular diagnosis in Allergology: application of the microarray tecnique J Investig Allergol Clin Immunol 19: 19–24.
13. Ott H, Baron JM, Heise R, Ocklenburg C, Stanzel S, et al. (2008) Clinical usefulness of microarray-based IgE detection in children with suspected food allergy. Allergy 63: 1521–8.
14. Sanz ML, Blázquez AB, Garcia BE (2011) Microarray of allergenic component-based diagnosis in food allergy. Curr Opin Allergy Clin Immunol 11: 204–9.
15. Renault NK, Mirotti L, Alcocer MJ (2007) Biotechnologies in new high-throughput food allergy tests: why we need them. Biotechnol Lett 29: 333–9.
16. Jahn-Schmid B, Harwanegg C, Hiller R, Bohle B, Ebner C, et al. (2003) Allergen microarray: Comparison of microarray using recombinant allergens with conventional diagnostic methods to detect allergen-specific serum immunoglobulin E. Clin Exp Allergy 33: 1443–9.
17. Mari A (2001) Multiple pollen sensitization: a molecular approach to the diagnosis. Int Arch Allergy Immunol 125: 57–65.
18. Scala E, Alessandri C, Bernardi ML, Ferrara R, Palazzo P, et al. (2010) Cross-sectional survey on immunoglobulin E reactivity in 23,077 subjects using an allergenic molecule-based microarray detection system. Clin Exp Allergy 40: 911–921
19. Wöhrl S, Vigl K, Zehetmayer S, Hiller R, Jarisch R, et al. (2006) The performance of a component-based allergen-microarray in clinical practice. Allergy 61: 633–9.
20. Sastre J, Landivar ME, Ruiz-García M, Andregnette-Rosigno MV, Mahillo I (2012) How molecular diagnosis can change allergen-specific immunotherapy prescription in a complex pollen area. Allergy 67: 709–11.
21. Cabrera-Freitag P, Goikoetxea MJ, Gamboa PM, Martínez-Aranguren R, Beorlegui C, et al. (2011) A study into the variability of the in vitro component-based microarray technique "ISAC CDR 103" J Invest Allergol Clin Immunol 21: 414–5.
22. Cabrera-Freitag P, Goikoetxea MJ, Beorlegui C, Gamboa PM, Gastaminza G, et al. (2011) Can component-based microarray replace fluorescent enzimoimmunoassay in the diagnosis of grass and cypress pollen allergy? Clin Exp Allergy 41: 1440–6.
23. Salcedo G, Díaz-Perales A (2010) Component-resolved diagnosis of allergy: more is better? Clin Exp Allergy 40: 836–8.
24. Villalta D, Asero R (2010) Is the detection of IgE to multiple Bet v 1-homologous food allergens by means of allergen microarray clinically useful? J Allergy Clin Immunol 125: 1158–61.
25. Prieto L, Lamarca L, Casado A (1998) La evaluación de la fiabilidad en las observaciones clínicas: el coeficiente de correlación intraclasse. Med Clin (Barc) 110: 142–45
26. Bravo G, Potvin L (1991) Estimating the reliability of continuos measures with Cronbach's alfa or the intraclass correlation coeficient: toward the integration of two traditions. J Clin Epidemiol 44: 381–390.
27. Fleiss JL (1986) Design and Analysis of Clinical Experiments. New York: John Wiley & Sons.
28. Hiller R, Laffer S, Harwanegg C, Huber M, Schmidt WM, et al. (2002) Microarrayed allergen molecules: diagnostics gatekeepers for allergy treatment. FASEB J 16: 414–6.
29. Canonica GW, Ansotegui IJ, Pawankar R, Schmid-Grendelmeier P, van Hage M, et al. (2013) A WAO - ARIA - GA2LEN consensus document on molecular-based allergy diagnostics. World Allergy Organ J 3; 6: 17.
30. Wang J, Godbold JH, Sampson HA (2008) Correlation of serum allergy (IgE) tests performed by different assay systems. J Allergy Clin Immunol 121: 1219–24.

Permissions

All chapters in this book were first published in PLOS ONE, by The Public Library of Science; hereby published with permission under the Creative Commons Attribution License or equivalent. Every chapter published in this book has been scrutinized by our experts. Their significance has been extensively debated. The topics covered herein carry significant findings which will fuel the growth of the discipline. They may even be implemented as practical applications or may be referred to as a beginning point for another development.

The contributors of this book come from diverse backgrounds, making this book a truly international effort. This book will bring forth new frontiers with its revolutionizing research information and detailed analysis of the nascent developments around the world.

We would like to thank all the contributing authors for lending their expertise to make the book truly unique. They have played a crucial role in the development of this book. Without their invaluable contributions this book wouldn't have been possible. They have made vital efforts to compile up to date information on the varied aspects of this subject to make this book a valuable addition to the collection of many professionals and students.

This book was conceptualized with the vision of imparting up-to-date information and advanced data in this field. To ensure the same, a matchless editorial board was set up. Every individual on the board went through rigorous rounds of assessment to prove their worth. After which they invested a large part of their time researching and compiling the most relevant data for our readers.

The editorial board has been involved in producing this book since its inception. They have spent rigorous hours researching and exploring the diverse topics which have resulted in the successful publishing of this book. They have passed on their knowledge of decades through this book. To expedite this challenging task, the publisher supported the team at every step. A small team of assistant editors was also appointed to further simplify the editing procedure and attain best results for the readers.

Apart from the editorial board, the designing team has also invested a significant amount of their time in understanding the subject and creating the most relevant covers. They scrutinized every image to scout for the most suitable representation of the subject and create an appropriate cover for the book.

The publishing team has been an ardent support to the editorial, designing and production team. Their endless efforts to recruit the best for this project, has resulted in the accomplishment of this book. They are a veteran in the field of academics and their pool of knowledge is as vast as their experience in printing. Their expertise and guidance has proved useful at every step. Their uncompromising quality standards have made this book an exceptional effort. Their encouragement from time to time has been an inspiration for everyone.

The publisher and the editorial board hope that this book will prove to be a valuable piece of knowledge for researchers, students, practitioners and scholars across the globe.

List of Contributors

Susanne Glaumann and Caroline Nilsson
Department of Clinical Science and Education, Södersjukhuset, Centre for Allergy Research, Karolinska Institutet, Stockholm, Sweden
Sach's Children's Hospital, Södersjukhuset, Stockholm, Sweden

Anna Nopp and S. G. O. Johansson
Department of Medicine, Clinical Immunology and Allergy Unit, Karolinska Institutet, Stockholm, Sweden

Magnus P. Borres
Thermo Fisher Scientific, Uppsala, Sweden
Department of Pediatrics, Institute for Clinical Sciences, The Sahlgrenska Academy at the University of Gothenburg, Sweden

Daniel Nilsson
Division of ENT Diseases, Department of Clinical Science, Intervention and Technology, Karolinska Institutet, Stockholm, Sweden
Biomedicine, Kristianstad University, Kristianstad, Sweden

Anand Kumar Andiappan
Department of Biological Sciences, National University of Singapore, Singapore, Singapore
Singapore Immunology Network (SIgN), Singapore, Singapore

Christer Halldén
Biomedicine, Kristianstad University, Kristianstad, Sweden

Chew Fook Tim
Department of Biological Sciences, National University of Singapore, Singapore, Singapore

Torbjörn Säll
Department of Cell and Organism Biology, Lund University, Lund, Sweden

De Yun Wang
Department of Otolaryngology, National University of Singapore, Singapore, Singapore

Lars-Olaf Cardell
Division of ENT Diseases, Department of Clinical Science, Intervention and Technology, Karolinska Institutet, Stockholm, Sweden

Gandhi Damaj
Service d'Hématologie, Centre Hospitalier Universitaire, Hôpital Sud; Amiens, France
Centre de Référence des Mastocytoses, Faculté de Médecine et AP-HP Necker-Enfants Malades, Paris, France
CNRS UMR 8147 and Institut Imagine, AP-HP, Hôpital Necker-Enfants Malades, Paris, France

Magalie Joris
Service d'Hématologie, Centre Hospitalier Universitaire, Hôpital Sud; Amiens, France

Olivia Chandesris
Centre de Référence des Mastocytoses, Faculté de Médecine et AP-HP Necker-Enfants Malades, Paris, France
Service d'Hématologie Adulte, Université Paris Descartes, Paris Sorbonne Cité, Faculté de Médecine et AP-HP Necker-Enfants Malades, Paris, France

Katia Hanssens, Erinn Soucie and Patrice Dubreuil
Inserm, U1068, CRCM, (Signaling, Hematopoiesis and Mechanism of Oncogenesis); Institut Paoli-Calmettes,Marseille; Aix-Marseille Univ; CNRS, UMR7258, Marseille, France

Danielle Canioni
Service d'Anatomo-pathologie, Université Paris Descartes, Paris Sorbonne Cité, Faculté de Médecine et AP-HP Necker-Enfants Malades, Paris, France

Brigitte Kolb
Service d'Hématologie, Centre Hospitalier Universitaire, Reims, France

Isabelle Durieu
Service de me´decine interne, Groupe Hospitalier Sud. Hospices Civils, Lyon, France

Emanuel Gyan
Service d'Hématologie et thérapie cellulaire, CIC INSERMU202, Centre Hospitalier Universitaire, Tours, France

Cristina Livideanu
Département de Dermatologie, Centre Hospitalier Universitaire, Toulouse, France

Stephane Chèze
Service d'Hématologie, Centre Hospitalier Universitaire, Caen, France

Momar Diouf
Département de bio-statistiques et de Recherche clinique, Centre Hospitalier Universitaire, Amiens, France

Reda Garidi
Service d'Hématologie, Centre Hospitalier, St Quentin, France

Sophie Georgin-Lavialle
Service de Médecine Interne, Hôpital Tenon, Assistance Publique-Hôpitaux, Université Pierre et Marie Curie, Paris, France

Vahid Asnafi and Ludovic Lhermitte
Laboratoire d'hématologie Biologique et UMR CNRS 8147, Université Paris Descartes, Paris Sorbonne Cité, Faculté de Médecine et Assistance Publique-Hôpitaux de Paris (AP-HP) Necker-Enfants Malades, Paris, France

Christian Lavigne
Service d'Hématologie, Centre Hospitalier Universitaire, Angers, France

David Launay
Service de Médecine Interne, CHRU, Lille, France

Michel Arock
CNRS UMR 8113, Laboratoire de Biologie et Pharmacologie Appliquée, Ecole Normale Supérieure, Cachan, France
Laboratoire Central d'Hématologie, Groupe Hospitalier Pitié-Salpetrière, Paris, France

Olivier Lortholary
Service de Me´decine Interne et de Maladie Infectieuses, Université Paris Descartes, Paris Sorbonne Cité, Faculté de Médecine et AP-HP Necker-Enfants Malades, Paris, France

Olivier Hermine
Centre de Référence des Mastocytoses, Faculté de Médecine et AP-HP Necker-Enfants Malades, Paris, France
CNRS UMR 8147 and Institut Imagine, AP-HP, Hôpital Necker-Enfants Malades, Paris, France
Service d'Hématologie Adulte, Université Paris Descartes, Paris Sorbonne Cité, Faculté de Médecine et AP-HP Necker-Enfants Malades, Paris, France

Ruo-Xi Chen, Wen-Min Lu, Lu-Ping Zhu, Mei-Ping Lu, Yun-Li Wang, Xin-Yuan Chen and Xin-Jie Zhu
Department of Otorhinolaryngology, The First Affiliated Hospital, Nanjing Medical University, Nanjing, China

Mei-Lin Wang and Zheng-Dong Zhang
Department of Molecular and Genetic Toxicology, School of Public Health, Nanjing Medical University, Nanjing, China

Min Yin and Lei Cheng
Department of Otorhinolaryngology, The First Affiliated Hospital, Nanjing Medical University, Nanjing, China
International Centre for Allergy Research, Nanjing Medical University, Nanjing, China

Camilla Rydberg Millrud, Terese Hylander, Susanna Kumlien Georen, Åsa Kågedal and Lars Olaf Cardell
Division of ENT diseases, Department of Clinical Science, Intervention and Technology, Karolinska Institutet, Karolinska University Hospital, Stockholm, Sweden

Ola Winqvist
Department of Medicine, Translational Immunology Unit, Karolinska Institutet, Stockholm, Sweden

Rosa Anna Iorio and Stefano Del Duca
Department of Biological, Earth and Environmental Sciences, University of Bologna, Bologna, Italy

Elisabetta Calamelli, Chiara Pula, Andrea Pession and Giampaolo Ricci
Department of Pediatric Allergology of the Women's, Children's and Adolescents' Health Gozzadini Children's Hospital Sant'Orsola-Malpighi, University of Bologna, Bologna, Italy

Magda Lodolini and Fortuna Scamardella
Laboratory Analysis Unit. Maggiore Hospital, Bologna, Italy

Prerna Sharma and Naveen Arora
Allergy and Immunology Section, CSIR-Institute of Genomics and Integrative Biology, Delhi, India

Shailendra Nath Gaur
Department of Respiratory Medicine, Vallabhbhai Patel Chest Institute, University of Delhi, Delhi, India

Galateja Jordakieva
Comparative Medicine, Messerli Research Institute of the University of Veterinary Medicine Vienna, Medical University of Vienna & University of Vienna, Vienna, Austria
Institute of Occupational Medicine, Department of Internal Medicine II, Medical University of Vienna, Vienna, Austria

Julia Wallmann and Thomas Nittke
Comparative Medicine, Messerli Research Institute of the University of Veterinary Medicine Vienna, Medical University of Vienna & University of Vienna, Vienna, Austria

René Schmutz, Patrick Lemell and René Zieglmayer
Vienna Challenge Chamber (VCC), Vienna, Austria

Michael Wegmann and Heinz Fehrenbach
Priority Area Asthma & Allergy, Leibniz Center for Medicine and Biosciences, Research Center Borstel, Airway Research Center North, Member of the German Center for Lung Research, Borstel, Germany

Martina Mittlböck
Section for Clinical Biometrics, Center for Medical Statistics, Informatics, and Intelligent Systems, Medical University of Vienna, Vienna, Austria

Jasminka Godnic-Cvar
Institute of Occupational Medicine, Department of Internal Medicine II, Medical University of Vienna, Vienna, Austria

Erika Jensen-Jarolim
Comparative Medicine, Messerli Research Institute of the University of Veterinary Medicine Vienna, Medical University of Vienna & University of Vienna, Vienna, Austria
Institute of Pathophysiology and Allergy Research, Center of Pathophysiology Infectiology and Immunology, Medical University of Vienna, Vienna, Austria

Stephanie Roll, Thomas Reinhold, Daniel Pach, Benno Brinkhaus, Katja Icke, Tanja Jäckel and Stefan N. Willich
Institute for Social Medicine, Epidemiology, and Health Economics, Charité University Medical Centre, Berlin, Germany

Doris Staab
Department of Paediatric Pulmonology and Immunology, Charité University Medical Centre, Berlin, Germany

Wegscheider
Department of Medical Biometry and Epidemiology, University Medical Centre, Hamburg-Eppendorf, Germany

Claudia M. Witt
Institute for Social Medicine, Epidemiology, and Health Economics, Charité University Medical Centre, Berlin, Germany
Centre for Integrative Medicine, University of Maryland School of Medicine, Baltimore, Maryland, United States of America

Surendran Thavagnanam
Paediatric Department, University Malaya Medical Centre, Kuala Lumpar, Malaysia

Jeremy C Parker, Grzegorz Skibinski and Liam G Heaney
Centre for Infection and Immunity, Queen's University Belfast, Belfast, Northern Ireland, United Kingdom

Michael E McBrien
Department of Anaesthetics, Royal Victoria Hospital, Belfast Health and Social Care Trust, Belfast, Northern Ireland, United Kingdom

Michael D Shields
Centre for Infection and Immunity, Queen's University Belfast, Belfast, Northern Ireland, United Kingdom
Department of Paediatrics, Royal Belfast Hospital for Sick Children, Belfast Health and Social Care Trust, Belfast, Northern Ireland, United Kingdom

Qiang Zeng and Sheng-Yong Dong
International Medical Center, Chinese PLA General Hospital, Beijing, China

Liu-Xin Wu
The Second Laboratory, PLA Air Force Institute of Aviation Medicine, Beijing, China

Hong Li
Health Management Center, Fujian Provincial Hospital, Fuzhou, Fujian, China

Zhi-Jian Sun
Health Management Center, Shandong Provincial Hospital, Jinan, Shandong, China

Jing-Bo Li
Health Management Center, Southwest Hospital, The Third Military Medical University, Chongqing, China

Hong-Xia Jiang
Health Management Center, Xiangya Hospital, Central South University, Changsha, Hunan, China

Zhi-Heng Chen
Health Management Center, The Third Xiangya Hospital of Central South University, Changsha, Hunan, China

Qi-Bin Wang
Health Management Center, Shandong Electric Power Center Hospital, Jinan, Shandong, China

Wei-Wei Chen
Treatment and Research Center for Infectious Diseases, 302 Hospital of PLA,
Beijing, China

Jenn-Ren Hsiao, Chun-Yen Ou, Hung-I Lo, Cheng-Chih Huang, Wei-Ting Lee, Sen-Tien Tsai and Fang-Ting Wang
Department of Otolaryngology, National Cheng Kung University Hospital, College of Medicine, National Cheng Kung University, Tainan, Taiwan

Jehn-Shyun Huang, Ken-Chung Chen and Tung-Yiu Wong
Department of Stomatology, National Cheng Kung University Hospital, College of Medicine, National Cheng Kung University, Tainan, Taiwan

Chia-Jui Yen and Shang-Yin Wu
Division of Hematology/Oncology, Department of Internal Medicine, National Cheng Kung University Hospital, College of Medicine, National Cheng Kung University, Tainan, Taiwan

Yuan-Hua Wu, Wei-Ting Hsueh and Ming-Wei Yang
Department of Radiation Oncology, National Cheng Kung University Hospital, College of Medicine, National Cheng Kung University, Tainan, Taiwan

Jang-Yang Chang and Kwang-Yu Chang
Division of Hematology/Oncology, Department of Internal Medicine, National Cheng Kung University Hospital, College of Medicine, National Cheng Kung University, Tainan, Taiwan
National Institute of Cancer Research, National Health Research Institutes, Tainan, Taiwan

Chen-Lin Lin
Department of Nursing, National Cheng Kung University Hospital, College of Medicine, National Cheng Kung University, Tainan, Taiwan

Yi-Hui Wang, Ya-Ling Weng, Han-Chien Yang and Jeffrey S. Chang
National Institute of Cancer Research, National Health Research Institutes, Tainan, Taiwan

Takeshi Yamamoto, Toshihisa Kodama, Jaemin Lee, Naho Utsunomiya, Shusaku Hayashi and Makoto Kadowaki
Division of Gastrointestinal Pathophysiology, Institute of Natural Medicine, University of Toyama, Toyama, Toyama, Japan

Hiroshi Sakamoto
Department of Physical Therapy, Health Science University, Fujikawaguchiko, Yamanashi, Japan

Hirofumi Kuramoto
Department of Applied Biology, Kyoto Institute of Technology, Kyoto, Kyoto, Japan

Ana Aranda
Allergy Research Laboratory, Carlos Haya Hospital, Málaga, Spain

Paloma Campo, Inmaculada Doña, Luisa Galindo and Miguel Blanca
Unidad de Gestión Clínica Allergy, Carlos Haya Hospital, Málaga, Spain

Arantxa Palacin, Cristina Gomez-Casado and Araceli Díaz-Perales
Biotechnology Department, Center for Plant Biotechnology and Genomics, Pozuelo de Alarcon, Madrid, Spain

Lucia Cazzoletti
Unit of Epidemiology and Medical Statistics, University of Verona, Verona, Italy

Angelo Guido Corsico
Department of Molecular Medicine, University of Pavia, Pavia, Italy

Federica Albicini, Eti Maria Giulia Di Vincenzo, Erica Gini, Amelia Grosso, Vanessa Ronzoni and Isa Cerveri
Division of Respiratory Diseases, Istituto di Ricovero e Cura a Carattere Scientifico "San Matteo" Hospital Foundation, University of Pavia, Pavia, Italy

Massimiliano Bugiani
Unit of Respiratory Medicine, National Health Service, Turin, Italy

Pietro Pirina
Institute of Respiratory Diseases, University of Sassari, Sassari, Italy

Antonios Patelis, Maria Gunnbjörnsdottir and Christer Janson
Department of Medical Sciences: Respiratory Medicine and Allergology, Uppsala University, Uppsala, Sweden

Magnus P. Borres
Immunodiagnostics, Thermo Fischer Scientific, Uppsala, Sweden
Department of Women's and Children's Health, Uppsala University, Uppsala, Sweden

Peter Burney
Respiratory Epidemiology and Public Health, Imperial College, London, United Kingdom

Thorarinn Gislason
University of Iceland, Medical Faculty and Department of Respiratory Medicine and Sleep, Landspitali University Hospital, Reykjavik, Iceland

Kjell Torén
Section of Occupational and Environmental Medicine, Institute of Medicine, University of Gothenburg, Gothenburg, Sweden

Bertil Forsberg
Division of Occupational and Environmental Medicine, Umeå University, Umeå, Sweden

Kjell Alving
Department of Women's and Children's Health, Uppsala University, Uppsala, Sweden

Andrei Malinovschi
Department of Medical Sciences: Clinical Physiology, Uppsala University, Uppsala, Sweden

Julie Barnett and Konstantina Vasileiou
Department of Information Systems and Computing, Brunel University, Middlesex, United Kingdom

M. Hazel Gowland
Allergy Action, Farnborough, United Kingdom

Monique M. Raats
School of Psychology, Faculty of Arts and Human Sciences, University of Surrey, Guildford, Surrey, United Kingdom

Jane S. Lucas
Clinical and Experimental Sciences, Faculty of Medicine, University of Southampton, University Hospital Southampton NHS Foundation Trust, Southampton, United Kingdom

Alemayehu Amberbir
Department of Infectious Disease Epidemiology, London School of Hygiene and Tropical Medicine, London, United Kingdom
Division of Epidemiology and Public Health, University of Nottingham, Nottingham, United Kingdom

Girmay Medhin
Aklilu Lemma Institute of Pathobiology, Addis Ababa University, Addis Ababa, Ethiopia

Charlotte Hanlon
Department of Psychiatry, Addis Ababa University, Addis Ababa, Ethiopia

John Britton and Andrea Venn
Division of Epidemiology and Public Health, University of Nottingham, Nottingham, United Kingdom

Gail Davey
Brighton & Sussex Medical School, University of Brighton, Brighton, United Kingdom

Xin Wei
Department of Otolaryngology, Head and Neck Surgery, Beijing Tongren Hospital, Capital Medical University, Beijing, PR China
Key Laboratory of Otolaryngology, Head and Neck Surgery (Ministry of Education of China), Beijing Institute of Otorhinolaryngology, Beijing, PR China,
Department of Otolaryngology, Head and Neck Surgery, People's Hospital of Hainan Province, Haikou, PR China

Yuan Zhang and Luo Zhang
Department of Otolaryngology, Head and Neck Surgery, Beijing Tongren Hospital, Capital Medical University, Beijing, PR China
Key Laboratory of Otolaryngology, Head and Neck Surgery (Ministry of Education of China), Beijing Institute of Otorhinolaryngology, Beijing, PR China

Zheng Fu
Department of Otolaryngology, Head and Neck Surgery, People's Hospital of Hainan Province, Haikou, PR China

Renata Curciarello, Angela M. Candreva and Guillermo H. Docena
Laboratorio de Investigaciones del Sistema Inmune-LISIN, Departamento de Ciencias Biológicas, Facultad de Ciencias Exactas, Universidad Nacional de La Plata, La Plata, Buenos Aires, Argentina
Centro de Investigaciones y Desarrollo en Criotecnología de Alimentos-CIDCA, Facultad de Ciencias Exactas, Universidad Nacional de La Plata, La Plata, Buenos Aires, Argentina

Paola L. Smaldini and Carlos A. Fossati
Laboratorio de Investigaciones del Sistema Inmune-LISIN, Departamento de Ciencias Biológicas, Facultad de Ciencias Exactas, Universidad Nacional de La Plata, La Plata, Buenos Aires, Argentina

Virginia González and Gustavo Parisi
Centro de Estudios e Investigaciones, Departamento de Ciencias y Tecnología Universidad Nacional de Quilmes, Quilmes, Buenos Aires, Argentina

Ana Cauerhff
Centro de Investigación y Desarrollo en Fermentaciones Industriales, CINDEFI (UNLP y CONICET) and Instituto de Investigaciones Bioquímicas de Buenos Aires
(IIBBA-CONICET), Fundacio´n Instituto Leloir, Buenos Aires, Argentina

Ivana Barrios and Luis Bruno Blanch
Cátedra de Química Medicinal, Departamento de Ciencias Biológicas, Facultad de Ciencias Exactas, Universidad Nacional de La Plata, La Plata, Buenos Aires, Argentina

Silvana Petruccelli
Centro de Investigaciones y Desarrollo en Criotecnología de Alimentos-CIDCA, Facultad de Ciencias Exactas, Universidad Nacional de La Plata, La Plata, Buenos Aires, Argentina

Nan Zhang, Koen Van Crombruggen, Gabriele Holtappels and Feng Lan
Upper Airway Research Laboratory, Ghent University Hospital, Ghent, Belgium

Michail Katotomichelakis
Department of Otorhinolaryngology, Medical School, Democritus University of Thrace, Alexandroupolis, Greece

Luo Zhang
Department of Otolaryngology Head and Neck Surgery, Beijing TongRen Hospital, Capital Medical University, Beijing, P.R.China

Petra Högger
Institute for Pharmacy and Food Chemistry, Julius-Maximilians-Universitity, Würzburg, Germany

Claus Bachert
Upper Airway Research Laboratory, Ghent University Hospital, Ghent, Belgium
Division of ENT Diseases, Clintec, Karolinska Institutet, Stockholm, Sweden

Ekaterina Maslova and Sjurdur F. Olsen
Centre for Fetal Programming, Department of Epidemiology, Statens Serum Institut, Copenhagen, Denmark
Department of Nutrition, Harvard School of Public Health, Boston, Massachusetts, United States of America

Marin Strøm
Centre for Fetal Programming, Department of Epidemiology, Statens Serum Institut, Copenhagen, Denmark

Thorhallur I. Halldorsson
Centre for Fetal Programming, Department of Epidemiology, Statens Serum Institut, Copenhagen, Denmark
Faculty of Food Science and Nutrition, School of Health Sciences, University of Iceland, Reykjavik, Iceland
Unit for Nutrition Research, Landspitali University Hospital, Reykjavik, Iceland

Juan Wang
Department of Medical Sciences, Uppsala University and University Hospital, Uppsala, Sweden
Key Laboratory of Three Gorges Reservoir Region's Eco-Environment, Ministry of Education, Chongqing University, Chongqing, China

Baizhan Li, Wei Yu, Qin Yang, Han Wang and Duchai Huang
Key Laboratory of Three Gorges Reservoir Region's Eco-Environment, Ministry of Education, Chongqing University, Chongqing, China

Jan Sundell
Key Laboratory of Three Gorges Reservoir Region's Eco-Environment, Ministry of Education, Chongqing University, Chongqing, China
Department of Building Science, Tsinghua University, Beijing, China

Dan Norbäck
Department of Medical Sciences, Uppsala University and University Hospital, Uppsala, Sweden

Kai-Jen Tien
Division of Endocrinology and Metabolism, Department of Internal Medicine, Chi Mei Medical Center, Tainan, Taiwan
Center of General Education, Chia Nan University of Pharmacy and Science, Tainan, Taiwan

Chien-Wen Chou, Shang-Yu Lee, Nai-Cheng Yeh, Chwen-Yi Yang and Feng-Chieh Yen
Division of Endocrinology and Metabolism, Department of Internal Medicine, Chi Mei Medical Center, Tainan, Taiwan

Jhi-Joung Wang
Department of Medical Research, Chi Mei Medical Center, Tainan, Taiwan

Shih-Feng Weng
Department of Medical Research, Chi Mei Medical Center, Tainan, Taiwan
Department of Hospital and Health Care Administration, Chia Nan University of Pharmacy and Science, Tainan, Taiwan

Rubén Martínez-Aranguren, María J. Goikoetxea, Paula Cabrera-Freitag and María L. Sanz
Department of Allergology and Clinical Immunology, Clínica Universidad de Navarra, Pamplona, Spain

María T. Lizaso and Blanca E. García
Allergology Service, Complejo Hospitalario de Navarra, Pamplona, Spain

Oswaldo Trellez
Department of Computer Architecture, Universidad de Málaga, Málaga, Spain

Index